# Surgical Education and Training in Pakistan:

## *Creating a Model*

# Surgical Education and Training in Pakistan:

*Creating a Model*


Edited by

Masood Umer, M. Hammad Ather and Syed Ather Enam



Cambridge Scholars Publishing

Surgical Education and Training in Pakistan: Creating a Model

Edited by Masood Umer, M. Hammad Ather and Syed Ather Enam

This book first published 2022

Cambridge Scholars Publishing

Lady Stephenson Library, Newcastle upon Tyne, NE6 2PA, UK

British Library Cataloguing in Publication Data
A catalogue record for this book is available from the British Library



ISBN (10): 1-5275-8658-8
ISBN (13): 978-1-5275-8658-1

# TABLE OF CONTENTS

# ACKNOWLEDGEMENTS

It gives us immense pleasure to share the book *Surgical Education and Training in Pakistan: Creating a Model* with our readers, published as an appurtenance of the Department of Surgery of Aga Khan University, Karachi, Pakistan.

This is the first book published by the Department. Our objective for this book is focused on improving surgery training Programmes in developing countries. Over the last 35 years we have strived to establish a surgical training Programme within our university that provides a balance between education and service. We have for the first time in Pakistan developed a residency structure with a fixed weekly, monthly and annual academic schedule across all surgical disciplines. Starting from induction to assessment and evaluation, imparting skills and evaluations, we have set very high standards in our country for others to follow and replicate within their own resources. This book will be a narrative of how we achieved all this and what the way forward is considering the resource constraints that we have in our lower-middle-income countries as compared to Western countries.

We would also like to take this opportunity to thank to all the contributors / authors of this book. We would like to appreciate Dr M. Shahzad Shamim, Neurosurgeon and Associate Professor in the Department of Surgery at Aga Khan University for the organizational structure of this book. We are also thankful to our university's departments: the President's Office, the Dean's Office, and the Legal, Communications, and Finance Departments. Front cover has been designed by Dr Rehan Nasir Khan. In the end we would also like to thank Ms Ayesha Jazib, Content Writer, and Mr Shariff Charania, Specialist in the Department of Surgery at Aga Khan University. They both worked tirelessly day and night and made this herculean task possible. We hope you will appreciate the quality of chapters in this book.

Happy reading,

Editorial Committee,

*Surgical Education and Training in Pakistan: Creating a Model*

# CHAPTER 1

# THE SURGICAL CLERKSHIP: THEORY AND PRACTICE OF SURGICAL EDUCATION IN MEDICAL SCHOOL

SADAF KHAN AND AMN SIDDIQI

The word surgery originates from the Latin word *chirurgia*, itself derived from the Greek words *cheiros* (meaning hand) and *ergon* (meaning work) (Haeger 1988). Since the beginning of time, man has had to deal with injuries, deformities, and pathologies requiring physical intervention, and these treatments have been undertaken by healers across the ages. Unfortunately, as our understanding of the human body and its afflictions advanced, surgery began to be regarded as a necessary evil in contrast to the more philosophical discipline of internal medicine. This resulted in the attitude that surgeons were a lesser caste of doctors, and stunted the development of surgical methods and philosophy. Out of Cordoba came the surgeon-educator Abul Qasim (936–1013), also known as Albucasis, and his book *Altasrif* ("Collection"). He provided detailed illustrations of surgical instruments and thorough descriptions of their use. The scope of the surgical chapters was vast, and ranged from the care of wounds to management of bladder stones. This text has been commonly cited in the Western world, where the evolution of the modern surgeon began.

Modern medical curricula are composed of basic sciences followed by the clinical sciences. For most programmes, the third year of instruction is a landmark in every aspiring doctor's career, as they transition from theoretical learning to clinical practice. The challenge is to develop the ability to apply fundamental principles of human biology to understand normal human function and behaviour across age and gender, and diagnose and manage a wide range of pathologies. At the same time, they practise the professional attitudes and behaviour required to become competent and empathetic healthcare providers. This initial clinical experience is vital in shaping a well-rounded doctor and is pivotal in the student's decision regarding future specialization. Practitioners of the primary clinical disciplines are tasked with the education of these novice learners. The hidden agenda in this process is the search for a learner who shows a passion and aptitude for that branch of medicine. Students on the postgraduate training programmes in North America depend on these initial exposures to select an area of interest for advanced training, thus necessitating high quality experiences as part of the curriculum. In Europe and Asia, the internship (or house job) year is an additional opportunity for exposure to varied clinical disciplines, prior to declaring a speciality of interest.

The surgical clerkship provides a glimpse into a variety of healthcare environments. Students participate in outpatient clinics, follow patients in the ward, contribute in the operating room, assess patients in the emergency room, and attend academic sessions and multidisciplinary meetings. This allows them to follow patients and the disease process over a period of time, while participating in care and decision making. Students also observe the mechanics of communication and team dynamics in high- and low-pressure scenarios. Traditionally, attributes of professionalism are imbibed through role-modelling, but there is a need to include instruction in the formal curriculum. Additionally, the surgical rotation allows medical students to learn and practise many basic technical skills required by a graduating doctor.

For students who wish to pursue surgery, a high-quality clerkship gives insight into the expectations and demands of a surgical career, allowing students to assess their fit for it and help tailor their course as they prepare for a surgical career. For the non-surgically inclined student, the surgical rotation has the enormous responsibility of providing a comprehensive and lasting understanding of surgical disease and its myriad presentations. An increasing volume of surgical care frequently necessitates participation from non-surgical physicians in some way, either when they consult surgeons, or when they are consulted by surgeons (McKinley et al. 2020). The surgical clerkship may be the only time in their career where they will have a meaningful exposure to this group of patients. Finally, the way students remember their surgical rotation can shape how they counsel future generations of students, either perpetuating or combatting misconceptions regarding a career in surgery.

## The challenges of undergraduate surgical education

The purpose of undergraduate medical education has been redefined over the years. Traditionally, graduating doctors were expected to have sound medical knowledge and the expertise to perform all tasks relevant to medical practice, including basic surgeries (Agha et al. 2005). With an ever-increasing body of knowledge, development of sub-specialties, and recognition of the importance of professionalism, there has been a reduction in curricular time devoted to technical subjects such as anatomy and surgery (Agha et al. 2005). This time has since been utilized for the instruction of essential generic skills and knowledge, such as communication skills, practice-based learning, system-based practice, and the medical humanities. The emphasis of teaching is now to produce a "pluripotent" doctor with the skill of self-directed learning, who can then dedicate a further six or seven years to becoming a specialist.

A new challenge presented itself with the institution of work-hour restrictions for postgraduate trainees (Acton 2015). These restrictions changed the structure of traditional surgical teams and altered the way in which teaching occurs. For almost a century, William Halsted's model of "see one, do one, teach one" formed the basic framework of surgical education. This relied on teaching the surgical team as a single cohesive unit consisting of medical students, interns, junior residents, and a chief resident. Each team spent a substantial (sometimes unreasonable) amount of time in the hospital and attended calls together. A significant portion of education took place in these ready-made groups during "down time," in which senior residents would teach junior residents and students. This, along with active participation in the operating room and ward, was considered sufficient for students to imbibe the knowledge, skills, and attitudes required for effective patient care. As resident work hour restrictions were implemented, teams became smaller as night floats and shifts were introduced to ensure uninterrupted patient care. Residents were responsible for more patients at a time, which left less time available for formal teaching within the team. To meet this challenge, programs have become more creative and specific about how and when to teach residents, and educating medical students is often relegated to a secondary level.

All academic clinicians balance four core activities: research, clinical practice, training residents, and teaching students (Agha et al. 2005). Academic institutions are perpetually on a quest for high-quality research output, translating to higher academic and clinical ratings, and subsequently greater funding opportunities. For the individual surgeon, research of an international calibre leads to professional recognition, larger grants, and career advancement. As a result, the academic surgeon spends more time and energy in the laboratory or designing and implementing clinical research, while clinical practice and teaching often become necessary distractions. Additionally, the demand to provide a high-quality patient experience and the intense competition between healthcare entities have led to a manifold increase in pressure on healthcare providers to reduce waiting times and provide rapid service for non-urgent service commitments. Since the consequences of not teaching medical students are less immediate than those of not fulfilling service requirements, training residents, research, and undergraduate education are often put at risk. In view of these realities, the need for physicians to become selective and develop a focus (clinical practice/research/teaching, alone or in combination) is advocated.

Finally, as the healthcare system is modernized, and as patients become more aware of quality and safety, students are becoming increasingly marginalized from active participation during surgical clerkships (Scally and Minter 2016). For example, while using an electronic medical record is undeniably advantageous for patient care, its implementation has limited students' opportunities to participate in clinical documentation. The loss of this active experience has a negative impact on their skill and efficiency, on documenting history and examination findings, procedure notes, and discharge summaries – skills that are essential as they enter residency. Similarly, a shift towards minimally invasive and laparoscopic procedures has reduced students' opportunities to "scrub in" and actively participate in surgical procedures. As a result, the surgical clerkship is increasingly resembling an "observership" with a less active role for medical students (Agha et al. 2005).

These challenges have resulted in an overall dissatisfaction amongst medical students regarding the quantity and quality of teaching within the surgical clerkship (ASiT Medical Student and Foundation Doctor Consensus Group 2020; Lee et al. 2016). Interest in surgical careers has been steadily declining, resulting in an impending shortage of general surgeons (Abbas et al. 2015; Peel, Schlachta and Alkhamesi 2018). Furthermore, graduating doctors have expressed under-confidence in their abilities, and concerns have been raised regarding their readiness to take on basic tasks expected of a surgical intern. This may cause potential safety issues and an increased reliance on senior members of the surgical team (Lee et al. 2016). This shortfall in training has resulted in programmes being obligated to spend a variable amount of time during the initial period of residency to prepare new interns for safely entering the workforce as healthcare providers (Scally and Minter 2016).

## Surgical education for contemporary medical students

The limitations discussed above highlight the need to create an environment that facilitates relevant, effective, and efficient teaching/learning. While developing a clear core curriculum and providing infrastructure and opportunity are essential interventions to improve education, the success of the education process is ultimately determined by the efforts of the two main parties involved: the surgeon and the student.

The modern medical student needs to be recognised as an adult learner (Agha et al. 2005). The commitment with which adult learners engage in education depends heavily on their own motivation. Factors that are associated with greater motivation include problem-based learning; learning content that is perceived to be relevant and applicable to practice; learning that can be tailored by the student; receiving regular feedback; and participating in an educational process that is founded on mutual respect. Surgeons need to take into account the characteristics of adult learning (Table 1-1) and adapt their teaching methods accordingly (Table 1-2). Fostering this modified role of the surgeon-teacher will take time and training to develop. Ideally, the shift must be nurtured and enabled at the level of the medical school.

**Table 1-1: The characteristics of adult learning (Hamdorf and Hall 2001)**

| Characteristics of adult learning |
|---|
| Clearly defined objectives<br>Voluntary participation<br>An active process<br>A desire for feedback<br>A need for reflection |

**Table 1-2: The shifting role of teachers (Hamdorf and Hall 2001)**

| Traditional | Future |
|---|---|
| Focus on teachers<br>Students subservient<br>Didactic teaching<br>Emphasis on what is taught | Focus on students and teachers<br>A partnership<br>Facilitator of learning<br>Emphasis on what is learned |

In 2019, a study conducted amongst medical students at three large academic hospitals assessed students' perceptions of what makes the surgical rotation a meaningful experience (McKinley et al. 2020). Positive predictors of a meaningful clerkship included active participation, such as closing skin with a stapler and performing electrocautery, receiving feedback and mentoring, establishing relationships with patients, and making a "real difference" in their health. These findings align with the characteristics of adult learning and the new role of a surgeon-teacher. Any interventions that enhance the frequency of these activities may result in better learning within the surgical clerkship.

## Objectives of the Surgical Clerkship

There is a perceived inconsistency in the terminal skills of medical graduates, a sentiment that is echoed across many governing medical bodies (Association of American Medical Colleges 2014; The Royal College of Surgeons of England 2015). To some extent, this is due to a varied exposure to the surgical specialty in terms of time and content of teaching (Lee et al. 2016). Further heterogeneity in the experience stems from clerkships being conducted in different hospital settings, and varying degrees of student involvement in patient care and decision making (Scally and Minter 2016). Utilizing a uniform surgical curriculum with clearly defined terminal objectives is a possible strategy to ensure appropriate baseline surgical knowledge and skills that are transferable to other interventional and non-interventional specialties.

The three domains that must be addressed by a medical curriculum (and that can be extrapolated to each discipline) are knowledge, skills, and attitude. Appropriate objectives for each domain must be formulated for the overall programme and each module. Each domain warrants the use of relevant teaching/learning and assessment methods. For instance, procedural skills cannot be assessed in a written format, and knowledge is poorly assessed by observation. Integrated novel teaching/learning modalities, such as simulation, have the added benefit of allowing learning and/or assessment across more than one domain.

The surgical curriculum consists of two components. The first component is the core curriculum which includes basic principles of surgery and common/essential surgical presentations. Students must have an understanding of the anatomy, physiology, pathology, investigations, differential diagnoses, management, and operative care relevant to each topic. For example, in 2015 the Royal College of Surgeons of England released a national undergraduate curriculum in surgery which covers the core surgical curriculum (Table 1-3) and defines the learning objectives for each topic. These topics are shared across other surgical national curricula (Association of American Medical Colleges 2014; Higher Education Commission, and Pakistan Medical & Dental Council 2011; Medical Council of India 2018). The second component of the surgical curriculum involves the necessary skills in which students must achieve a defined level of proficiency (Table 1-4). These include technical skills, such as basic suturing and catheterization of patients, as well as generic skills that all students must continue to develop, such as history taking and physical examinations.

**Table 1-3: Core topics to be covered in the surgery clerkship (adapted from the National Undergraduate Curriculum in Surgery by The Royal College of Surgeons of England 2015)**

| **Surgical Syllabus (General Surgery)** |
|---|
| Abdominal pain<br>Abdominal swelling<br>Change in bowel habit/rectal bleeding<br>Vomiting blood<br>Difficulty swallowing/dyspepsia/dysphagia<br>Jaundice<br>Lumps in groin<br>Breast lumps and nipple discharge<br>Consent for surgery including mental capacity<br>Caring for the postoperative patient, including nutrition, enhanced recovery, and the critically ill patient<br>Understanding wound healing<br>Trauma<br>Sepsis and infection<br>Surgical safety (WHO checklist, minimising complications, errors, communication and teamwork)<br>Caring for the patient before and after surgery, including fitness |

**Table 1-4: Skills emphasized in the surgical rotation**

| Skills emphasized in the surgical rotation |
|---|
| History taking, physical examination and case presentation |
| Interpreting labs and imaging |
| Performing nutritional assessments |
| Writing admission orders |
| Sterile technique - gowning and gloving, maintaining a sterile field |
| Basic knot tying |
| Basic suturing |
| Nasogastric tubes - placement and care |
| Foley catheterization |
| Surgical drains - care and removal |
| Basic airway management |
| Wound care and basic wound dressing |
| Venepuncture and peripheral IV |

## Teaching opportunities

> "What the eye doesn't see, and the mind doesn't know, doesn't exist"
> —D. H. Lawrence

Medical education requires that students have a basic understanding of the principles (knowledge) and practice (skills and attitudes) of the primary disciplines. The ideal clinical clerkship is one that provides relevant experiences and quality teaching, with efficiency of time and cost. Traditionally, clinical experience supplemented with didactic lectures was deemed sufficient for student education. With technological advancements and a better understanding of surgical pedagogy, surgical educators have developed teaching methods which align with the characteristics of adult learning (Table 1-1). Based on these principles, teaching opportunities are categorized as classroom based/didactic, inpatient and outpatient patient interactions, teaching/learning in the operating room, and simulation. Together these varied integrated exposures create the optimal student learning experience.

### "Classroom" teaching

While patient interactions are essential for the training of a medical professional, formal instruction remains an essential part of the curriculum. This prepares students for clinical experiences and for the development of clinical reasoning skills. This mode of instruction has multiple formats, ranging from the large class format or LCF (traditional lecture) to problem-based learning, with varying levels of interaction and collaboration between the facilitator and learner, and between the learners themselves. LCFs for large groups have traditionally been used as a method of medical content delivery. The ease of delivery, familiarity, and minimal resources required in terms of space, human resource, and technical support make it a popular method that is employed globally. Despite the popularity of this mode of instruction, it presents certain challenges. Within the classroom, traditional lectures and "death by bullet point" – as dubbed by Levinson (2010) – presents a teacher centred model which undermines an active role for students (Levinson 2010; Reis et al. 2015). Additionally, organizing LCFs is often made difficult due to faculty commitments and emergencies which lead to abrupt changes in scheduling, and medical students rotating at geographically distant sites (Cendan, Silver and Ben-David 2011). Further barriers to the use of didactic lectures include opportunity costs for faculty participation, and lack of consistency in the presented content and its applicability to learners (Lindeman et al. 2015).

Advances in medical education have introduced methods to circumvent the shortcomings of traditional lecture-based education. By using small group formats, online learning, workplace-based assessment and feedback techniques, and fostering environments that promote two-way communication between teaching faculty and students, the focus is shifting from "knowledge transmission to knowledge application."

A study at the University of Florida School of Medicine assessed the effectiveness of small group case-based teaching during the surgical clerkship (Cendan, Silver and Ben-David 2011). The didactic content was restructured from 33 large one-hour lectures to eight small group sessions consisting of four to five students, which would meet for two hours every week. Students reported spending more time preparing for these small group sessions compared to lectures. This was reflected in improved surgery examination scores. Faculty reported taking an hour or more to prepare for each session and the majority felt that such sessions were not disruptive to their workload. Additionally, faculty commented that it encouraged a two-way communication with the learner and created an environment which was ideal to assess student knowledge, judgement and reasoning.

Kaminski and colleagues (2019) assessed team based learning (TBL) strategies during an eight-week surgical clerkship. A class of 16 to 18 students was divided into smaller groups, each with a faculty leader. Students were to complete assigned readings prior to class. Sessions began with readiness tests followed by small group discussions on relevant clinical cases, guided by the faculty leaders. Finally, a faculty "topic-expert" would lead a large group discussion, further solidifying critical content. Students found that the anticipated discussions provided motivation to prepare in advance, which helped them stay on track for examination preparation. Overall, the TBL format was "educationally effective," "informative" and viewed as an "opportunity for interactive learning." Concerns were raised about the increased time students spent studying material that poorly correlated with the quizzes, and instructions and learning objectives were deemed as "unorganised." Furthermore, the extensive group work and interaction required all team members to participate, meaning that unprepared students placed the group dynamics and subsequent learning in jeopardy. They concluded that to ensure effective TBL, relevant learning material must be provided, and faculty should focus on clear communication, effective directions, and building diverse teams where all students are encouraged to be active participants.

Given the aptitude for technology of today's medical students and an increasing accessibility to the Internet, medical educators are harnessing technological resources to create online learning platforms. Lindeman and colleagues (2015) hypothesized that using a less faculty intense, blended online curriculum in the surgery rotation could provide a similar or improved academic experience as compared to curricula delivered via in person lectures. Blended learning combines online delivery of content at a time suitable to the student with formal supervised instruction in a scheduled face-to-face interaction. This allows students to have control over the time, place, and pace of their individual learning. In this study, lectures that were consistently given poor ratings were chosen to be delivered as online modules. Analysis of feedback suggested that the blended online curriculum improved students' academic performance and student satisfaction with the surgery clerkship, without any differences in students' rating of faculty clerkship involvement or teaching quality.

Moodle (Modular Object-Oriented Dynamic Learning Environment) is an online learning resource commonly used by medical schools. Leonardo Oliveira Reis and colleagues (2015) studied the use of Moodle to teach students, rotating through urology, two topics: haematuria and urological emergencies. The Moodle module was set up to provide an online interface with continuous access to audio lectures with slides, videos of operations, and electronic urology clinical cases. They observed a strong level of student engagement, with about 50% of students accessing the platform on weekends and holidays. By allowing online chat and open discussion, students were encouraged to interact with each other and with supervising faculty. Compared to traditional didactic lectures, faculty received more student inquiries, suggesting in-depth learning.

The flipped classroom paradigm has been proposed as an alternative educational approach. This approach combines blended online learning with interactive small group discussions, skills sessions, and continuous assessment and feedback. Its effectiveness in the surgery clerkship has been studied at Stanford University School of Medicine with promising results (Liebert et al. 2016). The shift to the flipped classroom was made to create a standardized curriculum that could be repeated in every clerkship block, to minimize the students' time away from clinical activities, to increase time spent using active learning strategies, and to allow more time for surgical skills training. Students reviewed material and watched online lectures asynchronously before class. Each session was conducted in a small group setting, and consisted of a pre-test, interactive case-based clinical reasoning discussion, skills session, and a post-test. A faculty member and surgical education fellow supervised each class. Students perceived that their time commitment remained the same as during lectures, with a larger proportion dedicated to active learning. A significant increase in the mean rating of career interest in surgery was also noted. Furthermore, faculty time dedicated to teaching decreased by 43%. The flipped classroom paradigm is flexible and can be applied to a variety of teaching environments. Its use in simulation labs for medical students has been shown to facilitate the acquisition of surgical skills such as laparoscopic suturing and knot tying (Chiu et al. 2018).

## Clinical teaching

Surgery is a high-volume service that offers a rich milieu of clinical learning opportunities. Active student participation in the outpatient, inpatient, operative, and emergency settings within the surgery clerkship cater to developing the knowledge, skills, and attitudes that are required of graduating medical students. Studies have shown that the time spent on activities involving direct patient contact is positively related to students' perceptions of the quality of their learning environment (Hinojosa-Gonzalez et al. 2020; McKinley et al. 2020).

A patient's first encounter with a member of the surgical team is often in the out-patient clinic, where an eager medical student waits, ready to take a thorough history and perform a detailed examination. Surgical patients frequently present with clear histories and prominent physical signs, which makes them suitable for developing these skills in novice medical practitioners (Agha et al. 2005). This first patient encounter initiates a doctor (medical student)-patient relationship which solidifies the student's role as a professional and active member of the surgery team. Furthermore, students are introduced to surgical pathology at its initial presentation and are given the chance to develop assessment and management plans and follow the disease process in detail during the course of their clerkship. The clinic also allows students to develop confidence in undertaking low-risk technical activities such as removing staples and sutures, simple wound dressings, drain management, and drain removal.

While an effective surgery clerkship is highly dependent on a cohesive team of students, residents and surgeons, it is ultimately supervising faculty that is responsible for overall student learning and evaluation. The relatively low-pressure environment and fewer number of team members in the clinic allow better student-faculty interaction in outpatient clinics than in the inpatient areas and operating room. There are several well-described strategies for efficient, patient-based teaching. These include the one-minute preceptor which is an easy to learn set of 5 "microskills" (Table 1-5) that can be utilized by busy faculty to teach students and trainees during the workday (Neher et al. 1992). The SNAPPS model is a student-centred model that encourages students and faculty to work together to achieve learning objectives (Wolpaw, Wolpaw and Papp 2003). Clinical faculty are able to provide students with immediate feedback after every patient presentation, identifying areas that need improvement and setting learning objectives for individual students to focus on. Subjective faculty evaluations, which make a significant portion of students' final surgery grade, typically reflect recollections of case presentations, write-ups, and observations of brief patient encounters (Butler et al. 2017). Hence, out-patient clinics are a valuable resource for monitoring student progress and informing final evaluations.

**Table 1-5: The five-step "microskills" model (Neher et al. 1992)**

| **Five-step "microskills" model** |
|---|
| Microskill 1: Get a commitment<br>Microskill 2: Probe for supporting evidence<br>Microskill 3: Teach general rules<br>Microskill 4: Reinforce what was done right<br>Microskill 5: Correct mistakes |

Ideally, the duration of the surgical clerkship allows students to cover the entire spectrum of care from admission and first clinical encounter to long term follow up. A significant portion of this takes place in the inpatient setting, where students follow the progress of two to four patients at a time. In the ward, students learn about post-operative complications, the need for regular observation, contingency planning, and discharge criteria (Agha et al. 2005).

Including students as active members of the surgery service is necessary for their training. Cortez and colleagues (2019) studied predictors of medical students' success on the surgery clerkship and found that according to students, the most highly rated active learning opportunities are presenting patients on rounds, developing assessment/plans, seeing individual consults, and answering directed questions. Passive learning activities that make a positive impact include bedside "on the fly" teaching (during rounds, in-between patients) and listening to patient care discussions.

Students as part of the surgical team do not necessarily guarantee that their involvement in patient care will allow them to practise clinical reasoning, patient management skills and procedural tasks. Programmes often depend on simulation strategies for the acquisition of these skills. However, Marie Catherine Morris and colleagues (2015) noted that medical students who have acquired a skill in a simulated setting often find it challenging to transfer this skill to the workplace. They hypothesized that a fully immersive experience requiring actual performance of an intern role (what is often referred to as a "subintern") would benefit students by allowing them to learn "on the job". They assigned fifth year students to surgical teams as subinterns for two weeks, and compared their learning experience with students who were shadowing interns. The subinterns were given clearly defined roles on the surgery team by senior residents. It is important to note that every subintern was supervised and empowered to not accept any responsibilities he/she felt incapable of handling. Each subintern was assigned to an intern as an apprentice and was provided a designated pager. Results showed that students who undertook the subinternship had a more valuable learning experience than those who just observed interns. The subintern role was an opportunity for student centred learning. The students were able to identify gaps in knowledge and skills in a safe, supervised setting, prompting them to seek remediation and practise. In the subintern group, students managed complete cases and entire patient episodes. Taking the roles of communicator, professional, and patient advocate proved a rewarding experience for the subinterns. This was in contrast to the “intern-shadow” group that reported a more fragmented experience. Furthermore, the subinterns identified their supervising interns and residents as good role models and valued the teaching they provided.

The in-house call is an essential component of training in many medical disciplines. For trainees, this is the setting where they develop many of the skills necessary for the discipline. For students, the purpose is slightly different. Most clinical rotations have students assigned to “elective” interactions (outpatient clinic, scheduled procedures) during the course of the workday. The surgery call experience exposes students to the care of patients presenting with acute pathology, allows them to assist in the on-going management of admitted patients, and provides exposure to high-stakes situations. They have a chance to experience the nuances of inpatient care, and the impact that attention to detail (or lack thereof) in this setting has on patient outcomes.

The traditional surgery clerkship call lasts 24-hours and occurs at least once a week. However, the ideal frequency of calls for medical students has not yet been established. Too few, and medical students will have limited exposure to the rigors of call and acute emergencies that arise on a surgery service. Too many, and students experience a decline in cognitive function which negatively impacts other vital academic and clinical requirements (Halbach, Spann and Egan 2003; Perez-Olmos and Ibáñez-Pinilla 2014). A study performed at a medical school in Mexico compared students taking surgical calls every three days to students taking calls every four days (Hinojosa-Gonzalez et al. 2020). They found that students who took call every third day had a higher prevalence of burnout syndrome than those who took call every fourth day. Meanwhile, students who took call every fourth day had a higher lecture attendance and academic performance than students who took call every third day. Therefore, student calls should be established in a manner that gives them the necessary on-call experience but has minimal impact on other clerkship commitments. This decision can vary from service to service and be informed by the level of on-call activity, patient acuity, length of work days, and patient load.

In 2020, the Association of Program Directors in Surgery released a consensus statement regarding the ideal senior medical student preparedness for general surgery internship (LaFemina et al. 2021). They concluded that the general surgery rotation should mirror the working environment of a surgical intern and strongly encouraged surgery clerkships to require a night, holiday and/or weekend shift experience for medical students. In addition to the obvious learning related to the discipline, such experiences encourage students to develop strategies for durability, resilience, fatigue mitigation, and burnout. This gives them insight into the requirements of a surgical career and empowers them to make an informed decision about their choice to pursue it.

Concerns regarding the value of student calls have also emerged in programs where students do 24 hour calls while residents follow a night float set up (Connelly et al. 2016). Different call schedules prevent team cohesion and result in a disconnect between students and residents on both the primary "day" team and night float. Residents play an important part in mentoring medical students. Disconnect between the two dilutes the overall educational value of the student rotation. One proposed solution is to eliminate calls for students to ensure that they remain on the same schedule as the primary team. However, this may lead to a gap in the student learning experience despite fostering team cohesion. Alternatively, students could be assigned to the night float for a period of time during which they would focus solely on call related activities. The remaining time within the clerkship would be spent on the primary surgical service, without any post-call day interruptions. Connelly and colleagues (2016) explored the effect of a night float week for students in a surgical clerkship and found that it led to improved morale, a better sense of belonging, and overall cohesion with the surgery team, without negatively impacting academic performance.

## Teaching in the operating room

The primary workplace of a surgeon is the operating room (OR). While a crucial part of every hospital, medical students often perceive the OR as a remote, somewhat daunting, separate entity. Behind those doors lies a new world with its own set of rules, code of conduct, and etiquette. In most programmes, students are introduced to the OR during their third year, and this experience is perhaps the hallmark of their surgical clerkship.

The OR presents a chance for students to observe the operative management of common and uncommon surgical diseases. They learn to appreciate the physical and emotional implications of surgery (Lyon 2003). Integrating tactile sensations of normal versus abnormal tissue and visualising real anatomy, aids students in creating a long term "clinical memory." For many, the OR also presents the chance to gain some technical surgical skill (O'Neill, Shapiro and Merchant 2018). Furthermore, the social environment of the OR allows students to develop insight into the importance of a well-functioning multidisciplinary team (Zundel et al. 2015).

Jennifer L. Irani and colleagues (2010) evaluated the quantity, quality, strategies, and content of OR teaching during the surgical clerkship at Brigham and Women's Hospital. They found that teaching residents technical aspects of the operation consumed a mean 55% of total case time, while only 9.8% of time was directed towards addressing the objectives of the surgery clerkship for students. Content that was addressed frequently was anatomy, communication skills, pathophysiology, professionalism, disease management, and post-operative care. The teaching and learning strategies most commonly employed were active student participation (e.g., placing a Foley catheter, cutting sutures), giving/following commands (e.g., "come in with the camera so you can see") and lectures (e.g., "the stenosis rate is 5-15%"). Results showed that surgeons perceive the educational value of the OR for students to be much higher than students do, a finding which mirrors other literature (McKinley et al. 2020; O'Neill, Shapiro and Merchant 2018). A better understanding of this discrepancy will allow surgical educators to improve the OR learning experience in the surgical clerkship.

In any hospital, the OR is a place of work which functions irrespective of the presence or absence of medical students. All operations are a serious matter and include an element of risk. Any education that occurs in the OR depends on the individual efforts of the surgeon and student. Lyon concluded that in order for students to have a truly effective educational experience, they must manage their learning across three related domains: managing the demands of the work environment and emotional aspects of surgery; managing educational tasks; and managing the social relations of work in the OR (Lyon 2003).

The first domain involves learning to navigate the physical environment of the OR. Students must familiarize themselves with OR protocols and the working culture, while coping with tensions that may arise during complications or during long procedures that require intense concentration (Lyon 2004). Feelings of intimidation and anxiety regarding the appropriate behaviour in the OR have been reported across the literature (O'Neill, Shapiro and Merchant 2018; Zundel et al. 2015). These feelings stem from fear of making a mistake that may cause harm to the patient, as well as fear of appearing foolish and being humiliated in the workplace. A proposed solution is to include an interactive orientation for all new students, which teaches OR protocols, hand washing, gowning and gloving, and an introduction to commonly used instruments and equipment. Studies have shown that an OR orientation has favourable results on the knowledge, skills and attitudes needed by the students (Patel et al. 2012). This also allows the surgeon a degree of comfort in knowing that they can trust students to competently play an active role during the operation, and more importantly, cause no harm.

Lyon’s second domain of managing educational tasks, involves setting clear learning objectives and goals to be achieved in the OR (Lyon 2003). The lack of clear objectives, especially in a setting where there is no defined role for the student, reduces the ability of using the OR as an effective educational setting. Students with a keen interest in surgery are motivated to develop their own goals in the OR, which largely involve gaining technical skills and procedural experience (O'Neill, Shapiro and Merchant 2018). However, these do not align with the expectations of the surgeons, who believe that learning the principles associated with surgical disease is more relevant to the students’ level than details of the operative procedure itself. Both students and surgeons agree that basic suturing and working under sterile conditions are objectives all students should achieve (Zundel et al. 2015). A proposed mechanism to ensure that students learn and participate in the OR is for programmes to develop log books or checklists that outline technical skills and procedures students must participate in (McKinley et al. 2020). Furthermore, faculty and students should share their expectations at the beginning of the clerkship, in order to develop goals that are agreed upon by both parties. Often students assigned to be in the operating room feel that unless they are part of the operating team, the experience is a poor use of their time. In a procedure where active teaching is not anticipated (usually due to the complexity of the procedure or the acuity of the patient), the surgeon should discuss this with the student beforehand. In these situations, if the student chooses to scrub in, it is understood that they are willing to maintain a strictly observational role. With the increasing utilization of laparoscopic and robotic surgery, students can be immersed in the surgical procedure without being scrubbed in, and indeed where the technology is available, they may observe the procedure remotely.

Negotiating the social relations of work and finding a legitimate role to play is Lyon's third and perhaps most important domain in determining a student's motivation to be an active participant (Lyon 2003). Medical students are at the end of the training queue, behind fellows, residents and interns. While there is no denying that students are legitimate learners in the OR and as such, they have a right to participate, many students believe they must promote themselves in the training queue to earn this right. They "size up" the OR environment (the surgeon's willingness to teach, number of people involved, responsiveness of the team, nurses' attitudes and the emotional climate) and reflect on these cues to determine the safety of initiating interaction with the team and asking for responsibility. Students who see an environment that is not fruitful to learning prefer to play the observer. Once scrubbed in, students report feeling pressured and rushed to keep up with the OR team, which hampers their engagement with the task at hand, and any learning that results from it (Zundel et al. 2015). One solution is to brief the OR team in advance regarding the time and importance of a teaching episode so as to encourage the learning process and not rush and pressure students as they perform tasks. In a study that evaluated student experience during a surgical clerkship, Berman and colleagues (2008) proved that students who are given the opportunity to actively participate in the operating room are much likelier to opt for surgical careers.

## Simulation-based teaching

The earliest use of simulation-based training in medicine can be traced back to approximately the sixth century BC. *The Sushruta Samhita*, a Sanskrit textbook written by Indian physician and surgeon Sushruta, was translated to English in 1907 (Acton 2015; Owen 2012). In it, he described lessons for students to develop their skills using natural objects that mimicked body parts, for example, making excisions on leather pouches and animal bladders filled with fluid, suturing on pieces of cloth and hides, and cauterizing pieces of meat. Between the $14^{th}$ and $17^{th}$ centuries, Chinese physicians employed bronze and clay dolls to teach students acupuncture points and meridians. Similarly, in Europe, life-size human wax models were used to teach anatomy. In response to a rising incidence of birth mortality, $18^{th}$ century Italy saw Giovanno Antonio Galli develop a birthing simulator using a glass uterus and flexible foetus to educate midwives and surgeons. Students were required to deliver the foetus blindfolded. This illustrates the key principles of effective simulation curricula: a needs assessment, an appropriate training method to teach the desired skill, and an assessment to verify learning.

Simulation-based training is a valuable tool in medical education. It allows users of all levels, from novice to expert, to practise and develop skills in a safe, supportive, educational environment, with comfort in the knowledge that mistakes will not cause harm to an actual patient (Acton 2015; Bradley 2006). By creating a realistic situation and contextual environment, simulation encourages the acquisition of skill through actual experience, thus facilitating skill transferral to the real clinical setting. Creating a standardized simulation-based training method also allows for effective assessment of skills to ensure that students have reached the desired proficiency level, before being allowed to actively participate in patient care. Simulation-based training can be applied to a number of scenarios in medicine and surgery. It is commonly employed to teach basic clinical and communication skills, simple technical skills and procedures, and teamwork and interprofessional learning.

Simulators can be divided into four broad categories: part-task trainers, simulated patients, computer-based systems, and integrated procedure simulators (Bradley 2006; Michael et al. 2014). Other characteristics used to classify simulators include animate/inanimate, virtual/real, and partial task trainer/procedural (Acton 2015).

Medical schools must consider a number of factors to conclude whether investing in a simulator is educationally worthwhile (Michael et al. 2014). Michael and colleagues summarize these key factors to include feasibility (degree of practicality of the task being performed), face validity (similarity between simulation and reality), content validity (assessment of the simulated task), construct validity (the ability to differentiate between levels of expertise), concurrent validity (similarity in outcomes between the simulation task and gold standard task), predictive validity (degree to which the task can indicate future performance in a specific skill), educational impact (degree to which the task improves performance), reliability (ability to reproduce results regardless of alteration in the subjects), acceptability (degree to which the subjects are accepting of the task), and cost effectiveness.

Part-task trainers are typically benchtop models that represent only a part of human anatomy. These trainers are often used to assist in the acquisition of technical, procedural or psychomotor skills (Bradley 2006). Abstract part-task trainers, such as knot tying boards, foam suture models, or simple laparoscopic box trainers, are reusable simulators that aid in teaching repetitive, simple tasks and are relatively inexpensive (Acton 2015). Physical anatomic trainers such as silicone, plastic, or foam replicas of human body parts are beneficial in teaching procedures with multiple steps. These include simulators for venepuncture and catheterization. Part-task trainers are very useful for teaching skills and techniques to novices, i.e., medical students. By using a simple representation of one body part to learn an isolated skill, students are able to compartmentalize the information and practise it repeatedly, without worrying about the other cognitive and procedural skills that may be required to conduct the task in reality. This allows for a better understanding of the task at hand and an improved retention of skill.

Simulated Patients (SPs) are used extensively in medical education, particularly to teach history taking, physical examinations and communication skills. A trained SP can realistically mimic clinical scenarios in a standardized, reliable manner (Bradley 2006). Furthermore, SPs can make valuable contributions to the assessment and feedback of the practised clinical encounter (Acton 2015). The departments of surgery at two large academic centres evaluated the impact of using simulated patients to teach and evaluate abdominal examinations and breast examinations to medical students during their surgical clerkship (Sachdeva et al. 1997). All medical students were shown a short instructional video developed by faculty experts demonstrating various components of each examination. They were given relevant textbook information and checklists to study from. The students in the intervention group attended a 70-minute teaching programme, conducted solely by trained SPs, who served as subject, instructor and evaluator. At the end of the clerkship, all students participated in a post-test and were assessed in four areas: breast examination skills, professionalism during the breast examination, abdominal examination skills, and professionalism during the abdominal examination. The intervention group performed better than the control group in all four categories. Furthermore, students in the intervention group also had higher scores on specific tasks such as palpation of the axillary tail, palpation of the axillary lymph nodes, and palpation of the liver and spleen, tasks that the authors believe are not performed well by most students.

Hybrid simulation combines SPs with anatomic task trainers. This adds a human element to the technical skills, which allows educators to emphasize the non-technical/communication skills that are necessary in patient care. Shariff and colleagues (2019) incorporated a hybrid abdominal wound simulation patient to teach medical students surgical drain removal, staple removal, and Steri-Strip application. Students were given relevant study material two weeks prior to a workshop where a hybrid simulation clinical scenario was first demonstrated, and then used to assess each student. A simulated patient was paired with recycled laparotomy pads which had approximated midline incisions closed with staples and a Jackson Pratt drain secured with silk sutures. Students were introduced to a two-part clinical scenario. The first was in the inpatient setting which required students to introduce themselves to the "post-op" patient, take a history, perform an abdominal exam, review the patient's chart, assess the suitability of removing the drain, and communicate plans with the nurse. On being told he had a drain, the patient acted surprised, and during removal, asked the students for a brief explanation of the procedure, if it would hurt, and whether they had any prior experience. Students then removed the drain and disposed of it in a biohazard bin. The second part emulated a follow up visit a week later in the outpatient setting, where students removed staples and applied Steri-Strips. Results showed that all students achieved proficiency in all three technical skills and scored well on communication skills.

Computer-based models use multimedia, interactive systems and virtual reality technology that allows real time human interaction within a virtual matrix (Michael et al. 2014). The LAP Mentor™ (Simbionix, Israel) virtual reality trainer consists of a screen, VR camera, two working instruments and foot pedals. The instruments and pedals are calibrated to translate any movement onto a screen depicting an intra-abdominal environment. Lucas and colleagues (2008) evaluated the effect of training medical students on the LAP Mentor to improve their virtual reality surgical performance. Students were divided into two groups. The first trained in eight tasks on the LAP Mentor, aimed at camera manipulation, hand eye coordination, clipping, grasping and clipping, two handed manoeuvres, cutting, fulguration, and object translocation. The second received no training. Both groups performed a laparoscopic cholecystectomy and were assessed using the Objective Structured Assessment of Technical Skills format. Group 1 achieved a significantly higher mean score than group 2.

Integrated procedure simulators combine a mannequin with computer controls that can result in physical (such as pulse rate or respiratory movements) or electrical (monitor readouts) outputs (Bradley 2006). U-Medic is a computer program that pairs with Harvey® The Cardiopulmonary Patient Simulator to emulate any cardiac disease by varying blood pressure, pulses, heart sounds, and murmurs. Together, the program and mannequin create a high fidelity simulator that has been shown to improve students' cardiac examination skills much more effectively than students who learn using simulated patients only (Kern et al. 2011). This system may be adapted for simulating the acute management of surgical patients.

The use of simulation as an integral part of undergraduate medical education is not up for debate. In order to use simulation effectively, medical schools must develop a simulation curriculum based on a comprehensive needs assessment. The question remains about the breadth and depth of speciality-related skills that a medical student is expected to acquire. As far as surgery is concerned, basic skills related to history taking and physical examination must be mastered. Simple procedural skills such as suturing a laceration, IV cannulation, and catheterization are a part of most programmes. Complex tasks, such as laparoscopic skill or advanced trauma care, are attractive for students with an interest in pursuing surgery as a career. However, to strive for all students to be proficient in such skills is neither necessary nor feasible.

## Summary

The global burden of surgical disease ranges between 28 to 32%, accounting for 11% of deaths annually. Five billion people do not have access to surgical care (Meara et al. 2015). There is much progress to be made to bridge this gap. However, till the deficit for specialist physicians (especially across lower-middle income countries [LMICs]) is met, it is essential that the undifferentiated doctor be well-trained in the basics related to all primary specialties. With this principle in mind, medical programmes must develop a surgical curriculum that recognizes the likelihood that the newly minted physician's ability to diagnose, triage, and to some extent, manage surgical conditions may be the key deciding factor for a favourable clinical outcome. Once the desired competencies are determined, teaching/learning and assessment strategies suited to the modern learner, the busy surgeon, the multifaceted health system, and the discerning patient must be adopted. In addition to providing substrate and instruction, programmes must be engaging and adaptive. Student engagement in patient care across multiple settings is essential. Programmes must strive to mitigate the real or perceived high-stress environment on surgical services in order to optimize learning. All this, because in the end, the surgical rotation is the nursery for tomorrow's surgeon.

## Bibliography

Abbas, Paulette, Juliet Holder-Haynes, Deborah J. Taylor, Bradford G. Scott, Mary L. Brandt, and Bindi Naik-Mathuria. "More than a Camera Holder: Teaching Surgical Skills to Medical Students." *Journal of Surgical Research* 195, no. 2 (May 2015): 385–89. DOI: https://doi.org/10.1016/j.jss.2015.01.035.

Acton, Robert D. "The Evolving Role of Simulation in Teaching Surgery in Undergraduate Medical Education." *Surgical Clinics of North America* 95, no. 4 (August 2015): 739–50. DOI: https://doi.org/10.1016/j.suc.2015.04.001.

Agha, R. A., A. Papanikitas, M. Baum and I. S. Benjamin. "The Teaching of Surgery in the Undergraduate Curriculum. Part II - Importance and Recommendations for Change." *International Journal of Surgery* 3, no. 2 (2005): 151–57. DOI: https://doi.org/10.1016/j.ijsu.2005.03.016.

Agha, R. A., A. Papanikitas, M. Baum and I. S. Benjamin "The Teaching of Surgery in the Undergraduate Curriculum - Reforms and Results." *International Journal of Surgery* 3, no. 1 (2005): 87–92. DOI: https://doi.org/10.1016/j.ijsu.2005.03.017.

Association of American Medical Colleges. "Core Entrustable Professional Activities for Entering Residency Faculty and Learners' Guide, 2014", Accessed December 10, 2020. URL: www.aamc.org/91514/reproductions.html.

ASiT Medical Student and Foundation Doctor Consensus Group, Authorship consensus group, Steering group, Writing group, Consensus exercise participants and External advisory group "Core Content of the Medical School Surgical Curriculum: Consensus Report from the Association of Surgeons in Training (ASIT)." *International Journal of Surgery* 84 (December 2020): 186–93. DOI: https://doi.org/10.1016/j.ijsu.2019.12.036.

Berman, Loren, Marjorie S. Rosenthal, Leslie A. Curry, Leigh V. Evans, and Richard J. Gusberg. "Attracting Surgical Clerks to Surgical Careers: Role Models, Mentoring, and Engagement in the Operating Room." *Journal of the American College of Surgeons* 207, no. 6 (December 2008): 793–800. DOI:

https://doi.org/10.1016/j.jamcollsurg.2008.08.003.

Bradley, Paul. "The History of Simulation in Medical Education and Possible Future Directions." *Medical Education* 40, no. 3 (March 2006): 254–62. DOI: https://doi.org/10.1111/j.1365-2929.2006.02394.x.

Butler, Kathryn L., David A. Hirsh, Emil R. Petrusa, D. Dante Yeh, Dana Stearns, David E. Sloane, Jeffrey A. Linder, Gaurab Basu, Lisa A. Thompson, and Marc A. de Moya. "Surgery Clerkship Evaluations Are Insufficient for Clinical Skills Appraisal: The Value of a Medical Student Surgical Objective Structured Clinical Examination." *Journal of Surgical Education* 74, no. 2 (March-April 2017): 286–94. DOI: https://doi.org/10.1016/j.jsurg.2016.08.018.

Cendan, Juan Carlos, Michele Silver and Kfir Ben-David. "Changing the Student Clerkship from Traditional Lectures to Small Group Case-Based Sessions Benefits the Student and the Faculty." *Journal of Surgical Education* 68, no. 2 (March-April 2011): 117–20. DOI: https://doi.org/10.1016/j.jsurg.2010.09.011.

Chiu, Hsin Yi, Yi No Kang, Wei Lin Wang, Hung Chang Huang, Chien Chih Wu, Wayne Hsu, Yiu Shun Tong, and Po Li Wei. "The Effectiveness of a Simulation-Based Flipped Classroom in the Acquisition of Laparoscopic Suturing Skills in Medical Students—A Pilot Study." *Journal of Surgical Education* 75, no. 2 (March-April 2018): 326–32. https://doi.org/10.1016/j.jsurg.2017.07.007.

Connelly, Christopher R., Phillip M. Kemp Bohan, MacKenzie R. Cook, Alexis M. Moren, Martin A. Schreiber, and Laszlo N. Kiraly. "A Night Float Week in a Surgical Clerkship Improves Student Team Cohesion." *American Journal of Surgery* 211, no. 5 (May 2016): 913–18. DOI: https://doi.org/10.1016/j.amjsurg.2016.01.011.

Cortez, Alexander R., Leah K. Winer, Young Kim, Dennis J. Hanseman, Krishna P. Athota, and R. Cutler Quillin. "Predictors of Medical Student Success on the Surgery Clerkship." *American Journal of Surgery* 217, no. 1 (January 2019): 169–74. DOI: https://doi.org/10.1016/j.amjsurg.2018.09.021.

Halbach, Melissa M., Cyril O. Spann and Glen Egan. "Effect of Sleep Deprivation on Medical Resident and Student Cognitive Function: A Prospective Study." *American Journal of Obstetrics and Gynecology* 188, no. 5 (May 2003): 1198–1201. DOI: https://doi.org/10.1067/mob.2003.306.

Hamdorf, Jeffrey M. and John C. Hall. "The Development of Undergraduate Curricula in Surgery: I. General Issues." *Australian and New Zealand Journal of Surgery* 71, no. 1 (January 2001): 46–51.

DOI: https://doi.org/10.1046/j.1440-1622.2001.02029.x.
Higher Education Commission, and Pakistan Medical & Dental Council. "Curriculum of MBBS (Revised 2011)." Accessed December 10, 2020. URL: https://hec.gov.pk/english/services/universities/RevisedCurricula/Documents/2010-2011/MBBS-Draft-2010-11.pdf.
Hinojosa-Gonzalez, David Eugenio, Juan S. Farias, Valeria Cecilia Tellez-Giron, David Aguirre-Villarreal, David Brenes-Castro, and Eduardo Flores-Villalba. "Lower Frequency of Call Shifts Leads to Higher Attendance, Higher Academic Performance, and Less Burnout Syndrome in Surgical Clerkships." *Journal of Surgical Education* (August 2020): 1–7. DOI: https://doi.org/10.1016/j.jsurg.2020.07.043.
Irani, Jennifer L., Jacob A. Greenberg, Maria A. Blanco, Caprice C. Greenberg, Stanley Ashley, Stuart R. Lipsitz, Janet Palmer Hafler, and Elizabeth Breen. "Educational Value of the Operating Room Experience during a Core Surgical Clerkship." *American Journal of Surgery* 200, no. 1 (July 2010): 167–72. DOI: https://doi.org/10.1016/j.amjsurg.2009.06.023.
Kaminski, Ashley D., Katherine M. Babbitt, Mary C. McCarthy, Ronald J. Markert, Melissa P. Roelle and Priti P. Parikh. "Team-Based Learning in the Surgery Clerkship: Impact on Student Examination Scores, Evaluations, and Perceptions." *Journal of Surgical Education* 76, no. 2 (March-April 2019): 408–13. DOI: https://doi.org/10.1016/j.jsurg.2018.07.031.
Kern, Donna H., Arch G. Mainous, Maura Carey, and Anne Beddingfield. "Simulation-Based Teaching to Improve Cardiovascular Exam Skills Performance among Third-Year Medical Students." *Teaching and Learning in Medicine* 23, no. 1 (January 2011): 15–20. DOI: https://doi.org/10.1080/10401334.2011.536753.
Knut, Haeger. *The Illustrated History of Surgery.* Jon van Leuven ed. Gothenburg, Sweden: AB Nordbok, 1988.
LaFemina, Jennifer, Vanita Ahuja, Adnan Alseidi, Marcus Balters, Karen Brasel, Clarence Clark, Keith A. Delman, et al. "APDS Consensus Statement: Ideal Senior Medical Student Experiences for Preparedness for General Surgery Internship." *Journal of Surgical Education* 78, no. 1 (January-February 2021): 69–75. DOI: https://doi.org/10.1016/j.jsurg.2020.07.015.
Lee, Matthew J., Thomas M. Drake, Tom A. M. Malik, Timothy O'Connor, Ryad Chebbout, Ahmed Daoub, and Jonathan R. L. Wild. "Has the Bachelor of Surgery Left Medical School? A National Undergraduate Assessment." *Journal of Surgical Education* 73, no. 4

(July-August 2016): 655–59. DOI: https://doi.org/10.1016/j.jsurg.2016.01.005.
Levinson, Anthony J. "Where Is Evidence-Based Instructional Design in Medical Education Curriculum Development?" *Medical Education* 44, no. 6 (June 2010): 536–37. DOI: 10.1111/j.1365-2923.2010.03715.x
Liebert, Cara A., Dana T. Lin, Laura M. Mazer, Sylvia Bereknyei and James N. Lau. "Effectiveness of the Surgery Core Clerkship Flipped Classroom: A Prospective Cohort Trial." *American Journal of Surgery* 211, no. 2 (February 2016): 451-457.e1. DOI: https://doi.org/10.1016/j.amjsurg.2015.10.004.
Lindeman, Brenessa M., Joanna K. Law, Pamela A. Lipsett, Trisha Arbella, Miloslawa Stem and Anne O. Lidor. "A Blended Online Curriculum in the Basic Surgery Clerkship: A Pilot Study." *American Journal of Surgery* 209, no. 1 (January 2015): 145–51. DOI: https://doi.org/10.1016/j.amjsurg.2014.10.003.
Lucas, Steven, Altug Tuncel, Karim Bensalah, Ilia Zeltser, Adam Jenkins, Margaret Pearle, and Jeffrey Cadeddu. "Virtual Reality Training Improves Simulated Laparoscopic Surgery Performance in Laparoscopy Naïve Medical Students." *Journal of Endourology* 22, no. 5 (2008): 1047–51. DOI: https://doi.org/10.1089/end.2007.0366.
Lyon, Patricia. "A Model of Teaching Learning in the Operating Theatre." *Medical Education* 38, no. 12 (December 2004): 1278–87. DOI: https://doi.org/10.1111/j.1365-2929.2004.02020.x.
Lyon, Patricia M. A. "Making the Most of Learning in the Operating Theatre: Student Strategies and Curricular Initiatives." *Medical Education* 37, no. 8 (August 2003): 680–88. DOI: https://doi.org/10.1046/j.1365-2923.2003.01583.x.
McKinley, Sophia K., Douglas J. Cassidy, Arian Mansur, Noelle Saillant, Arundhati Ghosh, Amy Evenson, Reza Askari, Alex Haynes, Nancy Cho, Benjamin C. James, Jaisa Olasky, Erika Rangel, Emil Petrusa and Roy Phitayakorn. "Identification of Specific Educational Targets to Improve the Student Surgical Clerkship Experience." *Journal of Surgical Research* 254 (October 2020): 49–57. DOI: https://doi.org/10.1016/j.jss.2020.03.066.
Meara, John G., Andrew J. M. Leather, Lars Hagander, Blake C. Alkire, Nivaldo Alonso, Emmanuel A. Ameh, Stephen W. Bickler, et al. "Global Surgery 2030: Evidence and Solutions for Achieving Health, Welfare, and Economic Development." *The Lancet* 386, no. 9993 (September 2015): 569–624. DOI: https://doi.org/10.1016/S0140-6736(15)60160-X.

Medical Council of India. “Competency Based Undergraduate Curriculum for the Indian Medical Graduate, Volume III, 2018”. Accessed December 10, 2020. URL: https://www.nmc.org.in/wp-content/uploads/2020/01/UG-Curriculum-Vol-III.pdf.

Michael, Michael, Hamid Abboudi, Jean Ker, Mohammed Shamim Khan, Prokar Dasgupta, and Kamran Ahmed. “Performance of Technology-Driven Simulators for Medical Students - A Systematic Review.” *Journal of Surgical Research* 192, no. 2 (December 2014): 531–43. DOI: https://doi.org/10.1016/j.jss.2014.06.043.

Morris, Marie Catherine, Martina Hennessy, Kevin C. Conlon, and Paul F. Ridgway. “Evaluation of a ‘Subintern’ Role: Action over Observation for Final-Year Medical Students in Surgery.” *Journal of Surgical Education* 72, no. 5 (September-October 2015): 862–67. DOI: https://doi.org/10.1016/j.jsurg.2015.03.003.

Neher, J. O., K. C. Gordon, B. Meyer, and N. Stevens. “A Five-Step ‘Microskills’ Model of Clinical Teaching.” *The Journal of the American Board of Family Practice / American Board of Family Practice* 5, no. 4 (July 1992): 419-424. DOI: https://doi.org/10.3122/jabfm.5.4.419.

O’Neill, Rebecca, Michael Shapiro, and Aziz Merchant. “The Role of the Operating Room in Medical Student Education: Differing Perspectives of Learners and Educators.” *Journal of Surgical Education* 75, no. 1 (January-February 2018): 14–28. DOI: https://doi.org/10.1016/j.jsurg.2017.06.013.

Owen, Harry. “Early Use of Simulation in Medical Education.” *Simulation in Healthcare* 7, no. 2 (April 2012): 102–16. DOI: https://doi.org/10.1097/SIH.0b013e3182415a91.

Patel, Vishal, Rajesh Aggarwal, Elizabeth Osinibi, Dave Taylor, Sonal Arora, and Ara Darzi. “Operating Room Introduction for the Novice.” *American Journal of Surgery* 203, no. 2 (February 2012): 266–75. DOI: https://doi.org/10.1016/j.amjsurg.2011.03.003.

Peel, John K., Christopher M. Schlachta and Nawar A. Alkhamesi. “A Systematic Review of the Factors Affecting Choice of Surgery as a Career.” *Canadian Journal of Surgery* 61, no. 1 (February 2018): 58–67. DOI: https://doi.org/10.1503/cjs.008217.

Pérez-Olmos, Isabel and Milcíades Ibáñez-Pinilla. “Night Shifts, Sleep Deprivation, and Attention Performance in Medical Students.” *International Journal of Medical Education* 5 (March 2014): 56–62. DOI: https://doi.org/10.5116/ijme.531a.f2c9.

Reis, Leonardo Oliveira, Osamu Ikari, Khaled A. Taha-Neto, Antonio Gugliotta and Fernandes Denardi. “Delivery of a Urology Online

Course Using Moodle versus Didactic Lectures Methods." *International Journal of Medical Informatics* 84, no. 2 (February 2015): 149–54. DOI: https://doi.org/10.1016/j.ijmedinf.2014.11.001.

Sachdeva, Ajit K., Philip J. Wolfson, Patrice Gabler Blair, Diane R. Gillum, Edward J. Gracely, and Miriam Friedman. "Impact of a Standardized Patient Intervention to Teach Breast and Abdominal Examination Skills to Third-Year Medical Students at Two Institutions." *American Journal of Surgery* 173, no. 4 (April 1997): 320–25. DOI: https://doi.org/10.1016/S0002-9610(96)00391-1.

Scally, Christopher P. and Rebecca M. Minter. "Medical School Training for the Surgeon." *Surgical Clinics of North America* 96, no. 1 (February 2016): 1–13. DOI: https://doi.org/10.1016/j.suc.2015.08.007.

Shariff, Faiz U., Adeline M. Deladisma, Josué W. Menard, Patricia A. Shewokis, and D. Scott Lind. "Use of a Hybrid-Abdominal Wound Simulated Patient in the ACS/ASE Medical Student Simulation Skills Curriculum." *American Journal of Surgery* 217, no. 2 (February 2019): 250–55. DOI: https://doi.org/10.1016/j.amjsurg.2018.07.039.

The Royal College of Surgeons of England. "National Undergraduate Curriculum in Surgery 2015." *RCSENG – Professional Standards and Regulation*, 2015. Accessed December 10, 2020. URL: https://www.rcseng.ac.uk/library-and-publications/rcs-publications/docs/national-undergraduate-curriculum-in-surgery/

Wolpaw, Terry M., Daniel R. Wolpaw, and Klara K. Papp. "SNAPPS: A Learner-Centered Model for Outpatient Education." *Academic Medicine* 78, no. 9 (September 2003): 893–98. DOI: https://doi.org/10.1097/00001888-200309000-00010.

Zundel, Sabine, Isabella Wolf, Hans-Juergen Christen, and Sören Huwendiek. "What Supports Students' Education in the Operating Room? A Focus Group Study Including Students' and Surgeons' Views." *American Journal of Surgery* 210, no. 5 (November 2015): 951–59. DOI: https://doi.org/10.1016/j.amjsurg.2015.03.011.

# CHAPTER 2

# BECOMING AN ACADEMIC SURGEON

HINA INAM AND ADIL HAIDER

## Beginning of academic surgery

Whilst surgery, as a practice, goes back thousands of years, gone are the days of the "barber-surgeons," famous for their bloodletting and amputations (Hindle and Hindle 2001). With the advent of modern science, and understanding of human anatomy and physiology, surgeons became specialists who knew both medicine and could "cut," and by the 19th century a new definition of surgeons emerged, as individuals specializing in performing complex operations, conducting high end research and teaching the next generation of surgeons.

Dr William Stewart Halsted, the father of modern surgery, epitomized this concept of the "triple threat" medical caregiver: he was a researcher, clinician, and teacher. Through his "Halstedian" training model, his goal was to train "not only surgeons but surgeons of the highest type." Given the number of his trainees who went on to become leaders in surgery, and in fact create new sub-specialities, he has left an incredible legacy and is proof that academic surgeons can be "triple threats," who use their clinical experience both to inform cutting edge research and as a means to educate students and trainees.

This model has been repeated in Pakistan in just the past few decades. At The Aga Khan University Hospital, Professors such as Dr Farhat Moazam and Dr Mushtaq Ahmed have shown what it means to be an astute clinician, an inspiring surgeon and a charismatic teacher. Like Halsted, they have trained prominent academic surgeons who are great assets to the country and have made great strides in advancing clinical care, and in understanding and curing disease through research and in training, both at the undergraduate and postgraduate level. In the following few pages, we hope to give readers practical tips on how they can potentially become the next Dr Farhat Moazam or Dr Mushtaq Ahmed of their generation.

## An academic surgeon

*"The chief legacy which a surgeon can bequeath is a gift of spirit. To inspire many successors with a firm belief in the high destiny of our calling...and to practise the knowledge so acquired with lofty purpose, high ideals and generous heart for the benefit of humanity — that is the best that a man can transmit".*
*Sir Berkeley Moynihan*

An academic surgeon or a triple threat is a surgeon who operates, and is both educator and researcher. They are an all-rounder, a unique bridge, extremely driven by practical surgery combined with academic research. She is a keen observer, an intellectual; she makes use of every chance and prospect provided, gains the proficiency of her mentors and eventually leads others (Balch 1986; Soybel 2001; Staveley-O'Carroll et al. 2004).

Aside from technical skills, compassion towards their work and a commitment to studying the basis of disease and disease processes are imperative for all surgeons. Surgeons hold a vital position: to make important contributions to understanding the biology of surgical diseases. Breakthrough achievements of past surgeon-scientists are an important example of this. Till date, the fields of science have nurtured nine Nobel Laureates who have made outstanding contributions in the fields of chemistry, physics, literature, peace, physiology and medicine.

One may ask why developing nations like Pakistan would need academic surgeons.

"We have so great a clinical burden; can we afford this luxury?"

The answer is a resounding, *yes*.

Only by doing original research and developing solutions to the local manifestations of clinical diseases, will we be able to provide patient cantered and culturally appropriate care – which all patients deserve. Similarly, by training more and more specialists we will be able to improve access to the millions of patients who need our help. In short, it's not a luxury; it's a necessity.

# Roadmap

Here, we present a very brief roadmap for trainees and young faculty to facilitate them in becoming an academic surgeon. Being an academic surgeon involves imagination, a deep understanding of the literature, and the ability to generate new ideas to solve clinical problems. Just like an athlete requires persistent training, dedication, and hard work, the aspiring academic surgeon also has to develop their skills not only in performing intricate surgical procedures, but also in research and grant writing. They need to be trained not only as a clinician but also as a researcher; thus, they require both surgical expertise and an investigating mind.

**The first step: find your passion**

*"Every great dream begins with a dreamer. Always remember, you have within you the strength, the patience, and the passion to reach for the stars to change the world".*
*Harriet Tubman*

Finding a career you love is equal to striking a jackpot. A career should make you wake up in the morning with enthusiasm and look forward to the day ahead. So how can you include yourself among people who can honestly say that they love what they do?

Luck has very little role to play here; it involves a mixture of career planning, hard work and persistence. Think what you're passionate about; what you would want to do day in, day out, without getting bored, something you could continue working on with the same drive and passion throughout your life. It could be general surgery, and you find your passion in the ED (Emergency Department) caring for and operating on trauma patients; it could be cardiothoracic surgery, where you love operating on the heart day in and day out without getting bored. It could be neurosurgery, where all you want to do all day is operate on the brain and see your patients make miraculous recoveries, thus, hinting towards your field of choice. Be open and listen for your passion; when you find it just go for it.

**Step two: developing mastery at your craft**

If you are not skilled, it will be difficult to love what you do. So it's important to use all your strengths and assets and chalk out a way to develop mastery in what you do. Train yourself to up your game, and once you have a strong standing to start with, additional training should be much simpler. In the case of the academic surgeon, not only do you do wonders by being the best clinician but you train yourself in research and writing grants, thus securing the essential skills necessary for success as an academic surgeon.

**Step three: find your caravan**

Once you have found your niche, it is extremely important to choose a supervisor and a mentor who can provide better training and teaching for a better career. A mentor is a companion as well as a counsellor, a coach, a role model and an advocate (Brock and Bouvet 2010; Goldstein et al. 2019). A good mentor is one who is qualified, respected in her/his field, is always available, is driven to inspire excellence, provides opportunities for collaboration and networking, and is enthusiastic to educate, direct, and counsel mentees (Bassam 2017; Cerullo and Lipsett 2017). It is similarly important to be an obedient mentee. The mentor and mentee relationship, like any other, will be more fruitful if both are dedicated to the success of the relationship. A mentor can be successful only if the mentee is proactive about meeting, open to listening, open to constructive criticism, listens to advice, is fully devoted, and is engrossed in their work. Thus, it is encouraged to seek out mentors and supporters in diverse fields for the best results.

The next step is to find likeminded people who have the same passion and love for the work you do. Being part of a group of dependable and unfailing individuals who will work with you and be there in times of need is another step towards achieving a successful academic surgery career.

While employing faculty dedicated to research is imperative, supporting new and existing faculty in the department is also essential for success. To do so, the department should form a small cohort of faculty across multiple specialties, an alliance that permits the sharing of ideas and continuous feedback and which supports its staff as they balance the equally demanding roles of surgeon and scientist.

Once you have all the necessary expertise, next you have to find a place to work that is strongly supportive of research; one should work in a department that is dedicated to research and basic sciences as discussed above. A dedicated working environment with likeminded individuals, all working towards the same goal, is definitely a sure shot recipe for success.

**Step four: perseverance and determination**

> *"Being a surgeon-scientist is a lot like playing a game of Tetris. All of the pieces have to fit together. You have to rotate them into position, and you can't stop them from dropping no matter what. If you don't get it all just right, your work continues to build up. As you progress, things get harder, not easier, and everything comes at you faster. The reward for playing the game—it's that you get to keep playing."*
> *Dr Kirk*

Academic surgery is a long road, with light at the far end of the tunnel. You may conduct research and it may be turned down a thousand times; you may carry out an experiment and end up in failure. The key here is not giving up and eventually you start enjoying the fruits of all your hard work. Perseverance, determination, and the ability to learn from failures are traits that help one during this early career period. Academic surgeons are distinctively positioned to make lasting contributions to scientific discovery through experiential expertise, which in turn will lead to improved patient care.

**Step five: teach**

"See one, do one, teach one" are famous lines in surgery. In this day and age you not only need to do one, but also get skilled at what you do, demonstrate proficiency, provide high quality care and – once you are self-dependent – you should teach your skills to the budding new surgeons. Inculcate in them the passion for their work and mentor them to success.

Joseph E. Murray, a Nobel Prize holder and first to carry out a successful kidney transplant in identical twins, notes that, "The life of a surgeon-scientist will never be a life for the faint-hearted. But with curiosity, imagination and persistence, a clinical surgeon can be a productive scientist."

Hence, educating a surgeon scientist is of the utmost importance if a surgeon wants to continue being the torch bearer of the field. The surgeon's skillset should not only be confined to the sterile field of the operating theatre but he should continue to have a standing in contemporary conversations of change. Without science at her back, a surgeon is a mere technician while others shape the future of the profession.

Thus…

*"Lesson number one is to be open for your passion, and when you feel it, pursue it. Sometimes your passion choses you…Lesson number two: be humble. And I know this is a surgeon saying 'Be humble!' Be humble, acknowledge your gaps, and address them to truly master the terrain you're trying to conquer. Now, that being said, passion and manic mastery are not enough…Lesson 3: find your caravan and don't let go. Some days you'll lead and some days you'll follow. Your caravan of teammates will aid you on your journey."*
*Dr Adil Haider (Commencement address at Washington University School of Medicine in St Louis's in 2018)*

## Bibliography

Balch, C. M. "The academic surgeon as a clinical investigator." *J. Surg. Res.* 40, no. 5 (May 1986): 413-20. DOI: 10.1016/0022-4804(86)90208-8.

Bassam, N. "Kane C in Memoriam: Michael E. Debakey." Foundation for Biomedical Research. July 11, *2017*. URL: https://fbresearch.org/memoriam-michael-e-debakey-md/.

Cerullo, M. and P. A. Lipsett. "Assessing the magnitude of a surgical career through his trainees: the John L. Cameron legacy factor." *Ann. Surg.* 265, no. 5 (May 2017): 866–868. DOI: 10.1097/SLA.0000000000002105.

Brock, M. V. and M. Bouvet. "Writing a successful NIH Mentored Career Development Grant (K award): hints for the junior faculty surgeon." *Ann. Surg.* 251, no. 6 (June 2010): 1013-7 DOI: 10.1097/SLA.0b013e3181deb4ef.

Goldstein, A. M., A. B. Blair, S. G. Keswani, A. Gosain, M. Morowitz, J. S. Kuo, M. Levine, N. Ahuja and D. J. Hackamet. "A Roadmap for Aspiring Surgeon-Scientists in Today's Healthcare Environment." *Ann. Surg.* 269, no. 1 (January 2019): 66-72. DOI: 10.1097/SLA.0000000000002840.

Hindle, K. S. and S. J. Hindle. "A History of Surgery." *J. R. Soc. Med.* 94, no. 8 (August 2001): 423. DOI: https://doi.org/10.1177/014107680109400819.

Soybel, D. I. "The education of an academic surgeon." *J. Surg. Res.* 97, no. 1 (May 2001): 1-8. DOI: 10.1006/jsre.2000.6076.

Staveley-O'Carroll, K., M. Pan, A. Meier, D. Han, D. McFadden and W. Souba. "Developing the young academic surgeon." *J. Surg. Res.* 118, no. 2 (May 2004): 109-13. DOI: https://doi.org/10.1016/j.jss.2005.09.006.

# CHAPTER 3

# FINDING A MENTOR, EASIER SAID THAN DONE!

RUKHSANA ZUBERI

> *Some are born mentors, some develop into mentors, and some have mentorship thrust upon them!*
> *(William Shakespeare)*

Mentoring is derived from a Greek word which means enduring. In Homer's *Odyssey*, Odysseus' friend Mentor was chosen to educate his son Telemachus, and Mentor's name endured through the centuries to become the term we use today. Mentor is used as a noun, as in an experienced and trusted advisor, and also as a verb, as in to advise. A mentor is traditionally defined as an influential senior person who provides help and advice over a period of time, especially at work or school, to a younger or less experienced person (Collins and Cambridge English Dictionaries), and who can hold up a mirror to us (Merriam-Webster Dictionary).

Mentoring does not mean the same thing to all people, as all people do not have the same mentoring needs, and do not need the same kind of mentor or the same kind of mentoring. Each mentor relationship has individual needs which may need individualised solutions. Effective mentorship is a careful blend of the science and the art of mentoring. This chapter will focus more on the science of mentoring; the art has to be developed by repeated deliberate practice, reflection and on-the-job learning, leading to the development of mentorship wisdom. There is one basic fundamental requirement: the mentor must truly care for the development of the mentee.

There are two kinds of mentoring. Informal mentoring, also called natural mentoring, develops on its own between a mentee and a mentor, as they may choose each other or just naturally enter a mentoring relationship.

Formal mentoring, also called planned mentoring, is where the mentees are assigned to a mentor through a mentorship programme. There is often a debate about which kind of mentoring to adopt; the informal or the formal. Informal mentoring is spontaneous and longer lasting, and may often be more successful than formal mentoring (Ragins and Cotton 1999). Mentees have a greater ownership of the mentors as they chose them, and mentors feel flattered to be chosen. Studies report that in informal mentoring, mentees were happier with their relationships and benefited from better career outcomes than those in formal relationships. However, marginalized groups, for example, minorities, those from underprivileged areas, and women, face significant challenges in establishing informal mentoring relationships (Entzami, Franzblau and Chung 2012). Rose and Rukstalis (2008) state it is unrealistic to expect that one-on-one mentoring relationships will come about by themselves if only the students can "find" the right faculty mentor. Ragins and Cotton (1999) recommend that formal mentorship programmes should be used as a foundation and a platform for developing informal mentoring relationships.

Formal mentoring is more often used and is in place for undergraduate students. In the case of graduate students, it is more often implicit in the advising/supervision function rather than explicitly written down. However, in the case of faculty, formal mentoring is often absent (Lunsford et al. 2017).

When mentors and mentees have opportunities to choose each other, formal planned mentoring takes on many aspects of natural informal mentoring.

## Why all the fuss about mentoring?

Mentoring leads to the personal, intellectual, educational and professional development of both the mentee and the mentor, and leads to the growth and enrichment of the nebulous and oft neglected institutional learning environment. Zhang et al. (2017) reported that mentoring by faculty reduced the high stress levels and exhaustion in surgical residents, resulting in happier and satisfied residents.

The Royal College of Surgeons of England strongly advocates that surgeons be mentored throughout their educational period and their career, as they are exposed to many special stresses. Residents have to endure shorter hours in relatively non-flexible residency programmes. Many newly qualified surgeons find their first steps as consultants challenging and need guidance in how to advance and how to manage, while mid-career and senior surgeons have to reach higher and higher targets, provide education to younger colleagues, change their communication styles, resolve conflicts and adapt to complicated clinical situations. Women and those from diverse backgrounds need particular support in surgery (Rashid, Narra and Woo 2015).

Hoover (2005) recommends that mentorship is not only needed for surgeons in academic practice but also for those working privately. The mentor may be a senior in the same group practice or a surgeon elsewhere. Young surgeons in private practice may need advice in negotiating contracts, avoiding sexual harassment and advice regarding fiscal and professional restraints, while senior surgeons may need advice and support on lack of hobbies, mid-life crises and diminishing skills.

In academic life, the mentoring needs of an assistant professor may be different from those of an associate professor and those again different from those of a professor (Hoover 2005). It has been said that the traditional Halstedian method of mentoring, "See one, do one, teach one," no longer serves all of the surgeon's needs.

## Who is a mentor?

A mentor is different from a supervisor. Although both have overlapping roles, both are needed in surgical training. A mentor provides a structure for educational, professional and personal developmental interactions, over a period of time (Rashid, Narra and Woo 2015).

Successful mentors in surgery are exceptional role models, demonstrate professionalism (accountability and honesty) and excellence in their field, accept responsibility for the development and achievement of their mentees, and demand the best patient care. They are innovative and reflective, self-assessing for improvement. Mentoring is crucial to professional identity formation (Warren 2005).

There are different mentorships and different mentorship traits and skills.

a. **Mentorship traits.** These include being caring, reliable, showing up on time, being committed to mentee goals and taking out time accordingly, being patient and tolerant, and having a sense of humour. There is often a greater interaction with mentors who are knowledgeable, who provide guidance and have broad perspectives (Sands et al. 1991).

*"If I have seen further it is by standing on the shoulders of giants." (Isaac Newton)*

On the other hand, it may be wise to watch out for and exclude those with some negative qualities from the mentoring programmes. These are individuals who do not wish to give time, who hold mentorship as a low priority area, who hold rigid views, who wish to mentor for the status of being called a mentor and do not maintain confidentiality. They may be sexist or violate boundaries, they may be unwilling to learn, unwilling to support, unwilling to let the mentee try new things and/or unwilling to challenge them when needed. Other negative qualities are being directive or being in competition with the mentee, especially in faculty-to-faculty mentorship, both at the same level or in senior-junior peer mentorship.

b. **Mentorship skills.** A good mentor should be an advocate for the mentee and must also portray several skills (Northouse 2018), many of which can be developed. They should show:
   - managerial skills providing structure to the mentorship process: these include scheduling meetings and defining mentor-mentee roles and responsibilities;
   - specialty-related technical skills in the relevant area of the mentee's need; and
   - people skills to work with people, to *build relationships*, trust, respect and liking between the mentor and mentees, and between mentees. In the latter case, mentees have an additional subgroup of peer mentors to rely on and become self-reliant.

The mentor should be caring, a good listener, non-judgmental, should maintain a high level of confidentiality, and have the skills to know when to push, when to just listen (most of the time) and when to back off. A mentor should judiciously challenge mentees to reach new heights. The trick is to help guide mentees through issues and highlight different options, but not offer them solutions. This hones the mentees' decision-making skills and enables them to grow.

Lastly, wanting the mentee to do better than the mentor is implicit in the relationship.

- Mentorship skills are situational; they require a balancing act. At one end of the spectrum, the mentee may seem not to need any advice and the mentor may feel redundant while at the other end, the mentee may become over-dependent on the mentor.

Situational mentorship comes into its own as the mentor needs to switch roles from mentee to mentee, and even towards the same mentee depending on the mentee's previous knowledge and experience of the task at hand. This is akin to the "Situational Leadership Style" where one's style may change from directing and coaching, to supporting and delegating with less and less direct involvement, as the mentees become more and more empowered and the mentor sits back and observes, ready to step in as needed (Blanchard, Zigarmi and Zigarmi 2013). This useful approach has been used in developing the adaptive mentorship model (Ralph and Walker 2013).

## Mentor-mentee trust relationship

**Building a trusting relationship is vital to the mentorship process.** There is a cyclical development to the mentoring relationship (Hunt and Michael 1983). Successful mentoring relationships go through four phases: initiating and negotiating, relationship cultivation, enabling, and closure; very similar to small group functional stages of storming, norming, performing and disbanding. These sequential phases build on each other and often vary in length. The point is not to get upset with the mentees at the negotiating phase of mentorship; it is a norm!

**A prequel to the four phases is the Preparation Phase.** Each potential mentor and mentee should be oriented to the Mentorship Programme. These are usually the processes for

a. orientation: finding out the responsibilities, available policies, support services and resources, as well as where to meet and how to meet;
b. mentor development: developing as an educated and enabled mentor through mentorship development sessions, workshops and programme(s); and
c. finding out the mentee's and mentor's background.

## Initiation and negotiating (the first phase)

With scheduled regular meetings (Lumkin 2011), mentors can attain a close presence in the life or work of the mentee. This is usually helped by having a structured mentorship programme, through which the first meeting(s) can be initiated.

**Step 1:** The mentee's needs have to be the point of focus.

**Step 2:** Mentors must get to know the mentees as persons in their own environments, as integral parts of their own families and their own friends, in their own habitat. The mentor must determine where the mentees need help, where they enjoy themselves, and what their strengths are.

**Step 3:** Mentors do not replace family or friends; they are in addition to them.

**Negotiating:** During the initiating phase discuss the initiative/control/direction with the mentees, as to who will manage the meeting(s). Several options may be tried out to find which work(s) best for each mentee and the mentor. This is also called the negotiating stage.

- The mentor leads throughout; the mentee follows the lead.
- The mentee does all the initiating, and the mentor lets them lead.
- Both the mentor and the mentee may share instigating and responding to the other's lead, nearly equally.
- The mentor may initiate and direct the initial meetings and then gradually let the mentee take over the direction.

Ask the mentee to choose one of the above options and test it out for at least three meetings. At the conclusion of every meeting, discuss if the option worked or not. Discuss the strengths of the option and determine if it helps the mentee or not. Honest discussion and feedback are essential. Even if the previous option feels right, the two may like to try out other options to find out whether they are better or worse. It provides additional practice for the mentee. Again, it must be followed up with honest feedback on how both the mentor and the mentee felt with the different options. The mentors should note and reflect on their own responses to the different options – it helps mentors grow. Find the option that works best and use it as the usual method of interaction. Discuss how the chosen option may differ from what others favour around them.

Both mentees and mentors need feedback. The mentor must consistently provide the mentees with steady constructive feedback on their performance, and ask for reactions to their own role.

**Crucial relationship cultivation (the second phase)**

Also called the mentor-mentee trust building phase, this stage is also largely dependent on the mentor.

Cultivation involves the building of mutual respect and trust, and the most successful mentoring occurs where such a relationship develops. It is very similar to trust building in the patient-doctor relationship, except that in this case the mentee is an empowered healthy adult, they know where they wish to go and may need the mentor's help in thinking things out or guidance only, and may occasionally need a more active role from the mentor.

While building the mentor-mentee relationship it is good to be aware of the changing face of mentorship. The older models were more authoritative, controlling, directive, paternalistic and rigid, while the newer models have a friendlier reciprocal relationship with non-judgmental, supportive, and active listening. The aim is to develop, inspire and empower the mentees.

> "The greatest good you can do for another is not just to share your riches but to reveal to him his own." (Benjamin Disraeli)

Several frameworks for the mentor-mentee or mentor-protégé relationship have been reported. Frameworks report the importance of context, the attributes desired by the mentor and the mentee in each other, and the developmental steps in the mentor-mentee relationship. If both belong to the same department, for example surgery, it is easier to understand the issues and suggestions, situating the issues within the department's and the mentees' needs. The relationship is sometimes affected by the genders of the mentor and mentee.

**Enabling (the third phase)**

This is the phase of most growth and is most beneficial for both mentee and mentor.

Once a strong mentor-mentee trust relationship has developed, it is likely to have a positive impact on the growth of the mentee, the mentor and the organization. The opposite is also true; a negative relationship may be detrimental to both parties and the institution (Hunt and Michael 1983).

The relationship may be strong and may even border on familial. This is where the mentor can do no wrong in the eyes of the mentee and is the time to be most careful, ethical, truthful, and open, the time at which to portray the highest level of integrity (Milton 2004). The actions and words of the mentor are picked up subconsciously by the mentee and internalized. Therefore, it is imperative the mentor "walks the talk" of portraying the highest professional values (Spiers 2020).

During the interactions, the mentors must hold back and not try to change the mentee into a replica of themselves; if the mentees wish to emulate the mentors, they will do so themselves. As Steven Spielberg said, "Mentoring is not creating them in your own image, but giving them the opportunity to create themselves."

This is the phase where the mentees, with philosophical discussions, guidance and some fun together, find themselves, reach their aspirations and may outperform themselves. Mentoring is not only a "*brain to pick, an ear to listen, and a push in the right direction,*" as quoted by John Crosby, but must fulfil "*our chief want in life ... somebody who will make us do what we can*", to quote Ralph Waldo Emerson.

*A mentee may need multiple mentors for multiple goals or at multiple stages,* and should be encouraged to find a variety of mentors, each with different strengths relevant to the different mentee needs. Surgical residents should be exposed to many types of role models and mentors, to learn surgery, management and communication skills, and to be able to make correct career choices and aim for a work–life balance (Rashid, Narra and Woo 2015). This is also called "mosaic mentoring" (Economopoulos et al. 2014). It not only ensures the mentees grow in all areas, but also exposes the mentees to different mentors with different mentoring styles.

**Closure (the fourth phase)**

After the mentoring is over, when mentees no longer need their mentors or when the mentee moves away, comes the separation stage. It may be painful and joyful: painful because a nurturing relationship is ending and joyful because the mentor did a great job; both have been transformed, and the mentee is now confident and empowered. However, the relationship need not end but may go through a redefinition towards a more collegial relationship of a lasting friendship and the mentors may continue to hold a special place in their mentees' lives.

## Peer mentorship

**Peer mentoring among students** has its own history of successes and risks. Five peer mentor roles have been reported as being appreciated by mentees; they can be: (a) a link to other students; (b) a leader in motivating and guiding them; (c) a coach to help identify their own strengths and areas needing strengthening; (d) an advocate and liaison between the mentee student and faculty members; and (e) a trusted friend (Colvin and Ashman 2010).

Student peer mentors also gain multiple benefits. These include developing the ability to offer student support, strengthening of their own life concepts and how to deal with adversity in their own lives, developing stronger links with faculty, and gaining appreciation and recognition (Colvin and Ashman 2010). Student peer mentors can also develop strong links with other student mentors and the support systems.

Relatively fewer risks have been reported. The main risks to peer mentors are lack of time and over-commitment, and the risk to peer mentees was becoming over-dependent on their peers.

**Peer mentoring among postgraduate residents** has been successful in PhD students (Lewinski et al. 2017) and in senior to junior resident mentoring, where the senior residents volunteered and were prepared for mentoring through mentoring workshops (Eisen et al. 2014). Decreasing in frequency, the areas under discussion centred around career development, accessing learning opportunities, work-life balance and performance issues, examinations, clinical skills, colleague relationships, time management, communication skills, and lastly, personal issues and ill health.

The senior resident peer mentor reported improvement in their own coaching and communication skills, in understanding issues faced by juniors and in building networks. There was a positive impact on their professionalism and they also gained a framework for solving problems (Eisen et al. 2014).

**Faculty to faculty peer mentorship** within the profession is an essential relationship. Despite knowing how important mentoring is for personal and professional development of juniors and for nurturing members of a discipline, faculty often have a laissez-faire approach to it.

In intra-departmental mentoring, the proximity of being seated together or working together aids stronger mentee-mentor relationships. When both are in the same discipline it is easier to help in their teaching, service or research roles, as well as help them through institutional and departmental issues.

Peer mentoring is critical for aiding recently qualified junior consultants and in helping those who may be facing problems and issues. In surgery, it is vital in developing future competent surgeons and surgical leaders. The desirable attributes or competencies have to be identified and carefully nurtured and enhanced by challenges, discussions and encouragement (Milton 2004). The essential qualities of a successful peer mentor include knowledge about the department or institution and knowledge about career advancement, competence in their specialty, influential status within the department, and the will to aid the growth of others. The best mentors protect, guide, coach, and challenge their mentees. They provide feedback and open doors for them. They are also role models and counsellors who provide inspiration and advice. Junior mentors can be as successful as senior mentors (Lumpkin 2011). New and creative ideas should be initiated, explored and discussed. This leads to improvement of the junior and senior faculty members, and also of the department, the institution and the profession (Milton 2004).

The secret is that the gains to both should be determined, verbalized and openly discussed. This needs to be the point of focus as more than one person gains during the mentorship relationship. Mentors have reported multiple gains ranging from extrinsic rewards (such as help in their projects, publicity and exposure) to intrinsic rewards (such as increasing their effectiveness, their experiences, and their wisdom by developing multiple perspectives of a problem). Achievement of self-actualization – reaching the apex of Maslow's hierarchy – is a tremendously powerful gain for the mentor.

Several newer directions were reported by Economopoulos et al. (2014). They advocate that the most experienced surgeons should mentor the most inexperienced, as professors have the most experience and probably the most time, and also recommend both mentoring in the Simulation Lab and "scrub-sink" mentoring. In the latter approach, questions like, "what is the procedure, why is it being done, how should it be done, and what is the evidence for doing it?" should be asked.

An important area, often missed, is being aware of the difficulties of women advancing in surgery. Women residents and women junior surgeons are often overlooked. They may prefer or need senior women surgeons as mentors, but there are few women in surgical leadership positions (Entzami, Franzblau and Chung 2012). All mentors of women mentees must introspect whether they carry an implicit bias for or against them. The women should be encouraged to find and live their true value, and to accept nothing less (Lillemoe 2017).

Group peer mentorship has been tried. It saves time and has been more successful than one-on-one mentoring for fulfilling the mentoring needs of the junior and mid-career faculty members (Bussey-Jones et al. 2006; Pololi and Evans 2015). Faculty at the same academic level, with diverse strengths and interests, come together in a structured format to provide mentorship to each other (Bussey-Jones et al. 2006) in professional development, research and education. However, competing demands of acute patient care and competition for research grants remain a challenge. A senior faculty member may advise and guide the peer mentoring group to keep them going.

The newer paradigm of "mosaic group mentoring" has emerged to fulfil the professional, discipline-based, procedural, career development and personal needs of the mentee (Economopoulos et al. 2014). This is particularly true for faculty members. The reasons are many, the commonest being that in a pyramidal departmental with a hierarchical structure, there are not enough senior faculty members to provide mentorship to all junior members in the department on a one-to-one basis (Bussey-Jones et al. 2006). Occasionally, the senior mentor may not have strengths in all the areas needed by the mentee. Thus, multiple, diverse and mutually beneficial mentoring relationships come into their own (Zellers, Howard and Barcic 2008).

## Mentorship ethics

Although multiple benefits have been reported from successful mentoring programmes for students, graduate students and residents, as well as for faculty members, it is vital to be aware of a variety of ethical issues which may ensue from the multiple roles and close mentoring relationships to negatively impact the mentoring process (Warren ES 2005). On a cautionary note, mentors must refrain from asking mentees to perform personal errands. Secondly, the double relationship of being in a strong mentoring relationship as well as an assessor may also have serious ethical concerns. Therefore, it is preferable if the mentor is not the assessor in summative assessments. Thirdly, to avoid any kind of romantic involvement in a close mentoring relationship, it is better not to have social one-to-one meetings with mentees. Group social events are fine. Lastly, the mentor's own biases must be faced, acknowledged and dealt with.

This area needs careful introspection and it is imperative to include it in mentee and mentor development programmes.

## Mentorship programme, structure and policies

Mentorship does not work without a programme. It may spurt up here and there on an individual basis but benefits only a few. A mentorship programme is needed to benefit *all.*

**The mentorship programme needs a structure.** A little structure goes a long way. While providing a framework for mentors and mentees to work within, it should provide enough flexibility to tweak their individual relationships as needed. The programme structure should include resources where the mentor can touch base and consult with others without breaking confidence. It must also include additional resources, policies, reporting and support structures which may be needed by the mentors or by the mentees (MENTOR/National Mentoring Partnership, 2005).

- **a. The mentorship programme needs a creative vision and mission**[1] for mentoring with an inspiring and powerful slogan! "*Help Others and Grow*!" The vision should be clear, concise and realistic, aligned to the institutional vision, and reflect the institutional values and beliefs. The mission should state what is to be accomplished, how it's to be done, and for whom – the target audience. It should also address the needs of those who are to be mentored.
- **b. The mentorship philosophy** must be clearly documented, as should the benefits to the mentees, the mentors and the institution. For example, "collegial, non-judgmental encouragement of the mentees to attain their full potential."
- **c. The goals and objectives** of the programme must follow from the vision and mission. They must be clear and explicit, Specific, Measurable, Achievable, Relevant and Time-bound (SMART).
- **d. Programme guidelines and policies**. There are different kinds of mentorships and the institution must identify which kind of mentoring will be part of the mentorship programme. It may be one of the following or a combination thereof:

**One-to-one** mentoring where:

---

[1] Adapted from The Abell Foundation. *Mentoring Manual: A Guide to Program Development* and Implementation. Abell Foundation, 1990.

- an elder person mentors a younger person or learner; or
- peers mentor each other.

**Group mentoring**: one adult mentors four to ten younger people, or a peer group mentor each other, with a senior advisor looking on.

**Team mentoring:** several adults mentor small teams and consult with each other. The mentees can access the other mentors for different aspects or issues – a variant of mosaic mentoring.

**The programme must clarify criteria and processes.**

**Mentor qualifications and attributes** should be explicitly documented and shared in the orientation and mentoring development programmes, and posted in the university or institutional domain. Finding mentors will require advertising, soliciting, and screening for recruitment. Some large scale programmes require written applications, interviews and signed agreements.

**The programme should preferably match** the mentors to mentees according to background, life experiences and race. Sometimes they may need to be re-matched if the mentee and/or mentor so desire. The programme coordinator should meet with the two together and also separately, to find out what went wrong. It is recommended to try mediation first. If it does not work out, then the programme coordinator should help them achieve closure and change.

**The process of mentoring** may be done through face-to-face meetings, via email and/or web-based, or any combinations or permutations of these. The mentoring site may be either the workplace and/or a recreational site for face-to-face meetings. The structures and options should be provided.

A **mentorship office** and **additional resources** must be available to mentors and regular communication has to be part of the programme. The mentorship office is needed for consultation in case of trouble-shooting and a mentorship helpline is useful in times of crises.

The mentorship programmes can guide all departments to ensure that their new incoming faculty members enter the support programmes and get connected early.

Mentors need to be supported throughout their mentorship career.

**The criteria for identifying outstanding mentor and/or mentee efforts** and their rewards and recognition should also be explicitly documented. It has also been recommended to recognize, announce, and applaud publicly and in writing, the departments with more mentors and/or more institutional role models as exemplary mentors in the institution.

### Mentorship advisory group

A mentorship advisory group has been strongly recommended to oversee the programme and identify SMART goals and objectives for the mentorship programme (Lumpkin 2011). The group should identify the philosophy, the aspirations and the vision. It must establish policies and processes, identify and/or delineate and develop resources for the programme, and implementation strategies for beginning an institution-wide or department-wide mentoring programme. The advisory group should also be responsible for interviewing potential mentors, preparing informational material to disseminate, creating a handbook for quick reference, and advising mentorship development programmes, as well as monitoring and planning for mentorship programme evaluation (Lumpkin 2011).

**It should also determine structures** to monitor and reduce costs, increase visibility, and conserve resources.

The advisory group should hold mentor-mentee and department recognition events. It has been recommended that the media be invited to the recognition event, and the match of the month or other forms of recognition should be announced as well as recognized in the written form. Running stories of successful mentors helps the cause.

The advisory group must disseminate, communicate and advertise the programme.

## A mentorship development programme to initiate and regularly refresh mentorship

*The mentor also grows from novice to competent to master mentor!*

All mentors need a development programme. Just as learners go through a process of developing from a novice, to an advanced learner, to become competent and then an expert, similarly mentors go through a developmental process from novice mentor, to advanced beginner mentor, to competent and then master mentor.

Mentor development programmes must provide knowledge regarding the department or institution, about career advancement and share how to initiate and develop a mentor-mentee trust relationship. It should emphasise the mentors' roles of student advocacy, academic tutoring and/or helping mentees access resources for academic tutoring, and counselling if needed. It is important for mentors to know how to defuse situations and the steps for crisis prevention if the mentee is overwhelmed. They should also know the different methods of resolving mentee grievances and conflicts.

Special attention should be given to ethics and ethical implications in the mentoring practices. Mentors must be asked to explore their own biases towards women and people from dissimilar backgrounds, to reflect and write them down and work out ways to minimize them.

Attention should also devoted to handling situations when mentees face common and/or serious problems, and should include knowledge of the available guidelines, policies, support and resources. The development programme should also develop the mentor's communication skills including non-judgmental listening and providing constructive feedback skills, with emphasis on the deafening power of silent open listening.

Both the mentees and the mentors should be provided on-going professional development.

The programme should empower mentors on how to define and develop mentee goals, and develop the mentee's skills in decision-making, value clarification and long term planning. The most important feeling to inculcate is that they belong to a great cause and the cause is theirs – developing their feeling of "ownership and belonging."

**Orientation programmes:** The mentorship orientation programmes should be held separately for the mentors and the mentees (Colvin and Ashman 2010). Invite media to the orientation event and include:

1. the mentorship programme structure, its governance and policies, how it will be monitored and evaluated;
2. responsibilities of the mentors and of mentees, before they join;

3. expected processes of mentorship, the responsibilities and time commitments;
4. qualities of a successful mentor and expectations from a mentee;
5. effective communication skills (listening skills, non-judgmental for mentors, and non-defensive for both);
6. the mentor recruitment process;
7. the mentorship development programme;
8. the resources available to the mentors;
9. the grievance handling process; and
10. the rewards and recognition of outstanding mentor and/or mentee efforts.

## Plan for monitoring and programme evaluation

The most meaningful outcomes to be targeted for effectiveness should be identified and selected.

On-going supportive monitoring is essential, not to penalize if any are falling short, but to enable all to meet the requirements and targets. Formative evaluations for feedback should be scheduled regularly (Lumpkin 2011). The programme coordinator may meet with the mentees and mentors periodically on a regular basis to monitor the meetings and the interaction, and find out about any issues before they escalate. Rose and Rukstalis (2008) advocate inclusion of monitoring of the mentoring process within the curriculum, as that would help to nurture and develop the medical student and resident mentees.

The benchmarks for programme evaluation and how to determine the impact and effectiveness of the mentorship programme should be defined early. The method for programme evaluation, for example the CIPP Model (Context, Input, Process and output or Product) or an alternative should also be identified early and personnel educated in it.

## Beware the pitfalls!

It is essential to avoid the pitfalls. A number of them have been taken into account in the sections above.

**Beware of the systemic/institutional flaws**. A lack of culture of mentoring! There may be a lack of emphasis of mentoring as a mission or too little value set on mentoring by the institution. Mentoring should be mandatory for all and included in the letter of expectations, and mentors must have protected exclusive time for mentoring.

**Lack of orientation and/or education and development of mentors and/or mentees** may prove to be a disaster, as they would not know how to set goals or make them explicit; they would have little idea of establishing the mentee-mentor relationship. If mentorship development programmes are optional, one ends up preaching to the choir!

**All incoming faculty want the Chairs to be their mentor.**

**Be careful regarding issues with gender and ethnicity** – sometimes they need to be matched like-for-like and sometimes with others.

**Generational gap and cultural differences** can sometimes be barriers to good mentoring (Entzami, Franzblau and Chung 2012).

**Mentor-mentee difficulties.** Recruiting clinical faculty is difficult and mentees sometimes may not wish for basic science faculty as mentors. On the other hand encouraging students to engage and maintain such relationships may be also be a challenge.

## Summary

Classically, a mentor is defined as an influential senior person who provides help and advice over a period of time, especially at work or school, to a younger or less experienced person. While informal mentoring has often proved to be more successful than formal mentoring, it provides unequal opportunities for women and people from disadvantaged backgrounds. It is more equitable to initiate formal mentorship programmes that may be used as a base for developing informal mentoring relationships.

The creation of a close mentee-mentor trust relationship is crucial to effective mentoring and can be transformational; it can change and transform both the mentees and the mentors. It leads to increased motivation, aspirations and achievements for both. Wishing the mentee does better than the mentor is implicit in the relationship.

A mentorship programme needs a structure, an office, an advisory group, policies, strong advertising and dissemination, mentee and mentor orientation, and development programmes, with due recognition and rewards. The programme must be monitored regularly and evaluated periodically. Ethics in mentorship should be given due cognizance as should the common challenges and pitfalls. All mentors and mentees need training and constant support.

Mentors should be chosen for their role modelling of professional behaviour, excellence in their fields, reliability, and commitment to developing others. The newer models of mentorship advocate non-judgmental supportive active listening and letting mentees find themselves, explore their values and build decision-making skills in their professional and personal lives. Mosaic mentoring, a subset of group mentoring, holds great promise, as mentees often need more than a single mentor for advancement as a professional, as a researcher, as an educator, as a manager and administrator, and for career advancement.

Mentorship has come a long way in many fields and there is a great tradition in mentorship in surgery, but there is also a plea to do it better in advancing the careers of the underprivileged and the increasing number of women surgeons (Lillemoe 2017).

A strong case is made that mentorship is needed in surgery at all levels. It is needed by medical students and residents, and by junior, mid-career, and senior faculty members, both in academic and private practices.

## Bibliography

Blanchard, K., P. Zigarmi and D. Zigarmi. *Leadership and the one minute manager: Increasing effectiveness through Situational Leadership II*. New York: William Morrow, 2013.

Bussey-Jones, J., L. Bernstein, S. Higgins, D. Malebranche, A. Paranjape, I. Genao, B. Lee and W. Branch. "Repaving the Road to Academic Success: The IMeRGE Approach to Peer Mentoring." *Acad. Med.* 81, no. 7 (July 2006): 674–679. DOI: 10.1097/01.ACM.0000232425.27041.88.

Colvin, J. W. and M. Ashman. "Roles, Risks, and Benefits of Peer Mentoring Relationships in Higher Education." *Mentoring & Tutoring: Partnership in Learning* 18 no. 2 (May 2010): 121–134. DOI: 10.1080/13611261003678879.

Economopoulos, K. P., R. C. Sun, E. M. Garvey, J. Hogan and A. Bazzarelli. "Coaching and mentoring modern surgeons." *Bulletin Am. Coll. Surg.;* 99, no. 8 (August 2014): 30-35. URL:

https://www.researchgate.net/profile/Raphael-Sun/publication/264991161_Coaching_and_mentoring_modern_surgeons/links/54f9db630cf29a9fbd7c5669/Coaching-and-mentoring-modern-surgeons.pdf#page=30).

Eisen, S., S. Sukhani, A. Brightwell, S. Stoneham and A. Long. "Peer mentoring: evaluation of a novel programme in paediatrics". *Arch. Dis. Child.* 99, no. 2 (October 2014): 142–146. DOI: 10.1136/archdischild-2013-304277.

Entezami P., L. E. Franzblau and K. C. Chung. "Mentorship in surgical training: a systematic review." *Hand* 7, no. 1 (March 2012): 30–36. DOI: DOI: 10.1007/s11552-011-9379-8.

Hoover E. L. Mentoring Surgeons in Private and Academic Practice. *Arch. Surg.* 140, no. 6 (June 2005): 598-608. DOI: 10.1001/archsurg.140.6.598.

Hunt, D. M. and C. Michael. "Mentorship: A Career Training and Development Tool." *Academy of Management Review* 8, no. 3 (July 1983): 475-485. DOI: https://doi.org/10.5465/amr.1983.4284603.

Lewinski, A. A., T. Mann, D. Flores, A. Vance, J. P. Bettger and J. Hirschey. "Partnership for development: A peer mentorship model for PhD students." *J. of Professional Nursing* 33, no. 5 (Sep-Oct 2017): 363-369. DOI: 10.1016/j.profnurs.2017.03.004.

Lillemoe, K. D. "Surgical Mentorship. A Great Tradition, But Can We Do Better for the Next Generation?" *Annals of Surgery* 266, no. 3 (November 2017): 401-410. DOI: 10.1097/SLA.0000000000002374.

Lumpkin, A. "A Model for Mentoring University Faculty." *The Educational Forum* 75 no. 4 (August 2011): 357-368. DOI: org./10.1080/00131725.2011.602466.

Lunsford, L. G., G. Crisp, E. L. Dolan and B. Wuetherick B. "Mentoring in Higher Education." In *The SAGE Handbook of Mentoring,* edited by David A. Clutterbuck, Frances K. Kochan, Laura Lunsford, Nora Dominguez and Julie Haddock-Millar, 316-334. London: SAGE Publishing Ltd, 2017.

MENTOR/National Mentoring Partnership. *How to build a Successful Mentoring Program Using the Elements of Effective Practice. A step by step toolkit for Program Managers*. Alexandria, VA: MENTOR/National Mentoring Partnership, 2005. URL: www.mentoring.org/eeptoolkit.

Milton, C. L. "The Ethics of Personal Integrity in Leadership and Mentorship: A Nursing Theoretical Perspective." *Nursing Science Quarterly* 17, no. 2 (April 2004): 116-20. DOI: https://doi.org/10.1177/0894318404263261.

Northouse, P. G. "Chapter 3 Skills Approach," in *Leadership Theory and Practice 8th Edition*, 100-134. California: SAGE Publications Inc., 2018.

Pololi, L. H. and A. T. Evans. "Group Peer Mentoring: An Answer to the Faculty Mentoring Problem? A Successful Program at a Large Academic Department of Medicine." *Journal of Continuing Education in the Health Professions* 35, no. 3 (Summer 2015): 192–200. DOI: 10.1002/chp.21296.

Ragins, B. R. and J. L. Cotton. "Mentor functions and outcomes: A comparison of men and women in formal and informal mentoring relationships." *Journal of Applied Psychology* 84, no. 4 (August 1999): 529-550. DOI:10.1037/0021-9010.84.4.529.

Ralph, E. G. and K. Walker. "The Efficacy of the Adaptive Mentorship© Model." *Open Journal of Leadership* 2, no. 2 (January 2013): 21-26. DOI: http://dx.doi.org/10.4236/ojl.2013.22003.

Rashid, P., M. Narra and H. Woo. "Mentoring in Surgical Training". *ANZ J. Surg.* 85, no. 4 (February 2015): 225–229. DOI: org/10.1111/ans.13004.

Rose, G. L. and M. R. Rukstalis. "Imparting medical ethics: the role of mentorship in clinical training." *Mentoring & Tutoring: Partnership in Learning* 16, no. 1 (February 2008): 77-89. DOI: 10.1080/13611260701801031.

Royal College of Surgeons of England. "Mentoring." Accessed January 26, 2021. URL: https://www.rcseng.ac.uk/standards-and-research/support-for-surgeons-and-services/professional-support-for-surgeons/mentoring/.

Sands, R. G., Parson, L. A., & Duane, J. Faculty Mentoring Faculty in a Public University. The Journal of Higher Education. 1991 62, no. 2 (March-April 1991): 174-193. DOI: doi.org/10.1080/00221546.1991.11774114.

Spiers, H. "Mentorship and its role in surgical training." *Urology News* 25, no. 1 (November-December 2020): para 3. URL: ww.urologynews.uk.com.

Warren, E. S. "Future Colleague or Convenient Friend: The Ethics of Mentorship." *Counseling and Values* 49, no. 2 (January 2005): 82-160. DOI: https://doi.org/10.1002/j.2161-007X.2005.tb00260.x.

Zellers, D. F., V. M. Howard and M. A. Barcic. 2008. "Faculty Mentoring Programs: Reenvisioning Rather Than Reinventing the Wheel." *Review of Educational Research* 78, no. 3 (September 2008): 552-558. DOI: 10.3102/0034654308320966

Zhang, H., A. Isaac, E. D. Wright, Y. Alrajhi and H. Seikaly. "Formal mentorship in a surgical residency training program: a prospective interventional study." *Journal of Otolaryngology – Head and Neck Surgery* 46, no. 1 (February 2017):13. DOI 10.1186/s40463-017-0186-2.

# CHAPTER 4

# TELEMENTORING IN SURGERY

NOMAN SHAHZAD AND TABISH CHAWLA

## Global burden of surgical diseases

Global surgery aims to provide safe, affordable and in time surgical care to all, by eliminating inequity in the distribution of surgical resources throughout the world irrespective of geographic or demographic bounds. Though initially surgery was neglected in global health initiatives, recently there has been increasing recognition of the global burden of surgical diseases and strategies are being developed to overcome the disparities in surgical care (Farmer and Meara 2013). Despite the efforts, most low- and lower-middle-income countries give low priority to surgical services in their health budgets, due to competing health priorities and financial constraints. Surgical care in these regions remains non-uniform.

About 30% of the global burden of disease is surgical (Shrime et al. 2015). Overall worldwide, two billion people lack access to surgical care (Funk et al. 2010). Only 25% of the estimated 234 million operations performed annually occur in low- and lower- middle-income countries, which constitute 70% of the world population (Weiser et al. 2008). Lack of access to surgery often results in preventable death and disability.

Surgery is likely to play an increasing role in the future, in the management of both acute and chronic illnesses due to shifting patterns of diseases, aging populations, increase in global population and improvement in surgical techniques and modalities (Weiser et al. 2008). This rising burden of surgical diseases is mostly to be shared by low and low-middle income countries due to their high population growth rates (Hofman et al. 2005).

However, issues regarding access to healthcare are not limited to low-income countries. In high-income countries, centralization of care has been shown to improve outcomes across a number of conditions (Birkmeyer 2002). Centralization typically concentrates specialist surgery in metropolitan hubs and an unintended consequence of this is the restriction of access to surgery in remote areas (Shively and Shively 2005).

**Obstacles to effective surgical care in remote areas and low- and lower-middle-income countries**

Major contributors to the lack of access to surgical care in low and lower-middle income countries are the lack of trained surgeons and non-availability of adequate operation facilities (Jamison et al. 2006).

Furthermore, due to ever changing needs of surgical care, continuing surgical education is required to keep the knowledge and skills of the trained surgeons up to date. A major barrier to keeping surgical skills in line with the latest developments for those working in resource constrained environments is the availability of training opportunities. Where they are available, access and affordability become a significant challenge.

Telementoring, being able to deliver training across borders (hence alleviating the need for travel), and simultaneous training at multiple centres, can overcome many of these obstacles.

**Traditional surgical training**

The training of surgeons has evolved remarkably over time since the inception of the art of surgery. Historically surgeons were not qualified doctors, rather they evolved from the "barber-surgeon," – which required no formal training, qualification, or degree – whereas physicians were referred to as "doctors". In some parts of the world the title of surgeons is still "mister" instead of doctor. They used to learn the art of surgery through apprenticeships. This apprenticeship model of training has persisted throughout the history of surgical training and is still considered to be the backbone of surgical education.

In the most basic form of this model, the student directly observes the procedure and then copies the actions of a skilled mentor (Dunnington 1996). In a way, this is the origin of the "see one, do one, teach one" mentality (Walter 2006).

The modern structured surgical training currently in practice in many parts of the world is influenced by Dr William Halstead and Dr William Osler and their work towards the end of nineteenth century. They advocated, for instance, the concept of resident training in United States (Nguyen 2012; Rankin 2006). Though standardization has refined surgical training, the apprenticeship model remains the central mode of surgical education.

## Minimal Access Surgery (MAS) and surgeons' training

The introduction and adaptation of laparoscopy, owing to proven advantages over traditional surgery in certain procedures, raised concerns about the adequacy of training practising surgeons in new techniques. This was especially true of the surgeons without access to means of keeping their surgical skills up to date.

Laparoscopic cholecystectomy was developed in the late 1980s (Litynski 1999). As it had several advantages over the traditional open approach, it rapidly became the standard method for cholecystectomy (Giurgiu and Roslyn 1997). Since the introduction of laparoscopic cholecystectomy, there has been an increase in the number of surgical procedures that can be performed laparoscopically and more recently robotically, and the term Minimal Access Surgery (MAS) has evolved to describe it (Sackier 1998). This evolution has created an ongoing continuing educational need among practising surgeons to train in these new techniques.

## Role of short courses in surgical training

Increasing the need to train surgeons in advanced MAS skills has been met with short courses developed by surgeons already experienced with the new procedures (Cuschieri 1993). Despite concerns of the adequacy of these courses to sufficiently train a surgeon to practise the skills, these courses have continued to expand (Dent 1991; Wright and O'Dwyer, 1998).

## Continuing medical education

To keep the practising surgeons up to date with the new developments, continuing medical education in surgery has been established. Guidelines have been developed by various regulatory authorities and surgical societies primarily for certification purposes to guide the privileges for minimal access procedures (SAGES 2021). Experience as an assistant and satisfactory performance under a supervision, in addition to taking a course, are generally requirements to attain the certification. The recommendations of the Society of American Gastrointestinal and Endoscopic Surgeons (SAGES) are an example of such guidelines.

According to a survey by SAGES, the lack of training opportunities, the cost of the training, and the lack of experienced colleagues are major reasons for the failure of practising surgeons to meet all the requirements of SAGES to keep their skills up to date (Escarce, Shea and Schwartz 1997). Longer interactive programmes with opportunity for practice are known to be more effective than short courses lasting only a day.

### Simulation based training

Simulation based training is used as an initial step to familiarize surgeons with actual surgery. Simulation based training in MAS has been shown to improve performance (Fried et al. 1999).

## Surgical training and general motor skills

Surgical skills training shares many characteristics with general motor skills training, thus suggesting several ways of improving continuing medical education in technical skills (Ericsson and Charness 1994), and this appears to apply to both experienced surgeons and trainees. The approach of teaching a complex surgical skill by dividing it into simpler component tasks, a strategy described in the motor skills literature (Lane 1987), has been validated.

A learning curve is a graphic representation of the relationship between experience with a procedure and clinical outcome, such as operative time. Increasing experience is known to lead to decreases in operative time, the complication rate, and conversions to the standard procedure from the minimal access approach (Meehan and Georgeson 1997; Soot et al. 1999).

The general shape of surgical learning curves is similar to the "performance curve" described in the general motor skills literature (Magill 1993). Improvement occurs rapidly during early experience as demonstrated by the early steep curve (Ohlsson 1996) (Fig. 1). With further experience, the improvement in outcome with each additional experience is smaller, resulting in the flattening of the curve. This demonstrates the importance of early simulation based training and short courses to familiarize surgeons with the procedure to bring about an early rapid improvement in its outcome.

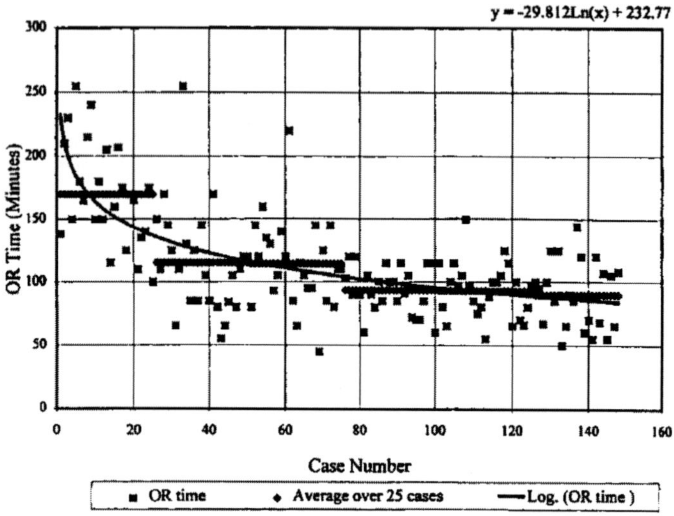


Figure 5-1: A learning curve showing the relationship between operative time and experience for laparoscopic fundoplication in children (Meehan and Georgeson 1997)

The fact that surgical learning curves are similar to motor performance curves provides additional evidence that what is known of the psychology of learning motor skills should be applied to teaching surgical skills.

## The Fitts and Posner three-stage model of motor skills acquisition

Fitts and Posner (Fitts and Posner, 1967) described a three-stage model of motor skills acquisition which can be replicated to acquire surgical skills (Kaufman, Wiegand and Tunick 1987). The first stage, called the cognitive phase, involves understanding of the task through explanations and demonstrations. In the second stage, called the associative phase, the learner practises the task to eliminate errors from the performance supervised by an experienced instructor, who provides regular feedback about corrective actions. In the last stage, autonomous learning, experience with the task makes the actions automatic without any cognitive input.

## Evolution of robotics and telesurgery

The first generation of surgical robot was notable for performing image-guided precision tasks, but was limited by the need for preoperative planning and basic computer interfaces. The evolution of surgical robots has led to a current generation of real-time telemanipulators.

The development of telesurgery arose in the 1970s with the da Vinci® Surgical and Zeus® systems. The routine use of telesurgical applications is still under development. In addition to technical challenges, there are many medico-legal and liability issues that must be resolved to enable wide adaptation of telesurgery. Despite current limitations, the potential of surgical robotics and telesurgery is enormous. The ability to deliver surgical expertise to distant locations will benefit patients worldwide.

## Modes of telementoring

Telementoring provides a unique solution to increasing both quality and access to surgical care. Telementoring is defined as "a relationship, facilitated by telecommunication technology, in which an expert (Mentor) provides guidance to a less experienced learner (Mentee) from a remote location" (Micali et al. 2000).

### Telementoring versus traditional mentoring

As opposed to traditional mentoring, telementoring is largely dependent upon telecommunication. Principles of skills acquisition remain the same in both modes of mentoring as proposed by Fitts and Posner. Traditional mentoring can be challenging due to the disproportion between the number of trained experts and the number of surgeons in need of training, as well as the significant time and resources required when surgeons are travelling from remote locations. Telementoring is an innovative strategy to overcome these challenges.

There are various methods of telementoring. In its most basic forms telementoring can be carried out via online courses to provide a good understanding of the basic concepts.

Sharing videos of the procedures performed, of simulators, or of actual procedures performed on patients to get feedback from the experienced surgeons, is another way of distant mentoring. In this way the experienced surgeon gives specific feedback for improvement which is incorporated in the later stages of the procedure or subsequent procedures. In this way, a new skill is acquired through distant learning, even if it lacks live corrective actions and feedback, which is known to be more effective.

The evolution of robotics and use of robots for telesurgery have helped to bridge this gap. Live feedback can be given on the procedures being performed. Though on-site mentoring is preferred by trainees (given both the options), due to observation of hand movements alongside the procedure on screen, telementoring is beneficial to address training needs in remote areas.

Various studies comparing clinical outcomes between telementoring and traditional mentoring have shown no difference in operative time, blood loss, postoperative pain management, recovery time, hospital stay and complications (Challacombe et al. 2005; Docimo, Moore and Kavoussi 2006; Sawyer et al. 2000).

Technology has been used to overlay the mentor's instruments onto a trainee's screen, thus providing trainees the opportunity to correlate the movement of instruments with the actions on screen. This allows a choreography of operations, including the positioning of the patient and assistant, along with identifying planes of dissection, and the chronological steps. Patients' benefits from telementoring include delivery of subspecialized care locally as well as the reduced need for travel for procedures and subsequent follow ups. It has been demonstrated to be a safe method of telementoring (Vera et al. 2014).

### Tele-education and tele-proctoring

As part of a structured programme, trainees can be signed off for specific procedures once they have acquired sufficient skill to perform the specific operation safely and do not need continuous supervision. This is also termed teleproctoring. Several studies have been performed demonstrating the equivalence of in person versus virtual training of simple surgical techniques to medical students, more complex laparoscopic procedures to residents, and even competence-based assessment of residents performing laparoscopic procedures.

## Virtual Interactive Presence and Augmented Reality (VIPAR)

Use of Augmented Reality in telementoring can potentially overcome many of the barriers in distant surgical education. This recently developed technology allows a surgeon at a remote location to deliver real time virtual assistance and training. This has been called Virtual Interactive Presence and Augmented Reality (VIPAR). With the help of this technology, remote surgeons can digitally reach the operative field, delineate anatomy, demonstrate surgical techniques and provide live feedback. Though VIPAR is in its infancy, reports of its use in various surgical disciplines including neurosurgery and orthopaedic surgery have been promising. Virtual reality games have been shown to improve laparoscopic skills as they use the same technology; developing motor skills to navigate in games is thus translated while performing laparoscopic skills, especially in an augmented reality environment.

## Practical implementation of telementoring in surgery

Telementoring programmes are highly dependent on telecommunication systems, and involve mentorship from remote locations which may be across borders. This makes implementation of telementoring systems complex, as the unreliability of telecommunication programmes can affect patient outcome (Marescaux and Rubino 2003). In addition, an ethical and legal framework needs to be in place for the involvement of mentors from remote locations (Senapati and Advincula 2005).

### Technical aspects of telementoring systems

Telementoring requires secure transmission of video and audio signals between the mentor and mentees' working stations. Telementoring systems provide real-time video streaming of the laparoscopic camera view, an audio communication link and a video view of the operating theatre.

There are many factors that influence the quality of the signal transmission in terms of latency and resolution of display.

Latency is defined as the amount of time it takes a packet to travel from source to destination. High latency can significantly impact the performance. Delays of more than half a second (500 ms) are noticeable and can have detrimental effects on performance (Micali et al. 2000). Experimental data have demonstrated a higher potential for actual surgical delays and errors with a latency of more than 500 ms (Anvari et al. 2005). A high speed connection with sufficient bandwidth is needed to minimize the latency of transmission. A minimum bandwidth of 512 kbps is considered safe for telementoring purposes. Advances in telecommunication technology with Integrated Services Digital Network (ISDN) links has allowed transmission rates of more than 512 kbps, which improves speed of modern telecommunication systems bringing down the latency. The minimum necessary resolution at mentor and mentee telecommunication stations is considered to be 480p which can be achieved with the implementation of modern telecommunication systems.

**Telestration technology**

Mentoring a surgical resident can be conveyed at several levels (SAGES 2000): one of these is providing oral instructions (i.e., while watching a transmitted real-time video of the mentee surgeon, operating and guiding them using only one's voice). This method is considered inferior since it depends on the mentor's ability to verbally deliver his instructions accurately so the mentee will understand exactly what the intended action is (Williams Jr and Ellison 2008).

**Cyber security**

Cyber security plays a crucial role in developing telementoring programmes as sensitive patient information is transmitted across secure Internet connections. A framework needs to be in place for the encryption of personal information.

**Legal framework**

Professional collaboration and mentoring across borders pose another challenge as the legal framework varies from country to country and in certain instances there are no clear policies about how to manage telesurgical and telementoring aspects, where dealing with patients is involved.

## Experience and evidence of telementoring in surgery

In an early experience, Cubano and colleagues (Cubano et al. 1999) reported an initial telemedicine and telementoring programme on an aircraft carrier. Surgeons were on the shore and they provided telementored assistance to perform hernia operations on the aircraft carrier. Five laparoscopic inguinal hernia repairs were successfully performed. Recently there has been a growing interest in telementoring in the surgical field. Schlachta and colleagues (Schlachta et al. 2009; Schlachta et al. 2010) reported the success of a telementoring programme for laparoscopic colon resections in a community hospital. It was a combined programme involving a laparoscopic course, on-site visit, and telementoring. The success rate of telementored procedures was 33%.

Canadian experience of telementoring in surgery has demonstrated that surgeons without any formal advanced laparoscopic training could perform laparoscopic colorectal procedures (Sebajang et al. 2005).

## Advantages of telementoring

Travel cost and time off from work can be minimized through implementation of structured telementoring programmes. This is true not only for mentors and mentees but for patients as well.

Combined with short courses, a telementoring programme may result in a gradual incorporation of demanding laparoscopic procedures in the surgical practice of less experienced surgeons.

Adoption of telementoring systems by modern institutions enhances professional collaboration and promotes advanced laparoscopic surgery in remote areas.

## Cost of surgical telementoring systems

Only a few studies have reported the costs of implementing telementoring systems. The initial installation cost generally varies from US$50,000 to US$80,000 (Singh et al. 2016), whereas annual costs for equipment maintenance and broadband services hosting reach approximately US$15,000 (Antoniou et al. 2012). The cost-effectiveness (Ohinmaa et al. 2002) and safety (Schulam et al. 1997) of telementoring systems have been discussed but more evidence is needed for educational outcomes to be solidified.

## Clinical and ethical considerations

A fail safe mechanism needs to be in place for the safe completion of procedures in case of a technical failure. Mentees should be able to complete the procedure by conventional ways in case telementoring is not successful. Patient information about the mentoring and risk associated with it should be complete and documented. The issue of patient privacy also represents a significant concern and presents a challenge for the clinical implementation of telementoring projects.

## Surgical mentoring and the COVID-19 pandemic

Since the outbreak of COVID-19 and the resulting pandemic in 2020, on-site mentoring opportunities have been restricted to avoid social contact as much as possible. This has resulted in the inadequate training of junior doctors. Telementoring provides a unique solution to overcome this challenge by providing training without an increased risk of infection to surgeons and patients.

## Summary

The outcome of surgical diseases is remarkably different across different regions of the world. This contrast is starker when the outcomes from remote/rural areas are compared with tertiary care centres. This reflects that access to surgical care is not uniform across various geographic/socioeconomic regions. Skilled surgeons constitute a major component of surgical care delivery. Challenges to equip surgeons with up-to-date surgical skills include time and resource limitation. Availability of training opportunities, and the travelling capacity of training institutions, trainers and their resources have been a few of the major limitations. Use of technology in terms of remote training of surgeons using teleconferencing and telerobotics is promising but is not without its own technical and ethical challenges; it is, however, the way forward.

## Bibliography

Antoniou, Stavros A., George A. Antoniou, Jan Franzen, Stefan Bollmann, Oliver O. Koch, Rudolf Pointner and Frank A. Granderath. "A comprehensive review of telementoring applications in laparoscopic general surgery." *Surg. Endosc.* 26, no. 8 (August 2012): 2111-2116. DOI: 10.1007/s00464-012-2175-x.

Anvari, Mehran, Tim Broderick, Harvey Stein, Trevor Chapman, Moji Ghodoussi, Daniel W. Birch, Craig Mckinley, Patrick Trudeau, Sanjeev Dutta and Charles H. Goldsmith. "The impact of latency on surgical precision and task completion during robotic-assisted remote telepresence surgery." *Comput. Aided Surg.* 10, no. 2 (March 2005): 93–99. DOI: 10.3109/10929080500228654.

Birkmeyer, John D., Andrea E. Siewers, Emily V. A. Finlayson, Therese A. Stukel, F. Lee Lucas, Ida Batista, H. Gilbert Welch and David E. Wennberg. "Hospital volume and surgical mortality in the United

States." The *New England Journal of Medicine* 346, no. 15 (April 2002): 1128-1137. DOI: 10.1056/NEJMsa012337.

Challacombe, B., R. Kandaswamy, P. Dasgupta and N. Mamode. "Telementoring facilitates independent hand-assisted laparoscopic living donor nephrectomy." *Transplant Proc.* 37, no. 2 (March 2005): 613-616. DOI: DOI: 10.1016/j.transproceed.2005.01.065.

Cubano, M., B. K. Poulose, M. A. Talamini, R. Stewart, L. E. Antosek, R. Lentz, R. Nibe, M. F. Kutka and M. Mendoza-Sagaon. "Long distance telementoring. A novel tool for laparoscopy aboard the USS Abraham Lincoln." *Surg. Endosc.* 13, no. 7 (July 1999): 673–678. DOI: 10.1007/s004649901071.

Cuschieri, A. "Reflections on surgical training" [editorial]. *Surgical Endoscopy* 7, no. 2 (March 1993): 73–74. DOI: 10.1007/BF00704380.

Debas Haile T., Richard Gosselin, Colin McCord and Amardeep Thind. "Surgery." In *Disease Control Priorities in Developing Countries 2nd edition,* eds. Dean T. Jamison, Joel G. Breman, Anthony R. Measham, George Alleyne, Mariam Claeson, David B. Evans, Prabhat Jha, Anne Mills, and Philip Musgrove. Washington, DC: World Bank, 2006.

Dent, Thomas L. "Training, credentialing, and granting of clinical privileges for laparoscopic general surgery." *The American Journal of Surgery* 161, no. 3 (March 1991): 399–403. DOI: https://doi.org/10.1016/0002-9610(91)90607-F.

Docimo, Steven G., Robert G. Moore and Louis R. Kavoussi. "Telerobotic surgery is clinical reality: current experience with telementoring in adults and children." *PRESENCE: Virtual and Augmented Reality* 6, no. 2 (March 2006): 173-178. DOI: https://doi.org/10.1162/pres.1997.6.2.173.

Dunnington, G. L., "The art of mentoring." *The American Journal of Surgery* 171, no. 6 (June 1996): 604–607. DOI: https://doi.org/10.1016/S0002-9610(95)00028-3

Ericsson, K. Anders and Neil Charness. "Expert performance: Its structure and acquisition." *American Psychologist* 48, no. 8 (August 1994): 725–747. DOI: https://doi.org/10.1037/0003-066X.49.8.725.

Escarce, Jose J., J. A. Shea and J. S. Schwartz. "How practicing surgeons trained for laparoscopic cholecystectomy." *Medical Care* 35, no. 3 (March 1997): 291–296. DOI: 10.1097/00005650-199703000-00009

Farmer, Paul and John G. Meara. "Commentary: the agenda for academic excellence in 'global' surgery." *Surgery* 153, no. 3 (March 2013): 321-322. DOI: 10.1016/j.surg.2012.08.047.

Fitts, Paul Morris and Michael I. Posner. *Human Performance*. Belmont, CA: Brooks-Cole, 1967.

Fried, G. M., A. M. Derossis, J. Bothwell and H. H. Sigman. "Comparison of laparoscopic performance in vivo with performance measured in a laparoscopic simulator." *Surgical Endoscopy* 13, no. 11 (November 1999): 1077–1081. DOI: 10.1007/s004649901176.

Funk, Luke M,, Thomas G. Weiser, William R. Berry, Stuart R. Lipsitz, Alan F. Merry, Angela C. Enright, Iain H. Wilson, Gerald Dziekan and Atul A. Gawande. "Global operating theatre distribution and pulse oximetry supply: an estimation from reported data." *The Lancet* 376, no. 9746 (September 2010): 1055-1061. DOI: https://doi.org/10.1016/S0140-6736(10)60392-3.

Giurgiu, D. I. and J. L. Roslyn. "Calculous biliary disease." *In Greenfield's Surgery: Scientific Principles and Practice, 2nd ed.*, eds. Michael W. Mulholland, Ronald V. Maier, Keith D. Lillemoe, Diane M. Simeone and Gerard M. Doherty. Philadelphia: Lippincott-Raven, 1997: 1033–1056.

Hofman, Karen, Aron Primack, Gerald Keusch and Sharon Hrynkow. "Addressing the growing burden of trauma and injury in low-and middle-income countries." *American Journal of Public Health* 95, no. 1 (January 2005): 13-7. DOI: 10.2105/AJPH.2004.039354.

Kaufman, H. H., R. L. Wiegand and R. H. Tunick. "Teaching surgeons to operate: principles of psychomotor skills training." *Acta Neurochirurgica* 87, no. 1 (August 1987): 1–7. DOI: 10.1007/BF02076007.

Lane, Norman E. *Skill Acquisition Rates and Patterns. Issues and Training Implications*. New York: Springer-Verlag, 1987.

Litynski, Grzegorz S. "Profiles in laparoscopy: Mouret, Dubois, and Perissat: the laparoscopic breakthrough in Europe (1987–1988)." *Journal of the Society of Laparoscopic & Robotic Surgeons* 3, no. 2 (April-June 1999): 163–167. PMID: 10444020.

Magill, Richard A. *Motor Learning Concepts and Applications, 4th ed.* Indianapolis: WCB Brown and Benchmark, 1993.

Marescaux, Jacques and Francesco Rubino. "Telesurgery, telementoring, virtual surgery and telerobotics." *Current Urology Reports* 4, no. 2 (March 2003): 109–113. DOI: 10.1007/s11934-003-0036-9.

Meehan, J. J. and K. E. Georgeson. "The learning curve associated with laparoscopic anti-reflux surgery in infants and children." *Journal of Pediatric Surgery* 32, no. 3 (March 1997): 426–429. DOI: https://doi.org/10.1016/S0022-3468(97)90597-2.

Micali, S., G. Virgili, E. Vannozzi, N. Grassi, T. W. Jarrett, J. J. Bauer, G. Vespasiani and L. R. Kavoussi. "Feasibility of telementoring between

Baltimore (USA) and Rome (Italy): the first five cases." *J. Endourol.* 14, no. 6 (August 2000): 493-496. DOI: 10.1089/end.2000.14.493.

Nguyen, Liz, F. Charles Brunicardi, Daniel J. Dibardino, Bradford G. Scott, Samir S. Awad, Ruth L. Bush and Mary L. Brandt. "Education of the modern surgical resident: novel approaches to learning in the era of the 80-hour workweek." *World Journal of Surgery* 30, no. 6 (May 2006): 1120–1127. DOI: 10.1007/s00268-005-0038-5.

Ohinmaa, Arto, Saija Vuolio, Kari Haukipuro and Ilkka Winblad. "A cost minimization analysis of orthopaedic consultations using videoconferencing in comparison with conventional consulting." *J. Telemed. Telecare* 8, no. 5 (October 2002): 283-289. DOI: 10.1177/1357633X0200800507.

Ohlsson, S. "Learning from performance errors." *Psychol. Rev.* 103, no. 2 (April 1996): 241–246. DOI: https://doi.org/10.1037/0033-295X.103.2.241.

Rankin, J. Scott. "William Stewart Halsted: a Lecture by Dr Peter D Olch." *Annals of Surgery* 243, no. 3 (March 2006): 418-425. DOI: 10.1097/01.sla.0000201546.94163.00.

Sackier, J. M. "Evaluation of technical surgical skills. Lessons from minimal access surgery [editorial]". *Surgical Endoscopy* 12, no. (September 1998): 1109–1110. DOI: https://doi.org/10.1007/s004649900794.

Shively, Eugene H. and Susan A. Shively. "Threats to rural surgery." *The American Journal of Surgery* 190, no. 2 (August 2005): 200-205. DOI: https://doi.org/10.1016/j.amjsurg.2005.05.012.

SAGES. "Guidelines for Granting of Privileges for Laparoscopic and/or Thoracoscopic General Surgery". January, 26, 2021. URL: https://www.sages.org/publications/guidelines/guidelines-for-institutions-granting-privileges-utilizing-laparoscopic-andor-thoracoscopic-techniques/

SAGES. "Framework for Post-Residency Surgical Education and Training. A SAGES Guideline". January, 26, 2021. URL: https://www.sages.org/publications/guidelines/framework-for-post-residency-surgical-education-training/

Sawyer, Michael A. J., Robert B. Lim, Sean Y. T. Wong, Paul T. Cirangle and Deborah Birkmire-Peters. "Telementored Laparoscopic Cholecystectomy: A Pilot Study". *Stud. Health Technol. Inform.* 70, no. 1 (January 2000): 302-308. DOI: 10.3233/978-1-60750-914-1-302.

Schlachta, Christopher M., A. Kent Sorsdahl, Kevin L. Lefebvre, Marcie L. McCune and Shiva Jayaraman. "A model for longitudinal mentoring and telementoring of laparoscopic colon surgery." *Surg. Endosc.* 23, no. 7 (July 2009): 1634–1638. DOI: 10.1007/s00464-008-0221-5.

Schlachta, Christopher M., Kevin L. Lefebvre, A. Kent Sorsdahl and Shiva Jayaraman. "Mentoring and telementoring leads to effective incorporation of laparoscopic colon surgery." *Surg. Endosc.* 24, no. 4 (April 2010): 841–844. DOI: 10.1007/s00464-009-0674-1.

Schulam, P. G., S. G. Docimo, W. Saleh, C. Breitenbach, R. G. Moore and L. Kavoussi. "Telesurgical mentoring. Initial clinical experience." *Surg. Endosc.* 11, no. 10 (October 1997): 1001-1005. DOI: 10.1007/s004649900511.

Sebajang, H., P. Trudeau, A. Dougall, S. Hegge, C. McKinley and M. Anvari. "Telementoring: an important enabling tool for the community surgeon." *Surg. Innov.* 12, no. 4 (December 2005): 327–331. DOI: 10.1177/155335060501200407.

Senapati, S. and A. P. Advincula. "Telementoring and robotics: paving the way to the globalization of surgery." *International Journal of Gynaecology and Obstetrics* 91, no. 3 (December 2005): 210–216. DOI: 10.1016/j.ijgo.2005.08.016.

Shrime, Mark G., Stephen W. Bickler, Blake C. Alkire and Charlie Mock. "Global burden of surgical disease: an estimation from the provider perspective." *The Lancet Global Health* 3, no. 3 (April 2015): S8-9. DOI: 10.1016/S2214-109X(14)70384-5.

Singh, Suresh, Vivekanand Sharma, Pinakin Patel, Gajendra Anuragi and Raj Govind Sharma. "Telementoring: an overview and our preliminary experience in the setting up of a cost-effective telementoring facility." *Indian J. Surg.* 78, no. 1 (February 2016): 70-73. DOI: 10.1007/s12262-015-1429-y.

Society of American Gastrointestinal Endoscopic Surgeons (SAGES). Guidelines for the surgical practice of telemedicine. *Surg. Endosc.* 14 (October 2000): article number 975-979. DOI: 10.1007/s004640000290.

Soot, Scott J., Nihnam Eshraghi, Mehrdad Farahmand, Brett C. Sheppard and Clifford W. Deveney. "Transition from open to laparoscopic fundoplication: the learning curve." *Arch. Surg.* 134, no. 3 (March 1999): 278–281. DOI: 10.1001/archsurg.134.3.278.

Vera, Angelina M., Michael Russo, Adnan Mohsin and Shawn Tsuda. "Augmented reality telementoring (ART) platform: a randomized controlled trial to assess the efficacy of a new surgical education technology." *Surg. Endosc.* 28, no. 12 (December 2014): 3467-3472. DOI: 10.1007/s00464-014-3625-4.

Verguet, Stéphane, Blake C. Alkire, Stephen W. Bickler, Jeremy A. Lauer, Tarsicio Uribe-Leitz, George Molina, Thomas G. Weiser, Gavin Yamey and Mark G. Shrime. "Timing and cost of scaling up surgical services in low-income and middle-income countries from 2012 to 2030: a modelling study." *The Lancet Global Health* 3, no. 3 (April 2015): S28-37. DOI: https://doi.org/10.1016/S2214-109X(15)70086-0.

Walter, Andrew J. "Surgical Education for the Twenty-first Century: Beyond the Apprentice Model." *Obstetrics and Gynecology Clinics of North America* 33, no. 2 (June 2006): 233-236. DOI: 10.1016/j.ogc.2006.01.003.

Weiser, Thomas G., Scott E. Regenbogen, Katherine D. Thompson, Alex B. Haynes, Stuart R. Lipsitz, William R. Berry and Atul A. Gawande. "An estimation of the global volume of surgery: a modelling strategy based on available data." *The Lancet* 372, no. 9633 (July 2008): 139-144. DOI: 10.1016/S0140-6736(08)60878-8.

Williams Jr, Thomas E. and E. Christopher Ellison. "Population analysis predicts a future critical shortage of general surgeons." *Surgery* 144, no. 4 (October 2008): 548-54; discussion 554-6. DOI: 10.1016/j.surg.2008.05.019.

Wright, David and P. J. O'Dwyer. "The Learning Curve for Laparoscopic Hernia Repair." *Semin. Laparosc. Surg.* 5, no. 4 (December 1998): 227–232. DOI: 10.1177/155335069800500405.

# CHAPTER 5

# ROTATIONS IN SURGICAL TRAINING

MUHAMMAD SHAHID SHAMIM
AND NIDA WAHID BASHIR

*"Learning the art of surgery is a process that takes time, patience and reflection over diverse experience."*

## Acknowledgement

The authors thank Dr Kiran Bana for her assistance in the literature review and development of the initial draft of this chapter.

## Need for rotations in surgical training

This chapter discusses the role of rotations in surgical training and factors that can enhance their effectiveness in developing competent surgical specialists.

The purpose of surgical training is to develop a competent surgeon enabled with the required attributes – including knowledge, skills, and attitude – and the wisdom to use these attributes appropriately to diagnose and treat surgical ailments independently. The quest to achieve the attributes and the accompanying wisdom has always been a tedious task for trainee surgeons. It requires during their training process a constant thirst for experience with supervisors who can provide the correct learning environment and guidance.

Rotations in surgical training are one way a surgical trainee is provided with the opportunities to quench the thirst for more knowledge and skills, and become a competent, autonomous surgeon. Rotations in surgical training can be described as the part of the training that a trainee spends away from her/his primary supervisor, to gain the knowledge and experience required in areas beyond the primary supervisor's expertise.

Historically, surgeons in training have visited other experienced surgeons to observe and learn from them (Amr and Tbakhi 2007; Polavarapu et al. 2013). Additionally, young surgeons have frequently gained experience during wartime by operating on injured patients, a method which allowed several of the fathers of surgery to progress in the field (Williams, O' Connell and McCaskie, eds. 2008). Many of these founding fathers travelled far and wide to learn the art of healing through surgery. The primary driving force behind the intense urge to gain more knowledge, skills and attitude, was to achieve the highest degree of competence as an independent surgeon and to become capable of managing diverse surgical conditions. They also understood that for proper training, they needed a mentor. Therefore, they would spend as much time learning with a mentor before moving on to the next learning journey or returning to their hometown to practise what they had learned – a process that can be well-identified now as an apprenticeship model.

The availability of multiple specialists and development of time-bound, structured training programmes altered these training journeys to surgical rotations. The remains of these journeys can still be found in electives or travelling fellowships, where surgeons travel to far off regions to gain knowledge and skills in areas that are not available in their country or region. However, several of the training programmes are now self-reliant and structured to fulfil the training requirements for developing autonomous surgical specialists optimally. In order to achieve this self-reliance, the programmes incorporate rotations within their training structure.

Interestingly, the objectivity in planning these rotations to optimise trainees' learning is highly variable globally. It has been (and still is) frequently questioned and debated upon and remains unclear even in well-recognised training programmes (Johnson, Travis and Shupp 2019; Michie and Bevan, 1978; O'Neill et al. 2012; Robinson et al. 2020). Additionally, the Accreditation Council for Graduate Medical Education (ACGME) does not define criteria for some of the established rotations such as surgical critical care (Napolitano et al. 2016). It is even more intriguing to explore the spectrum and ideas tried worldwide in an attempt to find the ideal combination. Rotations providing exposure to critical care or cross rotations between anaesthesia and surgery to nurture a better institutional environment are a few such examples (Webber et al. 2016).

## Goals and objectives of surgical rotations

A few decades ago, all surgeons, irrespective of their choice of surgical speciality, were supposed to acquire the competencies to become "general surgeons." Once they had mastered the knowledge and skills required as a general surgeon, they would (or would not) choose their surgical speciality. Typical general surgery training would have included ample time and training in trauma, urology and orthopaedic surgery, along with exposure in paediatric surgery, plastic surgery and neurosurgery. At that time a general surgeon would choose any of the specialities for further practice or may even decide to do several of the specialities. These "general surgeons" would fix broken femurs, excise brain tumours, resect prostate cancers and perform radical mastectomies, all in a day's work. It is hard to imagine for many now that such surgeons existed some decades ago!

Contemporary surgical practice has changed tremendously. Individual disciplines have become highly specialised and technically progressive. An explosive amount of information and evidence is available to gain insight. Therefore, one cannot keep pace with the progressing knowledge and technical advancements in several surgical specialities. Additionally, the development of surgical sub-specialities in practice has eradicated the need for multi-speciality surgeons, i.e., the previous model of training the "general surgeons."

In today's day and age, surgical training programmes are needed to develop surgical specialists with the in-depth knowledge and skills to manage surgical ailments pertinent to their specific speciality. These surgeons should be experts in their speciality who can perform as proficient surgeons, assist in the progress of knowledge and instruct others to become competent surgeons.

The goals of rotations through various surgical specialities in a surgeon's training have also progressed accordingly. The emphasis has shifted from developing a "general surgeon" capable of operating on all types of surgical problems to enhanced trainee effectiveness in a specific speciality. Any training activity that does not serve to develop a competent surgical specialist in her/his speciality is mostly considered a waste of time. For example, a neurosurgical trainee may not benefit from attending a urology operating room, or a hepato-biliary trainee would not be interested in spine fixation.

Having said that, it is important to recognise the need for a "global surgeon" capable of providing holistic surgical care, in some resource-constraint regions. The need has to be identified as a valid choice. It should be the choice of an individual or a training programme in such regions.

Therefore, the goals and objectives of rotations in surgical training must be developed with a thoughtful understanding of the following factors.

**Competencies required by the trainee for her/his surgical speciality**

The trainees rotating through a speciality may belong to various primary disciplines. This can create challenges for the rotating speciality, as it may not be feasible to develop different training pathways. A broad and similar goal with a trainee-specific set of objectives can help the supervisors/mentors in dealing with rotating trainees in such a scenario.

The level of the trainee may need to be considered for planning her/his training through the rotation. For example, a first-year trainee will have different rotation objectives than trainees towards the end of their training.

**Timeframe of the rotation**

In a structured time-bound training programme, the proper placement of a particular rotation and adequate use of trainees' working hours are of paramount importance. In general, rotations meant to provide comprehensive exposure to the trainee to facilitate their choice of speciality are scheduled in the initial two years of training. Simultaneously, rotations that are meant to enhance their sub-speciality exposure and expertise are placed towards the end of the training years, where the trainees are mature-enough to choose their future career pathway.

At present, this exposure is often beyond the control of the trainee and the trainers. The rotations are mostly decided by the training programme authorities, without any input from the trainees. Therefore, one important consideration in this process is the need for flexibility, ensuring the trainees can have a say in the choice of rotations. This flexibility can be coupled with the regular evaluation of trainees, identifying their weaknesses and strengths, and discussing future choices. The process will facilitate the trainees at various levels in enhancing their strengths, combatting their weaknesses and providing exposure for making appropriate future choices.

Every activity that a surgical trainee is involved in during a rotation must be focused on her/his ultimate goals and objectives of becoming a competent specialist surgeon. For instance, an orthopaedic surgery trainee on rotation will benefit from involvement in the surgical management of urinary bladder injuries. The acquired exposure will benefit the trainee in understanding the complexities that he/she may face while managing pelvic fractures. However, the same trainee may not benefit much from involvement in surgical procedures like pyelolithotomies or gastro-jejunostomies. Hence the time spent in various activities during rotation should be balanced with the rotating trainee's benefits.

These requirements point to the need for close collaboration between the trainee and the supervisor, and two-way communication between the primary supervisor/mentor and the supervisor in rotation. The agreed statement of objectives of rotations and pre-planned evaluation at the end of rotation can facilitate this collaborative process and help in catering to the needs of those involved.

**Available resources within the speciality where rotation is planned**

Any surgical rotation would not fulfil the demands of quality training without the availability of resources like skilled trainers or the adequate type and amount of workload and technical support for managing the training process. The responsibility for ensuring these resources' availability falls onto the shoulders of the primary supervisor in collaboration with the primary training institute. This is the "ownership" of the training process that is often missing in essence. For the successful completion of rotations with stated goals and objectives, this has to be a shared responsibility between the trainee, the supervisor and the institute(s) involved in the process.

The availability of resources may also impinge on the balance between training and service provision. The trainees on rotation form a vital part of the workforce required to provide services to patients in any clinical unit. While the training programme should not get derailed due to the service requirements, patient care must not become compromised due to training.

Finally, it is of utmost importance that rotations' goals and objectives are shared with all those involved in the training programme. The awareness of programme goals and objectives has shown to enhance training and increase trainees' and trainers' satisfaction (Robinson et al. 2020).

## Rotations for specialist surgical trainees

Traditionally, during a typical training programme, a surgical trainee rotates through several core specialities, specialised surgical units and non-operating specialities during the early years of their training. The core specialities usually include general/gastro-intestinal surgery, orthopaedics, paediatric surgery and urology. The specialised units may include breast/endocrine surgery, neurosurgery, plastic-reconstructive surgery and transplantation. The non-operating rotations usually incorporate emergency/trauma and intensive care. The early year rotations are considered to serve several purposes:

- To acquire basic knowledge about speciality care to improve upon the decision-making and holistic care of the patient of their speciality
- To acquire skills for the preoperative and postoperative care of surgical patients
- To learn the skills of teamwork, communication, ethics and research
- To acquire basic surgical skills used in the outpatient, wards, emergency and operating rooms
- To learn the basic management of emergency surgical patients requiring intensive care
- To be exposed to various surgical specialities, which may help them in taking decisions regarding their choice of specialities

In the later years of training, the trainees should rotate through their specific discipline sub-specialities to get a focused experience of their speciality. These rotations should:

- Provide the trainee with opportunities to practise the evidence-based day-to-day management of patients of common cases
- Expose them to dealing with difficult situations and unusual cases
- Provide them with insight into technical advancements and further opportunities for progress in their specialities

## Optimum duration for rotations

The duration of rotations within a surgical training programme has been under intense debate lately. Rotations in North American training programmes are frequently of 4 to 12 weeks duration, while in the United

Kingdom and Australia the duration of rotations is 6 months on average (Robinson et al. 2020). The proponents of a longer duration of rotations, especially at a senior level of training, suggest it is congruent with a better supervisor-trainee relationship. The continuity of the learning process enhances trainees' confidence to make knowledgeable decisions and augments their learning. The longer rotations also allow the supervisors to observe their trainees' development over time and modify their training as per their needs. However, on the flip-side, long rotations may reduce the breadth of trainees' experiences and limit the learning process due to the smaller variety of cases and the supervisors' ability.

Therefore, the optimum duration of rotations should be variable for different specialities, depending on the objectives to be achieved from a given rotation. This may not be easy for some training programmes, where to run the programme smoothly the rotations are kept to a similar duration and the trainees are moved from one rotation to the other at the same time. However, the programme directors need to revisit the duration of rotations in their programme. The "one-size-fits-all" approach may not be the best policy for the education of all trainees in a programme or the achievement of the programme's objectives.

## Effect of exposure of rural and state of the art centres in surgical training

There is an increasing trend among trainees for taking elective rotations beyond their workplace during or after their surgical training. Several trainees volunteer to work in less developed areas, while others opt to gain experience at advanced centres, within their country or abroad. The experience can have a profound effect on the trainees.

Trainees who choose to work in resource-constrained areas gain exposure and insight into varied conditions and cost-conscious care with greater reliance on medical history and physical examination. Trainees that opt for state of the art centres get the opportunity to experience the technical advancements in their field. The benefits of electives are well established. We see them as remains of the historic journeys taken by the forefathers of surgery to expand their knowledge and skills. However, in most programmes, the electives have largely been voluntary, not formally linked with structured training.

## Trainees as "global surgeons"

The Amsterdam Declaration of 2015 emphasised the need for essential surgical care to be available across borders regardless of age, race, gender, ethnicity, demographic location, religious and political affiliation and financial status (Dare et al. 2014). The era of global surgery intends to improve health outcomes and equity in essential surgery care for populations in crisis by incorporating research, study, practice and advocacy (Dare et al. 2014). There are fully funded elective rotations available under the global surgery programmes that aim at providing surgery, trauma, obstetric and anaesthesia care (Wilkinson et al. 2021).

It is possible that some of the trainees may feel the urge to be a part of this process and may gain confidence, self-esteem, exposure and expertise as a result of it. Usually, a resident undertaking a higher level of training can gain from it if given the option. This again calls for the consideration of flexibility while designing a programme structure.

## Challenges of rotations in surgical training

### Value of rotations in a surgical training programme

Surgical training has evolved, influenced by many different variables, including developing other specialities, the trend towards sub-specialisation with a growing body of knowledge and technological advancements, and evolving medical education concepts at postgraduate level. Designing a structure as per local needs and resources requires an in-depth analysis of these factors.

This becomes even more important when this process becomes strictly time-bound, with the limited duration of rotations in the initial years of training. Achieving the critical need for exposure to all the essential areas, making the final choice of specialisation, and acquiring the basic knowledge, skills, attitude and wisdom for the future, become an impossible task for the trainees and programme directors.

### Alignment with goals/objectives

Defining the goal/objective as per the individual and local needs seems to be the most important component of the process. The spectrum of surgical practice and the trainee surgeon's aspiration can range from practising in a rural setting to academic positions in specialised setups (Webber et al. 2016).

To cater for these aspirations, the trainees need to acknowledge their goals at the beginning of the training and be allowed flexibility in their choice of rotations with regard to the speciality and the setup (Klingensmith et al. 2015). It is an uphill task for a novel trainee to have this kind of insight and access to the places of rotations. Supervisors, residency programme directors, training institutes and accreditation bodies need to provide adequate counselling and facilitate the process.

This facilitation also demands a clear-cut understanding of the knowledge and the skills that an individual trainee will gain from each rotation. For example, rotations that provide the trainees with exposure and experience in critical care or emergency surgery can be useful at all training levels. An attempt needs to be made to ensure that it occurs.

**Unstructured rotations**

As identified earlier, the lack of well-defined objectives and inappropriate use of the trainee's time as per the level of rotating trainee reduces the effectiveness and efficacy of the whole process. This situation is further compounded by a general lack of commitment towards structured training with time-bound competency acquisition.

Therefore, adequate utilisation of resources (including the workforce) and a balance between service delivery and training become possible only if a trainee enters a rotation with pre-defined objectives at a time when he/she has acquired the basic attitude and background knowledge to gain the most from it.

The impact of this lack of structure on the standard and standardisation of surgical training needs to be investigated with a robust research plan to identify deficits and take some corrective action to improve upon the delivery of surgical care to the community (Chirdan et al. 2010).

**Lack of ownership of the responsibility of rotations by the primary supervisor and the training institute**

The issue of unstructured rotation is further compounded by the lack of ownership of these rotations by the primary institute or speciality. The issue is a recognised global phenomenon. In countries where structured surgical training is not a norm, the possibility of obtaining training outside the primary training institute in the area of choice or need depends on the "personal motivation and generosity of the hospital" (Drossard, 2019). An expectation of service provision in terms of on-call duties in the primary institution even while rotating outside is common and generally considered acceptable in many training setups.

With the current movement beyond the apprenticeship model and rising sub-specialisation alongside working hours restrictions, learning opportunities have become quite a challenge. This challenge is further enhanced when training programmes do not identify their weaknesses in providing these opportunities (and thus are not able to take proactive measures to fix these weaknesses), and do not facilitate their residents in the process.

**Disconnect from a primary speciality**

It is a well-documented fact that rotations within a single institution with close interaction with the primary supervisor result in better workplace productivity (Robinson et al. 2020). The task of setting up standards of training such as workplace-based assessments and operative and academic productivity monitoring also becomes easier when the training is happening within a single institution. Nevertheless, this is only possible when the institute either has the capacity to offer these rotations with the right kind of expert supervision or acquires it over time as a result of regularly evaluating the programme and identifying its weaknesses.

This calls for greater integration at national, local and institutional levels with standardisation of the surgical training in the areas mentioned above. The general agreement on standards of training can help with external rotations by making this a shared responsibility between the institutions and trainees.

**Appropriately planned duration of rotation**

The level of training and the trainee's ultimate goal are the two main determinants of the duration of the rotation. Spending eight weeks in a highly specialised rotation such as neurosurgery without an actual interest in the field can be an absolute waste of time for a trainee who aims to be a urologist or colorectal surgeon in future. However, the same rotation can be extremely useful for a trainee who later aims to be a trauma surgeon or a neurosurgeon.

### Supervision/supervisors' role

A rotation in surgical training is meaningful only in the presence of committed supervision. The agreed-upon objectives can only be met with a supervisor who is eager to train as per the trainee's need. Most often, the quality of supervision in a rotation is affected by the supervisor's level of ownership. Tools that can ensure and assess it are essential. An evaluation form, which is filled in as a mere requirement, may not achieve that.

### Adequacy of exposure

All the challenges mentioned above serve as the determinants of the adequacy of exposure. The number of cases alone does not ensure the required learning and any monitoring process that is only looking at numbers of cases in a rotation cannot serve to enhance training standards. However, it does serve as one of the many parameters and should be taken into account. A minimum number of cases in a rotation and a specific number of procedures at a particular level of training need to be defined and ensured.

## Conclusion

Most of the discussion in this chapter is contextual to the modern surgical training concept in a sub-specialisation era. The concept may not be practically relevant to some regions with limitations of resources and a trained workforce. These regions may still need the classic "general surgeons" to run the show. Similarly, disaster struck regions worldwide create a regular demand for the breed of global-general-surgeons.

In most of the existing scenarios, rotations during surgical training have an extremely important role in developing autonomous, competent surgeons, provided that it is thoughtfully planned with the trainees' benefit in mind. Pre-defined written objectives with clear goals, the inherent flexibility to accommodate young aspiring minds, and a well-defined monitoring process can help get the best out of a rotation. The effectiveness of each rotation in a surgical training programme is the shared responsibility of the trainee, supervisor, the training institute and the regulatory/accrediting body. All the stakeholders need to contribute to the process to enhance its quality and standards.

Taking the considerations discussed in this chapter into account while designing the rotations through various surgical specialities will provide surgical trainees with the opportunities to acquire the required attributes (knowledge, skills, attitude), and the wisdom to use these attributes appropriately to diagnose and treat surgical ailments independently within their primary discipline.

## Bibliography

Amr, S. S. and A. Tbakhi. "Abu Al Qasim Al Zahrawi (Albucasis): Pioneer Of Modern Surgery." *Annals Of Saudi Medicine* 27, no. 3 (May 2007): 220-221. DOI: https://doi.org/10.5144/0256-4947.2007.220.

Chirdan, L. B., E. A. Ameh, F. A. Abantanga, D. Sidler and E. A. Elhalaby. "Challenges Of Training And Delivery Of Pediatric Surgical Services In Africa." *Journal Of Pediatric Surgery* 45, no. 3 (March 2010): 610-618. DOI: https://doi.org/10.1016/j.jpedsurg.2009.11.007.

Dare, A. J., C. E. Grimes, R. Gillies, S. L. Greenberg, L. Hagander J. G. Meara and A. J. M. Leather. "Global Surgery: Defining An Emerging Global Health Field." *The Lancet* 384 no. 9961 (December 2014): 2245-2247. DOI: http://dx.doi.org/10.1016/ S0140-6736(14)60237-3.

Drossard, S. "Structured Surgical Residency Training In Germany: An Overview of Existing Training Programs in 10 Surgical Subspecialties." *Innovative Surgical Sciences* 4, no. 01 (May 2019): 15-24. DOI: https://doi.org/10.1515/iss-2018-0033.

Johnson, L. S., T. E. Travis and J. W. Shupp. "What Is The Value Of A Burn Surgery Rotation In Surgical Residency?" *The American Surgeon* 85, no. 12 (December 2019): 1314-1317. DOI: http://dx.doi.org/10.1177/000313481908501222.

Klingensmith, M. E., M. Awad, K. A. Delman, K. Deveney, T. J. Fahey III, J. S. Lees, P. Lipsett, J. T. Mullen, D. S. Smink and J. Wayne. "Early Results from the Flexibility in Surgical Training Research Consortium: Resident and Program Director Attitudes Toward Flexible Rotations in Senior Residency." *Journal Of Surgical Education* 72, no. 06 (December 2015): E151-E157. DOI: https://doi.org/10.1016/j.jsurg.2015.05.007.

Michie, W. and P. G. Bevan. "Surgical Training In The European Economic Community." *Annals Of The Royal College Of Surgeons Of England* 60, no. 04 (July 1978): 350. URL: https://www.ncbi.nlm.nih.gov/pmc/articles/PMC2492125/pdf/annrcse01489-0069.pdf.

Napolitano, L. M., T. W. Biester, G. J. Jurkovich, J. Buyske, M. A. Malangoni, F. R. Lewis Jr, R. M. Albrecht, K. J. Brasel, E. M. Bulger and M. A. Croce. “General Surgery Resident Rotations In Surgical Critical Care, Trauma, And Burns: What Is Optimal For Residency Training?” *The American Journal Of Surgery* 212, no. 04 (October 2016): 629-637. DOI: https://doi.org/10.1016/j.amjsurg.2016.07.016.

O’Neill, B. J., S. O’heireamhoin, A-M Byrne, S J O’Flanagan, P Keogh and P J Kenny. “Research In Higher Surgical Training: Which Rotation?” *Irish Journal Of Medical Science* 181, no. 04 (December 2012): 535-539. DOI: https://doi.org/10.1007/s11845-012-0812-y.

Polavarapu, H. V., A. N. Kulaylat, S. Sun and O. H. Hamed. “100 Years Of Surgical Education: The Past, Present, And Future.” *Bull. Am. Coll. Surg.* 98, no. 07 (July 2013): 22-27. PMID: 24010218.

Robinson, D., L. Hopkins, O. James, C. Brown, A. Powell, S. Hemington-Gorse, T. Abdelrahman, W. Lewis and R. Egan. “Surgical Training Rotation Design: Effects Of Hospital Type, Rotation Theme And Duration.” *BJS Open* 4, no. 05 (October 2020): 970. DOI: https://doi.org/10.1002/bjs5.50326.

Webber, E. M., A. R. Ronson, L. J. Gorman, S. A. Taber and K. A. Harris. “The Future Of General Surgery: Evolving To Meet A Changing Practice.” *Journal Of Surgical Education* 73, no. 03 (May 2016): 496-503. DOI: https://doi.org/10.1016/j.jsurg.2015.12.002.

Wilkinson, K. H., A. N. Bowder, M. I. Goldblatt, L. Olson and C. M. Dodgion. “General Surgery Applicants Are Interested In Global Surgery, But Does It Affect Their Rank List?” *Journal Of Surgical Research* 257, no. 01 (January 2021): 449-454. DOI: https://doi.org/10.1016/j.jss.2020.08.025.

Williams, N., P. R. O’Connell and Andrew McCaskie (eds.). *Bailey & Love’s Short Practice Of Surgery*. Florida, United States: CRC Press, 2008.

# Chapter 6

# Initiation and Establishment of a New Residency Program

Syed Murtaza Raza Kazmi, Humayun Kaleem Siddiqui and Farhan Raza Khan

The residency programme for postgraduate specialty training is defined as "a course with specific pre-defined competencies to be achieved in a set duration of time." Most residency programmes have identified the significance of inculcating the desired competencies in their product (graduating residents) so that the programme graduates can predictably perform their intended task of patient care to the highest standards (Harden 2007).

## How to assess the need of initiating a residency programme?

Initiating a new residency/training programme is an exciting but challenging task. The ever-increasing demand and need for specialty training positions require a process which includes development of the infrastructure, educational development, accreditation, marketing, and recruitment of an institution (Hasnain et al. 2014). But the important question here is, why do we need a residency programme and how can the need of such a programme be assessed?

There are over 50 specialties in medicine and surgery and nearly 9 specialties in dentistry, but still a big number of medical or dental graduates remain general practitioners and do not seek advanced specialty education. Though serving as a general clinician is on no account a lesser undertaking, building one's capacity to become a specialist practitioner has always been considered a noble mission. Residency programmes can be seen as factories that receive raw material (the general medical/dental graduate or intern) and process them into the refined final product (a trained specialist). In this process, the programme director acts as the quality control supervisor, who closely monitors and mentors the raw graduate to transform them into a polished specialist.

In many institutions, the enhancement of ongoing residency programmes is primarily dictated by the patient volume, space available to deliver the education, and other physical and logistical constraints. What should a prospective residency programme director do to initiate a residency programme? Very little has been published on this topic. The foremost thing is to objectively assess why a residency programme is needed in the first place.

If there is an increase in patient load that cannot be managed with the simple induction of medical officers, then one must explore if residents can fill up the service delivery gap. Residents being enrolled in an educational and training programme are academically more sound service providers compared to their non-academic counterparts (medical officers). Since the residents are on a career pathway and are involved in all domains of learning, they are expected to manage the complexities associated with the patients more efficiently than the medical officers. Another reason for initiating a residency programme is to fill the need of a specialist workforce in a particular field of study. This is especially true if new institutions are being set up for which consultants and faculty are needed. In this case, the existing specialists are being asked to initiate residency programmes by serving as programme director and to start mentoring the trainees under their supervision to provide a workforce who could in some years fill up the existing vacancies.

The future faculty building of a teaching hospital can be managed best if residency programmes in the hospital are tailored in a manner that provides the trained faculty with the right set of competencies (Sciarretta et al. 2019; Winters et al. 2019).

## How to initiate a new residency programme, a step- by-step guide

### Formal approvals

The challenges while initiating a new residency programme are multiple. The foremost step is to understand the hierarchy of the stakeholders and offices involved in the decision-making of initiating a residency programme. The office of the dean, office of the chair, the postgraduate education committee, the medical director's office, and the leadership of the finance department should be on-board, and written approvals from the relevant offices must be sought beforehand. The most important buy-in should be from the faculty members of the discipline in which the new residency programme is being considered; without their support, no programme could run successfully. Having faculty members on the same page would help them contribute towards the residency programme and inculcate the desirable skills in the future residents. Communication and cooperation among faculty members are of paramount importance.

**Building the infrastructure**

This is an essential requirement. The prospective programme has to ensure smooth and efficient healthcare settings that are conducive for education at a postgraduate level. There is now more than ever a need for physically designated areas of work, assignments, on-call rooms, technology support, library books, and access to online healthcare databases.

**Establish a primary site**

Ensure that the hospital/clinics have desirable infrastructure for the programme, alongside the vision to develop more secondary sites for having different settings for the residents and possibly catering to different cohort of patients. The primary site will remain a key place where all meetings, major assignments, data management and records will be kept and protected. The primary site will also be responsible for key educational and professional activities.

**Develop and ensure funding**

This would require help from the departmental managers to frame a realistic budget (Winters et al. 2019). The prospective programme director could explore the existing residency programmes in the institution to help in this matter. Appropriate budget allocation can be made for stipends, procuring equipment for resident training and for instruments used in healthcare. It is a key role of the finance department to ensure that all budgetary allocations are aligned with the vision and mission of the institution.

## Timeline

Developing a timeline for the programme ensures a timely execution of the project. The prospective programme director must play the role of captain of the ship in this task.

## Meetings for the specialty programme

Regular time-bound meetings are necessary with the institutional authorities and other programme directors to evaluate the programme's progress and further direction in due course. It is better to have formal meetings with the writing of minutes to ensure all the agenda is met and followed up on in subsequent meetings.

## On-board faculty

It is important to ensure that on-board faculty members have the appropriate qualifications, credentials and skills required to run a residency programme. It is important to have programme coordinators, and suitably trained and experienced faculty members in the department who are eligible or could become the future programme director. It is wise to encourage the programme faculty to attend special courses or workshops on medical education beforehand (Sciarretta et al. 2019).

## Educational development

### *Developing the vision*

The vision of the programme can be developed by considering the available resources, faculty members and available facilities. Other factors such as patient population, hospital organizational structure and positioning within the community should also be considered. Striking the right balance between patient service and delivery of advanced education is of paramount importance and should be planned at the beginning.

### *Curriculum and programme design*

The curriculum of the residency programme should be made in consultation with an educationist. Careful considerations on clinical rotations and didactic teaching should be implemented. For clinical rotations, competency-based goals and objectives for each clinical rotation should be defined and written in the document (programme handbook or residency manual). It is necessary to develop an overall educational map of teaching and assessment of each competency over time (Barajaz and Turner 2016).

The prospective programme director can seek help from existing residency manuals of other specialties for guidance but should compose the actual specialty manual of their discipline, in accordance with the programme requirements.

### *Time for research and other areas*

With an increasing emphasis on research, it is imperative that the prospective residency programme has the provision for inculcating research competence in the curriculum. Dedicated time for writing research protocols, ethics committee applications, grants and paper or thesis writing should be provided and documented. This would help in generating original research in the residency programme and the final product (specialist practitioner) will be moulded to act more as a scientist and researcher than just as a trained technician.

### Support regarding counselling and wellness

The programme director should explore the availability of counselling support and wellness programmes within the campus. Residents should feel that there are people on campus who will listen to them and will advise them on solving their personal and social issues. The names of such mentors and resource persons should be available in the programme handbook. One cannot predict the need of such support, as it may arise at any time (Katzung et al. 2019).

### Administrative support

For a successful programme, some form of electronic residency management evaluation system and a web-based educational platform are now a requirement by diploma or degree awarding institutions. Electronic evaluation and health records ensure easy entries are made by the residents, counter signed by the director and are accessible for quick reference.

### Memorandum of Understanding (MoUs) within the institution and outside

Developing a memorandum of understanding (MoU) with other departments and institutions for elective rotations within the campus or outside the campus is an important task. This will enhance cooperation among the departments as to when and how the residents will approach their objectives of rotations and what to expect from them. Additionally, there should be a feedback mechanism from the other departments about the resident. Finally, residents should be asked to document what they have learnt from such internal and external rotations in their logbooks.

**Programme accreditation**

After all the above-mentioned matters have been considered, the accreditation of the residency programme should be planned with the national/local accrediting body. In the case of Pakistan, the national accrediting authority is the College of Physicians and Surgeons of Pakistan.

The evaluation of a residency programme with reference to education and healthcare system is not an easy task (Tannenbaum et al. 2011). In the modern era, residency programmes are usually evaluated with reference to their final "product" or "outcome"; in simpler terms, the quality and impact of their graduates (Santos, Snell and Nunes 2017). There are two models for residency programme evaluation: Donabedian's model, which is based on "structure, process and outcome" and Stufflebeam's model, which is based on the "context, input, process and product" (Berwick and Fox 2016).

The primary objective of having accreditation is to ensure external oversight and thus maintain quality in an educational programme. Moreover, with accreditation, the new residency programme can be compared and calibrated with existing programme(s) in that discipline. Some important parameters that are evaluated in the accreditation process are: the working environment, the education vs service balance, mentorship, the academic curriculum, assessment procedures and the credentials of the programme directors (Tran et al. 2010).

In addition to the focus on quality of teaching, the accreditation bodies also probe into areas such as the research curriculum, patient safety and professional practice (Santos, Snell and Nunes 2017). The programme director in consultation with the associate programme director (if such a position exists) along with other programme faculty should work as a team to prepare the application for accreditation. There is a definite advantage to using the experience of reviewers from other residency programmes to build an impressive application. The next step is preparation for a visit. The accreditation body usually makes an informed visit to evaluate the infrastructure, faculty, and funding possibilities. There are different requirements of different accrediting bodies. The residency programme faculty must be prepared well before the visit. There must be a printed book/binding including the original application, prospective residency manual/programme handbook, credential of the faculty, statistics regarding patient volumes and any other related document(s). The "mock site visit" is advantageous and helps in preparation and management in the final inspection (Barajaz and Turner 2016). The next phase is a waiting period for final accreditation. In this period, no induction or marketing of the residency programme should be carried out without the final accreditation of the programme. After the final accreditation, the time for marketing and the induction of residents should be planned.

The recruitment of residents is an important milestone. Proper time should be given to the announcement and marketing of the residency programme to invite the best applicants, which can be helpful to uplift the programme (Barajaz and Turner 2016). As the newly initiated programme does not have any previous graduate outcomes, the credentials of the programme director, faculty members and departmental/institutional resources can be emphasised as a marketing tool to attract the best possible cohort of candidates from whom the most suitable ones can be shortlisted.

## Monitoring of the programme

This is the most important aspect for the supervising institute to ensure the merit, transparency, and quality of any residency programme. This should be done mainly to warrant smooth progress with the timely completion of the whole curriculum. The residents may be formatively assessed and/or assessed on a summative examination/interview.

A mechanism of internal and external monitoring of the residency programme should be devised. This may entail following the guidelines of the institutional department concerned with the postgraduate medical education or external accreditation bodies. Alternatively, the residency programme may decide to invite an external agency to evaluate it. Such a decision must be made in consultation with higher authorities such the Dean, Chief Executive Officer or Chief Medical Officer or Hospital Superintendent.

## Conclusion

The overall developing and successful running of residency programmes require thorough preparation, development of infrastructure, monitoring, and continuous evaluation. Without these, high quality clinicians cannot be produced. The national needs must always be kept in mind when starting a new residency programme along with the social and cultural sensitivity of a country. Lastly, initiating and establishing a residency programme consumes a substantial amount of time, energy, and resources. A residency programme can be beneficial only if it brings positive improvements in the lives of patients it aims to serve, and the people involved in the organized delivery of education and skills.

## Bibliography

Barajaz, M. and T. Turner. "Starting a new residency program: a step-by-step guide for institutions, hospitals, and programme directors." *Med. Educ. Online* 21, no. 1 (August 2016): 32271. DOI: 10.3402/meo.v21.32271.

Berwick, D. and D. M. Fox. "'Evaluating the Quality of Medical Care': Donabedian's Classic Article 50 Years Later." *Milbank Q.* 94, no. 2 (June 2016): 237-41. DOI: 10.1111/1468-0009.12189.

Gondal, K. M. and A. U. Qureshi. "Postgraduate trainee performance with structured assessment techniques in competency-based model of training." *J. Coll. Physicians Surg. Pak.* 21, no. 6 (June 2011): 338-41. DOI: 07.2011/jcpsp.338341.

Harden, R. M. "Outcome-based education: the future is today." *Med. Teach.* 29, no. 7 (September 2007): 625-9. DOI: 10.1080/01421590701729930.

Hasnain, M., L. Massengale, A. Dykens and E. Figueroa. "Health disparities training in residency programs in the United States." *Fam. Med.* 46, no. 3 (March 2014): 186-91. URL: https://fammedarchives.blob.core.windows.net/imagesandpdfs/pdfs/FamilyMedicineVol46Issue3Hasnain186.pdf.

Katzung, K. G., F. Ankel, M. Clark, L. E. Lawson, P. M. C. DeBlieux, M. A. Cheaito, E. A. Hitti, M. Epter and A. Kazzi. "What do program directors look for in an applicant?" *J. Emerg. Med.* 56, no. 5 (May 2019): e95-e101. DOI: 10.1016/j.jemermed.2019.01.010.

Santos, R. A. D., L. Snell and Maria do Patrocinio Tenorio Nunes. "The link between quality and accreditation of residency programs: the surveyors' perceptions." *Med. Educ. Online* 22, no. 1 (January 2017): 1270093. DOI: 10.1080/10872981.2016.1270093.

Sciarretta, J. D., C. D. Atchison, A. O. Onayemi and J. M. Davis. "Starting Line for Scholarly Activity in New Residency Programs: Lessons

Learned for Institutional Success." *J. Surg. Res.* 239 (July 2019): 136-141. DOI: 10.1016/j.jss.2019.02.008.

Tannenbaum D., J. Kerr, J. Konkin, A. Organek, E. Parsons, D. Saucier, L. Shaw and A. Walsh. "Triple C competency-based curriculum. Report of the Working Group on Postgraduate Curriculum Review – Part 1." Mississauga (ON): College of Family Physicians of Canada, 2011. URL: https://portal.cfpc.ca/resourcesdocs/uploadedFiles/Education/_PDFs/WGCR_TripleC_Report_English_Final_18Mar11.pdf.

Task Force on Residency Training Information, D. G. Perina, R. E. Collier, H. A. Thomas, E. A. Witt and M. A. Reinhart. "Report of the task force on residency training information (2008-2009), American Board of Emergency Medicine." *Ann. Emerg. Med.* 53, no. 5 (May 2009): 653-61. DOI: 10.1016/j.annemergmed.2009.03.009.

Tran, L., M. Giuliani, M. Masterson and R. Mungroo. Features of high-quality residency programs: a Canadian perspective. Ottawa (ON): Royal College of Physicians and Surgeons of Canada, 2010. URL: https://documents.cpdtoronto.ca/wp-content/uploads/2017/04/CPD-Final-5-Year-Report.pdf.

Winters, M. E., D. C. Devereaux, N. Goyal, J. P. Martinez, A. Mattu, P. L. Dyne, M. A. Cheaito, S. Lotfipour and A. Kazzi. "Combined Residency Programs in Emergency Medicine." *J. Emerg. Med.* 57, no. 6 (December 2019): e199-e204. DOI: 10.1016/j.jemermed.2019.06.001.

# CHAPTER 7

# DEVELOPING A COMPREHENSIVE HOUSE JOB OR INTERNSHIP PROGRAMME

QAMAR RIAZ
AND MUHAMMAD SHAHZAD SHAMIM

Internship is a term used for various on-training jobs wherein a graduate learns in the context of hands-on practice, acquiring skills under supervision so that he/she may become capable of functioning independently. In some countries, including Pakistan, 'intern' is a term that refers to a fresh medical graduate who has graduated from a medical school but does not have a license to practise independently as a physician. This position is also known as a "house-job" and such physicians are commonly referred to as "house officers" (Wall, Bolshaw and Carolan 2006).

The duration of an internship period varies in different countries. In Pakistan, each medical professional is mandated to complete a one-year supervised training period immediately after graduation but prior to being awarded licensure for practice by the Pakistan Medical and Dental Council (PMDC), the regulatory and registration authority for medical and dental education and practitioners in Pakistan. This one-year training period is also a pre-requisite for joining any formal residency programme.

As per the directives of the PMDC, this one-year internship or house job has to be completed in PMDC recognized hospital and requires six months rotations through both medicine and allied, and surgery and allied surgical specialties (Pakistan Medical and Dental Council 2008). This is irrespective of the graduate's specific area of interest. The aim is to provide quality exposure to each intern in the fields of medicine and surgery.

Medical students soon after graduation are not prepared for independently managing patients, both with regards to clinical and practical skills, and the more challenging communication skills. These freshly graduated physicians feel ill-prepared by their undergraduate medical student education and ill-equipped for their new role (Matheson and Matheson 2009). The internship, the transition from medical student to being an independent health professional, has long been considered a significant rite of passage and is therefore recognized as a critical period. The purpose of this one-year internship period is to aid the freshly graduated doctors in their professional development by providing them with clinical skills and experience of working with patients and in teams. During this period, the intern is supposed to master skills and consolidate his medical knowledge as well as deliver patient service under supervision. It is during this time when medical graduates apply what they have learned in medical school while taking responsibility for the continuity of care of their patients and continuing to learn real life applications of scientific knowledge (Brennan et al. 2010). During the course of the programme, interns improve their professional knowledge and acquire adequate hands-on experience and skills, so that they become functional members of their teams, which form the basic working and learning unit. Interns take part in various activities, including assessing patients, preparing case records and follow-up notes, and ordering investigations under the supervision of departmental faculty (Peluso et al. 2017). These activities are expected to improve the interns' clinical knowledge and skills and give them the opportunity to treat patients in a supervised environment. The interns may have variable clinical exposure but the overall aim of any internship programme is to provide diverse clinical experience in order to learn patient care, and gain confidence.

Additionally, the exposure to different disciplines in clinical medicine and surgery prepares the newly qualified doctor in deciding and entering their future specialty of choice (Aslam et al. 2011).

Internship also plays a significant role in the national health system. In many developing countries including Pakistan, the physicians graduating from an internship represent the majority of the physician workforce, serving as general and primary care physicians and points of access to the health system (Bakir and Abdel-Razig 2019).

Considering the role that an internship programme plays in the development of a medical professional, it is essential that deliberate efforts are made to reform and enhance the internship programme. This one-year period should be structured so that it does not follow the traditional apprenticeship model, thereby allowing interns to gain the necessary knowledge, skills and attitudes and develop appropriate medical ethics and practices (Cousins 1981; Al-Moamary, Mamede and Schmidt 2010). This would not only improve the quality of care delivered by the health system as a whole, but would also provide the optimum learning experience for interns for preparing for post-graduation.

Different medical schools have acknowledged the impact of this transition in terms of patient care, and devised different training programmes. At Aga Khan University, efforts were made to convert this one-year training period into a formally structured educational and training programme (Tariq et al. 2017). In this chapter we have provided an overview of the systematic approach and various educational interventions that could help develop a highly competitive internship programme.

## Internship programme at the Aga Khan University Hospital (AKUH)

The internship program at the Aga Khan University Hospital (AKUH) was initiated in 1988. Currently AKUH offers 82 internship positions for a one-year internship programme. Medical graduates, not just from the Aga Khan University (AKU) itself, but from institutes across the country apply for internship at AKUH with more than a thousand applicants each year.

## Governance

The internship programme at AKU is governed by the Postgraduate Medical Education Committee (PGMEC) of the University. The overall responsibility for all intern related activities rests with the Director and the Coordinator of the Internship Programme. The day-to-day issues are managed by the Internship Committee. This is headed by the internship director and has coordinators from the Departments of Medicine, Surgery, Paediatrics, Obstetrics/Gynaecology and Family Medicine as its members. The departmental coordinators are responsible for the internship-related issues in their specific departments.

## Induction process

In most hospitals, selection for the internship is primarily based on a graduate's scores in their medical school exams, and sometimes on their interviews (Patterson et al. 2016). This may be practical in hospitals that receive medical graduates from their own school, but since at AKUH we receive applicants from more than two dozen medical schools, the need for an independent induction process was imperative. We also decided to assess other attributes that we considered essential, and that enable a medical graduate to practise independently as a compassionate physician, such as communication skills, teamwork, professionalism, integrity, commitment, altruism, and empathy. We feel that this has made the induction criteria more holistic. Moreover, we involved other stakeholders in the selection process and each applicant shortlisted for selection is now interviewed by a group of physicians, senior residents, senior nurses, and representatives from human resources, making it a unique selection process. This also introduces the applicant to the team concept in healthcare delivery.

At AKUH, the induction into the internship programme is carried out in two stages:

i) A written clinical problem-solving test comprising 100 one-best type Multiple Choice Questions (MCQs) as per a Table of Specification (ToS) aimed at assessing knowledge expected from a freshly graduated medical student related to disciplines like surgery, medicine, obstetrics and gynaecology, emergency medicine, and paediatrics. The minimum passing cut off for the written test is 55%.

ii) This is followed by modified Multiple Mini Interviews (MMIs) for the shortlisted candidates. MMIs are a variant of Objective Structured Clinical Examinations (OSCE). The MMI stations simulate the situations that an intern is likely to encounter in the workplace (Wolf et al. 2018). MMIs comprise the essential clinical and procedural skills expected from a fresh medical graduate as well as soft or attitudinal skills pertaining to attributes of professionalism such as ethics, communication skills, teamwork, confidentiality, and time management, among others (Pau et al. 2013).

## Orientation programme

The orientation plays an important role in acclimatizing the new interns to the workplace and the systems in place. At AKU, a week-long orientation module was developed. It is comprised of formal sessions related to the policies, guidelines and protocols followed at AKU, as well as an orientation of the facilities at the institute. An "overlap" between the outgoing and incoming interns is also made part of the orientation module, allowing for a smoother handover and continuity of care. During this overlap period, for three full days the outgoing interns and recently enrolled interns work on the floor together. More emphasis is laid on ward orientation and maximizing exposure by putting them on call for a day prior to formally joining.

- **Boot camp:** The transition from medical student to active and responsible intern requires critical thinking, knowledge integration, and the application of that knowledge in clinical decision making. Interns are also expected to complete technical tasks without direct supervision (e.g., patient transport). This gap between the formal learning and actual expected performance is perceived as stressful by interns with over 90% of interns reporting to be not prepared for internship. This is also likely to compromise patient care. "Boot-camp" programmes have been identified as a means to better prepare interns for their first year of practice with emphasis on technical and clinical skills, and self-learning of protocols and procedures in a monitored, safe environment promoting experience and confidence gaining without jeopardizing patients' safety (Heskin et al. 2015). The boot camp at AKU focuses on providing hands-on training with employee and patient record related software being used at AKU. Hands-on training of Basic Life Support was also made part of the interns' orientation programme. This "just-in-time" timing of the boot camp has the highest effect on the trainees in enhancing their confidence and easing their acclimatization into the new work environment (Okusanya et al. 2012).
- **Internship manual:** A manual has been developed for interns and is shared with the new interns at the time of induction at AKU, and is available for reference on the website. It includes details related to clinical rotations, their respective learning objectives, and mandatory activities related to interns, job descriptions and expectations. It also provides information on the policies and regulations related to the internship programme.

## Education and training

Patient care in most hospitals is heavily dependent on interns. Of all the physicians in the hospital, the intern spends the most time with patients and his/her family. The aim of the internship programme is to provide a quality learning experience during the year-long transition from medical college to specialty training for interns. A number of interventions have been made in order to enhance knowledge and skills acquisition and retention during this internship period, and a thorough analysis of the impact of these interventions has revealed improvement in the on-job learning and job-satisfaction of interns (Subhan et al. 2021). The formal, structured clinical programme comprises classroom-based teaching, hands-on workshops, career counselling, formative assessment, and graduation, among other things. These interventions are briefly described below.

- **Formal academic sessions:** Internship training offers an important opportunity for personal development and career planning. The internship year in Pakistani hospitals is a stressful year in terms of workload, and the interns use it to pass their pre-residency exams and narrow down the course of their careers, while still trying to acquire basic clinical skills. The academic sessions at AKU are structured in such a way that they contribute to interns' endeavour to enhance their knowledge and skills while developing their professional skills. Weekly tutorials and core lectures are conducted covering medical and surgical topics and workshops are arranged regularly, thus providing them the opportunity to develop personal and professional skills.
- **Skills workshop:** Simulation based workshops have been reported to be effective in rapid acquisition of technical and surgical skills, improving the confidence levels and readiness of the interns to meet the daily skills they require, thus improving their student to doctor transition (Neylan et al. 2017).

Half day simulator-based, hands-on surgical workshops are conducted twice a year as part of the teaching schedule on topics like instrument handling, suturing, fracture immobilization and plastering, urinary catheterization, chest tube insertion, wound care and aseptic dressing, and taking care of stomas. These workshops are organized at the commencement of each 6 months' surgical rotation, i.e., in January and June, and address important surgical skills for interns which are difficult to teach otherwise. The surgical skills workshop not only allow an opportunity for interns to learn the basics of surgical procedures, but also allow close interactions with surgical faculty that can later contribute to improving the work environment in wards.

Some other workshops are also arranged with the aim of developing general interpersonal skills such as handling difficult patients, conflict management, anger management, presentation and communication skills, career counselling and personal effectiveness etc.

- **Clinical rotations:** The rotations during the internship period of one year have been arranged such that all the interns get a chance to work in medical and surgical specialties while aligning with the requirements of the PMDC and the departmental workforce needs. Allocation of rotation is based purely on merit, i.e., on the performance of candidates in the entrance test and MMIs. The expectations and responsibilities are delineated for all rotations and the learning objectives for every rotation are described. The departmental coordinators are made responsible for ensuring each rotating intern's weekly exposure to clinics and operating rooms thus allowing them adequate clinical hands-on opportunities.

## T-Half

This is the name given to a mid-year casual gathering of interns, chief residents and faculty over snacks and tea. The event is run by the interns, who make skits and commentaries about their experience as part of the programme.

## Formative assessments

- **Logbook:** In most institutes, the internship programme follows the apprenticeship model of training, with the intern largely dependent on the rotation they are assigned to. In general, the programmes lack a system for formative assessment, and learning is primarily achieved through the residents. Interns who are more eager enjoy more hands-on exposure and learning opportunities, whereas many can go through the entire year without learning essential clinical skills (Cousins 1981). To ensure achievement of adequate competence in the essential skills, a skills logbook was developed and implemented as a mandatory requirement for completion of the internship. This logbook was developed on the principle of workplace-based assessments (McLeod, Mires and Ker 2012). Interns are required to perform all the essential clinical and procedural skills listed in the logbook a specific number of times under supervision. Each time the intern is performing a skill, s/he will be observed by a supervisor, who may be an attending, a senior nurse or a chief resident, who will sign the logbook according to the defined rubrics for each skill. It is the responsibility of the intern to get the logbook completed, thus motivating them to take on the responsibility of their own learning.

- **Continuous assessments:** Continuous assessments evaluate a learner's progress throughout a prescribed course and are often preferred over the annual examination. At AKU, all interns are evaluated by the supervising faculty members of their respective teams at the end of each rotation using an online modality. These evaluations take into account their self-directed learning, knowledge application, and performance as a team member. Input is also taken from their chief/senior residents. These continuous assessments are easily accessible by the interns and serve as feedback on their performance, appreciating strengths and identifying areas for improvement.

## Summative assessment – EXIT examinations

Generally, there is no end of training exam or assessment in the internship programme, and thus no mechanism to gauge the gain in knowledge of the interns during the one-year training period. At AKU however, the graduating interns are tested at the end of the one-year internship, through a written test comprising 100 one-best type MCQs. Interns, having completed the one-year internship at AKU, are exempted from the entrance test for postgraduate programmes (if they apply within 2 years of completing internship), and the scores of the summative exit examinations are used in place of the entrance tests scores.

## Awards and appreciations

Recognizing learners for their performance increases self-confidence, offers a sense of accomplishment, and generates respect among their peers. At AKU, the intern who has accrued the highest scores from attendance in formal academic lectures and workshops, continuous assessments and the exit exam is recognized as the "Best Intern" and given an award at the annual graduation ceremony. The next four interns on the merit list are also awarded special recognition certificates. Giving such recognition develops a sense of accomplishment and spurs improvement.

## Graduation

The interns graduate through a formal ceremony that is organized for the entire batch of graduating interns, residents and fellows. The ceremony is held almost exactly on the lines of a university convocation, complete with regalia, anthem, university academic procession comprising of university leadership and clinical faculty, chief guests, valedictorian speeches, etc. All interns are awarded their certificates by the Dean and the best interns are also announced. Parents and guests of graduating interns are also invited to attend this ceremony. Each graduating intern receives the lifetime status of Alumnus, and all associated perks of University Alumni.

## Programme evaluation

The literature suggests varied factors that affect the efficiency of training and thus an intern's satisfaction with the training. These factors differ widely across institutes and different clinical rotations. The underlying factors identified in the literature include quality of supervisors, effectiveness of supervision, adequacy of opportunities for experiential learning, the support system (hospital management, hospital staff, and academic opportunities), personal attributes, workload, maltreatment and abuse. All these factors in turn affect the environment in which the learning of an intern is expected to take place, and may result in the desired programme outcomes not being met. It is therefore essential to have a formal system in place for regular programme evaluation (Frye and Hemmer 2012). Feedback from medical interns is essential to assess their perceptions of internship training programmes and to identify any deficits, thereby helping to improve the quality of their medical education.

The current framework evaluates the internship experience from various dimensions and in different fora as a quality assurance mechanism. These are:

1. **Interns' Forum:** The Interns' Forum was introduced as a platform for the interns to share their experiences, issues and concerns, be they general or related to specific rotations, and allows the Internship Committee to address these as far as possible.
2. **Rotation evaluation:** All the interns evaluate each clinical rotation using the online evaluation forms. The anonymized evaluation reports are compiled and shared with the respective departmental coordinator as well as the internship committee director so as to be able to take action when needed.
3. **Evaluation of the learning environment:** The learners' perceptions regarding the learning environment provide very useful insights into various factors affecting the educational experience (Hutchinson 2003). While many tools are available to measure the learning environments, the postgraduate hospital educational environment measure (PHEEM), a globally reliable and valid tool (Roff,

McAleer and Skinner 2005; Chan et al. 2016), is administered electronically on an annual basis at AKU to evaluate the learning environment as perceived by interns. The items scoring less than or equal to 1 are evaluated further to explore their underlying weaknesses and measures are taken to address those areas.

4. **Job satisfaction survey:** The interns are also subjected to routine job satisfaction surveys. In fact, we have shown that minor interventions in the programme can improve the interns' job satisfaction. This was done by reviewing the surveys from a two-year period, and making changes within the programme as proposed by the graduating interns through open ended feedback and small group discussions. Once again, after surveying satisfaction rates, changes were implemented.

## Challenges and the way forward

The internship is a highly demanding phase of a medical graduate. It is one of the critical transitional points in medicine, when the observational apprentice becomes an active and accountable practitioner. We have described a systematic approach towards reforming this critical juncture in physician training for consideration by other medical schools and universities. Universities should plan for maximum utilization of this period as a learning opportunity and preparing young doctors for post-graduation. The potential barriers in such reform may include a structured curriculum, inadequate resources, expertise, physical facilities, and funds for training. This is because both the medical students and residents tend to stay within a programme for longer periods of time (minimum 5 years for medical students, 4-6 years for residents). On the other hand, the interns stay for only a year, and even in that year, tend to stay in one specialty for no longer than 3 months. This allows little time for a mentor-mentee relation to be established. In our experience, a dedicated internship committee, with representation from different specialties, can better supervise the interns, and can greatly overcome this barrier.

## Bibliography

Al-Moamary, M. S., S. Mamede and H. G. Schmidt. "Innovations in medical internship: benchmarking and application within the King Saud bin Abdulaziz University for Health Sciences." *Education for Health* 23, no. 1 (April 2010): 367. DOI: https://www.educationforhealth.net/text.asp?2010/23/1/367/101500.

Aslam, M., A. Ali, T. Taj, N. Badar, W. Mirza, A. Ammar, S. Muzaffar and J. R. Kauten. "Specialty choices of medical students and house officers in Karachi, Pakistan." *EMHJ-Eastern Mediterranean Health Journal* 17, no. 1 (January 2011): 74-79. DOI: https://apps.who.int/iris/handle/10665/118082.

Bakir, I. and S. Abdel-Razig. "The Internship Year: A Potential Missed Opportunity to Expand Medical Access in International Settings." *Journal of graduate medical education* 11, no. 4s (August 2019): 30-3. DOI: https://doi.org/10.4300/JGME-D-19-00117.

Brennan, N., O. Corrigan, J. Allard, J. Archer, R. Barnes, A. Bleakley, T. Collett and S. R. De Bere. "The transition from medical student to junior doctor: today's experiences of Tomorrow's Doctors." *Medical Education* 44, no. 5 (May 2010): 449-58. DOI: https://doi.org/10.1111/j.1365-2923.2009.03604.x

Butt A. S., Shamim M. S., Ali M. A., Qamar F., Khan I. Q., Tariq S., Hashmi S. A., Hafeez Q., Tariq M. "Applying a mixed-method approach to improve on-the-job learning and job satisfaction in a cohort of interns at a university hospital." *Cureus* 13, no. 6 (June 2021): e15905. DOI: https://doi.org/10.7759/cureus.15905.

Chan, C. Y., M. Y. Sum, W. S. Lim, N. W. Chew, D. D. Samarasekera and K. Sim. "Adoption and correlates of Postgraduate Hospital Educational Environment Measure (PHEEM) in the evaluation of learning environments–a systematic review." *Medical teacher* 38, no. 12 (December 2016): 1248-55. DOI: https://doi.org/10.1080/0142159X.2016.1210108.

Cousins, N. "Internship: preparation or hazing?" *JAMA* 245, no. 4 (January 1981): 377. DOI: 10.1001/jama.1981.03310290045025.

Frye, A. W. and P. A. Hemmer. "Program evaluation models and related theories: AMEE guide no. 67." *Medical Teacher* 34, no. 5 (May 2012): e288-99. DOI: https://doi.org/10.3109/0142159X.2012.668637.

Heskin, L., E. Mansour, B. Lane, D. Kavanagh, P. Dicker, D. Ryan, K. Gildea-Byrne, T. Pawlikowska, S. Tierney and O. Traynor. "The impact of a surgical boot camp on early acquisition of technical and nontechnical skills by novice surgical trainees." *The American Journal of Surgery* 210, no. 3 (September 2015): 570-7. DOI: https://doi.org/10.1016/j.amjsurg.2014.12.046.

Hutchinson, L. "Educational environment." *BMJ* 326, no. 7393 (April 2003): 810-2. DOI: https://doi.org/10.1136/bmj.326.7393.810.

Matheson, C. and D. Matheson. "How well prepared are medical students for their first year as doctors? The views of consultants and specialist registrars in two teaching hospitals." *Postgraduate Medical Journal* 85, no. 1009 (November 2009): 582-9. DOI: http://dx.doi.org/10.1136/pgmj.2008.071639.

McLeod, R., G. Mires and J. Ker. "Direct observed procedural skills assessment in the undergraduate setting." *The clinical teacher* 9, no. 4 (August 2012): 228-32. DOI: https://doi.org/10.1111/j.1743-498X.2012.00582.x.

Neylan, C. J., E. F. Nelson, K. R. Dumon, J. B. Morris, N. N. Williams, D. T. Dempsey, R. R. Kelz, C. S. Fisher and S. R. Allen. "Medical school surgical boot camps: a systematic review." *Journal of surgical education* 74, no. 3 (May 2017): 384-9. DOI: https://doi.org/10.1016/j.jsurg.2016.10.014.

Okusanya, O. T., Z. N. Kornfield, C. E. Reinke, J. B. Morris, B. Sarani, N. N. Williams and R. R. Kelz. "The effect and durability of a pregraduation boot camp on the confidence of senior medical student entering surgical residencies." *Journal of surgical education* 69, no. 4 (July 2012): 536-43. DOI: https://doi.org/10.1016/j.jsurg.2012.04.001.

Pakistan Medical and Dental Council. "HOUSE JOB OR INTERNHSIP." Accessed February 25, 2021. URL: https://www.uhs.edu.pk/mcat/pmdcregulations30052019.pdf.

Patterson, F., A. Knight, J. Dowell, S. Nicholson, F. Cousans and J. Cleland. "How effective are selection methods in medical education? A systematic review." *Medical education* 50, no. 1 (January 2016): 36-60. DOI: https://doi.org/10.1111/medu.12817.

Pau, A., K. Jeevaratnam, Y. S. Chen, A. A. Fall, C. Khoo and V. D. Nadarajah. "The multiple mini-interview (MMI) for student selection in health professions training–a systematic review." *Medical teacher* 35, no. 12 (December 2013): 1027-41. DOI: https://doi.org/10.3109/0142159X.2013.829912.

Peluso, M. J., R. Luckett, S. Mantzor, A. G. Bedada, P. Saleeb, M. Haverkamp, M. Mosepele, C. Haverkamp, R. Maoto, D. Prozesky and N. Tapela. "Strengthening medical training programmes by focusing on professional transitions: a national bridging programme to prepare medical school graduates for their role as medical interns in

Botswana." *BMC medical education* 17, no. 1 (December 2017): 1-1. DOI: https://doi.org/10.1186/s12909-017-1102-1.

Roff, S., S. McAleer and A. Skinner. "Development and validation of an instrument to measure the postgraduate clinical learning and teaching educational environment for hospital-based junior doctors in the UK." *Medical Teacher* 27, no. 4 (June 2005): 326-31. DOI: https://doi.org/10.1080/01421590500150874.

Tariq, M., M. S. Shamim, A. Subhan, S. Saeed, Z. Rehman, B. Virani, A. Ashraf, I. Qamar, F. Qamar, R. Mohsin and S. Tariq. "Re-structuring a University Hospital's Internship Program Using Kern's Six-Step Model of Instructional Design." *MedEdPublish* 6, no. 1 (February 2017): Article 38. DOI: https://doi.org/10.15694/mep.2017.000038.

Wall, D., A. Bolshaw and J. Carolan. "From undergraduate medical education to pre-registration house officer year: how prepared are students?" *Medical teacher* 28, no. 5 (January 2006): 435-9. DOI: https://doi.org/10.1080/01421590600625171.

Wolf, S. J., T. M. Lockspeiser, J. Gong and G. Guiton. "Identification of foundational non-clinical attributes necessary for successful transition to residency: a modified Delphi study with experienced medical educators." *BMC medical education* 18, no. 1 (December 2018): 150. DOI: https://doi.org/10.1186/s12909-018-1247-6.

# CHAPTER 8

# EVIDENCE BASED MEDICINE AND ITS IMPACT ON SURGICAL TRAINING

CAMERON EDWIN ALEXANDER, JELIZAVETA PERECA, AMBREEN SHAKIL AND MUHAMMAD IMRAN OMAR

## What is evidence based medicine?

In 1996, Professor David Sackett, who is widely regarded as "the father of evidence based medicine," published an article entitled, "Evidence based medicine: what is it and what it isn't" in the *British Medical Journal* (Sackett et al. 1996). This represented a landmark moment, in which he laid out his views on what he felt was meant by this now frequently used phrase. Within this, evidence based medicine (EBM) was defined as:

> the conscientious, explicit, and judicious use of current best evidence in making decisions about the care of individual patients. The practice of evidence based medicine means integrating individual clinical expertise with the best available external clinical evidence from systematic research. (Sackett et al. 1996)

What was crucial about this explanation was that it relied on the amalgamation of two key components: clinical experience and understanding from direct patient exposure, in combination with the use of data generated from medical research performed in a way which is reliable and valid. The view of Sackett and colleagues was that EBM was not simply a prescriptive way of dictating clinical practice which relied on data generated explicitly from "gold standard" randomised controlled trials, systematic reviews or meta-analyses, but that it was more broadly about being able to identify and use the best evidence alongside clinical judgement. Fundamentally, EBM looks to improve patient care through the use of clinical decision making that is grounded in the objective assessment of available scientific data, rather than assuming that a specific decision might be right because it has "always been that way," or because that is the way that it is most commonly practised (Alexander, Dahm and Omar 2016).

## History of evidence based medicine

The concepts which underpin EBM evolved from a number of famous examples of work done by pioneering physicians through the 18th and 19th centuries (Greenstone 2009). This included the works of:

- Dr James Lind (1716-1794), a naval surgeon on HMS Salisbury, who conducted a controlled trial on the use of oranges and lemons in the treatment of scurvy in 12 men on board a navy ship.
- Dr Pierre-Charles Alexandre Louis (1787-1872), a French physician who examined the efficacy of bloodletting in the treatment of acute pneumonia, and was able to conclude through his study of 77 patients that the effect of this procedure "was actually much less than has been commonly believed" (Morabia 1996).
- Dr Ignaz Semmelweis (1818-1865), an Austrian physician who was able to demonstrate a reduction in maternal death through the introduction of handwashing with chlorinated lime solution in clinicians who performed an autopsy prior to examination of women in labour.

The introduction of randomised controlled trials (RCTs) by the United Kingdom Medical Research Council (MRC) in the 1940s represents one of the most important experimental advances in EBM (Keating 2017). The first RCT to be completed (and therefore also the first RCT to be published) in 1948, was run by the MRC and compared streptomycin and bedrest to bedrest alone in patients with pulmonary tuberculosis (Medical Research Council 1948). This was a landmark study because of the way in which it implemented the randomisation process, and due to its use of systematic enrolment criteria and data collection (Bhatt 2010).

In 1972, the Scottish doctor Archibald Cochrane's book, *Effectiveness and Efficiency: Random Reflections on Health Services*, sought to demonstrate the necessity of using better evidence to inform healthcare services, and highlighted, in particular, the crucial role of RCTs. The subsequent formation of The Cochrane Database of Systematic Reviews (CDSR) and the formation of The Cochrane Collaboration in 1993 by Ian Chalmers, acted as a direct response to Cochrane's key conclusion in this piece of work, where he confirmed the need for "a critical summary, adapted periodically, of all…relevant randomised controlled trials" (Cochrane 1972).

The Cochrane Collaboration has subsequently evolved to represent a symbol of the success of EBM and a global independent network. It is made up of collaborators from more than 130 countries which act to summarise the best evidence from research to facilitate informed treatment decisions. At the time of writing, there are over 7,500 published Cochrane Systematic Reviews, and the standard of these reviews is recognised as the benchmark for high quality information about the effectiveness of healthcare (Cochrane 2021a).

The phrase "evidence based medicine" was first used by Gordon Guyatt, the Programme Director of Internal Medicine at McMaster University, Canada, from 1990 to 1997, and a mentee of Professor Sackett (Thoma and Eaves 2015). Clearly, whilst this modern definition of EBM was first developed by a group of McMaster epidemiologists at this time, it can be seen that the principles that underpinning it have been present for a much longer period. In Professor David Sackett's *BMJ* obituary, it is noted that he believed EBM, "took off like wild-fire," for two main reasons: it was supported by senior clinicians who were secure in their practice and happy to be challenged and it empowered young doctors – and subsequently nurses and other clinicians (Smith 2015).

## The hierarchy of evidence based medicine

The concept of different levels of evidence was first described in a report produced in 1979 by the Canadian Task Force on the Periodic Health Examination. In this, they provided an explicit system which could be used to classify the level or grade of evidence according to its perceived "quality" (Table 8-1) (Burns, Rohrich and Chung 2011). However, the central underpinning feature was that those studies that offered the highest level of evidence were those employing methodology which was at a lower risk of bias or results which systematically deviated from the truth.

**Table 8-1: Classification of quality of evidence to allow assessment of the effectiveness of intervention (adapted from: Canadian Task Force on The Periodic Health Examination 1979).**

| Level of evidence | Description |
|---|---|
| I | Evidence obtained from at least one properly randomised controlled trial |
| II-1 | Evidence obtained from well-designed cohort or case-control analytic studies, preferably from more than one centre or research group |
| II – 2 | Evidence obtained from comparisons between times or places with or without the intervention. Dramatic results in uncontrolled experiments (such as the results of the introduction of penicillin in the 1940s) could also be regarded as this type of evidence |
| III | Opinions of respected authorities based on clinical experience, descriptive studies or reports of expert committees |

In 1989, Professor Sackett went on to offer his own modifications and interpretation of the levels of evidence and integrated this approach with a system that subsequently allowed for differing grades of recommendation as related to anti-thrombotic agents (Sackett 1989). Since this time, individual organisations and journals have gone on to further modify and describe their own versions of this tool, with different tools applied to different types of studies. For example, it may be appropriate to use a different tool for studies related to therapy, prognosis, and diagnosis or economic/decision analyses. Whilst there has subsequently been no universally agreed upon tool to describe the levels of evidence, the underlying principles are broadly comparable. The Oxford Centre of Evidence Based Medicine has developed one such system which has been widely adopted (Table 8-2).

**Table 8-2: Simplified version of the Oxford Centre for Evidence Based Medicine's Levels of Evidence (March 2009); as applied to studies assessing therapy/prevention/aetiology/harm (Oxford Centre for Evidence Based Medicine 2021).**

| Level of evidence | Description |
|---|---|
| 1a | Systematic review of RCTs (with homogeneity of RCTs) |
| 1b | Individual RCTs (with narrow confidence intervals) |
| 2a | Systematic review of cohort studies (with homogeneity of cohort studies) |
| 2b | Individual cohort studies (includes low quality RCTs; e.g. <80% follow-up) |
| 2c | "Outcomes" research; ecological studies |
| 3a | Systematic review of case-control studies (with homogeneity of case-control studies) |
| 3b | Individual case-control studies |
| 4 | Case series (and poor-quality cohort and case-control series) |
| 5 | Expert opinion without expert critical appraisal, or based on physiology, bench research or "first principles" |

## RCTs

In an RCT, participants are assigned to an intervention or control group at random. The process of randomisation serves theoretically to create groups which only differ in terms of their exposure to the intervention. This means that any known or unknown determinant of outcomes should be equally distributed between groups, and acts to minimise the risk of selection bias, which occurs where there are systematic differences between the baseline characteristics of the groups being compared (Higgins et al. 2020).

RCTs are prospective, comparative, quantitative studies that are undertaken under controlled conditions, with pre-specified outcomes measured at specific time points, and differences in the response between groups determined statistically. They represent a study design which is well suited to the assessment of the effectiveness of one or more interventions. The need for protocol development, ethical approval, and equipoise – where there is sufficient uncertainty surrounding the utility of the intervention – represents essential pre-requisites. They can be undertaken across single or multiple enrolled sites (Bhide, Shah and Acharya 2018).

The randomisation process represents an essential component of RCTs, and the integrity of this process underpins the ability of the study to truly consider itself an RCT. It is essential that participants have an equal chance of being assigned the control or intervention group, and that investigators cannot predict which group each participant will be assigned to (Cochrane Consumers and Communication Review Group 2013). One appropriate method of randomisation would be the production of computer-generated sets of random allocations by a research support unit in advance of the study, which can be subsequently sealed in consecutively numbered opaque envelopes. It may also be appropriate in larger multi-centre RCTs to make use of a remote randomisation facility which the clinician can contact at the time of randomisation (Kendall 2003). Two other key methods of randomisation include:

- Blocked randomisation: making use of "blocks" of sequences to ensure that approximately the same number of participants are assigned to each group within these blocks. It may be of particular use in studies with small to moderate sample sizes
- Stratified randomisation: typically used in order to ensure that certain variables or confounding factors are equally balanced between groups; it makes use of separate randomisation procedures within subsets of participants based on pre-defined key characteristics or strata (e.g., disease severity)

The process of analysing patients to the group which they were allocated, irrespective of whether they received the intended intervention – also known as intention to treat analysis – represents another key feature of RCTs which aims to reduce selection bias (Sibbald and Roland 1998).

The process of blinding, by which knowledge of the allocated intervention is withheld from the participant and/or investigator, is a key method to reduce performance bias in RCTs and aims to avoid systematic differences between groups in terms of care provided or exposure to other treatment-related factors. Blinding of those involved in outcome assessment is also important in minimising systematic differences between groups in how outcomes are determined (detection bias) (Higgins et al. 2020).

## Real world evidence, big data and artificial intelligence: their roles in evidence based medicine

Big data refers to datasets that are considered too large or complex to analyse with traditional methods, but instead are reliant on self-updating algorithms that build predictive models by finding patterns in data (artificial intelligence) (Dhindsa, Bhandari and Sonnadara 2018; Omar et al. 2020). Whilst it can be argued that the role of artificial intelligence in healthcare research is still rapidly developing and is still in its infancy, the expansion in the ability of researchers to collect large volumes of healthcare data has been one component of a "digital revolution" in clinical research. This has occurred alongside the rise of international research collaboratives, including a growing number which are focused on developing large scale multi-centre audit and clinical trials in surgery. Within the field of urological surgery, British Urology Researchers in Surgical Training (BURST) is one such example of successful international research collaboration (BURST 2021). The power of such collaborations lies in their ability to increase recruitment so that large numbers of patients can be included in studies in a short time span, which can often be a challenge in most single centre studies. The subsequent result is the development of research projects which are more generalisable and are adequately powered to answer the question of interest. In turn, such projects can be used to inform clinical decision making and guidelines, and therefore will have a pivotal role in evidence-based practice in surgery in the future.

## Systematic reviews including differences between systematic review and traditional narrative review

Reviews of the existing literature have always played an important role in medical education. Historically, experts in their field have collated existing knowledge and published summaries of the evidence. Whilst **traditional reviews** (also called literature reviews, narrative reviews or critical reviews) provide useful overviews of the topic, they may be biased, selectively citing appropriate studies to support the personal views of the authors, and sometimes provide different conclusions looking at the same topic (Teagarden 1989).

Only 30 years ago the inadequacies of traditional reviews became clear and the need for a systematic approach was emphasised. Crucial papers by Antman, Lau and their colleagues showed that the traditional approaches to reviews failed to extract the necessary knowledge from the existing literature, and that the secondary research (in this case, the review itself) should be as rigorous as the primary research (Antman et al. 1992; Lau et al. 1992).

A **systematic review** aims to identify, appraise and synthesise all empirical evidence that meets pre-specified eligibility criteria to answer a specific research question (Knoll et al. 2018). The search strategy for systematic reviews should be comprehensive, reproducible, and include all relevant databases. After the relevant studies and reports are selected, they should be evaluated to determine whether they meet the inclusion criteria. The relevant data are extracted from the eligible studies along with risk of bias assessment, meta-analysed (if appropriate), and the certainty of the evidence is assessed (Knoll et al. 2018).

**Table 8-3. Differences between a systematic review and traditional review (adapted from Knoll 2018).**

| Criteria | Systematic reviews | Traditional narrative reviews |
|---|---|---|
| Review question | Focused, well-defined clinical question formulated with PICO framework (Population, Intervention, Comparison and Outcome) | Question is usually broad and not well defined, might include an overview |
| Protocol | A peer-reviewed protocol or plan which is developed and published before the review | No protocol or plan included |
| Methods | Well-defined and explicitly stated with formulated inclusion and exclusion criteria, stated before the review is conducted | Not well-defined |
| Literature search strategy | Comprehensive, systematic, without language or other restrictions | Not explicitly stated/not always comprehensive or systematic; the review is confined to well-known articles often supporting the authors' views |
| Critical appraisal | Internal validity of the individual studies included in a systematic review is vetted by various tools | Usually not performed |

| | | |
|---|---|---|
| Synthesis | Qualitative (sometimes quantitative with meta-analysis): may answer a clinical question which may not be answerable by individual studies | Usually a qualitative summary |
| Findings/conclusion | Reproducible | Not reproducible. Authors' personal beliefs may influence the overall conclusion |

The value of any systematic review depends on the quality of the included studies. The quality of the systematic reviews can be assessed using different tools, such as AMSTAR (A Measurement Tool to Assess Systematic Reviews).

## AMSTAR (a measurement tool to assess systematic reviews) and AMSTAR-2

The first version of AMSTAR was developed by Shea and colleagues in 2007 (Shea et al. 2007). This was a popular instrument for critically appraising systematic reviews. However, it only allowed the appraisal of reviews of randomised controlled clinical trials. Systematic reviews including studies that assess the effects of healthcare interventions often include non-randomised studies, and therefore AMSTAR had to undergo further development.

The revised instrument, named AMSTAR-2, contains 16 different domains, seven of which are critical, and can significantly affect the validity of a review and its conclusions (Shea et al. 2017):

- Protocol registered before commencement of the review
- Adequacy of the literature search
- Justification for excluding individual studies
- Risk of bias from individual studies being included in the review
- Appropriateness of meta-analytical methods
- Consideration of risk of bias when interpreting the results of the review
- Assessment of presence and likely impact of publication bias

The responses to the AMSTAR-2 items should not be used to derive the overall score, but rather focus on identification of weaknesses or flaws in critical domains, which may weaken the confidence that can be placed in a systematic review. If there are no non-critical weaknesses or one non-critical weakness, the overall confidence in the results of the review is **high**, and the review provides an accurate and comprehensive summary of the results of the available studies that address the question of interest. If there is more than one non-critical weakness, the confidence is considered **moderate**. If there is one critical flaw with or without non-critical weaknesses, the review has a **low** overall confidence. In cases where there is more than one critical flaw with or without non-critical weaknesses, the confidence level is **critically low**, and the review should not be relied on to provide an accurate and comprehensive summary of the available studies.

## The Appraisal of Guidelines for Research and Evaluation Instrument (AGREE II)

Clinical practice guidelines provide a framework for clinical decision making, intending to optimise healthcare provision and decrease the risk of preventable adverse events or harms. Modern health systems rely on clinical practice guidelines to deliver the best possible care to their patients (Graham et al. 2011).

Reliable guidelines are based on systematic reviews of the best available evidence, meticulously identifying all relevant studies and judging their scientific strength. A consensus on recommendations should be reached by a diverse group of experts. In reality, the quality of clinical practice guidelines often varies (Knoll et al. 2018).

In 2011, the Institute of Medicine released the report *Clinical Practice Guidelines We Can Trust*, which explored the quality of existing guidelines (Graham et al. 2011). It proposed new standards for developing trustworthy clinical practice guidelines: transparency; management of conflicts of interest; a systematic review-guideline development intersection; the establishment of an evidence foundation for (and rating the strength of) guideline recommendations; articulation of recommendations; external reviews; and frequent updating. This led to a dramatic reduction of nearly 50% in the publication of guidelines listed in the National Guideline Clearinghouse (NGC) between 2014 and 2018 (Shekelle 2018).

The AGREE (The **A**ppraisal of **G**uidelines for **Re**search & **E**valuation) instrument was developed in 2003 to address the issue of variability in guideline quality. An updated version, AGREE II (published in 2010), provides a framework to assess the quality of guidelines and a methodological strategy for the development of guidelines. It provides a checklist to assess various domains of guidelines, including its scope and purpose, stakeholder involvement, rigour of development, clarity of presentation, applicability and editorial independence (Brouwers et al. 2010).

## The Cochrane Collaboration and the Cochrane Library

Cochrane (previously known as The Cochrane Collaboration) was established in 1992. A global organization, its members come from more than 130 countries worldwide (Cochrane 2021a). Cochrane has pioneered the methodology used to conduct systematic reviews. Central to the ethos of Cochrane is the implementation of explicit, reproducible methodology in the development of evidence that can improve clinical decision making. Each Cochrane Review group is a member of one of the following eight networks:

1. Abdomen and Endocrine
2. Acute and Emergency Care
3. Cancer
4. Children and Families
5. Circulation and Breathing
6. Mental Health and Neuroscience
7. Musculoskeletal, Oral, Skin and Sensory
8. Public Health and Health Systems

More information about these Cochrane Networks can be found at the following link: https://www.cochranelibrary.com/about/cochrane-review-groups (Cochrane 2021b)

Cochrane represents a key international player in evidence based clinical decision making. Cochrane systematic reviews also play a key role in informing future research design, identifying literature gaps and making recommendations for future research, especially the development of adequately powered RCTs. The Cochrane Library contains The Cochrane Database of Systematic Reviews (CDSR), The Cochrane Central Register of Controlled Trials (CENTRAL) and Cochrane Clinical Answers (CCAs). The Cochrane Library is accessible at https://www.cochranelibrary.com/ (Cochrane 2021c). There are more than 7500 Cochrane systematic reviews in the Cochrane Library.

## GRADE Working Group and the GRADE process

The Grading of Recommendations, Assessment, Development, and Evaluation (GRADE) Working Group was established in 2000 (Grade Working Group 2021a). Members of the GRADE Working Group include health care methodologists, guideline developers, clinicians, health services researchers, health economists, public health experts and other stakeholders. The GRADE approach was developed to provide a framework that was transparent and reproducible in order to assess the certainty (previously known as quality) of evidence (Grade Working Group 2021b). According to the GRADE approach, there are four levels of certainty of evidence: high, moderate, low and very low (Knoll et al. 2018). More than 110 organisations have endorsed GRADE or are using it, and it has become the gold standard for developing trustworthy guidelines. By adopting the GRADE process the review author team can summarise their findings in a table. Table 8-4 illustrates an example of a Summary of Findings table (Alexander et al. 2019).

**Table 8-4: Summary of Findings table – Bipolar TURP compared to Monopolar TURP for lower urinary tract symptoms secondary to benign prostatic obstruction (Alexander 2019).**

| **BTURP compared to MTURP for lower urinary tract symptoms secondary to benign prostatic obstruction** | | | | | |
|---|---|---|---|---|---|
| **Patient or population:** men with lower urinary tract symptoms secondary to benign prostatic obstruction<br>**Setting:** hospital<br>**Intervention:** BTURP<br>**Comparison:** MTURP | | | | | |
| **Outcomes** | **№ of participants (studies) Follow-up** | **Certainty of the evidence (GRADE)** | **Relative effect (95% CI)** | **Anticipated absolute effects* (95% CI)** | |
| | | | | **Risk with MTURP** | **Risk difference with BTURP** |
| Urological symptoms (IPSS[a] at 12 months[a]) | 2531 (16 RCTs) | ⊕⊕⊕⊖ MODERATE[b] | - | Mean urological symptoms (IPSS at 12 months) was 6.4 Weighted mean = 6.4 | MD 0.24 lower (0.39 lower to 0.09 lower) |
| Bother (HRQoL[c] at 12 months) | 2004 (11 RCTs) | ⊕⊕⊕⊖ MODERATE[b] | - | Mean bother (HRQoL at 12 months) was 1.7 Weighted mean = 1.7 | MD 0.12 lower (0.25 lower to 0.02 higher) |
| TUR syndrome | 5745 (44 RCTs) | ⊕⊕⊕⊖ MODERATE[b] | RR 0.17 (0.09 to 0.30) | Study population | |
| | | | | 24 per 1000 Weighed mean number of events = 1.8 | 20 fewer per 1000 (22 fewer to 17 fewer) |

| | | | | | |
|---|---|---|---|---|---|
| Urinary incontinence at 12 months | 751 (4 RCTs) | ⊕⊕⊖⊖ LOW[b,d] | RR 0.20 (0.01 to 4.06) | Study population | |
| | | | | 5 per 1000 Weighted mean number of events = 0.5 | 4 fewer per 1000 (5 fewer to 16 more) |
| Blood transfusion | 5727 (38 RCTs) | ⊕⊕⊕⊖ MODERATE[b] | RR 0.42 (0.30 to 0.59) | Study population | |
| | | | | 48 per 1000 Weighted mean number of events = 3.7 | 28 fewer per 1000 (34 fewer to 20 fewer) |
| Re-TURP | 652 (6 RCTs) | ⊕⊕⊖⊖ LOW[b,d] | RR 1.02 (0.44 to 2.40) | Study population | |
| | | | | 34 per 1000 Weighted mean number of events = 1.8 | 1 more per 1000 (19 fewer to 48 more) |
| Erectile function (IIEF-5[e] score at 12 months) | 321 (3 RCTs) | ⊕⊕⊕⊖ MODERATE[b] | - | Mean erectile function (IIEF-5 score at 12 months) was 19.2 Weighted mean = 19.2 | MD 0.88 higher (0.56 lower to 2.32 higher) |

***The risk in the intervention group** (and its 95% confidence interval) is based on the assumed risk in the comparison group and the **relative effect** of the intervention (and its 95% CI).

BTURP: bipolar transurethral resection of the prostate; CI: confidence interval; HRQoL: health-related quality of life; IIEF-5: International Index of Erectile Function; IPSS: International Prostate Symptoms Score; MD: mean difference; MTURP: monopolar transurethral resection of the prostate; OR: odds ratio; RCT: randomised controlled trial; RR: risk ratio; TUR: transurethral resection; TURP: transurethral resection of the prostate.

**GRADE Working Group grades of evidence.**

**High certainty:** we are very confident that the true effect lies close to that of the estimate of the effect.

**Moderate certainty:** we are moderately confident in the effect estimate: the true effect is likely to be close to the estimate of the effect, but there is a possibility that it is substantially different.

| |
|---|
| **Low certainty:** our confidence in the effect estimate is limited: the true effect may be substantially different from the estimate of the effect.<br>**Very low certainty:** we have very little confidence in the effect estimate: the true effect is likely to be substantially different from the estimate of effect. |
| **Footnotes** |
| [a]IPSS questionnaire scores range from 0 to 35, with higher values signalling more severe lower urinary tract symptoms; the minimum clinically important difference was defined as 4. |
| [b]Downgraded by one level for study limitations: blinding of operating surgeon considered unlikely in all trials; method of randomisation, allocation concealment, and blinding of outcome assessment unclear in > 50% of included trials. |
| [c]HRQoL questionnaire scores range from 0 to 6, with higher values signalling poorer quality of life. |
| [d]Downgraded by one level for imprecision: wide confidence intervals, very small numbers of events for urinary incontinence and re-TURP. |
| [e]IIEF-5 questionnaire scores range from 5 to 25, with higher values signalling better erectile function; the minimum clinically important difference was defined as 4. |

## Evidence based clinical practice guidelines

According to the Institute of Medicine, clinical practice guidelines should be evidenced based. Evidence based clinical practice guidelines should assess both the benefits and harms of an intervention as well as alternative care options. The Institute of Medicine defines clinical practice guidelines as:

> [S]tatements that include recommendations, intended to optimize patient care, that are informed by a systematic review of evidence and an assessment of the benefits and harms of alternative care options (Graham et al. 2011).

This definition was also adopted by the National Guideline Clearinghouse (NGS). The National Guideline Clearinghouse was a database of evidence based clinical practice guidelines that was funded by the US Department of Health and Human Services. However, they lost their funding according to an announcement of Agency for Healthcare Research and Quality (AHRQ) on July 16, 2018, and the database is no longer accessible. However, the Guidelines International Network (G-I-N) has developed a new International Guideline Library that is powered by EBSCO (Guidelines International Network 2021). This repository contains around 3000 guidelines. The Guidelines International Network (G-I-N) is an international scientific organisation and its network includes more than 100 guidelines' developer groups worldwide. G-I-N was established in 2002 as a Scottish charity.

## Surgical education and training

Surgical training is designed to produce competent, confident, self-motivated professionals who are able to provide the highest quality of care for patients (Royal College of Surgeons of England 2021). Typically, the UK surgical training programme consists of two years of foundation training (FY1-2) followed by a competitive national selection process for a two-year "surgical core training" (CT1-2) programme. After that, there is a further national selection process for "speciality training" (ST3-8), during which trainees can have extra time for fellowships, research and academic work. The outcome of the training is a Certificate of Completion of Training (CCT) (Ashmore 2019).

Over the past few years, attempts have been made to improve the quality of surgical training, implementing a new pilot scheme of Improved Surgical

Training. It aims to provide surgical trainees with a greater quality and quantity of training through a variety of innovative initiatives. These include appropriate emphasis on clinical exposure supported by simulation, enhanced trainee-trainer interactions with dedicated training time and working with members of the surgical care team (Ashmore 2019; Royal College of Surgeons of England 2021).

Surgical training, as any craftsmanship, has traditionally been based on the apprenticeship model, when an experienced surgeon guides the training of a young surgeon in the operating theatre and outside it. The trainee acquires the "tips and tricks" of their trainer which is grounded in the trainer's personal experiences.

Over the past several decades, EBM has been introduced into surgery, and it is now crucial to include it in the clinical decision-making process. It has been gradually incorporated into surgical education in order to develop clinicians' critical appraisal skills. The basics of EBM are introduced during the undergraduate years and further developed with regular journal clubs and courses throughout surgical training. Moreover, these skills are required for progression of the trainee to consultant. For example, the national selection process may require candidates to critically appraise a journal paper, and points are awarded for writing peer-reviewed papers.

## Teaching evidence based medicine including barriers and challenges

Learning how to practise EBM is a core component of the modern medical education curriculum (Dawes et al. 2005). It is essential to teach the fundamentals of research and application of an evidence based approach in order to successfully implement evidence based healthcare. "The Sicily Statement" was a consensus statement published in 2005 and suggested the use of the term "Evidence Based Practice" to reflect the integration of EBM into clinical practice across disciplines. In order to conduct Evidence Based Practice, the Sicily Statement put forward a five part step-wise approach (Dawes et al. 2005):

1. Asking a clinical question
2. Collecting the most relevant evidence
3. Critically appraising the evidence
4. Integrating the evidence with one's clinical expertise, patient preferences and values to make a practice decision
5. Evaluating the change or outcome

The teaching of EBM requires skills that have not traditionally been a part of medical training. A systematic review of teaching of EBM for postgraduate students revealed that standalone teaching improves knowledge, but not skills, attitudes, or behaviour (Coomarasamy and Khan 2004). To achieve improvements in skills, attitudes and behaviour it is important to move the teaching of EBM from classrooms to clinical practice. Clinically integrated teaching on EBM can be delivered using various learning strategies that include journal clubs, bed-side teaching, and case-based discussions.

Despite the integration of EBM into clinical practice, its becoming established in the surgical field was initially a slow process. The reasons behind this vary and include issues with disseminating of evidence, attitudes of surgeons, complexity of cases and challenges of randomising surgical procedures. A major hurdle in the implementation of EBM is the dissemination of the summarised evidence. Significant efforts are still required to close the gap between research and clinical practice.

Several studies have suggested that previous experience and contradictory clinical judgements are major barriers to the integration of EBM by surgeons (Kitto et al. 2007; Kwann and Melton 2012). In addition to this, the surgical decision making process may vary significantly on a case-to-case basis and may be influenced by diagnostic uncertainty or patient comorbidities. Certain subgroups of patients may fall outside the established evidence based practices because they are not included in the available studies and clinical trials. Furthermore, it can be challenging to precisely define a surgical approach in the context of clinical research studies.

From the perspective of the surgical trainee, the main barriers to implementing EBM in practice are a lack of education, time constraints, and disapproval from their mentors or surgical trainers (Bhandari et al. 2003).

## Conclusion

Evidence based medicine is crucial for modern and safe clinical practice, including surgical training. This chapter has highlighted some of the key elements of evidence based medicine including the history of evidence based medicine, randomised controlled trials, levels of evidence, systematic reviews, and evidence based clinical practice guidelines. The chapter has also highlighted the barriers and challenges of evidence-based medicine in surgical training and identified some of the key sources which could be helpful not only for a surgical trainee but also a practising surgeon. Evidence based medicine will continue to act as a central pillar of everyday surgical practice, and as its dissemination and training improves, it will be more widely adopted on a global scale.

## Bibliography


Alexander, Cameron E., Philipp Dahm and Muhammad Imran Omar. "What is the role of evidence-based medicine in urology?" Accessed January 21, 2021. URL: https://www.urologynews.uk.com/features/features/post/what-is-the-role-of-evidence-based-medicine-in-urology.

Alexander, C. E., Malo Mf Scullion, Muhammad Imran Omar, Yuhong Yuan, Charalampos Mamoulakis, James Mo N'Dow, Changhao Chen and Thomas Bl Lam, TBL. "Bipolar versus monopolar transurethral resection of the prostate for lower urinary tract symptoms secondary to benign prostatic obstruction." *Cochrane Database of Systematic Reviews* 12, no. 12 (December 2019): 1-172. DOI: 10.1002/14651858.CD009629.pub4.

Antman, E. M., J. Lau, B. Kupelnick, F. Mosteller and T. C. Chalmers. "A comparison of results of meta-analyses of randomized control trials and recommendations of clinical experts. Treatments for myocardial infarction." *JAMA* 268, no. 2 (July1992): 240–248. DOI: 10.1001/jama.1992.03490020088036.

Ashmore, D. L. "Strategic thinking to improve surgical training in the UK." *Cureus* 11, no. 5 (May 2019): e4683. DOI: 10.7759/cureus.4683.

Bhatt, Arun. "Evolution of Clinical Research: A History Before and Beyond James Lind." *Perspect. Clin. Res.* 1, no. 1 (January-March 2010): 6 10. DOI: 10.4103/2229 3485.103599.

Bhandari, Mohit, Victor Montori, P. J. Devereaux, Sonia Dosanjh, Sheila Sprague and Gordon H. Guyatt. "Challenges to the practice of evidence-based medicine during residents' surgical training: a qualitative study using grounded theory." *Acad. Med.* 78, no. 11 (November 2003): 1183-90. DOI: 10.1097/00001888-200311000-00022.

Bhide, Amar, Prakesh S. Shah and Ganesh Acharya. "A simplified guide to randomized controlled trials." *Acta. Obstet. Gynecol. Scand.* 97, no. 4 (April 2018): 380-387. DOI: 10.1111/aogs.13309.

Brouwers, Melissa C., Michelle E. Kho, George P. Browman, Jako S. Burgers, Francoise Cluzeau, Gene Feder, Béatrice Fervers, Ian D.

Graham, Jeremy Grimshaw, Steven E. Hanna, Peter Littlejohns, Julie Makarski and Louise Zitzelsberger, for the AGREE Next Steps Consortium. "AGREE II: Advancing guideline development, reporting and evaluation in healthcare." *Can. Med. Assoc. J.* 182, no. 82 (December 2010): E839-E842. DOI: 10.1503/cmaj.090449.

Burns, Patricia B., Rod J. Rohrich and Kevin C. Chung. "The levels of evidence and their role in evidence-based medicine." *Plas Reconstr Surg* 128, no. 1 (July 2011): 305-310. DOI: 10.1097/PRS.0b013e318219c171.

British Urology Researchers in Surgical Training (BURST). "About Us." Accessed January 21, 2021. URL: https://www.bursturology.com/about/about-burst.

Canadian Task Force on the Periodic Health Examination. "The period health examination." *Can. Med. Assoc. J.* 121, no. 9 (November 1979): 1193-1254. URL: https://www.ncbi.nlm.nih.gov/pmc/articles/PMC1704686/.

Cochrane, Archibald. *Effectiveness and efficiency: Random reflections on health services*. London: Nuffield Trust, 1972.

Cochrane. "About us." Accessed January 21, 2021. URL: https://www.cochrane.org/about-us.

Cochrane. "Cochrane Review Groups and Networks." Accessed January 21, 2021. URL: https://www.cochranelibrary.com/about/cochrane-review-groups.

Cochrane. "Cochrane Library." Accessed January 21, 2021. URL: https://www.cochranelibrary.com.

The Cochrane Consumers and Communication Review Group. "Supplementary guidance for authors undertaking reviews with the Cochrane consumers and communication review group." Accessed January 21, 2021. URL: https://cccrg.cochrane.org/sites/cccrg.cochrane.org/files/public/uploads/Study_design_guide2013.pdf.

Coomarasamy, Arri and Khalid S. Khan. "What is the evidence that postgraduate teaching in evidence based medicine changes anything? A systematic review." *BMJ* 329, no. 7473 (October 2004): 1017. DOI: 10.1136/bmj.329.7473.1017.

Dawes, Martin, William Summerskill, Paul Glasziou, Antonino Cartabellotta, Janet Martin, Kevork Hopayian, Franz Porzsolt, Amanda Burls and James Osborne. "Second International Conference of Evidence-Based Health Care Teachers and Developers. Sicily statement on evidence-based practice." *BMC Med. Educ.* 5, no. 5 (January 2005): 1. DOI: 10.1186/1472-6920-5-1.

Dhindsa, Kiret, Mohit Bhandari and Ranil R Sonnadara. "What's holding up the big data revolution in healthcare?" *BMJ* 363 no. (December 2018): k5357. DOI: 10.1136/bmj.k5357.

Grade Working Group. "GRADE." Accessed January 21, 2021. URL: https://www.gradeworkinggroup.org.

Grade Working Group. "GRADE Handbook." Accessed January 21, 2021. URL: https://gdt.gradepro.org/app/handbook/handbook.html#h.9rdbelsnu4iy.

Graham, Robin, Michelle Mancher, Dianne Miller Wolman, Sheldon Greenfield and Earl Steinberg, eds. *Clinical Practice Guidelines We Can Trust. Institute of Medicine (US) Committee on Standards for Developing Trustworthy Clinical Practice Guidelines*. Washington DC: National Academies Press (US), 2011.

Greenstone, Gerry. "The roots of evidence-based medicine." *BCMJ* 51, no. 8 (October 2009): 342-344. URL: https://bcmj.org/premise/roots-evidence-based-medicine.

Guidelines International Network. "Guidelines International Network." Accessed January 21, 2021. URL: https://guidelines.ebmportal.com/guidelines-international-network?query=&catalog=ext.

Higgins, Julian, James Thomas, Jacqueline Chandler, Miranda Cumpston, Tianjing Li, Matthew Page and Vivian Welch, eds. "Cochrane Handbook for Systematic Reviews of Interventions version 6.1." Cochrane Training. Accessed January 21, 2021. URL: www.training.cochrane.org/handbook.

Keating, Conrad. "Introducing a history of key trials in The Lancet." *Lancet* 390, no 10107 (November 2017): 2025. DOI: 10.1016/S0140-6736(17)31452-6.

Kendall, J. M. "Designing a research project: randomised controlled trials and their principles." *Emerg. Med. J.* 20, no. 2 (March 2003): 164-168. DOI: 10.1136/emj.20.2.164.

Kitto, Simon, Elmer V. Villanueva, Janice Chesters, Ana Petrovic, Bruce P. Waxman and Julian A. Smith. "Surgeons' attitudes towards and usage of evidence-based medicine in surgical practice: a pilot study". *ANZ. J. Surg*. 77, no. 4 (April 2007): 231-6. DOI: 10.1111/j.1445-2197.2007.04022.x.

Knoll, Thomas, Muhammad Imran Omar, Steven Maclennan, Virginia Hernández, Steven Canfield, Yuhong Yuan, Max Bruins, Lorenzo Marconi, Hein Van Poppel, James N'Dow and Richard Sylvester, "Key Steps in Conducting Systematic Reviews for Underpinning Clinical

Practice Guidelines: Methodology of the European Association of Urology." *European Urology* 73, no. 2 (February 2018) : 290-300.
Kwaan, Mary R. and Genevieve B. Melton. "Evidence-based medicine in surgical education." *Clin. Colon. Rectal Surg.* 25, no. 3 (September 2012): 151-155. DOI: 10.1055/s-0032-1322552.
Lau, J., E. M. Antman, J. Jimenez-Silva, B. Kupelnick, F. Mosteller and T. C. Chalmers. "Cumulative meta-analysis of therapeutic trials for myocardial infarction". *N. Engl. J. Med.* 327, no. 4 (July 1992): 248–254. DOI: 10.1056/NEJM199207233270406.
Morabia A. "P.C.A. Louis and the birth of clinical epidemiology." *Clin. Epidemiol.* 1996; 49: 1327-1333.
MRC Streptomycin in Tuberculosis Trials Committee. "Streptomycin treatment of pulmonary tuberculosis." *BMJ* 2 (October 1948): 769–83. DOI: https://doi.org/10.1136/bmj.2.4582.769.
Omar, Muhammad Imran, Monique J. Roobol, Maria J. Ribal, Thomas Abbott, Paul-Michael Agapow, Sonia Araujo, Alex Asiimwe et al. "Introducing PIONEER: a project to harness big data in prostate cancer research." *Nat. Rev. Urol.* 17, no. 2 (May 2020): 351-362. DOI: 10.1038/s41585-020-0324-x.
Centre for Evidence-Based Medicine, University of Oxford. "Oxford Centre for Evidence-Based Medicine: Levels of Evidence (March 2009)." Accessed January 21, 2021. URL: https://www.cebm.ox.ac.uk/resources/levels-of-evidence/oxford-centre-for-evidence-based-medicine-levels-of-evidence-march-2009.
Royal College of Surgeons of England. "Improving Surgical Training." Accessed January 21, 2021. URL: https://www.rcseng.ac.uk/careers-in-surgery/trainees/ist/.
Sackett, D. L. "Rules of evidence and clinical recommendations on the use of antithrombotic agents." *Chest* 95, Suppl 2 (February 1989): 2S-4S. DOI: 10.1378/chest.105.2.647b.
Sackett, David L., William M. C. Rosenberg, J. A. Muir Gray, R. Brian Haynes and W. Scott Richardson. Evidence based medicine: what it is and what it isn't." *BMJ* 312 (January 1996): 71. DOI: https://doi.org/10.1136/bmj.312.7023.71.
Shea, Beverley J., Jeremy M. Grimshaw, George A. Wells, Maarten Boers, Neil Andersson, Candyce Hamel, Ashley C. Porter, Peter Tugwell, David Moher and Lex M. Bouter. "Development of AMSTAR: a measurement tool to assess the methodological quality of systematic reviews." *BMC Med. Res. Methodol.* 7, article number 10 (February 2007). DOI: https://doi.org/10.1186/1471-2288-7-10.

Shea, Beverley J., Barnaby C. Reeves, George Wells, Micere Thuku, Candyce Hamel, Julian Moran, David Moher, Peter Tugwell, Vivian Welch, Elizabeth Kristjansson and David A. Henry. "AMSTAR 2: a critical appraisal tool for systematic reviews that include randomised or non-randomised studies of healthcare interventions, or both." *BMJ* 358 (August 2017): j4008. DOI: https://doi.org/10.1136/bmj.j4008.

Shekelle, P. G. "*Clinical Practice Guidelines. What's next?*" JAMA 320, no. 8 (August 2018): 757. DOI: 10.1001/jama.2018.9660.

Sibbald, B. and M. Roland. "Understanding controlled trials. Why are randomised controlled trials important?" *BMJ* 316, no. 7126 (January 1998): 201. DOI: https://doi.org/10.1136/bmj.316.7126.201.

Smith, Richard. "David Sackett. Physician, trialist, and teacher." *BMJ* 350 (May 2015): H2639. DOI: https://doi.org/10.1136/bmj.h2639.

Teagarden, J. R. "Meta-analysis: whither narrative review?" *Pharmacotherapy* 9, no. 5 (September-October 1989): 274–281. DOI: https://doi.org/10.1002/j.1875-9114.1989.tb04139.x.

Thoma, A. and Felmont F. Eaves, "A brief history of evidence-based medicine (EBM) and the contributions of Dr David Sackett." *Aesthet. Surg. J.* 3, no. 8 (November 2015): N261-3. DOI: 10.1093/asj/sjv130.

# CHAPTER 9

# TEACHING ADVANCED SURGICAL SKILLS: STRUCTURED TRAINING FROM DRY SURGICAL MODELS TO ANIMAL MODELS

NADIA KHAN, SAAD AKHTAR KHAN, NAVEED ZAMAN AKHUNZADA, VIRAM KUMAR AND MUHAMMAD EHSAN BARI

Microsurgery is a highly demanding field requiring specialized skills. It is an advanced surgical field where surgeons perform complex surgical techniques under the microscope under magnification, using precision instruments thereby restoring anatomy and function partly or completely for the respective organ. These techniques are most common in vascular neurosurgery where arterial anastomoses help in preventing strokes, along with plastic and reconstructive surgery where tissue transplantation provides for organ restoration (Agrawal et al. 2020; Evgenii et al. 2018; Evgeniou, Walker and Gujral 2018).

Prior to the application of these techniques in the operating room, repeated and dedicated training in the lab is essential. Basic and advanced hands-on courses allow for orientation, familiarization, understanding, and appreciation of conditions that may present in a live operation theatre setting. These courses in the lab ensure exercising vessel dissection, working with micro-instruments, microscope handling at high magnification and micro suturing.

Furthermore, several anastomosis techniques can be practised. Such an exercise allows the development and reinforcement of good surgical microvascular skills. A wide range of surgical models and courses are available worldwide (Kang et al. 2017; Rodriguez et al. 2016; Shurey et al. 2014; Yonekawa et al. 1999). Developing such courses in a third world setting is challenging. We present an overview of the different practice models available and highlight the experience gathered and steady progress made during the past four years in establishing a structured microsurgery education and training course at the Aga Khan University Hospital in Karachi, Pakistan.

## How to train: from basic to advanced training

### Microsurgical training key concepts

Over the years several surgical institutions worldwide have established skills lab facilities for training in microsurgery along with their respective courses (Shurey et al. 2014; Yonekawa et al. 1999). These individual training courses provide both basic and advanced courses with variations in the curriculum in terms of trainees per course, days/hours of hands-on training, and specific techniques practised.

Structured step by step hands-on training is essential (Fig. 9-1).

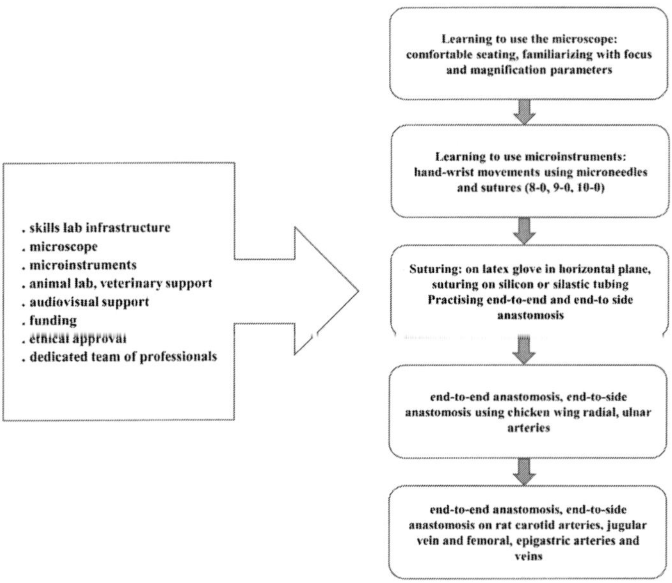


Fig. 9-1: A progressive model for advanced surgical skill training in developing countries: from essentials in logistics to structured step by step training from basic to advanced microsurgery.

This can be achieved by progressing form learning basic microsurgery techniques to the more advanced anastomosis, first on dry models and then followed by a gradual progression to the live animal model. Basic training should include an introduction to microsurgery, practice in basic suturing techniques, introduction to different types of vessel anastomosis and their applications.

Introduction to microsurgery involves first and foremost practice in working with a microscope. Understanding the importance of magnification from low (x4) to medium (x15) and maximum (x25), as well as the focussing process while performing surgical procedures, is essential. Hand-eye coordination can then be practised. Additional use of a microscope-mouthpiece, if available, or microscope-foot pedal to enable zoom and focus if necessary, is also recommended. Sitting comfortably while supporting the forearm without stress on the shoulder and back is essential. Suturing with micro-sutures (8-0, 9-0, and 10-0) is trained first by repeatedly picking up the respective microneedles with forceps and then a needle holder. Fluid hand and wrist movements enabling unity with the micro-instruments should be emphasized here. Not only working with micro-instruments but instrument cleaning and care is also vital. Advanced training includes practising an anastomosis on a live animal model, successively performing end-to-end and end-to-side anastomosis from larger vessels (>1mm) to micro-vessels (<1mm). Once the right degree of manual dexterity has been achieved and depending on the individual goals and level of expertise of the trainees a range of additional surgical procedures can also be accomplished during the period of a single live animal course, such as: nerve repair in hand surgery, free tissues flaps, and transfer in plastic surgery. 1:1 teaching and supervision during these courses is mandatory. Individual trainee evaluation is essential for their self-reflection and improvement.

## What to train on: simulation models

We differentiate between dry models, non-living and live animal simulation models. A variety of dry model simulations have been available and described in the literature (Alser et al. 2020; Belykh and Byvaltsev 2014; Mutoh et al. 2010). The most common non-living model is the chicken vessel model (Kang et al. 2017), while the rat model is the gold standard for advanced training in an animal simulation (Mikami et al. 2018; Shurey et al. 2014; Yonekawa et al. 1999).

**Dry model simulation**

Dry material is used to practise simple surgical knots; this can be a simple latex glove where sutures may be applied at different angles on the horizontal plane. The next step is the use of tubing material to enable the practice of end-to-end and end-to-side or even side-to-side anastomosis before moving on to live animal models. The tubing material may be silicone or Silastic tubes. At first, basic knotting is practised on the tube wall before embarking on performing an anastomosis using interrupted sutures. Silicon and Silastic tubes though easy to obtain are not very flexible or elastic. Tubes made of PVA (polyvinyl alcohol hydrogel) being closer to soft tissue or vessels offer a good anastomosis training model although they cost more and easily dry out when not kept moist at all times. To improve dexterity, the tube sizes can be changed from 0.5mm to 2mm.

**Chicken vessel model**

Once the students have shown dexterity in the dry model training they can proceed to the chicken vessel model which provides a range of vessels of different sizes and calibre. Depending on the level of specialization of the trainees attending, either the chicken upper extremity/wing model (with the brachial, radial, and ulnar arteries [external diameter of <0.8mm] and basilic vein [1-3mm]) or the chicken lower extremities/drumstick (i.e., thigh or lower leg with the ischiatic artery [1-2mm] and vein [2-3mm]) can be used. This model is less costly and the extra challenges of animal housing and disposal are absent.

**Rat vessel model**

This model has been around for several years and has been a major training prerequisite for all surgeons practising micro-anastomosis surgeries in their daily practice. Although this model is more costly and presents extra challenges in the approval of the institutional board of ethics, animal housing and disposal, its adaptability makes it a unique and indispensable simulation tool for all disciplines of microsurgery. Only once a trainee is well versed in the basic use of a microscope and micro-suturing techniques does the opportunity to work on a live animal become possible.

The vessels available are the carotid artery (1mm), jugular vein (1.6–2mm), femoral artery and vein (0.7–1 mm), and the epigastric artery (0.35mm) and vein (0.5mm).

The rat model can be used for practising vessel dissection and end-to-end, end-to-side, and side-to-side anastomotic techniques.

The dissection of vessels is especially important when it comes to veins. This allows for meticulous training in the careful use of micro-forceps and micro-scissors without injuring thin-walled veins and causing bleeding. Similarly, dissection of the adventitia of the arteries is another exercise that enhances dexterity in using controlled movements while handling micro-scissors. Once the vessels are dissected the use of temporary vessel clamps and/or clips can be practised and applied prior to the desired anastomosis. Arteriotomy or venotomy are also practised. The following end-to-end procedures can be applied: carotid artery end-to-end, femoral artery end-to-end, and femoral vein end-to-end. For an end-to-side anastomosis, the following can be performed: carotid to the jugular, femoral artery to a vein, and epigastric artery to femoral artery, among others. The main principle in every anastomosis is to apply single interrupted knots always equidistant to the 2 edges of the vessel end or the arteriotomy site or sutures already placed. The trainees learn to understand the handling of vessel walls of varying thickness and fragility by learning how much pressure needs to be applied while suturing these vessels. They learn how to focus under high magnification while applying each suture with appropriate inter suture distance and without suturing the front to the back wall or vice versa. The use of the rat model mimics real life surgery with real-time blood flow situations.

While assisting in learning various anastomotic techniques, lessons are learned in patience, endurance, keeping calm in any and every situation, and mastering all unforeseen mistakes and difficulties.

The length of a single microsurgery course may vary from 2-5 days. It is important to standardize these courses into basic and advanced courses and allow time for adequate practice for all trainees. Hence, prior to such courses the course applicants must be informed of the tasks to be introduced, taught, and repeated.

The idea of training is not only to learn and practise advanced microsurgery techniques like end-to-end or end-to-side vessel anastomoses but to fully prepare one for all the scenarios that may occur during real-time surgery on patients. It is the lessons learned from repeated training in the lab that gives us security and confidence. It is therefore crucial to master individual surgical techniques so that in challenging situations the surgeon is at their best and can carry out procedures with total calm and confidence.

Live animal model training must follow animal welfare and safety guidelines (Clevenger et al. 2018; Gross and Tolba 2015; National Research Council 2011).

On-site availability and presence of a dedicated veterinarian and their team are essential for proper animal handling, sedation and analgesia.

The trained veterinarian performs the necessary monitoring and recording of the animal under sedation while repeating the dose of anaesthesia and analgesia at all times. The dose of anaesthesia must be suitable for the duration desired for the animal to be without pain and distress. Animals should be placed on heating pads to maintain their body temperature. Personnel present in the area must observe strict cleanliness practices for both themselves and the animals. Practising microanastomosis technique for an extended duration requires using aseptic technique. Personnel involved in these procedures must wear protective clothing and gloves. On completion of surgical training protocol the animal is euthanized, commonly by a lethal dose of anaesthesia.

**Other biological simulation models**

Cadaveric brains with a preserved circle of Willis have been used for vessel anastomosis training purposes where the carotid and vertebral arteries could be cannulated, flushed, and fixed in formaldehyde (Olabe, Olabe and Sancho 2009). This may not be a readily available model in a developing country where local beliefs and practices must be respected. Similarly microsurgical practice on the human placenta (Evgenii et al. 2018; Magaldi et al. 2014) has also shown to be a beneficial model with vessels similar to cerebral arteries. The placenta can also be used many times by different trainees within a period of 1-2 weeks after which it should be discarded. The main limitation here is infection, hence the mandatory use of protective gear while training.

Training on dry and live animal models should not be a one-time practice. It must be followed in a structured manner from the time of being a medical student (with a future surgical career in mind), during one's surgical residency, and right up to the consultant, fellow and specialist level. Annual course attendance along with repeated self exercises in dry and live models must be continued throughout one's clinical practice (Fig. 9-2).

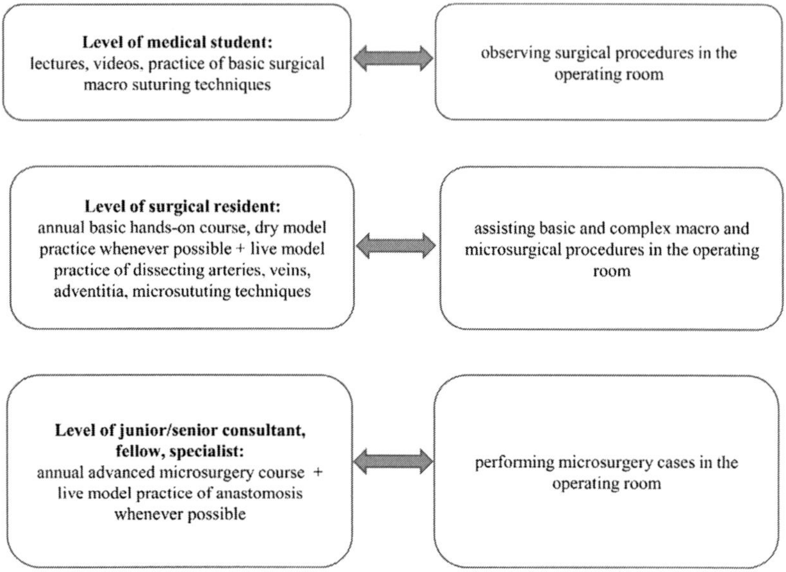


Fig. 9-2: Microsurgical skill training algorithm from medical students to specialists: from different levels of lab training to using microsurgery skills in the operating room.

Dry or live animal simulation courses should be conducted keeping in mind the need for training and the goals to be achieved (Bugaj and Nikendel 2016). Course validation should not only be based on the attendance of the trainee but also on a structured evaluation protocol (Chan, Paolo and Southern 2007; Mokhtari et al. 2019; Tolba et al. 2017). This motivates the trainees to persevere and revisit training on a regular basis.

## Logistics and challenges of creating a progressive microsurgery course model in a developing country

Creating an efficient and sustainable microsurgery course and practice in a developing country presents a range of challenges and difficulties.

For the past four years, we have been hosting a microsurgical workshop annually. It was initiated as a cerebrovascular workshop over one and a half days with a basic microsurgery course for neurosurgery residents. The course included practising the basic suturing technique using 10-00 sutures on silicon tubes. Successively the course was expanded to include advanced micro-anastomosis training on chicken wing arteries. With the acquirement of state-of-the-art microscopes and dedicated lab space recently we were able to hold the first live animal, i.e., rat anastomosis course in 2020. The availability and support of the institutional veterinary department were ground-breaking. The need for such a course has been validated by the positive response of its participants from all microsurgical fields including plastic and reconstructive surgery, ENT, orthopaedics and neurosurgery.

Here we summarise and address the standard logistical and infrastructure requirements essential for establishing a microsurgery training course and highlight the efforts undertaken to successfully conduct such workshops at the Aga Khan University Hospital, Karachi, Pakistan.

## Availability of infrastructure

This includes the presence of a functional skills lab where both dry models as well as live animal model training is possible. For live animal models the presence of veterinarian support is essential, fulfilling the institutional animal ethical guidelines.

The first two basic microsurgery courses were held in a skills lab space permitting only dry model simulation. These initial courses were essential in introducing the concept of training in the microsurgical field and in identifying the needs of local trainees. They also helped the authors in understanding the limitations and possibilities of expanding training towards advanced microsurgery.

With the recent availability of a skills lab space allowing for live animal training as well as local institutional veterinarian support the first advanced microsurgery course using the rat model was achieved.

## Availability of instrumentation

Microsurgical instruments are precision instruments essential for performing microscopic techniques in vessels of a micro calibre. The availability of high-quality instruments is pivotal to allow for quality training without trainee frustration and more successful performances. A single microsurgical set includes: jewellers forceps no. 3 and no. 5, or micro forceps with a fine tip and one with a blunt tip; straight and curved micro-scissors; vessel clamps/temporary aneurysm clips; and additional items such as 8-0, 9-0, and 10-0 nylon sutures. Various types of tubing and latex gloves are needed for dry practice. For live animal practice Sprague-Dawley Rats (300-500g) should be used. As well as anaesthetics, analgesics and muscle relaxants like Ketamine (75-95mg/Kg), Xylazine (5-8mg/Kg) and Pancuronium bromide (2mg/kg) or locally available substitutes are essential. Heparin for vessel flushing, syringes, retractors, and a surgical cauterization system are additionally required. Good quality double eyepiece microscopes are indispensable, as is the availability of a monitoring video camera attached to all stations for the direct projection of individual training. Adjustable seating is crucial to allow for the required focus and magnification.

A special microsurgery instrument set was acquired by the first author with private sponsoring and institutional support to meet the costs. This instrument set was tailor made to the demands of the basic and advanced course and included in addition to the microforceps and microscissors a set of bipolar forceps. Operating microscopes with automized zoom and focus for each individual trainee were essential for these workshops. While a few microscopes were acquired by the local department others were arranged on loan or demo models were requested from vendors. The non-availability of Xylazine in Pakistan was a major limitation. A combination of Xylazine and Ketamine is generally required for single-dose long term anaesthesia but due to the non-availability Sodium Thiopental had to be used as an alternative. This is a short-acting anaesthetic agent requiring multiple dosing, putting animals at risk of expiry during dissection.

**Funding**

Funding seems to be one of the major challenges in setting up and sustaining highly specialized courses in a developing country. While international courses aim for individual trainee fees ranging between 1500USD and 2500USD, such an amount can definitely not be asked from trainees of a developing country. Local institutional support plays a key role in making such an endeavour possible. Only with dedication and determination can such a course succeed to standards of excellence allowing perhaps in the future attendance of even international trainees.

**Lessons learned from the microsurgery workshop at the Aga Khan University Hospital, Karachi, Pakistan and future vision**

The collective dedication of the authors and their teams has allowed for a step by step development of a microsurgical course including both basic suturing techniques in dry models to more advanced microsurgical anastomosis practice in the live rat model. Major limitations included the availability of a dedicated lab space as well as funding and the acquirement of microsurgical instruments including state-of-the-art microscopes.

Our future vision encompasses making this annual course mandatory (with the respective certification of training for basic or advanced training) and increasing the days of each course to give more time to the participants. Additionally, the dry courses could be maintained annually on a quarterly basis for all neurosurgical residents. The following are the steps required to improve and expand our current know-how:

- Expand and improvise current teaching tools with the incorporation of dry models available in the market.
- Expand on written teaching material, hand-outs, and teaching videos.
- Introduce objective assessment of each trainee during the dry model and live training to increase individual responsibility and competency.
- Standardize the advanced microsurgery course to include hands-on training on
    - Vessel dissection
    - Vessel clamp/clip application
    - End-to-end anastomosis
    - End-to-side anastomosis on various rat arteries
    - Patency evaluation
- Increase the length of the advanced microsurgery live animal course to 4-5 days (minimum of 40 hours) with 3-4 full days of hands-on training and one final day of trainee assessment.
- Standardize the basic microsurgery course to include hands-on training on
    - Use of microscopes and micro-instrumentation
    - Micro-suturing on different dry practice material
    - Dissection of chicken vessels
    - Anastomosis training and practice
- Increase the length of the basic microsurgery non-live animal course to 3 to 4 days (minimum of 32 hours) with 2 to 3 days of hands-on training and one day of trainee assessment.
- Achieve flawless animal handling including anaesthesia (procurement of substitute anaesthetics), and analgesia in a live animal model (rat model) for efficient training, i.e., longer hours of training per animal with the support of the institutional veterinarian team.

- Increase the visibility of the courses by introducing an annual budget for instrumentation: microscopes, micro-instruments, lab space with specific infrastructure at departmental level, etc.
- Increase awareness locally, nationally, and internationally.
- Specify a person/personnel to monitor the status of the course and the repair of instrumentation.
- Train a team of local institutional residents and fellows to first attend the basic and advanced courses and later assist in the annual course instructions to gain experience.
- Increase the frequency of the annual one-time course to at least 2 supervised courses by experienced instructors per year.

## Conclusion

The goal of microsurgical training in any geographical or institutional setting is not only to learn and practice advanced microsurgery techniques like end-to-end or end-to-side vessel anastomosis but to fully prepare surgeons in training for all the scenarios that may occur during real-time surgery on patients. The lessons learned from repeated training in the lab give us security and confidence. It is therefore crucial to master individual surgical techniques so that in challenging situations the surgeon can achieve their best work with total calm and confidence. Future vision must include improvement in the availability of dry and live animal models, easy availability and replacement of microsurgical instrumentation, and the dedicated involvement and participation of a highly specialized team. Institutional commitment to continuous economic support along with raising the awareness of the significance of acquiring microsurgical skills locally, nationwide, and regionally remain imperative.

## Bibliography

Agrawal, Nikhil, A. Turner, Luke Grome, Amjed Abu-Ghname, Matthew J. Davis, Edward M. Reece, Edward P. Buchanan and Sebastian Winocour. "Use of simulation in plastic surgery training." *Plast. Reconstr. Surg. Glob. Open* 8, no. 7 (July 2020): e2896. DOI: http://doi.org/10.1097/GOX.0000000000002896.

Alser, Osaid, Gehad Youssef, Simon Myers and Ali M. Ghanem. "A novel three-in-one silicone model for basic microsurgery training." *European Journal of Plastic Surgery* 43 (April 2020): 621-626. DOI: https://doi.org/10.1007/s00238-020-01666-4.

Belykh, Evgenii and V. Byvaltsev. "Off the job microsurgical training on dry models: Siberian experience." *World Neurosurgery* 82, no. 1-2 (July-August 2014): 20-24. DOI: http://doi.org/10.1016/j.wneu.2014.01.018.

Bugaj, T. J., and C. Nikendel. "Practical clinical training in skills labs: theory and practice." *GMS J. Med. Educ.* 33, no. 4 (August 2016): 1-21. DOI: https://doi.org/10.3205/zma001062.

Chan, Woan-Yi, Paolo Matteucci and Stephen J. Southern. "Validation of microsurgical models in microsurgery training and competence: a review." *Microsurgery* 27, no. 5 (June 2007): 494-499. DOI: https://doi:org/10.1002/micr.20393.

Clevenger, R. R., J. Bernal, M. Talcott, Teresa R. Gleason, Tracie Rindfield, and Robert F. Hoyt, Jr. "Surgery". In *Management of Animal Care and Use Programs in Research, Education, and Testing. 2nd edition* edited by, R. H. Weichbrod, G. A. H. Thompson and J. N. Norton, 807–826. Boca Raton (FL): CRC Press/Taylor & Francis, 2018. https://doi:org/10.1201/9781315152189-34.

Belykh, Evgenii, Michael A. Bohl, Kaith K. Almefty, Mark C. Preul and Peter Nakaji. "Biological models for neurosurgical training in microanastomosis." In *Comprehensive Healthcare Simulation: Neurosurgery,* edited by A. Alara, 91-102, Cham, Springer International Publishing, 2018. DOI: https://doi.org/10.1007/978-3-319-75583-0_7.

Evgeniou, Evgenios, Harriet Walker and Sameer Gujral. "The role of simulation in microsurgical training." *Journal of Surgical Education* 75, no. 1 (January-February 2018): 171-181. DOI: https://doi.org/10.1016/j.jsurg.2017.06.03.

Gross, D., and René H. Tolba. "Ethics in Animal-Based Research." *Eur. Surg. Res.* 55, no. 1-2 (August 2015): 43-57. DOI: https://doi.org/10.1159/000377721

Kang, Bo Young, Byung-Joon Jeon, Kyeong-Tae Lee and Goo-Hyun Mun. "Comprehensive analysis of chicken vessels as microvascular anastomosis training model." *Archives of Plastic Surgery* 44, no. 1 (January 2017): 12-18. DOI: https://doi.org/10.5999/aps.2017.44.1.12.

Magaldi, Marcelo Oliveira, Arthur Nicolato, Joao V. Godinho, Marcilea Santos, Andre Prosdocimi, Jose A. Malheiros, Ting Lei, et al. "Human placenta aneurysm model for training neurosurgeons in vascular microsurgery." *Operative Neurosurgery* 10, no. 4 (September 2014): 592–601. DOI: https://doi.org/10.1227/neu.0000000000000553.

Mikami, Takeshi, Hime Suzuki, Ryo Ukai, Katsuya Komatsu, Yusuke Kimura, Y. Akiyama, Masahiko Wanibuchi and Nobuhiro Mikuni.

"Surgical anatomy of rats for the training of microsurgical anastomosis." *World Neurosurgery* 120 (December 2018): 1310-1318. DOI : https://doi.org/10.1016/j.wneu.2018.09.071.

Mokhtari P., A. Tayebi Meybodi, A. Benet and M. T. Lawton. "Microvascular Anastomosis: Proposition of a Learning Curve." *Oper. Neurosurg. (Hagerstown)* 16, no. 2 (February 2019): 211-216. DOI: https://doi.org/10.1093/ons/opy072.

Mutoh, Tatsushi, Tatsuya Ishikawa, Hidenori Ono and Nobuyuki Yasui. "A new polyvinyl alcohol hydrogel vascular model (KEZLEX) for microvascular anastomosis training." *Surgical Neurology International* 1, no. 74 (November 2010): 74-77. DOI: https://doi.org/10.4103/2152-7806.72626.

National Research Council. *Guide for the Care and Use of Laboratory Animals: Eighth Edition.* Washington, DC: The National Academies Press, 2011. DOI: https://doi.org/10.17226/12910.

Olabe, Jon, Javier Olabe and Vidal Sancho. "Human cadaver brain infusion model for neurosurgical training." *Surgical Neurology* 72, no. 6 (December 2009): 700-702. DOI: https://doi.org/10.1016/j.surneu.2009.02.028.

Rodriguez, J. R., R. Yañez, I. Cifuentes, J. Varas and B. Dagnino. "Microsurgery Workout: A Novel Simulation Training Curriculum Based on Non-living Models." *Plast. Reconstr. Surg.* 138, no. 4 (October 2016): 739e-747e. DOI: https://doi.org/10.1097/PRS.0000000000002456.

Shurey, Sandra, Yelena Akelina, Josette Legagneux, Geardo Malzone, Lucian Jiga and Ali Mohmoud Ghanem. "The rat model in microsurgery education: classical exercises and new horizons." *Archives of Plastic Surgery* 41, no. 3 (May 2014): 201-208. DOI: https://doi.org/10.5999/aps.2014.41.3.201.

Tolba, Rene H., Zoltán Czigány, Suzanne Osorio Lujan, Mihai Oltean, Michael Axelsson, Yelena Akelina, Antonio Di Cataldo, et al. "Defining Standards in Experimental Microsurgical Training: Recommendations of the European Society for Surgical Research (ESSR) and the International Society for Experimental Microsurgery (ISEM)." *Eur. Surg. Res.* 58, nos. 5-6 (December 2017): 246-262. DOI: https://doi.org/10.1159/000479005.

Yonekawa, Yasuhiro, Rosmarie Frick, Peter Roth, Ethan Taub and Hans-Georg Imhof. "Laboratory training in microsurgical techniques and microvascular anastomosis." *Operative Techniques in Neurosurgery* 2, no. 3 (September 1999): 149-158. DOI: https://doi.org/10.1016/S1092-440X(99)80007-3.

# CHAPTER 10

# ACADEMIC SESSIONS DURING THE TRAINING

HASNAIN ZAFAR AND SABAH UDDIN SAQIB

"Postgraduate medical education is a unique educational environment with its emphasis on work-based learning, clinical supervision as a predominant method of training, performance-based assessment and the challenge of simultaneously delivering education, training, and service."
(Dr Yvonne Steinert 2011)

Academic medicine is like a tripod, standing on three legs: one leg is patient care; one is research; and the last is education (Gunderman 2006). Conventionally, the stability to this tripod is largely provided by the medical faculty at teaching hospitals, who take on three different roles: that of the skilled clinician delivering quality healthcare to his or her patients; that of the researcher, looking after innovations and methods of cure for ailments; and that of the educator, largely responsible for the transformation of trainees into the role of clinician, researcher and educator (and so the cycle goes continuously on). This cycle ensures the attainment of competencies among trainees that not only includes technical knowledge and skills related to medicine but also encompasses attributes of professionalism and scholarship.

## Teaching and learning methods in postgraduate training

Postgraduate medical education (PGME), also known as residency education, is mainly focused on the learner in both clinical and non-clinical settings. Academic sessions during medical training can be broadly classified into those happening in the inpatient care area and outside the patient care area (Figure 10.1).

Figure 10.1: Academic sessions in training broadly take place in a patient care area and outside patient care area.

As the trainees, also known as residents, advance along the path of their education, their learning and academic activities evolve to meet the demands of a practising doctor with an increasing level of autonomy. Much of the learning and experience in one's postgraduate medical education or residency is obtained at the workplace where a resident is simultaneously involved in healthcare provision and performing necessary clinical tasks. Alongside work-based learning, residents' education also occurs in non-clinical settings through journal clubs, academic core sessions, and formal lectures. Clinical supervisors and lead consultants use various academic tools to formally train their residents to enhance knowledge and master the skills to acquire a professional identity. These tools comprise a wide range of academic activities and sessions, some that happen with real patients and others that are formally tutorial or presentation-based discussion sessions taking place outside the workplace usually in seminar rooms, auditoriums, or in skill labs (Table 10.1).

**Table 10.1: Different types of academic sessions in postgraduate medical education and training.**

| Academic sessions in clinical settings | Academic sessions in non-clinical settings |
|---|---|
| Bedside teaching | Academic core sessions |
| Morning follow-ups and attending rounds | Journal clubs |
| Morbidity and Mortality meetings | Grand rounds |
| Mini-CEX and DOPS | Research conferences |
| Multidisciplinary team meetings | Training through simulators |

This chapter will mainly focus on academic sessions in residency with special emphasis at the end, on in-service assessment tools after the acquisition of desired clinical knowledge and skills, yet maintaining the quality of care and patient safety in its supreme form.

## Academic sessions in training

Academic hospitals are mainly involved in the medical education of postgraduate fellow residents and interns. The curriculum of postgraduate training varies both from country to country and within individual countries, with distinct approaches among different teaching hospitals. However, all over the world postgraduate medical education heavily relies on academic sessions both in clinical and non-clinical settings. In various PGME programs, there is an effort to balance clinically based education with reserved time for formal educational activities and novel methods of training. Our next discussion will be on the various methods of teaching applied in each setting.

## A. Academic sessions in clinical settings

Learning in a clinical setting is also known as patient-centred learning as patients are the best teachers and they link the pursuit of knowledge to the real goal of the medical profession. Academic sessions based on this approach enable residents to apply their core knowledge to understand disease processes and better formulate management plans. In the clinical setting, different academic activities are conducted and some of them are described below.

### I) Bedside teaching

Bedside teaching lies at the heart of postgraduate medical training. Didactic bedside sessions enable trainees to acquire the skills of history taking, physical examinations, and effective and empathetic communication. Bedside teaching provides an excellent opportunity for the trainees to understand patients and their problems, clinical reasoning, performing or witnessing procedures, and above all, professionalism. According to a study conducted at the University of Washington School of Medicine (Shetty, Magazine and Chogtu 2021), not just students but teachers too perceive a profound positive impact on their clinical skills from teaching students at the bedside. This teaching-learning strategy can be utilized in outpatient clinics, hospital wards, and emergency rooms. Bedside teaching and learning form the basis of the acquisition of clinical reasoning skills, by which the student learns to generate a differential diagnosis and management plan based on the information they gather while interacting with patients. Despite the unique benefits of this very important training tool, several studies have highlighted that with the advancement in medical technology and explosion of modern tools of training, bedside teaching has seen a decline in its popularity in many teaching institutes. Several factors of this decline have been listed in the literature, such as time constraints on the part of senior clinicians (Jayakumar 2016), availability of suitable patients, and lack of interest among both trainees and consultants. Surgeons involved in the training of their residents often feel conflicted owing to the ever-increasing "time crunch" (Kim and Mellinger 2020). This is because of several external pressures on faculty to meet performance metrics in terms of clinical and research productivity which results in decreased faculty-resident interactions. It is a necessity to build a culture of reserving time for bedside teaching at all possible clinical venues, including both emergency and elective settings, and redeem this effective and antediluvian method of medical teaching.

**II) Morning follow-ups and attending rounds**

Morning reports and follow-ups in a teaching hospital serve as an excellent tool to identify any new problem that has occurred during the night. They set out the first academic meeting of the day and are best held at 7AM to ensure the delivery of excellent patient care. Morning rounds allow discussing patients admitted to the hospital in the last 24 hours and also those who were already admitted. All new problems and their possible solutions are discussed in these rounds, and a decision is arrived at the following day (after discussion with the attending). The chief resident is responsible for initiating the morning round and making it an academic activity for students and postgraduate trainees. Caring for patients in such a way has many possible benefits (Figure 10.2).

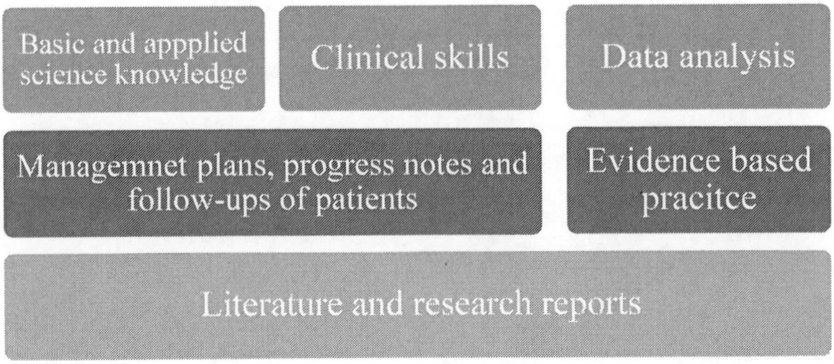


Figure 10.2: Items that are emphasized during morning reports and attending rounds.

One of the greatest by-products of morning rounds is that trainees detect the concerns of chief residents for patient care and teaching. They also encourage the development of self-learning, solidifying the commanding abilities in the chief to lead his or her team and to identify patients for further discussions at other teaching sessions. The morning rounds of chief residents are mostly followed by attending clinicians. Attending rounds allow the senior clinician to assess the history taking and physical examination skills of a trainee. Didactic attending rounds are the hallmark of a tertiary care hospital where problem-based scenarios are discussed given recent advances and in light of current literature. Daily attending rounds, when done effectively, provide numerous opportunities for high-impact teaching in a setting where trainees are likely to be motivated, engaged, and able to make immediate use of the new skills or knowledge they acquire. When conducted ineffectively, attending rounds can be lengthy, redundant, and provide little educational content for learners (Merritt et al. 2017).

### III) Morbidity and Mortality meetings

The Morbidity & Mortality (M&M) meeting is a weekly or monthly gathering of surgeons, postgraduate residents, fellows, nurses, and medical students to discuss unwanted or, in some settings, avoidable outcomes of surgical patients. M&M meetings allow improving patient safety, healthcare delivery, and raising the standards of education among clinical staff. This opportunity for improvisation has a direct impact on the overall surgical outcomes of the patient (Figure 10.3).

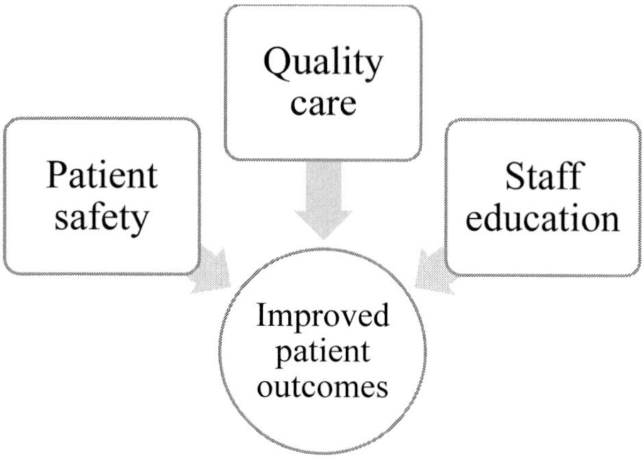


Figure 10.3: The process through which M&M meetings have the potential to improve patient outcomes.

M&M meetings assure from an administrative point of view in any hospital that the adverse outcome of a patient is being monitored and addressed. Such meetings permit an open discussion which allows healthcare providers to critically analyse lapses and weaknesses in thought processes, decision making, and the technical aspects of surgery. This in return favours the better outcomes of surgical patients in the future. These meetings are now a mandatory requirement in the United States and should also be attended by all UK surgeons according to Good Surgical Practice. A systematic review presented at the Royal Australasian College of Surgeons Annual Scientific Congress 2017, highlighted enabling and barrier factors that have an impact on the conduct of M&M meetings (Vreugdenburg et al. 2018).

This systematic review concluded that a structured meeting format, structured case identification and presentation, and a systems focus have a positive impact on the conduct of M&M meetings. The absence of key personnel from meetings, lack of education regarding the meeting process, poor perceptions of the process, logistical issues, and heterogeneity in case evaluation were identified as barriers to effective M&M meetings.

**IV) Mini-CEX and DOPS**

Medical training is a very dynamic field, where the acquisition of new knowledge and skills has a direct impact on the overall care of the patient and sometimes even on outcomes. To get through the growing responsibilities as physicians and to develop new skills safely and effectively, trainees must receive feedback on their performance. Most such activities and performances are clinically based and occur in the inpatient care area, just after performing the particular clinical task. The Mini-Clinical Evaluation Exercise (Mini-CEX), whether it takes place in an outpatient or inpatient setting, allows the trainee to learn the correct clinical examination methods of patients. Similarly, the Direct Observation of Procedural Skills (DOPS) is an academic exercise in which a trainee performs a particular skill under the observation of a senior or his or her trainer. These academic activities are usually a feature of well reputable training institutes, where there are structured postgraduate training programmes. Both Mini-CEX and DOPS allow constructive feedback of the trainees and are increasingly used as methods of formative assessment, to shape and support trainees' learning. However, this feedback process is heavily influenced by complex relationships between the feedback recipient, the feedback provider, and the training institution. Ideally, the trainee should show active feedback-seeking behaviour and the supervisor must show active feedback-providing behaviour at the end of this very valuable academic activity.

**V) Multidisciplinary team meetings**

Multidisciplinary team (MDT) working is widely accepted as the "gold standard" of quality care delivery across the world. MDTs in teaching hospitals now serve as very valuable academic tools for enhancement of knowledge among trainees, besides their chief aim of formulating a management plan for patients. Such MDTs are now an integral part of cancer care and also very common in other specialties like vascular surgery, cardiac medicine, neuroscience and in paediatric medicine. Most of these meetings occur in seminar rooms of clinical areas and allow evidence-based discussion among the lead consultants, trainees, and nursing staff of the various departments. Such collaborative effort promises a very fruitful academic activity that aims to establish an evidence-based medicine. Several issues will influence the benefits from an MDT meeting, such as participation from qualified and effective experts, case selection, access to relevant information, discussion format and structure, leadership, health professionals' interactions, technical equipment, and administrative processes (Rosell et al. 2018). Despite all this, if MDT meetings are conducted in a structured manner they serve as a very effective training session for residents and other trainees alongside their chief aim of provision of quality healthcare to patients.

## B. Academic sessions in non-clinical settings

Medical teaching has greatly evolved from the "see one, do one, teach one" ideology over the years. In most postgraduate medical training, residents get trained in the patient-centred approach but several other didactic training methods in non-clinical settings also enhance their core knowledge and skills. These academic sessions, either in the form of formal tutorial-based sessions or learning through skill labs and simulators, serve as a very valuable tool for continuing medical education (CME) and training. Some important academic sessions in non-clinical settings are listed below.

### I) Academic core sessions

Academic core sessions in a teaching hospital lay the foundation of concepts related to a trainee's pertinent specialty. As trainees rotate from specialty to specialty in different years, they take on the relevant core specialty modules. Academic core sessions ameliorate knowledge and concepts which trainees in clinical placement must acquire, regardless of their specialty of choice. These modules align with the quality indicators suggested by the postgraduate medical education (PGME) department associated with a teaching hospital and mostly are supervised by lead consultants. Academic core sessions enable trainees to discuss and improve their fundamental concepts of basic and clinical science. The format of academic core sessions varies in different programmes from lecture-based sessions to problem-based discussion among trainees of different levels under the supervision of faculty. It is one of the responsibilities of programme directors of residency programmes to ensure reserved time for this session every week (including both elective and emergency patients' responsibilities) in which a specific group of trainees is free from their clinical activities. Although not patient-centred, these academic sessions allow for the discussion of various clinical scenarios and diseases in light of the current practice of evidence-based medicine. Later trainees use this core knowledge in maintaining good standards of patient care.

### II) Journal clubs

Possibly the earliest reference to a journal club is in the biography of Sir James Paget from 1835 to 1854, in which it is noted that a group of students met in a room over a baker's shop near St. Bartholomew's Hospital to read journals or play cards (Linzer 1987). Since this early description, journal clubs have become ubiquitous in postgraduate medical education training programmes and one of the learning techniques which come under the peer-assisted learning (PAL) strategy. Journal club sessions are academic activities organised by trainees themselves in which they select a recent article from any index journal and formally criticise its application, strengths, and shortcomings. Although these academic sessions are mostly supervised by trained specialists, such academic activities highly encourage PAL. Essentially, it is a proven fact that the great potential of trainees to assist in the learning of their peers has been recognised and encouraged via informally organised teaching and mentoring programmes. The best advantage of the journal club is that it gives trainees an opportunity to discuss current evidence-based medicine and remain updated with recent literature. The selection of the article is a crucial step in effective conduction of a journal club and sometimes the article might be very good in a particular setting, but its role and conclusions may not apply to another setting. Since trainees mostly select the article for a journal club, after surveying the table of contents of a journal or by using search engines designed for medical research, as a result, an article that is very current and shows a good level of evidence may not focus on solving the patient's problem. Therefore, concepts shared and discussed in journal clubs may be forgotten by the trainees, including those who presented the article; because they are not trying to solve a problem and not using new information in their day to day work. It is clear from this literature review that an ideal journal club format does not exist (Alguire 1998). Rather, the format depends on the goals of the journal club, the parameters used to define success, and the available resources. The clear articulation of goals of a journal club, selecting the appropriate formats, and the direct presence of senior faculty are a few common steps that must be incorporated into the PGME curriculum to increase the effectiveness of this very important academic session

### III) Grand rounds

Trainees at all levels of their medical training and education, find some difficulty in analysing, integrating and correlating data which they extract from patients. Even after gathering data, they have trouble presenting them in front of their colleagues and senior consultants. A grand round in any teaching hospital provides an exciting opportunity to overcome this problem. This academic activity ensures the production of analytical skills and presentation of data extracted in a more didactic way. There are various kinds of grand rounds formats prevalent in different countries. In some centres it is lecture-based, which brings some unity to the service, while in some academic institutions it is largely a teaching activity that promotes some exciting debates and arguments. Medical grand rounds are a well-established form of postgraduate medical education and are a component of most UK hospital teaching programmes. Worth mentioning here is the grand round format at the Hammersmith Hospital London (Hurst 1992), which is very interesting as it involves trainees, students, and consultants in very intellectual discussion. Their grand rounds are patient-oriented in which younger trainees mostly start with case presentations and they give all information related to the patients' history, physical examination, and all investigations conducted during their stay. Later treatment options are discussed among trainees and finally, faculty members are asked to share their research work which is related to the particular problem. In the authors' institute trainees are involved in weekly as well as annual grand rounds. The former are mostly patient-oriented where actual cases are discussed with specialists in light of current literature and research, and occur in almost all disciplines, while the latter is an annual activity of a trainee which is more research-based and prominently seen in the department of surgery. In our annual surgical grand round, the trainee has to present a research study conducted in the preceding year after proper approval of the ethical board of the hospital. After the formal presentation, the forum opens for the audience which consists of medical students, postgraduate trainees, and consultants. They all give constructive feedback and ask questions if they want further clarity. Such a research-based activity develops scholarly characteristics amongst trainees and demands good communication skills. Annual surgical grand round presentation is now an essential criterion set for surgical trainees to meet so they can progress to the next year in our institute.

## IV) Research conferences

National and international conferences are valuable media to exchange views and opinions on standards of care and novel methods of treatment. Attending a conference during training is itself a very good academic activity which provides many opportunities to learn and embark on as a professional in future. Research conferences are basically of two types: clinical and basic science. Clinical research conferences are mostly attended by faculty, fellows, and residents engaged in clinical research. They promote the acquisition of new clinical skills and are based on studies done on patients. Basic research conferences, on the other hand, are attended by scientists as they mainly focus on the molecular basis of diseases (Hurst 1992). Regardless of their types, postgraduate training programmes greatly encourage the participation of trainees at medical conferences in their training years to enhance their expertise in healthcare.

### V) Training through simulators

Medical simulators are training tools that fall into the broad context of simulation-based medical education (SMBE). The concept of SMBE is not new; however, its adoptions have changed in recent years from simple mannequins to high-tech patient simulators. SMBE is broadly classified into two main families, low-tech and high-tech simulation modalities, and each has its different types (Figure 10.4).

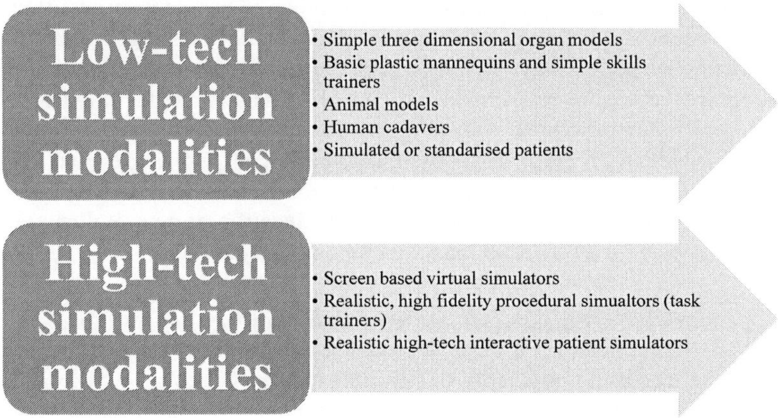


Figure 10.4: The two main families of simulation-based medical education and their characteristics.

Worldwide, SMBE is now recognised as an increasingly powerful complementary teaching modality in medical training. However, most novel methods of teaching and learning strategies, like training with the help of high-tech simulators, are in their infancy in low- to middle-income countries. The Centre of Innovation in Medical Education (CIME) at the Aga Khan University is the first simulation-based educational institute in South Asia and is utilised for medical and nursing education at both undergraduate and postgraduate levels. Recognition of these novel methods of training in all teaching hospitals is a necessity and trainees must be given an allocated time to use simulators under the supervision of an experienced trainer.

## Residents as teachers

Teaching is an intrinsic part of any healthcare professional's role. Clinicians are often involved in teaching medical students, residents, nursing staff, and even patients and their families. Residents regularly contribute to the education of medical students and their fellow residents, and may spend up to one-fourth of their time supervising, instructing, and evaluating students and junior colleagues (Seely et al. 1999). Those residents who possess good teaching skills and teach on a regular basis tend to have better knowledge acquisition. Residents with efficacious teaching abilities may also have a positive impact on patient care. Resident involvement in teaching activities has been shown to have a positive effect on the resident's communication skills (Bulte et al. 2007) and good patient communication skills play a vital role in the good outcomes of patients. Among the various levels of residency, the chief resident is the one who is the central figure among the entire team of residents. The job description of chief residents, regardless of their disciplines, must include effective teaching of their junior colleagues. Their abilities to lead a team and contribute constructively to the learning and education of other colleagues ensure they remain a powerful leader and mentor in the future.

## In-service assessment, promotion, and certification

Despite the increasing popularity of performance and workplace assessment, written assessments are still probably the most widely used assessment methods in medical training. Multiple modalities are utilised across various institutions for this purpose and include multiple choice questions (MCQs,) essay type questions, short answer questions and extended matching questions. Clinical examination assessments are also widely used, where students demonstrate clinical examination and clinical reasoning skills while interacting with patients. Communication skills are taught and assessed formally. Skills assessments include lab-based assessments, objective structured practical examination (OPSE), viva-voce, and objective structured clinical examination (OSCE). In-service terminal assessments allow local institutional regulatory bodies, like PGME, to promote trainees to their subsequent stages and finally help them graduate in different disciplines. In addition to registration with local institutes and governing bodies at the national level, trainees may wish to apply for some international courses, training, and certificates to embark on their careers in more revolutionised healthcare systems.

## Patient safety and quality of care

Patient safety is defined as the avoidance of inadvertent harm or injury to patients. The aim of patient safety is the prevention of harm, not the elimination of errors. Training in healthcare quality and patient safety must be based on an understanding of developing and maintaining complex systems of healthcare and the role of healthcare providers in the provision of quality care within those systems (Dent, Harden and Hunt [eds.] 2007). A good healthcare system is not entirely dependent on the dedicated activities of its staff but also relies on the ability of the health system to capture errors before they reach patients and cause hazards. Healthcare organisations have their root cause analysis (RCA) committees identify medical errors and find solutions to minimise them to ensure patient safety, all the while maintaining good standards of training. In most RCAs, the serious adverse events in healthcare are related to failure in communication. One of the areas of focus of academic sessions in training is that the training residents or fellows develop an ability to communicate in a more effective and intelligible way which reduces medical errors and maintains the highest standards of quality care.

## Summary

The purpose of academic sessions in any training institute is to facilitate the learning and acquisition of sufficient skills by the trainee, who is required to deliver safe and quality care to patients. With time these academic sessions always need reform(s), in terms of the curriculum, the role of trainers, interactive supervision, and many newer methods of training. Hence, academic sessions are one of the fundamental components of the postgraduate training programme which eventually gives strength to the tripod of academic medicine.

## Bibliography

Alguire, P. C. "A review of journal clubs in postgraduate medical education." *J. Gen. Intern. Med.* 13, no. 5 (May 1998): 347-53. DOI: 10.1046/j.1525-1497.1998.00102.x.

Bulte, C., A. Betts, K. Garner and S. Durning. "Student teaching: views of student near-peer teachers and learners." *Med. Teach.* 29, no. 6 (September 2007): 583-90. DOI: 10.1080/01421590701583824.

Dent, John, Ronald Harden and Dan Hunt (eds.) *A practical guide for medical teachers*. USA: Elsevier, 2007.

Gunderman, Richard B. *Achieving excellence in medical education.* Indiana University Indianapolis USA: Springer, 2006.

Hurst, Wilis J. *The Bench and Me: Teaching and Learning Medicine.* Emory University School of Medicine Atlanta, Georgia: IGAKU-SHOIN Publishers, 1992.

Jayakumar, N. "Bedside teaching with unwell patients: Can it ever be appropriate?" *Med Teach.* 39, no. 3 (November 2016): 323-324. DOI: 10.1080/0142159X.2016.1248922.

Kim, Roger H. and John D. Mellinger. "Educational strategies to foster bedside teaching." *Surgery* 167, no. 3 (March 2020): 532-534. DOI: doi.org/10.1016/j.surg.2019.06.007.

Linzer, M. "The journal club and medical education: over one hundred years of unrecorded history." *Postgrad. Med. J.* 63, no. 740 (June 1987): 475-478. DOI: 10.1136/pgmj.63.740.475.

Merritt, F. W., M. N. Noble, A. V. Prochazka, E. M. Aagaard and C. R. Stickrath. "Attending rounds: What do the all-star teachers do?" *Med Teach.* 39, no. 1 (January 2017): 100-104. DOI: 10.1080/0142159X.2017.1248914.

Rosell, L., N. Alexandersson, O. Hagberg and M. Nilbert. "Benefits, barriers and opinions on multidisciplinary team meetings: a survey in Swedish cancer care." *BMC Health Serv Res.* 18, no. 1 (April 2018): 249. DOI: 10.1186/s12913-018-2990-4.

Seely, A. J., M. P. Pelletier, L. S. Snell and J. L. Trudel. "Do surgical residents rated as better teachers perform better on in-training examinations?" *Am. J. Surg.* 177, no. 1 (January 1999): 33-7. DOI: 10.1016/s0002-9610(98)00306-7.

Shetty, Pritam A, Rahul Magazine and Bharti Chogtu. "Patient outlook on bedside teaching in a medical school." *Journal of Taibah University Medical Sciences* 16, no. 1 (February 2021): 50-56. DOI: doi.org/10.1016/j.jtumed.2020.10.002.

Vreugdenburg, Thomas D., Deanne Forel, Nicholas Marlow, Guy J Maddern, John Quinn, Richard Lander and Stephen Tobin. "Morbidity and mortality meetings: gold, silver or bronze?" *Medical teacher* 88, no. 10 (October 2018): 966-974. DOI: doi.org/10.1111/ans.14380.

# CHAPTER 11

# EVIDENCE-BASE FOR PROMOTION AND GRADUATION: FORMATIVE AND SUMMATIVE ASSESSMENT OF SURGICAL SKILLS

TASHFEEN AHMAD

## Abstract

On-the-job teaching accounts for much of the training in surgery. Hence, judgement about the competence of trainees is primarily done by the supervising trainers subjectively. The trend now is to move towards objective assessment methods, both for feedback and promotion, to decrease subjectivity and potential inaccuracy in the estimation of competency. For disciplines such as surgery, competence in technical skills is of prime concern during decision-making about academic progression; thus objective tools for assessment of skills have received substantial interest in recent literature. As a result, various tools such as Direct Observation of Procedural Skills, Procedure Based Assessment, Objective Structured Assessment of Technical Skills, and Entrustable Professional Activities are becoming increasingly popular. This chapter describes their advantages and limitations, implementation and obstacles, and the expected programme-level outcomes with the utilization of these tools.

## Introduction

Surgical training programmes face challenging yet rewarding responsibilities: to train a novice to become a safe and competent surgeon, and to certify the achievement of a sufficient fund of knowledge and skills for an independent surgical practice.

Training in surgical specialties spreads across multiple domains of learning, broadly categorized as cognitive, affective, and psychomotor domains. As much of the training in surgery is received on-the-job by observing and performing, judgement on achievement of a satisfactory level of competency has historically been largely left to the trainer. Although knowledge is usually assessed in an objective manner through exams, technical competence in surgical skills is often evaluated subjectively by clinical supervisors. Surgical high-stakes “exit exams” such as those of the Royal Colleges in the UK and their counterparts across the world comprise a knowledge exam and a practical exam which includes clinical and diagnostic skills, communication skills and minor procedural skills. For surgical skills, however, they rely on certification from the academic programmes at training institutes. Thus, the onus to provide society with competent surgeons rests mainly on the training institutes, and partly on examining/licensing bodies. Thus, institutes need to have robust systems to reliably assess surgical competence.

For surgical training programmes, surgical skills form an important and distinctive component of the curriculum. Hence, objectivity is desirable in assessment of these skills. The trend now is to move towards objective methods of assessment for feedback, for estimation of progression, and to decrease subjectivity and potential inaccuracies in the estimation of competency. Tools to aid the objective assessment of the cognitive domain are robust and well established, with multiple-choice questions dominating in reliability and practicality. However, tools for assessment in the affective and psychomotor domains continue to evolve.

Many validated tools for assessment of skills are in practice across the world and these tools have been developed with the intention of achieving the desired objectivity (Table 11-1).

# Table 11-1: Overview of workplace-based assessment tools identified in the literature.

**Table 1:** Overview of workplace-based assessment tools identified in the literature

| |
|---|
| Short-practice observations (Table S4A) |
| Mini-Clinical Evaluation Exercise (Mini-CEX)[20-38] |
| Handoff Mini-Clinical Evaluation Exercise (Handoff Mini-CEX)[39] |
| Professionalism Mini-Evaluation Exercise (P-MEX)[40] |
| Electronic problem-specific Clinical Evaluation Exercise (eCEX)[41] |
| Just In Time Medicine (JIT) Clinical Evaluation Exercise[42] |
| Ophthalmic Clinical Evaluation Exercise[43,44] |
| Teamwork Mini-Clinical Evaluation Exercise[45] |
| Personal Digital Assistant (PDA)-based Mini-Clinical Evaluation Exercise[46] |
| Outpatient Clinic Evaluation (OPC)[57] |
| Systematically Observed Medical Encounters[90] |
| Mini-assessed Clinical Encounter[48] |
| Assessment of Clinical Expertise[48] |
| Case Presentation (CP)[48] |
| Minicard[67] |
| Direct Observation Clinical Encounter Examination (DOCEE)[84] |
| Acute Care Assessment Tool (ACAT)[56] |
| Direct Observation of Clinical Skills (DOCS)[68] |
| Structured Clinical Observation (SCO)[96] |
| Unnamed – Analysis of videotaped patient interactions[52] |
| Davis Observation Code (DOC)[63] |
| Case Conference Assessment Tool (cCAT)[71] |
| Standardized Direct Observation Tool (SDOT)[73] |
| Unnamed scoring form – global rating form[72] |
| Unnamed – group assessment tool[91] |
| Unnamed – one minute mentor[92] |
| Long Case[77,78] |
| Video Communication Assessment and Feedback (Video-CAF)[80] |
| **Procedural short-practice observations (Table S4B)** |
| Procedure-Based Assessment (PBA)[49,86,95] |
| Direct Observation of Procedural Skills (DOPS)[28,31,37,38,47,48] |
| Direct Observation of Procedural Skills in Surgery (SDOPS)[95] |
| Objective Structured Assessment of Technical Skills (OSATS)[85,86] |
| Non-Technical Skills for Surgeons (NOTSS)[86] |
| Structured Assessment of Microsurgical Skills (SAMS)[87] |
| Hopkins Assessment of Surgical Competency (HASC)[88] |
| Procedure Feedback Form (PFF)[98] |
| Global Rating Index for Technical Skills (GRITS)[89] |
| Zwisch Scale[50] |
| Global Evaluative Assessment of Robotic Skills (GEARS)[83] |
| Global Operative Assessment of Laparoscopic Skills[77,82] |
| **Unnamed assessment tool to measure competence in video-assisted thoracoscopic surgery[70]** |
| Operative Performance Rating Scale (OPRS)[51] |
| Unnamed scoring form – checklist for task-specific items[72] |
| **Long-practice observations (Table S5)** |
| Multi-Source Feedback (MSF)[38,52] |
| Sheffield Peer Review Assessment Tool (SPRAT) (based on MSF)[53] |
| Team Observation Tool (based on MSF)[54] |
| Ward Evaluations (WE)[57] |
| Preceptor Evaluations (PE)[57] |
| Mini-Peer Assessment Tool[48] |
| Patient Satisfaction Questionnaires (PSQ)[48] |
| Patient Survey (PS)[56] |
| **In-training Assessment (ITA)[93]** |
| **Clinical Work Sampling (CWS) for In-Training Evaluation[76]** |
| **McGill Electronic Evaluation Portfolio (MEEP)[97]** |
| **Consultation And Relational Empathy (CARE)[52]** |
| **Specifically, monthly performance evaluations[63]** |
| **Ambulatory Care Competency Assessment Tool[81]** |
| **Case-based discussion (Table S5)** |
| Case-based discussion[48,56] |
| **Simulation tests (Table S6)** |
| Objective Structured Clinical Examination (OSCE)[57,65] |
| Unnamed – based on OSCE[66] |
| Integrated Procedural Performance Instrument[69] |
| **Product evaluation (Table S7)** |
| Audit Assessment[56] |
| Criterion Audit[53] |
| Assessment of referral letters[52] |
| Significant Event Analysis (SEA)[52] |
| Clinical Learning Electronic Portfolio System[94] |
| Vanderbilt Learning Portfolio (VLP)[75] |

Based on Miller's pyramid (Miller 1990) which depicts a hierarchy of clinical assessment, the highest "level" is *action* where the trainee *does* the task in the actual setting, rather than performing in a simulated or exam setting (Figure 11-1).

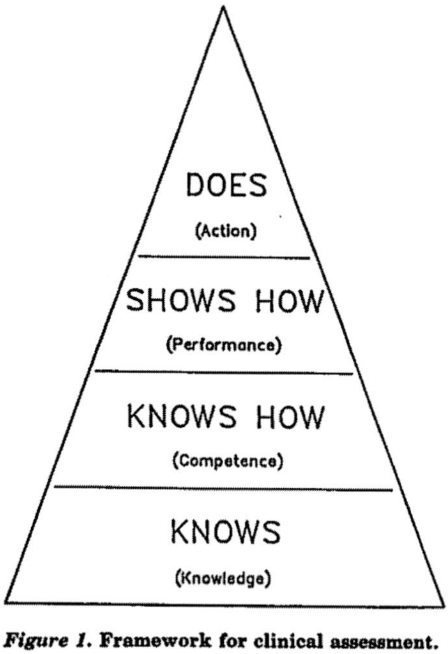


Figure 11-1: Miller's pyramid showing a framework for clinical assessment. Workplace-based assessments belong to the highest level.

Thus, workplace-based assessments stand at the highest level according to Miller's pyramid (Table 11-2).

This review focuses on tools for workplace-based assessment to assess surgical and procedural skills for providing objective data permitting evidence-based decisions on promotion and graduation.

**Table 11-2: Overview of assessment methods aligned with Miller's pyramid.**

Table 1. Overview of assessment methods aligned with Miller's pyramid[a].

| Stage | Corresponding methods to assess performance |
|---|---|
| Does | Chart/electronic medical record review (e.g. medical decision-making, cost-effective care, documentation) |
| | "Collective perspective"/clinical competency committee/residency education committee decisions |
| | Direct observation in clinical environments |
| | Efficiency data |
| | End-of-rotation evaluations |
| | Multi-source feedback/360-degree |
| | Patient outcomes data, including patient-reported outcome measures |
| | Portfolio[b] |
| | Procedure or case log with reflection and/or assessment |
| | Product review (e.g. splint, laceration repair) |
| | Project review (e.g. evidence-based medicine project, quality improvement project) |
| | Video review from clinical environments |
| Shows how | Objective structured clinical examination/standardized patient encounter |
| | Oral case presentation |
| | Simulated case |
| | Skills station |
| | Virtual reality/computerized patient management problem |
| Knows how | Chart-stimulated recall |
| | Development of individualized learning plan |
| | Mock oral boards examination/progressive case disclosure |
| | Oral questioning targeting patient management |
| | Written assignment/essay test |
| Knows | Multiple-choice questionnaire/short-answer test/audience response system |
| | Oral questioning targeting fact recall |

## What is the purpose of assessment?

A fundamental question needs to be answered when considering assessment methods: is the intention assessment *of* learning, or assessment *for* learning (Mayne, Wilson and Kennedy 2020)? Although assessments are generally done to determine whether the intended learning has been achieved by the learner or not, assessment itself has a well-known effect of driving the learning. Thus, students tend to study and learn what is assessed. Moreover, assessments can be used to provide feedback, and when feedback is given appropriately, it has consistently proven to be a reliable method to improve subsequent performance. This inclusion of feedback in the assessment without a direct bearing on pass or fail decisions is called formative assessment. It is intended to improve learning, and is therefore termed assessment *for* learning. On the other hand, when assessment is used for determining the achievement of desired learning in exam settings or for the purpose of decision on progression, it is termed summative assessment, also known as assessment *of* learning.

Establishing the purpose of assessment is important when developing or employing a particular tool for assessment because the selected tools must be validated for the intended purpose. If a tool is designed and validated for formative assessment, its use for summative assessment would technically be erroneous. In practice, though, there are many examples of formative tools being used for summative purposes (Massie and Ali 2016; Shalhoub 2014). This generally takes place in the setting of multiple formative assessments performed over time and collated at the end of the training/rotation period to get a total number of assessments done and/or an average score. These indices contribute to a defined proportion within the overall summative assessment components. Direct use of the formative tools for pass or fail decisions in one-time exams is not advisable as evidence on their validity for such use is lacking.

One major concern has arisen. As workplace-based assessments are gaining popularity, they are becoming incorporated in the overall assessment scheme of training programmes in the form of one of the "numbers" or "scores" to be added to the rest; their main role, as tools for structured formative feedback to improve performance, is being misunderstood (Aryal et al. 2020; Massie and Ali 2016).

An aspect which has recently gained interest in workplace-based assessments is entrustment decision. Certifying a trainee as being competent in a particular surgery does not always imply that the trainer can entrust the trainee with the procedure unsupervised. An entrustment decision considers factors including but not limited to reliability and integrity, apart from the capability to perform the procedure (ten Cate and Chen 2020a). Thus, if the purpose of a particular assessment is entrustment, tools specifically designed for entrustment decisions need to be employed.

Looking ahead, once competence has been assessed, and the decision to entrust made, the logical expectation would be to expect educational impact. Donald and James Kirkpatrick (1959) have defined a four-level model for evaluating training programmes for their outcomes, and this has formed the basis for many programme evaluations, some using Barr's modification (Barr et al. 2000). The Joint Committee for Surgical Training evaluated the Intercollegiate Surgical Curriculum Programme (ISCP) using this model, and found that workplace-based assessments perform well at levels 1 and 2, i.e., reaction and learning, but for levels 3 and 4, i.e., performance and impact (on patient outcomes), there is a lack of evidence in the published literature (ISCP Management Group 2012). Similar findings were reported in a prospective multicentre study on surgical skills assessment methods (Beard et al. 2011) and a systematic review (Barrett et al. 2016). This does not undermine the utility of workplace-based assessments, but highlights the need for further studies on performance and impact post-training.

## Tools for assessment – the good and the not-so-good

Learning during surgical specialty training spreads across multiple learning domains, broadly categorized under cognitive, affective, and psychomotor skills. Tools to aid objective assessment in the cognitive domain are robust and well established, with multiple-choice questions dominating in reliability and feasibility. However, for the affective and psychomotor domains, tools continue to evolve.

In clinical settings such as outpatient and inpatient bedside settings, clinical skills and communication skills, including counselling, professionalism and ethics, become the major assessment areas, falling into the affective domain (and to a lesser extent the psychomotor one). Some of the tools which have gained popularity due to their validity and reliability for such domains include the Mini-Clinical Evaluation Exercise (Mini-CEX) (Norcini et al. 1995), Mini-Peer Assessment Test (Mini-PAT) (Archer et al. 2008) and Multi-Source Feedback (Violato 2003). However, technical skills for surgery and other procedures have a different set of tools for assessment, which focus on more elements from the psychomotor compared to the affective domain. Some of the popular tools, their method of use and caveats are summarized below.

### Direct Observation of Procedural Skills (DOPS)

Technical skills require a different scheme for assessment, distinct from clinical skills. The latter focuses on a diagnosis and planning of treatment, while the former focuses on knowledge of procedures and performance in a safe, technically sound manner. One of the tools to assess procedural skills is the Direct Observation of Procedural Skills (DOPS) tool. DOPS was developed in the UK as a method to assess technical competence of specialist registrars (Wragg et al. 2003). In the original paper, the acronym stood for "directly observed assessment of practical skills," thus, its usage has evolved to the current one above. DOPS has been shown to have acceptable reliability and validity (Khanghahi and Azar 2018; Mayne, Wilson and Kennedy 2020). This tool is comprised of a generic form for procedures which can be used for minor procedures such as those performed at the bedside or clinic setting as well as surgical procedures in the operating room. A sample DOPS form is downloadable from the ISCP website (Joint Commission on Surgical Training 2015a). It is also presented in the following table.

**Table 11-3: DOPS from used by the Intercollegiate Surgical Curriculum programme.**

ISCP INTERCOLLEGIATE SURGICAL CURRICULUM PROGRAMME

## Direct Observation of Procedural Skills (DOPS)

| Trainee | Assessor |
|---|---|
| Name / GMC/GDC/IMC number: | Name / GMC/GDC/IMC number: |
| Assessment date: | Hospital DOPS took place: |

| FEEDBACK: |
|---|
| Verbal and written feedback is a mandatory component of this assessment. |
| General |
| Strengths |
| Development needs |
| Recommended actions |

| TRAINEE REFLECTIONS ON THIS ACTIVITY (optional) |
|---|
| What did I learn from this experience? |
| What did I do well? |
| What do I need to improve or change? How will I achieve it? |

**RATINGS**
Your ratings should be judged against the standard laid out in the syllabus for the trainee's stage of training.
**N** = Not observed **D** = Development required, **S** = Satisfactory (no prompting or intervention required) **O** = Outstanding

| Domain | Rating | Comments |
|---|---|---|
| 1: Describes indications, anatomy, procedure and complications to assessor | | |
| 2: Obtains consent, after explaining procedure and possible complications to patient | | |
| 3: Prepares for procedure according to an agreed protocol | | |
| 4: Administers effective analgesia or safe sedation (if no anaesthetist) | | |
| 5: Demonstrates good asepsis and safe use of instruments and sharps | | |
| 6: Performs the technical aspects in line with the guidance notes | | |
| 7: Deals with any unexpected event or seeks help when appropriate | | |
| 8: Completes required documentation (written or dictated) | | |
| 9: Communicates clearly with patient and staff throughout the procedure | | |
| 10: Demonstrates professional behaviour throughout the procedure | | |

| GLOBAL SUMMARY<br>Level at which completed elements of the PBA were performed on this occasion | | Tick |
|---|---|---|
| Level 0 | Insufficient evidence observed to support a summary judgement | |
| Level 1a | Able to assist with guidance (was not familiar with all steps of procedure) | |
| Level 1b | Able to assist without guidance (knew all steps of procedure and anticipated next move) | |
| Level 2a | Guidance required for most/all of the procedure (or part performed) | |
| Level 2b | Guidance or intervention required for key steps only | |
| Level 3a | Procedure performed with minimal guidance or intervention (needed occasional help) | |
| Level 3b | Procedure performed competently without guidance or intervention but lacked confidence | |
| Level 4a | Procedure performed confidently to a high standard without any guidance or intervention | |
| Level 4b | As 4a and was able to anticipate, avoid and/or deal with common problems/complications | |

| DOPS DETAILS | |
|---|---|
| **Name of Procedure:** | |
| **No. times procedure previously performed:** | **Emergency / Elective** (please circle) |
| **Performed in a simulated setting** ☐ **Description of the simulation:** | |
| **DOPS performed while on a course** Yes / No **If yes, please give details:** | |
| **Difficulty of procedure: Easier than usual** ☐ **Average difficulty** ☐ **More difficult than usual** ☐ | |
| **Trainee's signature:** | **Assessor's signature:** |

JUL 2015

Some other forms are available in the AMEE Guide no. 31 (Norcini and Burch 2007) and Jonathan Beard's article (Beard et al. 2009). It contains multiple areas to be rated, covering indication, anatomy, consent, pre-op preparation, analgesia, technical ability, aseptic technique, seeking help, post-procedure management, communication skills, and professionalism.

DOPS is administered at the trainee's initiative. The trainee identifies an upcoming procedure, informs the surgeon trainer of his or her intention to be assessed through DOPS on that procedure, and hands the DOPS form to the trainer. The trainer reviews the form to recap which aspects to observe. After completion of the procedure, the trainer completes the form to rate the different domains of competency listed, and also writes areas of strength and suggestions for development. Then the trainee meets the trainer who discusses the assessment with the trainee and provides structured verbal feedback according to the DOPS form face-to-face. This is a powerful method to convey strengths and weaknesses, and has been proven to lead to improvement in performance (Khanghahi and Azar 2018). The form is then collected by the trainee, counter signed, with comments, if any are recorded, and eventually submitted to the programme office. As for the frequency, there is an overall recommendation of all workplace-based assessments (e.g. DOPS + PBA + OSATS) amounting to 40 forms altogether in a year (JCST 2015a).

Like all assessments, DOPS has its limitations (Khanghahi and Azar 2018). It is highly dependent on the adequacy of training of both the assessors and trainees about DOPS. Despite training, assessor bias and dissimilarity in perception of their role in the DOPS process may affect the feedback and the scores. It requires substantial coordination by the trainee, and demands a short but definite time commitment from the trainers on an on-going basis.

Notably, a subjective, generic assessment by the trainer at the end of the procedure about the trainees' performance may not identify specific areas of competence or weakness to permit reflection and improvement. A generic DOPS tool does not provide separation of components of procedures to enable dissection of the technical learning needs. Two commonly used tools enabling in-depth assessment of technical competence are the Procedure Based Assessment and the Objective Structured Assessment of Technical Skills.

## Objective Structured Assessment of Technical Skills (OSATS)

A commonly used tool to assess competence in specific components of a surgical procedure is the Objective Structured Assessment of Technical Skills (OSATS). This tool focuses on different technical components of procedures. The assessor instead of interpreting complex psychomotor behaviour observes and rates specific domains which render the assessment objective (Okoro, Sirianni and Brigden 2010). The use of OSATS in surgical training was reported initially by Martin in 1997 (Martin et al. 1997). It has been shown to be reliable and valid in assessing surgical procedures (Bernard et al. 2016; Hatala et al. 2015). OSATS is now in use for assessment of competence in procedures in most surgical and procedural specialties (Hatala et al. 2015).

The OSATS form is comprised of three main sections, a procedure-specific technical checklist, a general checklist for generic portions of procedures, and a pass/fail judgement (Table 11-4). For administration of OSATS, the trainee informs the trainer before the procedure and undergoes observation while performing the procedure. After the procedure, the trainee first performs a self-rating on the OSATS checklist then gives it to the trainer for rating. Then, the trainee is provided structured feedback face-to-face according to the checklist. The comparison of self-rating and trainer rating helps the trainee understand the biases in self-perception and clarifies the reality of their competence.

Similar to DOPS, OSATS data provide information about competence in specific domains. Progress of competence over time for some procedures can be demonstrated graphically. Analysis of OSATS data can differentiate novice learners of varying performance levels undergoing training in complex technical tasks (Wilson et al. 2021). OSATS requires training, and reports show novice raters, after training, achieve a high agreement with ratings by experts (Asif et al. 2021) and greater reliability (Robertson et al. 2020).

Whether performance, as assessed by OSATS, corresponds to the quality of surgical result has also been a topic of research. Anderson et al. (2016) showed that articular surface restoration quality as assessed by post-procedure CT or laser scan did not correlate with OSATS score. Visual assessment, which the raters rely upon during surgery, may not be as accurate as a CT scan. Moreover, the OSATS checklist may not discern the finer details of surgery in order to achieve accurate scores reflecting the quality of surgery. When technically complex procedures are being assessed, a more exhaustive checklist is required which specifies the technical steps considered important for learning by the trainees. To address this need, Procedure Based Assessment has been developed.

Table 11-4: Detailed global 5-point rating scale and pass/failure score for OSATS.

**Please rate the candidate's performance on the following scale:**

| | 1 | 2 | 3 | 4 | 5 |
|---|---|---|---|---|---|
| **Respect for tissue** | Frequently used unnecessary force on tissue or caused damage by inappropriate use of instruments. | | Careful handling of tissue but occasionally caused inadvertent damage. | | Consistently handled tissues appropriately with minimal damage. |
| **Time and motion** | Many unnecessary moves. | | Efficient time/motion but some unnecessary moves. | | Economy of movement and maximum efficiency. |
| **Instrument handling** | Repeatedly makes tentative or awkward moves with instruments. | | Competent use of instruments although occasionally appeared stiff or awkward. | | Fluid moves with instruments and no awkwardness. |
| **Knowledge of instruments** | Frequently asked for the wrong instrument or used an inappropriate instrument. | | Knew the names of most instruments and used appropriate instrument for the task. | | Obviously familiar with the instruments required and their names. |
| **Use of assistants** | Consistently placed assistants poorly or failed to use assistants. | | Good use of assistants most of the time. | | Strategically used assistant to the best advantage at all times. |
| **Flow of operation and forward planning** | Frequently stopped operating or needed to discuss next move. | | Demonstrated ability for forward planning with steady progression of operative procedure. | | Obviously planned course of operation with effortless flow from one move to the next. |
| **Knowledge of specific procedure** | Deficient knowledge. Needed specific instruction at most operative steps. | | Knew all important aspects of the operation. | | Demonstrated familiarity with all aspects of the operation. |

**Overall, on this task, should this candidate: ☐Pass ☐ Fail ?**

## Procedure Based Assessment (PBA)

Since surgical procedures depend heavily on accurate technical performance of the procedure, achievement of a satisfactory competence level in the technical steps is required of trainees. Procedure Based Assessment includes identification of key technical steps in specific procedures and observation of the trainee while performing those steps, and thus enables the rater to assess and give feedback on the steps considered crucial for that procedure by those who develop the forms. Thus, it differs from DOPS by being specific to a list of selected procedures.

PBA was originally developed by the Orthopaedic Competence Assessment Project for Trauma and Emergency Surgery (Pitts et al. 2006) but has subsequently been adopted by multiple surgical specialties. A sample generic PBA form developed by the British Orthopaedic Association is available from the General Medical Council website

(Training Standards Committee of the British Orthopaedic Association 2015) and is presented in Table 11-5.

**Table 11-5: Generic PBA form developed by the British Orthopaedic Association and used by the General Medical Council.**

**Generic pba tool**

**[Specialty] PBA: [Procedure] APPROVED SURGICAL**

| | | |
|---|---|---|
| **Trainee:** | **Assessor:** | **Date:** |
| Start time: | End time: | Duration: |
| Operation more difficult than usual? Yes / No (If yes, state reason) | | |

**Score: N = Not observed or not appropriate D= Development required S = Satisfactory**

| **Competencies and Definitions** | | **Score N / D / S** | **Comments** |
|---|---|---|---|
| | **Consent** | | |
| C1 | Demonstrates sound knowledge of indications and contraindications including alternatives to surgery | | |
| C2 | Demonstrates awareness of sequelae of operative or non-operative management | | |
| C3 | Demonstrates sound knowledge of complications of surgery | | |
| C4 | Explains the perioperative process to the patient and/or relatives or carers and checks understanding | | |
| C5 | Explains likely outcome and time to recovery and checks understanding | | |
| | **Pre-operative planning** | | |
| PL1 | Demonstrates recognition of anatomical and pathological abnormalities (and relevant co-morbidities) and selects appropriate operative strategies/techniques to deal with these e.g. nutritional status | | |
| PL2 | Demonstrates ability to make reasoned choice of appropriate equipment, materials or devices (if any) taking into account appropriate investigations e.g. x-rays | | |
| PL3 | Checks materials, equipment and device requirements with operating room staff | | |
| PL4 | Ensures the operation site is marked where applicable | | |
| PL5 | Checks patient records, personally reviews investigations | | |

Page **163** of **232**

Approved 10 July 2017 for implementation in August 2018

| | | | |
|---|---|---|---|
| | **Pre-operative preparation** | | |
| PR1 | Checks in theatre that consent has been obtained | | |
| PR2 | Gives effective briefing to theatre team | | |
| PR3 | Ensures proper and safe positioning of the patient on the operating table | | |
| PR4 | Demonstrates careful skin preparation | | |
| PR5 | Demonstrates careful draping of the patient's operative field | | |
| PR6 | Ensures general equipment and materials are deployed safely (e.g. catheter, diathermy) | | |
| PR7 | Ensures appropriate drugs administered | | |
| PR8 | Arranges for and deploys specialist supporting equipment (e.g. image intensifiers) effectively | | |
| | **Exposure and closure** | | |
| E1 | Demonstrates knowledge of optimum skin incision / portal / access | | |
| E2 | Achieves an adequate exposure through purposeful dissection in correct tissue planes and identifies all structures correctly | | |
| E3 | Completes a sound wound repair where appropriate | | |
| E4 | Protects the wound with dressings, splints and drains where appropriate | | |

| Competencies and Definitions | | Score N / D / S | Comments |
|---|---|---|---|
| | **Intra operative Technique** | | |
| IT1 | Follows an agreed, logical sequence or protocol for the procedure | | |
| IT2 | Consistently handles tissue well with minimal damage | | |
| IT3 | Controls bleeding promptly by an appropriate method | | |
| IT4 | Demonstrates a sound technique of knots and sutures/staples | | |
| IT5 | Uses instruments appropriately and safely | | |
| IT6 | Proceeds at appropriate pace with economy of movement | | |
| IT7 | Anticipates and responds appropriately to variation e.g. anatomy | | |
| IT8 | Deals calmly and effectively with unexpected events/complications | | |
| IT9 | Uses assistant(s) to the best advantage at all times | | |
| IT10 | Communicates clearly and consistently with the scrub team | | |
| IT11 | Communicates clearly and consistently with the anaesthetist | | |
| | **Post-operative management** | | |
| PM1 | Ensures the patient is transferred safely from the operating table to bed | | |
| PM2 | Constructs a clear operation note | | |
| PM3 | Records clear and appropriate post-operative instructions | | |
| PM4 | Deals with specimens. Labels and orientates specimens appropriately | | |

Page **164** of **232**

Approved 10 July 2017 for implementation in August 2018

| Trainer feedback | |
|---|---|
| Trainee Reflection | |

## Global summary

| Level at which completed elements of the PBA were performed | | Tick as appropriate |
|---|---|---|
| **Level 0** | Insufficient evidence observed to support a judgment | |
| **Level 1** | Unable to perform the procedure under supervision | |
| **Level 2** | Able to perform the procedure under supervision | |
| **Level 3** | Able to perform the procedure with minimum supervision (would need occasional help) | |
| **Level 4** | Able to perform the procedure unsupervised (could deal with complications) | |

## Signatures:

| Trainee: | Assessor(s): |
|---|---|
| | |

A specific PBA form for total knee replacement spread over 12 pages is also provided in the same document, and another procedure-specific sample is available from Beard et al. (2009).

This assessment method involves direct observation of trainee performance of a defined set of "index" procedures of the specialty which the trainees are expected to perform in their level of training. It covers pre-operative, intra-operative and post-operative care related skills. Detailed guidance is available from several resources, including the Intercollegiate website (JCST 2015b). Some competencies are generic while some are specific to the procedure. Like DOPS, the trainee identifies an upcoming procedure, informs the surgeon trainer of his or her intention to be assessed through PBA on that procedure, and hands the PBA form to the trainer for review of what aspects are to be observed. During the procedure, the performance should be natural and the supervision standard. The only difference recommended is that the trainee verbalise his/her thinking and planning as the procedure proceeds. After completion of the procedure, the trainer completes the form and gives a rating according to the standard expected at the completion of training. Then, the trainee meets the trainer and obtains structured verbal feedback face-to-face.

PBA has been demonstrated to have high reliability, validity and acceptability (Marriot et al. 2011). Use of PBA is recommended every time the index procedures are performed, though practices may vary. A minimum number of required PBAs has not been established, as is the case with DOPS, except for the overall recommendation of 40 forms for all workplace-based assessments in a year (JCST 2015b). PBA is an elaborate tool and therefore requires more time to complete than DOPS and OSATS; hence, there may be a tendency by busy programmes to prefer the latter two over PBA. However, PBA has the ability to assess procedure-specific skills in detail which the other two do not. Thus, programmes need to decide the level of detail in procedure-specific skills they intend to assess in order to select the appropriate tool. Although PBA does permit assessment of technical skills in general, aspects such as situation awareness, decision-making, team-work and leadership may not be adequately addressed (Beard et al. 2009). These, and other aspects of professional practice, may extend beyond the boundary-specific competencies. Thus a broader framework is required to assess the suitability of a trainee to become a professional. These considerations are addressed by Entrustable Professional Activities.

## Entrustable Professional Activities

Considering the culmination of surgical training as the certification of an independent surgeon, the role of the surgical trainers is to sufficiently develop the trainee to trust them with surgical management. The assessment methods described above aim to assess capability of the trainee to perform a technical procedure, but whether "passing" in these assessments means that the trainee can be trusted to independently practise the procedure is a different decision altogether. To aid such a decision, Entrustable Professional Activities (EPAs) were developed, described as

> … units of professional practice, defined as tasks or responsibilities that trainees are entrusted to perform unsupervised once they have attained sufficient specific competence. EPAs are independently executable, observable, and measurable in their process and outcome, and, therefore, suitable for entrustment decisions. (ten Cate 2014)

Notably the assessment tools described in the above sections are to a large extent objective, but the entrustment decision has a greater subjective element to it. The trainers responsible for the entrustment decision are assumed to have personal experience of the trainee exhibiting these elements, and base their judgement partly on their experience(s). A decision to entrust someone carries with it a subjective overview of multiple trainee characteristics, i.e. agency, reliability, integrity, capability and humility (ten Cate and Chen 2020a). Notably, these trainee characteristics, known as "a rich entrustment decision" (2020a) may already exist within continuous assessments performed over time by multiple trainers; but do all trainers have the chance to observe and remember all their trainees' performances in all the listed domains? As these forms are generally filled completely, raising doubts about them being 100% accurate, tools specifically designed to aid entrustment decisions are welcome. Thus, EPAs have evolved as a tool since their introduction in 2005 (ten Cate 2005) to become the main assessment method employed for entrustment decisions.

EPAs can be a single task or a bundle of tasks, but they need to have specific attributes as shown in the following box.

Features of entrustable professional activities. Adapted from ten Cate 2020b

- Has a clearly defined beginning and end
- Independently executable to achieve a defined clinical outcome
- Is specific and focused
- Observable in process and measurable in outcome
- Clearly distinguished from other EPAs in the framework
- Reflects work that is essential and important to the profession
- Leads to recognized output or outcome of labour
- Is restricted to qualified personnel
- Requires application of knowledge, skills, and/or attitudes acquired through training
- Involves application and integration of multiple domains of competence
- Describes a task, not qualities or competencies of a learner and avoids adjectives (or adverbs) that refer to proficiency

They provide a holistic assessment covering the overall knowledge, skills, attitudes and experiences required in the performance of a professional activity. Specialties need to decide a list of EPAs considered as critical, according to yearly progression. When this list is successfully completed by the trainee, it forms the grounds for considering the trainee for an entrustment decision, i.e., transformation from a trainee to a professional. The EPA differs significantly from DOPS, OSATS and PBA, in that it not only covers specific competencies, but also potential risks in case of failure; it requires information sources for progress assessment; it specifies the entrustment level expected at each stage of training, and sets an "expiry date" for practice. EPAs thus describe work which operationally defines a profession (ten Cate and Taylor 2020b). Progress assessment for specific competencies may be done using the above-mentioned workplace-based assessment tools, and these tools can provide data which feed into the relevant EPAs.

A sample EPA form is reproduced in Table 11-6.

## Table 11-6: Proposed full description of an EPA for ophthalmology residents.

**AMEE Guide 140 Appendix:**
**Proposed full description of an EPA for ophthalmology residents**

| | |
|---|---|
| 1. EPA Title | **Managing patients with cataract** |
| 2. Specifications and Limitations | *This activity contains or may contain the following elements:*<br>*Non technical:*<br>• Medical history<br>• Full ophthalmological examination<br>• Interpretation of specific investigations (such as biometry in relation to the refractive error)<br>• Diagnosis and determining indication for cataract surgery<br>• Informing the patient about the procedure, contraindications and possible complications, intraocular lens options, to guide expectations and guarded prognosis<br>• Indication of local anesthesia or indication for general anesthesia<br><br>*Technical:*<br>• Preparation of surgery before and in the OR, instruction of OR staff<br>• Administration of local anesthesia<br>• Performing phaco emulsification and intra ocular lens implantation<br>• Timely diagnosis and management of per-operative complications.<br>• Diagnosis and management of post-operative complications. |
| | *A summative entrustment decision for this EPA does not apply for:*<br>• Patients with high risk because of patient-related or eye-related comorbidity conditions |
| 3. Potential risks in case of failure | • Pre-operative risks (medication use, pseudoexfoliation, mature cataract, trauma, small pupil, high refractive errors, previous ocular surgery, ocular pathology requiring treatment prior to surgery)<br>• Intra-operative complications (posterior capsular rupture, iris prolaps, zonular dehiscence, suprachoroidal haemorrhage)<br>• Post-operative complications (posterior capsular opacification, raised intraocular pressure, corneal decompensation, cystoid macular oedema, retinal detachment, endophthalmitis, refractive surprise)<br>• Anxiety, loss of confidence and psychological stress to patients<br>• Undue financial costs and societal impact |
| 4. Most Relevant Competency Domains | X Medical Expert   X Communicator   X Collaborator<br>O Scholar   X Professional   O Health advocate<br>O Leader |
| 5. Required Knowledge, Skills, Attitudes and Experience | **Knowledge:**<br>• All aspects of disorders of the lens<br>• Risks, complications and indications for cataract surgery<br>• Guideline for cataract surgery of the Dutch Ophthalmological Society<br>• The different intra ocular lenses, multifocal, toric lenses<br>• The methods of anesthesia and indications<br>• The detailed anatomy of the anterior segment<br>• The technical features of the instruments, phaco machine, fluidics etc |

| | |
|---|---|
| | **Non technical Skills:**<br>• Signs and symptoms of cataract<br>• Expectation management<br>• Adequate communication with the patient pre-, per- and post-operatively<br>• Adequate communication with OR staff<br><br>**Technical skills:**<br>• Technical steps of phaco emulsification and IOL implantation<br>• Adequate eye – hand coordination during surgery<br>• Handling of the microscope and phaco machine<br><br>**Non technical skills:**<br>Attitudes related to task-specific trustworthiness, in addition to task-specific capability:<br>• Integrity (truthful, good intentions, patient-centered)<br>• Reliability (conscientious, predictable, accountable, responsible)<br>• Humility (observing limits, willing to ask help, receptive to feedback)<br>• Agency (self-confident, proactive toward work, team, safety)<br><br>**Experiences**:<br>• Completion of the simulation training program and/or<br>• Wetlab training program<br>• At least 250 supervised cataract surgeries before unsupervised practice can be considered |
| 6. **Information sources to assess progress and support summative entrustment** | • Three satisfactory brief observations (cf MiniCEX) of patient consultation in the (outpatient) clinic<br>• Videorecording of 80% of procedures<br>• One hundred supervised satisfactory full OSATS in the operation suite (19)<br>• Satisfactory entrustment-based discussions [31] |
| 7. **When is which entrustment-supervision level expected?** | The resident is expected to reach Level 4 (ready for unsupervised practice):<br>• In PGY 4 at the general hospital*<br>• In PGY 5 at the academic hospital<br>* adjusted to the local program |
| 8. **Expiry date** | Two months of non-practice of cataract surgery will require indirect supervision (level 3) |

## Implementing workplace-based assessment in surgical residency programmes

Formal discussions among the residency programme faculty, residents and programme officers are recommended before deciding which workplace-based assessments are practical and should be implemented. Once the tools have been decided, training of all stakeholders is required which may be followed by a pilot phase where implementation issues may be identified and subsequently addressed.

The formative role of workplace-based assessments is beneficial if it occurs at an appropriate frequency. Doing too many assessments becomes impractical, and too few meaningless. In general, the appropriate frequency is about 40 forms altogether in a year, or 10 in a quarter, or once a week, for each trainee (JCST 2015ab). The total number of forms filled can be counted in the rotation or end-of-year evaluations while a minimum number can be set as the cut-off for progression. The scores may also be used in the evaluations as a proportion within the total score, though reliance on these scores separately for decisions about promotion would become summative, which may be incorrect as these tools were designed for formative assessment.

Much as the theoretical concepts behind workplace-based assessments and published evidence of their effectiveness appear convincing, their implementation in residency programmes continues to be challenging. Resistance to such implementation occurs at all levels, among the trainees, the trainers and the programme management, regardless of the "go ahead" by academic leadership. Buy-in by key stakeholders for such programmatic changes is not smooth sailing, thus changes in management strategies are generally required, such as the "Switch" model (Heath and Heath 2010). A recent study demonstrated successful implementation using the Switch model for an interdepartmental EPA between emergency medicine and surgery (Collins et al. 2020). This model identifies the separation of the rational and the emotional minds, and builds on converging the two towards common aims to get acceptance. Thus the "riders" who readily accept the change are to be directed, the "elephants" who resist are to be motivated, and the path to change is to be deliberately shaped.

For the implementation of a new workplace-based assessment at an institution, acceptance by the faculty members of its need is a fundamental requirement, and may be facilitated by discussions on advantages over existing assessments and recent trends. As for practicability, most of these assessments do not consume a significant amount of faculty time. For DOPS, the time to complete the form and give feedback is about 15 minutes (Khanghahi and Azar 2018). Training of faculty members is required to familiarize them with the forms and represents the process to be followed to ensure consistency in following the prescribed method.

Trainees, who are the direct beneficiaries of the workplace-based assessments, also pose a challenge in terms of engagement. A training session, like for the faculty, is essential to ensure that all residents understand the purpose of the new assessments and the process to be followed, as well as ensuring they become familiar with the forms. At the outset, a new assessment method appears to them as an additional burden on their already exhaustive programmatic requirements. Requesting their supervisors to observe them, seeking their feedback after procedures, keeping forms safely and submitting them to the programme office in time all appear burdensome. Acceptance may be facilitated by highlighting the benefits of structured feedback, and the potential enhancement of their surgical portfolio with data from these assessments.

The programme management may also feel challenged in completing requirements for these assessments. When residents are lagging behind in submitting forms in a timely manner, reminders need to be sent to them. This requires active tracking of submissions against set expectations according to specified time durations. Faculty may also be engaged to remind trainees rotating with them for the forms. Data from the forms need to be in a database from which periodic custom reports can be generated.

Online forms are the norm now in many institutions which have a learning management system. Although this makes the task simpler, there may be a tendency for the trainer to defer the filling of forms to the evening or the next day following surgery due to their busy surgical routine, in order to complete the online forms at one's convenience. Physical presence of the trainee for feedback may become an issue in that case. Thus, it is recommended that the forms be filled in immediately after the procedure, or before the end of work that day. Delay to the next day or afterwards could lead to recall bias potentially rendering the feedback unreliable, or omission of the assessment altogether. A culture of timely filling of forms and giving verbal feedback needs to be developed. Paper-based forms work well because once in the hand, one feels compelled to fill them appropriately before filing or storing them. There are, however, practical issues with paper-based forms about where to keep the stock of multiple blank forms of the different assessment methods while facilitating ready access, the availability of printing stations in all procedure areas if stocks of paper forms cannot be kept, and keeping filled forms securely until submission to the programme office.

One of the strategies to improve compliance is to make these forms a mandatory programmatic requirement, for both the trainees and the trainers. However, the repercussions of defaulting need to be clearly defined, communicated and followed, for which an institutional level directive may be required.

## Programme level outcomes

Workplace-based assessments generate a substantial amount of training related data. Completion of a required number of forms can be used as a milestone. Performance of trainees in specific procedures can be tracked over time, and progress in specific sections listed in the forms may separately be visualized (JAG 2017) (Figure 11-2). Moreover, training conditions, such as case load, can be correlated to assessment scores. Thus, Hiemstra et al. (2011) demonstrated higher scores on OSATS for residents exposed to a higher case load on a specific procedure (Figure 11-3).

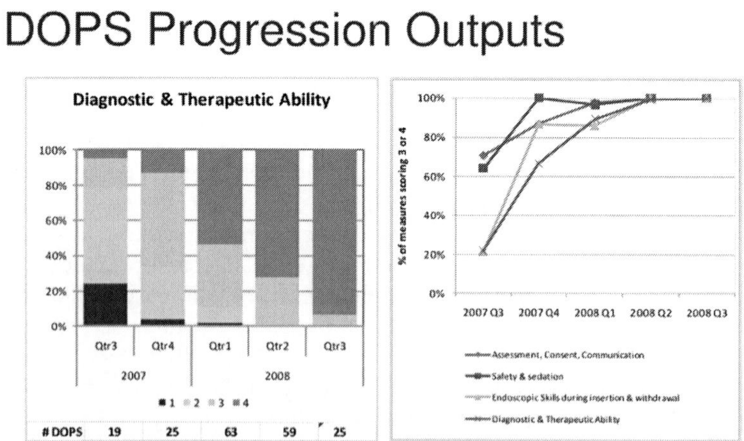


Figure 11-2: Trainee progression over time, as depicted by this JAG E-portfolio.

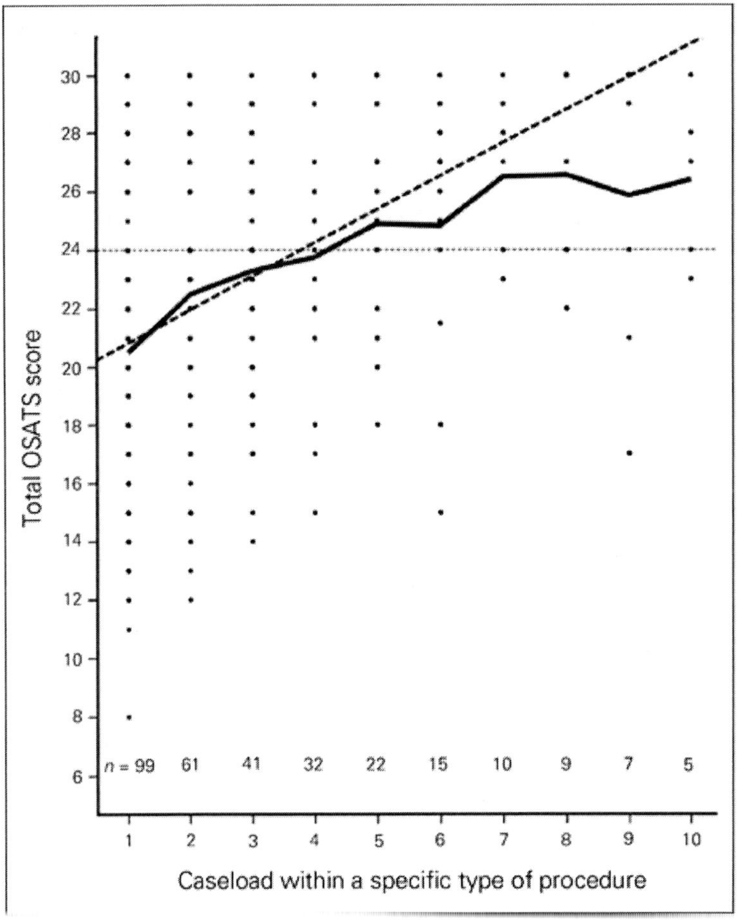


Figure 11-3: Average Objective Structured Assessment of Technical Skills (OSATS) scores plotted against a procedure-specific learning curve for the first 10 of a specific type of procedure.

Completion of entrustable activities may justify independent credentialing at appropriate stages of training. Not only can "strong" trainees be marked for promotion or graduation, but "weak" trainees can be flagged in order to develop a plan to improve their performance. Patterns of trainer bias in ratings can be statistically inferred. Post-graduation performance, if it's possible to obtain, can provide valuable information on the achievement of outcomes of the specific assessments, and the training programme in general.

## Summary

Workplace-based assessments have evolved to achieve a sufficient degree of validity, reliability and acceptability for the purpose of summative assessment. They have also proven to be effective in improving technical performance in procedures and surgery. Their use is recommended for objective assessments and improvement of skills. Collated scores and/or the completion record of workplace-based assessments is being used as a component of overall summative assessments, but their use for pass-or-fail decisions and exam purposes remains unsupported by the literature.

## Bibliography

Anderson, D. D., S. Long, G. W. Thomas, M. D. Putnam, J. E. Bechtold and M. D. Karam. "Objective Structured Assessments of Technical Skills (OSATS) Does Not Assess the Quality of the Surgical Result Effectively." *Clin. Orthop. Relat. Res*. 474, no. 4 (April 2016):874-81. DOI: 10.1007/s11999-015-4603-4.

Archer, J., J. Norcini, L. Southgate, S. Heard and H. Davies. "mini-PAT (Peer Assessment Tool): a valid component of a national assessment programme in the UK?" *Adv. Health Sci. Educ. Theory Pract*. 13, no. 2 (May 2008):181-92. DOI: 10.1007/s10459-006-9033-3.

Aryal, K. R., C. Currow, S. Downey, R. Praseedom and A. Seager. "Work-Based Assessments in Higher General Surgical Training Program: A Mixed Methods Study Exploring Trainers' and Trainees' Views and Experiences." *Surg. J. (N Y).* 9; 6, no. 1 (March 2020): e49-e61. DOI: 10.1055/s-0040-1708062.

Asif, H., C. McInnis, F. Dang, H. Ajzenberg, P. L. Wang, A. Mosa, G. Ko, B. Zevin, S. Mann and A. Winthrop. "Objective Structured Assessment of technical skill (OSATS) in the Surgical Skills and Technology Elective Program (SSTEP): Comparison of peer and expert raters." *Am. J. Surg.* S0002-9610, no. 21 (April 2021): 225-7. DOI: 10.1016/j.amjsurg.2021.03.064.

Barr, H., D. Freeth, M. Hammick, I. Koppel and S. Reeves. *Evaluations of interprofessional education; a United Kingdom review of health and social care*. London: CAIPE/BERA, 2000. Available from:

https://www.caipe.org/resources/publications/barr-h-freethd-hammick-m-koppel-i-reeves-s-2000-evaluations-of-interprofessional-education Accessed August 8, 2021.

Barrett, A., R. Galvin, Y. Steinert, A. Scherpbier, A. O'Shaughnessy, M. Horgan and T. Horsley. “A BEME (Best Evidence in Medical Education) review of the use of workplace-based assessment in identifying and remediating underperformance among postgraduate medical trainees: BEME Guide No. 43.” *Med Teach.* 38, no. 12 (September 2016):1188-1198. DOI: 10.1080/0142159X.2016.1215413.

Beard, J. D., J. Marriott, H. Purdie and J. Crossley. “Assessing the surgical skills of trainees in the operating theatre: a prospective observational study of the methodology.” *Health Technol Assess.* 15, no. 1 (January 2011):i-xxi, 1-162. DOI: 10.3310/hta15010.

Beard, J., D. Rowley, M. Bussey and D. Pitts. “Workplace-based assessment: assessing technical skill throughout the continuum of surgical training.” *ANZ J. Surg.* 79, no. 3 (March 2009):148-53. DOI: 10.1111/j.1445-2197.2008.04832.x.

Bernard, J. A., J. R. Dattilo, U. Srikumaran, B. A. Zikria, A. Jain and D. M. LaPorte. “Reliability and Validity of 3 Methods of Assessing Orthopedic Resident Skill in Shoulder Surgery.” *J. Surg. Educ.* 73, no. 6 (November-December 2016): 1020-1025. DOI: 10.1016/j.jsurg.2016.04.023.

Collins, E., C. Stahl, B. Schnapp, M. Westergaard, J. Greenberg, S. Jung, A. Rosser, R. Minter, A. Hamedani and A. Kraut. “Changing Medical Education When Change Is Hard: Implementing an Interdepartmental Entrustable Professional Activity.” *AEM Educ Train.* 5, no. 3 (December 2020): e10561. DOI: 10.1002/aet2.10561.

Duijn, C. C. M. A., E. J. van Dijk, M. Mandoki, H. G. J. Bok, and O. T. J. ten Cate. “Assessment Tools for Feedback and Entrustment Decisions in the Clinical Workplace: A Systematic Review.” *J. Vet. Med. Educ.* 46, no. 3 (Fall 2019): 340-352. DOI: 10.3138/jvme.0917-123r.

Hatala, R., D. A. Cook, R. Brydges, and R. Hawkins. “Constructing a validity argument for the Objective Structured Assessment of Technical Skills (OSATS): a systematic review of validity evidence.” *Adv. Health Sci. Educ. Theory Pract.* 20, no. 5 (December 2015):1149-75. DOI: 10.1007/s10459-015-9593-1.

Heath, C., and D. Heath. *Switch: How to change things when change is hard*. Waterville, Me: Thorndike Press, 2011.

Hiemstra, E., W. Kolkman, R. Wolterbeek, B. Trimbos and F. W. Jansen. “Value of an objective assessment tool in the operating room.” *Can. J. Surg.* 54, no. 2 (April 2011): 116-22. DOI: 10.1503/cjs.032909.

ISCP Management Group. “ISCP evaluation report; 2012.” Accessed August 8, 2021. URL: https://www.jcst.org/-/media/files/jcst/archive/full_evaluation_report.pdf.

JAG – Joint Advisory Group on Endoscopy. “JET User Guide for Trainees.” Accessed August 8, 2021. URL: https://www.thejag.org.uk/AboutUs/DownloadCentre.aspx?PageId=134.

Joint Commission on Surgical Training. “Direct Observation of Procedural Skills (DOPS): DOPS form.” Accessed August 8, 2021. URL: https://www.iscp.ac.uk/curriculum/surgical/assessment_dops.aspx.

Joint Commission on Surgical Training. “Procedure Based Assessment (PBA): PBA Guidance.” Accessed August 8, 2021. URL: https://www.iscp.ac.uk/curriculum/surgical/assessment_pba.aspx.

Kirkpatrick, D. L. “Techniques for evaluating training programs”. *J. ASTD.* 11 (1959): 1-13.

Khanghahi, M. Erfani, and F. Ebadi Fard Azar. “Direct observation of procedural skills (DOPS) evaluation method: Systematic review of evidence.” *Med. J. Islam. Repub. Iran.* 32 (June 2018):45. DOI: 10.14196/mjiri.32.45.

Lockyer, J., C. Carraccio, M-K Chan, D. Hart, S. Smee, C. Touchie, E. S. Holmboe, J. R. Frank and ICBME Collaborators. “Core principles of assessment in competency-based medical education.” *Medical Teacher* 39, no. 6 (June 2017): 609-616. DOI: 10.1080/0142159X.2017.1315082.

Massie, J., and J. M. Ali. “Workplace-based assessment: a review of user perceptions and strategies to address the identified shortcomings.” *Adv. Health Sci. Educ. Theory Pract.* 21, no. 2 (2016): 455-73. DOI: 10.1007/s10459-015-9614-0.

Mayne, A., L. Wilson and N. Kennedy. “The Usefulness of Procedure-Based Assessments in Postgraduate Surgical Training Within the Intercollegiate Surgical Curriculum Programme; A Scoping Review.” *J. Surg. Educ.* 77, no. 5 (May 2020): 1227-1235. DOI: 10.1016/j.jsurg.2020.03.005.

Miller, G. E. “The assessment of clinical skills/competence/performance.” *Acad. Med.* 65, Suppl 9 (September 1990): S63-7. DOI: 10.1097/00001888-199009000-00045.

Marriott, J., H. Purdie, J. Crossley and J. D. Beard. “Evaluation of procedure-based assessment for assessing trainees’ skills in the operating theatre.” *Br. J. Surg.* 98, no. 3 (March 2011): 450-457. DOI: 10.1002/bjs.7342.

Martin, J. A., G. Regehr, R. Reznick, H. MacRae, J. Murnaghan, C. Hutchison and M. Brown. "Objective structured assessment of technical skill (OSATS) for surgical residents." *Br. J. Surg.* 84, no. 2 (February 1997): 273-8. DOI: 10.1046/j.1365-2168.1997.02502.x.

Norcini, J. J., L. L. Blank, G. K. Arnold and H. R. Kimball. "The mini-CEX (clinical evaluation exercise): a preliminary investigation." *Ann Intern Med.* 123, no. 10 (November 1995): 795-9. DOI: 10.7326/0003-4819-123-10-199511150-00008.

Norcini, J., and V. Burch. "Workplace-based assessment as an educational tool: AMEE Guide No. 31." *Medical Teacher* 29, no. 9 (November 2007): 855-871, DOI: 10.1080/01421590701775453.

Okoro, T., C. Sirianni and D. Brigden. "The concept of surgical assessment: Part 2 – Available tools." *Ann. R. Coll. Surg. Engl. (Suppl)* 92, no. 9 (October 2010): 324–326. URL: https://publishing.rcseng.ac.uk/doi/pdf/10.1308/147363510X527682.

Pitts, D., D. I. Rowley, C. Marx, L. Sher, T. Banks and A. Murray. *A Competency Based Curriculum for Specialist Training in Trauma and Orthopaedics.* London: British Orthopaedic Association, 2006. URL: https://publishing.rcseng.ac.uk/doi/pdf/10.1308/147363510X527682.

Robertson, R. L., J. Park, L. Gillman and A. Vergis. "The impact of rater training on the psychometric properties of standardized surgical skill assessment tools." *Am. J. Surg.* 220, no. 3 (September 2020): 610-615. DOI: 10.1016/j.amjsurg.2020.01.019.

Shalhoub, J., A. T. Vesey and J. E. Fitzgerald. "What evidence is there for the use of workplace-based assessment in surgical training?" *J. Surg. Educ.* 71, no. 6 (November-December 2014): 906-15. DOI: 10.1016/j.jsurg.2014.03.013.

ten Cate, O. "Entrustability of professional activities and competency-based training." *Med. Educ.* 39, no. 12 (December 2005): 1176-7. DOI: 10.1111/j.1365-2929.2005.02341.x.

ten Cate, O. "Trusting graduates to enter residency: what does it take?" *J. Grad. Med. Educ.* 6, no. 1 (March 2014): 7-10. DOI: 10.4300/JGME-D-13-00436.1.

ten Cate, O., and H. C. Chen. "The ingredients of a rich entrustment decision." *Med Teach.* 42, no. 12 (December 2020a): 1413-1420. DOI: 10.1080/0142159X.2020.1817348.

ten Cate, O., and D. R. Taylor. "The recommended description of an entrustable professional activity: AMEE Guide No. 140." *Med. Teach* (November 2020b): 1-9. DOI: 10.1080/0142159X.2020.1838465.

Training Standards Committee of the British Orthopaedic Association. "Training Specialist Training in Trauma and Orthopaedics Curriculum."

Accessed August 8, 2021. URL: https://www.gmc-uk.org/-/media/documents/T_and_O_inc._Trauma_TIG_approved_Jul_17.pdf_72511367.pdf.

Violato, C., J. Lockyer and H. Fidler. "Multisource feedback: a method of assessing surgical practice." *BMJ.* 326, no. 7388 (March 2003): 546-8. DOI: 10.1136/bmj.326.7388.546.

Wilson, C. A., S. Chahine, J. Davidson, S. Dave, A. Sener, A. Rasmussen, D. H. Saklofske and P. Z. T. Wang. "Working Towards Competence: A Novel Application of Borderline Regression to a Task-Specific Checklist for Technical Skills in Novices." *J. Surg. Educ.* S1931-7204, no. 21 (June 2021): 122-7. DOI: 10.1016/j.jsurg.2021.05.004.

Wragg, A., W. Wade, G. Fuller, G. Cowan and P. Mills. "Assessing the performance of specialist registrars." *Clin. Med. (Lond).* 3, no. 2 (March 2003): 131-4. DOI: 10.7861/clinmedicine.3-2-131.

# CHAPTER 12

# INCORPORATING RESEARCH DURING SURGICAL RESIDENCY TRAINING

MUHAMMAD HAMMAD ATHER

## Introduction

The primary ambition of residency training in surgery is to be able to train surgeons in the diagnosis and management of surgical conditions, to teach the ability to "cut and sew," and manage post-surgical complications. Attainment of basic research skills, ability to share experience and ability to disseminate knowledge are considered imperative in the training of surgeons. The traditional surgery training models impose significant limitations in the pursuit of these goals and performing quality research during residency, creating a significant impediment in the formative years of a surgeon. Various modifications have been proposed in the residency training programmes to overcome this limitation. In a recent descriptive report Morbitzer et al. (2019) described the use of a flipped residency research model. In this model the authors attempted to better align research activities with residents' abilities at specific intervals during the year. They noted a discernable improvement in the quality and number of research projects. The introduction of a formal research track programme and core clinical rotations in research units are some of the other innovative ways of facilitating resident led research (Arbuckle et al. 2013). One of the fundamental grounding aspects of this endeavour is the provision of core training in research literacy and research opportunities for the residents, stimulating their interest during the formative years of residency training, so they are trained in research during their years in residency.

The governing bodies monitoring training require all accredited resident training programmes to incorporate active involvement in scholarly activities as training in academic units and university programmes adds a rather definite balance of practice and knowledge in further research and training.

Academic research not only ensures a sound résumé for future appointments but also helps in developing a thinking surgeon. It introduces the concept and improves residents' ability to comprehend the meaning of evidence-based medicine. It also allows residents to develop analytical and critical thinking, fostering reflection, introspection and the capacity for creativity. In order to develop "thinking surgeons" residency programmes around the world facilitate a research culture in their surgical departments. Dedicating time for research, conducting courses in research methodology, facilitating and ensuring availability of ancillary research staff including bio statisticians, epidemiologists etc., are some of the ways to promote a research culture.

The role of research during medical school lays the foundation of the research path in future life. In highly competitive residency programmes, the acceptance of international medical graduates can be improved with an extensive and astute background in research. In a survey conducted to study the impact of dedicated research in acquiring a categorical or preliminary residency position in the USA (in this instance, a general surgery residency) Jajja et al. (2019) noted a higher success rate for graduates from Aga Khan University, Karachi with a significant research background.

Various governing bodies overseeing residency training like graduate medical institutions in the States provide their residents opportunities of $\geq$1 year of dedicated research during a residency. In Pakistan the College of Physicians and Surgeons (CPSP) requires trainees to write a dissertation or two original papers in a peer reviewed indexed journal in order to sit the exit examination. In various survey conducted to assess programme-specific proportions of general surgery residents who had participated in $\geq$1 year of dedicated research ranged from 72–99% (Robertson, Klingensmith and Coopersmith 2007; Thakur et al. 2000). A recent study by Andriole et al. (2020) indicated that trainees who have participated in $\geq$1 year of dedicated research during their residency are now more likely due to academic faculty and federal research grants.

The skills to access and critically appraise synthesized evidence are essential. Teaching critical appraisal skills of published evidence is a mandatory component of surgical residency curricula and is well established in the first world; however, clinicians in the developing world are still in the process of training the new generation of surgeons, well equipped with concepts of evidence-based practice.

The current chapter analyses the concurrent evidence to support dedicated research during residency training, evaluating its impact, need, barrier and scope.

## Acknowledgments

M. Hasan Ather for providing a meticulous proof read of the chapter.

## Evidence-based medical practice

Sackett et al. over quarter of a century ago defined evidence-based medicine (EBM) as the "conscientious, explicit and judicious use of current best evidence in making decisions about the care of individual patients" (Sackett et al. 1996). Evidence-based decision-making in the management of surgical patients involves the integration of expertise and availability of resources in light of contemporary literature. The EBM loop involves defining the question, a systematic review and evaluation of the evidence, application of the evidence to the individual patient, and then auditing the results to close the loop.

Day to day decision making in the management of surgical patients historically tends to be empirical and based on a combination of anecdotal evidence, personal preference and local practices. Surgery has seen rapid change over the past three decades. Minimally invasive surgery (MIS) is fast replacing open surgery. Though MIS has its own set of issues, critical appraisal of any new intervention is necessary before it replaces other established and time-tested modalities (Ather et al. 2020). Therefore it is more important than in the past to use current best evidence to evaluate innovative management strategies. It is generally accepted that the half-life of any medical practice is no more than 5 years (Emanuel 1975). Wisdom that comes with age is important, but no more important than clinical judgment, common sense and a critical evaluation of new information, which essentially implies that contemporary knowledge is one part of clinical practice and cultivation of clinical judgment by self-evaluation and review of our everyday practice (Macgregor 1975) and a basic level of competence are the others.

In the past two decades EBM has gained popularity in clinical decision-making. Guidelines and clinical recommendations with a level of evidence are the cornerstones of modern clinical practice. This change in practice has improved safety and decreased morbidity (Kehlet and Wilmore 2008). In a review several authors stressed the incorporation of data from multinational, multicentre cohort studies, randomized studies, and meta-analyses; they noted how the concept of the "fast-track methodology" has positively impacted patient recovery, leading to shorter in-patient stay, and a consequent reduction in medical morbidity (although "surgery-specific" morbidity remained unchanged) (Andriole et al. 2020). In order for the surgeons to practise EBM, training in the critical appraisal of evidence is absolutely necessary. It is imperative that young surgeons are taught these skills in the earlier years of their training. There is considerable variation when specifically training the residents in critically analysing evidence. The tools for training these skills are also not well defined. Generally, the journal club is considered as the most effective way of teaching EBM. Ahmadi and colleagues (2012) conducted a systematic review to assess methods of teaching the EBM process. They noted that journal clubs seem to be the preferred method of teaching critical appraisal skills, however the authors attempt to determine the most effective format and components of a journal club in teaching critical appraisal skills to surgical residents was inconclusive. Studies have indicated that short courses in EBM are effective to enhance the knowledge of postgraduates (Fritsche et al. 2002). Ubbink et al. (2016) assessed the impact of two-day, evidence-based surgery courses and noted an improved EBM aptitude of surgical residents. They also noted significant improvement in the understanding and concepts of residents following the course.

Research is the cornerstone for innovations needed to improve quality of care. However, translation of new evidence into practice is less self-evident than expected. Many barriers have been identified in the implementation of EBM in surgery. These include time constraints and resource limitations, a lack of required skills, and a culture that continues to rely on an apprenticeship style of teaching. There are also obstacles including ethical and technical barriers in conducting randomized controlled trials (RCTs) in surgery. Surgeons are also resistant to change certain long-existing surgical practices (Meakins 2006). Changing a physician's existing ideas and habits can make implementation in behaviour subsequently difficult as well (Grol and Grimshaw 2003). Effective care of the surgical patient is a team effort. Surgical outcomes are heavily dependent on the pre-operative ward and special care management; nurses provide round the clock care to these patients. It is therefore important that the entire team involved in patient care is cognizant of the principles of EBM to be able to execute the methodology in a genuine manner.

Besides the general barriers such as time, culture issues and the surgeon's inherent approach, which is often based on anecdotal evidence, there are specific bridges that the residents may falter in trying to gap. One of the fundamental issues is time constraints, both for busy clinicians and for residents. Online teaching is an alternate way of bypassing this issue. RCTs have addressed the effectiveness of online teaching of EBM or online journal clubs versus in-person formats. Kulier and colleagues (2009) reported no significant difference in mean scores between the 2 groups who attended lectures given by tutors or completed the modules online over a 4 to 6 week period. Often clinical supervisors are not the ideal role models to emblematically follow in EBM clinical practice. This is particularly important in resource restrained set ups, like low-and middle-income countries (LMICs). The quality of data and information available is often far from the reality of actual clinical practice. This is restricted by funding, easy access to modern technology, cultural barriers in its application and the inured apathetic attitude of supervisors. The vast majority of surgical literature consists of cohort studies, with very few RCTs, which is quite low on the rung of the evidence ladder. In addition, high quality evidence coming from RCTs is farther from reality. The vast majority of grant-funded, high end research is reported from the western world, which lacks relevance in the rest of the world with significant logistic and financial constraints having very little ecological validity or reliability in the results of "time-tested procedures."

In order for surgeons to practise EBM, it has been suggested that critical appraisal skills be introduced to residents early in their training (Kitto et al. 2011). One of the best ways of teaching the critical appraisal of literature is the journal club. Regular journal clubs enhance resident skills in developing a critical mind. Supervisors and trainers should also share peer reviews of unpublished work to help the residents to develop skills in analysing literature with a scientific mind.

## Research during medical school

Contemporary research is competitive and requires a mastery of skills not only in the subject area and research methodology but also in basic statistics. Most clinical researchers find it difficult to grasp these skills. It is important that a basic understanding is developed early in their career. Most high school curricula are now formulated to teach these skills however they do so in a manner that can be described as most unintelligent. It is imperative that the earlier these skills are mastered the better, as a grounded understanding of basic methodologies at a younger age with a fresher perspective allows for a much smoother progression through medical school. Medical schools are also teaching basics in clinical and community research. These skills are honed and put to use during residency training. Medical schools and residency training programmes now support and expect completion of at least a few scholarly projects as part of postgraduate training. This has since seen an increase in the number of scientific publications during residency (Chen et al. 2015). There are multiple reports also showing that publications during residency and medical school are associated with better academic records in professional life (Dorsey et al. 2006; Rezek McDonald and Kallmes 2012; Yang et al. 2011). Evidence also suggests that student researchers are more likely to get onto competitive residency programmes and subsequently begin an academic career with prior experience and training (Gupta, Norris and Writer 2016). A report published by Kohlert et al. (2017) showed that in comparison to residents who did not publish prior to residency, otolaryngology residents who published at least once prior to residency were nearly six times as likely to publish in postgraduate training. The authors however noticed that there was a lack of evidence linking publication history with the success clinicians garner. In any case, lack of prior research experience is indicative of an early mentorship and formal training in research skills during residency training.

## Research during residency

The priority of actively incorporating research in the training curriculum of a residency varies between university and non-university programmes. The significance of clinician led research cannot be overemphasized. With their unique clinical perspective and scientific inquisitiveness, they are more likely to do translation research and develop innovative management strategies leading to improved healthcare outcomes. Clinician-scientist's research contributions are more likely to have early tangible outcomes and are therefore critical. However, there has been a significant and consistent decline in the amount of physician led research (Brown et al. 2018; Ley and Rosenberg 2005). In 2014, the Physician-Scientist Workforce Working Group of the National Institutes of Health (NIH) reported a gloomy prospect with only 1.5% of physicians who considered research to be their primary focus. Despite extensive advancements, translating science into clinical practice remains a perpetual and generational challenge. Proctor and colleagues (2009) noted a daunting, near two-decade gap between development of new knowledge and established standards for patient care. There are multitudes of reasons for this gap; however it is evident that highly trained clinicians and scientists are needed to bridge between the bench and the bedside.

Not all training programmes consider furthering the goal of teaching and the spread of knowledge by both commitment to research and teaching. Understandably not all surgical candidates are either inclined or suited to take up the academic surgery position. It is the responsibility of the training programme supervisors to identify and train the right person to take up academic surgery. In university or academic training programmes one of the major selection criteria for surgical trainees should be commitment to research and teaching. Trainees should be able to demonstrate objective evidence to research. The American Board of Orthopaedic Surgery mandates that their residents must complete a 5-year postdoctoral training programme accredited by the Accreditation Council for Graduate Medical Education (Hurwitz ed. 2012). The objective is to provide exposure to the evaluative sciences, clinical and/or laboratory research and promote the ability to synthesize research data.

## Dedicated research time

One of the biggest obstacles faced in research initiatives during residency is limited time. Surgical trainees are too busy to pursue research-training goals while meeting clinical training requirements. Andriole and colleagues (2020) studied the relationship between ≥1 year of dedicated research during general surgery residency and surgeons' career paths. They noted that general surgery graduates' medical education-research participation was independently associated with faculty appointment. This is a significant observation and serves as a benchmark and standard for residency programmes aiming to prepare trainees for life as academic surgeons. Not all trainees have either a proclivity or the required ethic to follow an academic path as a future career. It is important to identify candidates who have the potential, inclination and will to pursue academic surgery. Academic surgical training programmes are set to train future academicians, surgeon researchers and teachers. Beninato et al. (2016) studied Rank lists from an academic surgical residency programme from 1992 to 1997. They reviewed all ranked candidates' career paths following residency training to determine whether they stayed in academia, were university affiliated, or were now in private practice. The authors noted that graduates of a surgical residency ranked high at the time of the residency match were more likely to pursue an academic career.

Macknin et al. (2014) addressed some important questions concerning the course of trainees with research interests during their formative years. This included whether trainee surgeons who had an indexed publication during residency were more likely to publish during the rest of their career, or whether surgical trainees who had opted for a dedicated year in research were more likely to publish during their residency and have an academic-affiliated practice after graduation. They noted that 3/4 of trainees who published peer-reviewed research during their residency continued with peer-reviewed publications in their careers, compared to just over half of residents who did not publish during their residency ($p = 0.02$) (Proctor et al. 2009).

## Concluding remarks

Academic research is an integral part of residency training. Residents actively involved in research during their residency are more comfortable with the principles and practice of EBM. Research involvement helps in the development of critical thinking and enhances analytical skills while providing time for reflection and creativity. Residents who have regularly published in the formative years of their training have higher chances of success as postgraduates and in developing a career in academic surgery.

Claude Bernard (1865), a French physiologist credited with many landmark achievements, coined the concept of "blind experiments" (Daston 2005) bringing objectivity and transparency to scientific research and introducing the concept of the "*milieu intérieur*," later refined to the concept of homeostasis.

In his indelible words,

> In a word, I consider hospitals only as the entrance to scientific medicine; they are the first field of observation which a physician enters; but the true sanctuary of medical science is a laboratory; only there can he seek explanations of life in the normal and pathological states by means of experimental analysis (Bernard, 1957).

## Bibliography

Ahmadi, N., M. E. McKenzie, A. Maclean, C. J. Brown, T. Mastracci and R. S. McLeod. "Teaching evidence based medicine to surgery residents-is journal club the best format? A systematic review of the literature." *J. Surg. Educ.* 69, no. 1 (January-February 2012): 91-100. DOI: 10.1016/j.jsurg.2011.07.004.

Andriole, D. A., M. E. Klingensmith, R. C. Fields and D. B. Jeffe. "Is dedicated research time during surgery residency associated with surgeons' future career paths? A national study." *Ann. Surg.* 271, no. 3 (March 2020): 590-597. DOI: 10.1097/SLA.0000000000003015.

Arbuckle, Melissa R., Joshua A. Gordon, Harold A. Pincus and Maria A. Oquendo. "Bridging the Gap: Supporting Translational Research Careers Through an Integrated Research Track Within Residency Training." *Acad. Med.* 88, no. 6 (June 2013): 759-65. DOI: 10.1097/ACM.0b013e31828ffacb.

Ather, M. H., T. Ahmad, S. Akhtar, T. Chawla, A. Darbar, W. Rafaqat, S. Shahabuddin, N. Shahzad and S. Sami. "Latrogenic trauma following percutaneous and minimally invasive surgical interventions." *J. Pak. Med. Assoc.* 70, Suppl 1 (2) (February 2020): S83-S88. URL: https://www.jpma.org.pk/supplement-article-details/460.

Beninato, T., D. A. Kleiman, R. Zarnegar and T. J. Fahey III. "Can Future Academic Surgeons be Identified in the Residency Ranking Process?" *J. Surg. Educ.* 73, no. 5 (September-October 2016): 788-92. DOI: 10.1016/j.jsurg.2016.03.013.

Bernard, Claude. *An Introduction to the Study of Experimental Medicine.* New York: Dover Publications, 1957.

Brown, Abigail M., Teresa M. Chipps, Tebeb Gebretsadik, Lorraine B. Ware, Jessica Y. Islam, Luke R. Finck, Joey Barnett and Tina V. Hartert. "Training the next generation of physician researchers – Vanderbilt Medical Scholars Program." *BMC Med Educ.* 18, no. 1 (January 2018): 5. DOI: 10.1186/s12909-017-1103-0.

Chen, Jenny X., Elliott D. Kozin, Rosh K. V. Sethi, Aaron K. Remenschneider, Kevin S. Emerick and Stacey T. Gray. "Increased Resident Research over an 18-Year Period: A Single Institution's Experience." *Otolaryngol Head Neck Surg.* 153, no. 3 (September 2015): 350–6. DOI: 10.1177/0194599815587908.

Daston, Lorraine. "Scientific Error and the Ethos of Belief." *Social Research* 72, no. 1 (Spring 2005): 18. URL: www.jstor.org/stable/40972000.

Dorsey, E. R., B. A. Raphael, L. J. Balcer and S. L. Galetta. "Predictors of future publication record and academic rank in a cohort of neurology residents." *Neurology* 67, no. 8 (October 2006): 1335-7. DOI: 10.1212/01.wnl.0000240058.26740.22.

Emanuel, E. "A half-life of 5 years." *Can. Med. Assoc. J.* 112, no. 5 (March 1975): 572. URL: https://www.ncbi.nlm.nih.gov/pmc/articles/PMC1956300/.

Fritsche, L., T. Greenhalgh, Y. Falck-Ytter, H. H. Neumayer and R. Kunz. "Do short courses in evidence-based medicine improve knowledge and skills? Validation of Berlin questionnaire and before and after study of courses in evidence based medicine." *Br. Med. J.* 325, no. 7376 (December 2002): 1338–134. DOI: 10.1136/bmj.325.7376.1338.

Grol, R., and J. Grimshaw. "From best evidence to best practice: Effective implementation of change in patients' care." *Lancet* 362, no. 9391 (October 2003): 1225–1230. DOI: 10.1016/S0140-6736(03)14546-1.

Gupta, R., M. L. Norris and H. Writer. "Preresidency publication record and its association with publishing during paediatric residency." *Perspect. Med. Educ.* 6, no. 6 (December 2017): 388-395. DOI: 10.1007/s40037-017-0383-8.

Herkowitz, H. N. "American Board of Orthopedic Surgery (ABOS) Part II oral examination." *Spine (Phila Pa 1976)* 31, no. 20 (September 2006): 2277. DOI: 10.1097/01.brs.0000236130.74517.ad.

Jajja, Mohammad Raheel, Marvi Tariq, Salila Shoaib Hashmi, Thomas F. Dodson and Rashida Ahmed. "Value of Dedicated Research Time for IMGs in Obtaining Surgical Residency Training Positions: A 10-Year Review of Applicants from a Medical College in Pakistan." *J. Surg. Educ.* 76, no. 1 (January-February 2019): 43-49. DOI: 10.1016/j.jsurg.2018.06.003.

Kehlet, H., and D. W. Wilmore. "Evidence-based surgical care and the evolution of fast-track surgery." *Ann. Surg.* 248, no. 2 (August 2008): 189-98. DOI: 10.1097/SLA.0b013e31817f2c1a.

Kitto, S., A. Petrovic, R. L. Gruen and J. A. Smith. "Evidence-based medicine training and implementation in surgery: the role of surgical cultures." *J. Eval. Clin. Pract.* 17, no. 4 (August 2011): 819-826. DOI: 10.1111/j.1365-2753.2010.01526.x.

Kohlert, S., L. Zuccaro, L. McLean and K. Mcdonald. "Does medical school research productivity predict a resident's research productivity during residency?" *J. Otolaryngol. Head and Neck Surgery* 46, no. 1 (April 2017): 34. DOI: 10.1186/s40463-017-0202-6.

Kulier, Regina, Sjors F. P. J. Coppus, Javier Zamora, Julie Hadley, Sadia Malick, Kausik Das, Susanne Weinbrenner, et al. "The effectiveness of

a clinically integrated e-learning course in evidence-based medicine: A cluster randomised controlled trial." *BMC Med. Educ.* 9 (May 2009): 21. DOI: 10.1186/1472-6920-9-21/.
Ley, T. J., and L. E. Rosenberg. "The physician scientist career pipeline in 2005: build it, and they will come." *JAMA* 294, no. 11 (September 2005): 1343–1351. DOI: 10.1001/jama.294.11.1343.
Macgregor, A. J. "Letter: Half-life of medical knowledge." *Can. Med. Assoc. J.* 112, no. 10 (May 1975): 1165-6. URL: https://www.ncbi.nlm.nih.gov/pmc/articles/PMC1959111/.
Macknin, J. B., A. Brown and R. E. Marcus. "Does research participation make a difference in residency training?" *Clin. Orthop. Relat. Res.* 472, no. 1 (January 2014): 370-6. DOI: 10.1007/s11999-013-3233-y.
Meakins, J. L. "Evidence-based surgery." *Surg. Clin. North. Am.* 86, no. 1 (February 2006): 1-16. DOI: 10.1016/j.suc.2005.10.004.
Morbitzer, Kathryn A., Kamakshi V. Rao, Denise H. Rhoney, Ashley L. Pappas, Emily A. Durr, Said M. Sultan, Stephen F. Eckel, Scott W. Savage, B. Rowell Daniels and Nicole R. Pinelli. "Implementation of the flipped residency research model to enhance residency research training." *Am. J. Health-Syst. Pharm.* 76, no. 9 (April 2019): 608-612. DOI: 10.1093/ajhp/zxz064.
National Institutes of Health. "Physician scientist workforce working group report." Accessed February 17, 2021. URL. https://acd.od.nih.gov/documents/reports/PSW_Report_ACD_06042014.pdf.
Proctor, E. K., J. Landsverk, G. Aarons, D. Chambers, C. Glisson and B. Mittman. "Implementation research in mental health services: An emerging science with conceptual, methodological, and training challenges." *Adm. Policy Ment. Health* 36, no. 1 (January 2009): 24–34. DOI: 10.1007/s10488-008-0197-4.
Rezek, I., R. J. McDonald and D. F. Kallmes. "Pre-residency publication rate strongly predicts future academic radiology potential." *Acad. Radiol.* 19, no. 5 (May 2012): 632-4. DOI: 10.1016/j.acra.2011.11.017.
Robertson, C. M., M. E. Klingensmith and C. M. Coopersmith. "Long-term outcomes of performing a postdoctoral research fellowship during general surgery residency." *Annals of Surgery* 245, no. 4 (April 2007): 516-523. DOI: 10.1097/01.sla.0000245468.98852.42.
Sackett, D. L., W. M. Rosenberg, J. A. Gray, R. B. Haynes and W. S. Richardson. "Evidence based medicine: What it is and what it isn't." *Clin. Orthop. Relat. Res.* 455 (February 2007): 3-5.

Thakur, A., V. Thakur, E. W. Fonkalsrud, S. Singh and T. L. Buchmiller. "The outcome of research training during surgical residency." *J. Surg. Res*. 90, no. 1 (May 2000): 10-12. DOI: 10.1006/jsre.2000.5817.

Ubbink, D. T., D. A. Legemate and M. J. Koelemay. "The Merits of a Two-Day Evidence-Based Medicine Course for Surgical Residents." *World J. Surg.* 40, no. 8 (August 2016): 1809-14. DOI: 10.1007/s00268-016-3495-0.

Yang, Glen, Uwais B. Zaid, Bradley A. Erickson, Sarah D. Blaschko, Peter R. Carroll and Benjamin N. Breyer. "Urology resident publication output and future academic achievement." *J. Urol.* 185, no. 2 (February 2011): 642-6. DOI: 10.1016/j.juro.2010.09.097.

# CHAPTER 13

# CLINICAL DIAGNOSTIC REASONING ABILITY: WHY IT IS ESSENTIAL AND HOW IT CAN BE CULTIVATED

MUSHTAQ AHMED

## Introduction

Clinical Diagnostic Reasoning (CDR) is a learned cognitive ability that physicians can put to use to improve diagnostic accuracy and patient safety (Croskerry 2009; Rajkomar and Dhaliwal 2011). Yet, in clinical practice the reasoning required to arrive at an actionable diagnosis is frequently bypassed in favour of investigations; test results are accepted without questioning. More recently CDR has come under threat from another source: the perception that Artificial Intelligence (AI) will displace the clinician as diagnostician. Under the circumstances it is prudent that we first re-establish the case for CDR as an essential skill for physicians, before going on to explain how it works and how it may be taught.

## Acknowledgement

I would like to thank Dr Inam Pal for reviewing the chapter, along with Dr Sheeraz Siddiqui, Dr Abdaal Wasim Khan, Dr Athar Ali and Dr Adrian Njau for providing access to cases.

## Re-establishing the case for clinical diagnostic reasoning as an essential skill

In order to confirm the lasting importance of CDR as a skill for physicians, it is necessary to draw attention to the undermining effect of excessive dependence on investigations. In the same vein, we should review the truth about AI's diagnostic potential.

**The problem with inappropriate dependence on investigations**

In the majority of clinical situations it is possible to use CDR to arrive at a likely diagnosis; unfamiliar and highly complex presentations may be exceptions. Therefore asking for an investigation before reaching a plausible clinical diagnosis is inappropriate as it could lead to a false investigation or incorrect interpretation of a test result; these consequences would amount to cognitive failure which is a well-known cause of diagnostic error associated with morbidity and mortality (Graber, Gordan and Franklin 2002). Additionally, excessive testing leads to incidental findings, like incidentalomas, that can draw attention away from the main problem and result in overtreatment with its potential harmful effects and increased cost of healthcare (Brodersen et al. 2018).

This is not all. Undue dependence on investigations sets a bad example for medical students and trainee doctors, who are led to believe that CDR is unimportant. In this way, the bad habit of inappropriate testing is perpetuated. There is yet another facet of the problem that arises in low resource settings, such as district hospitals in developing countries, where investigations are hard to come by or are of unacceptable quality; in this situation CDR is indispensable but is found wanting. As a result even common clinical problems are frequently misdiagnosed and mismanaged (Das et al. 2018).

One of the manifestations of undue dependence on investigations is "the demise of the physical exam;" physicians in training consider the physical exam "arcane" in comparison with modern investigative technology (Jauhar 2006). It is easy to see how this happens but equally it is important to consider why this notion should be dispelled (Case 1).

**Case 1: Discouraging the tendency to forgo the physical exam in favour of investigation**

A 33 year old man, a truck loader by occupation, developed left sided abdominal pain 5 months ago which has been increasing in severity. He has noticed a swelling in the left side of the abdomen and has lost weight; his clothes fit him loosely. He has no urinary symptoms. On examination he does not appear pale and seems to be in reasonable physical shape despite losing weight. On abdominal examination he has a visible left sided intra-abdominal swelling. The tendency at this point is to ask for an abdominal Computerized Tomography (CT) scan. However, the attending surgeon insists that the resident should first characterize the abdominal swelling on physical examination. This is a firm swelling that extends from the midline to the left flank and from the left iliac fossa to under the left costal margin; the upper border cannot be reached. The swelling is bimanually palpable and moves with respiration which raises the possibilities of a left kidney or adrenal mass. After a brief discussion, hypernephroma is considered the provisional diagnosis. The attending persuades the resident to look again for associated features like fever, haematuria, anaemia and left varicoele; none are present.

A double contrast abdominal CT scan shows a large vascular mass with a necrotic centre, displacing the pancreas, splenic vessels and the spleen. It is anterior to the left kidney with a clear plane in between, except in the mid portion of the kidney where it appears to merge with the renal parenchyma. The left adrenal is not separately identifiable. An angiogram further shows a vascular tumour with arterial supply mainly from the left renal artery and the aorta. A Tru-cut biopsy reveals a clear cell carcinoma.

Was it important in this case to insist on characterizing the mass on physical examination prior to a CT scan? A CT scan could have been requested straightaway based on the presence of an abdominal swelling; after all the CT did a better job at characterizing the mass and enabling transcutaneous biopsy which established the diagnosis. Perhaps, that is the wrong question; what is really worth reflecting on is the importance of having done a sensitive and thoughtful physical examination as a means of developing clinical diagnostic reasoning ability. In this case for instance, the association of hypernephroma with an intra-abdominal mass of a certain physical description in a given clinical context will have been registered in the resident's memory for future use in pattern recognition which, as we shall see, is the basis for generating intuitive hypotheses. Failure to have used the teaching opportunity would have been a failure to develop the physician as a diagnostician.

## The truth about AI's diagnostic potential

The increasing use of AI for diagnosis demands a review of its current status in relation to physicians' clinical diagnostic reasoning. Is AI about to displace the physician as master diagnostician? Let us try and answer this question systematically.

First, AI currently bears little resemblance to the general intelligence of humans or animals. In particular, humans have a unique capacity for "understanding," which is associated with a higher level of consciousness; it enables them to analyse the minds of others, gain conceptual insights into complex problems, differentiate cause from effect, reflect on their thoughts and actions and plan the future (Norvig 2020). By contrast "understanding" and consciousness remain a dream in the development of Strong AI. This fact alone ought to give physicians comfort that their role as diagnosticians equipped with "understanding" is not at stake.

Moreover, AI operates solely on the basis of pattern recognition; either a pattern which the machine has been primed with or a pattern that the machine has itself learned from processing large amounts of data (Wooldridge 2020). Pattern recognition which amounts to observational inference is at the lowest rung on the ladder of cause effect reasoning; interventional inference is higher and counterfactual inference highest (Pearl and Mackenzie 2019). In graphic terms, an owl uses observational inference to pounce on a rat that it has observed scurrying between point A and point B; a chimpanzee uses interventional inference to probe a termite mound with a stick for extracting supper. By contrast, the highest level of cause-effect reasoning raises counterfactual questions attributable exclusively to human imagination. When in the course of clinical problem solving a physician asks, "What if the underlying pathophysiology is X? Would it explain the clinical finding Y?" she is in effect raising a counterfactual question.

Now coming to practical considerations, AI's approach to diagnosis is very different from CDR. Expert physicians need relatively little clinical information in a given context to arrive intuitively at a hypothesis; at this stage they use deduction to acquire some more data with a view to accept or reject the hypothesis. Furthermore experts can apply this form of hypothetico-deductive reasoning to a wide array of clinical conditions. In contrast AI needs substantial data from the outset. In the case of image recognition, all the data related to the problem must be immediately available as in diagnosing intracranial haemorrhage from a CT scan of the head; a mathematically fine-tuned algorithm (known as a deep neural network) processes the data sequentially to arrive at a diagnostic solution. Besides, AI can only process specific information related to a specific diagnostic task; for every new task it must start all over again to fine tune the algorithm using substantial data from a new training set (Pelaccia, Forrestier and Wemmert 2019; Rajkomar, Dean and Kohane 2018).[1]

We may conclude given the differences in diagnostic approach that in the foreseeable future AI will excel only at certain targeted tasks, e.g., reading various kinds of medical images for diagnosis;[2] for the most part AI will complement CDR rather than displace it.

## How clinical diagnostic reasoning works and how it may be taught

As a necessary skill of lasting importance, CDR should be habitually practised and deliberately taught. Considerable work has been done on the science of CDR which is worth reviewing briefly to get a grasp of the underpinning concepts. Through case illustrations we shall then review how it works in actual clinical practice and see how elements of it can be taught by seizing the right moment.

### The science behind clinical diagnostic reasoning

Research in cognitive aspects of clinical diagnostic reasoning has pursued two avenues: how knowledge is organised in long term memory and the nature of the reasoning process (Monteiro and Norman 2013). Knowledge gained through practical experience and glued together by relevant theory following a clinical encounter as in Case 1, is stored in long term memory; how well it is organised is important because this greatly facilitates recognition of a similar presentation in the future. There are many ways knowledge may be organised, one of which, known as illness script (Bowen 2006), is described later.

---

[1] There are other differences: a physicians' diagnostic error is mostly due to premature closure on a diagnostic hypothesis, whereas with AI diagnostic errors arise mostly as a result of problems with data in the training set; for the most part physicians can explain how they came to a diagnosis, whereas, AI's processes remain a black box. Physicians' performances are affected by internal and external influences, whereas AI's performance is highly consistent for a given diagnostic task (Pelaccia, Forrestier and Wemmert 2019).

[2] Examples of diagnoses based on medical images that AI currently excels at are an intracranial haemorrhage based on a CT scan of head and metastatic disease based on a digitized pathology slide of a sentinel lymph node.

Regarding the reasoning process, sensory input from a history, physical examination and test results is capable of stimulating two pathways leading to a pathophysiological hypothesis (Croskerry 2009; Pelaccia et al. 2011). The first pathway results intuitively in recognition of a pattern previously experienced and leads quickly and effortlessly to a pathophysiological hypothesis; only part of the information available need be picked up to make an assessment of the overall situation, which makes it at once clever and dangerous because it could lead to error. This is system 1 that Kahneman alludes to in his popular book, *Thinking Fast and Slow* (Kahneman 2011). The second pathway is analytic and is brought into play when the case is unfamiliar or complex; it is slow and requires mental effort by means of which pre-existing biomedical concepts are used to arrive at a pathophysiological hypothesis. More commonly it is used for deductive reasoning when there is doubt about the intuitive hypothesis. This is Kahneman's system 2. Dual process theory explains the combined use of the two pathways or systems (Fig. 13.1) as when system 2 overrules system 1 to avoid diagnostic error from bias (Croskerry 2009; Pelaccia et al. 2011).

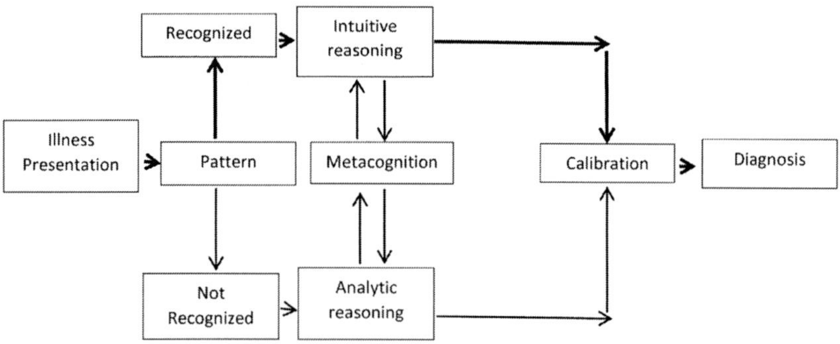


Figure 13.1: Dual processing involved in diagnostic reasoning: bold arrows indicate the intuitive pathway to the hypothesis more commonly used by experts in familiar cases; however, there is room for appeal to analytic reasoning upon sensing that "there is something wrong." The analytic pathway is the preferred route in unfamiliar and complex cases. Metacognition is being aware of one's thoughts; calibration means measuring against a standard, in this case the product of analytic reasoning (Modified from Croskerry 2009).

## Teachable elements of clinical diagnostic reasoning

From the standpoint of facilitating teaching-learning, it is more useful to divide clinical diagnostic reasoning into smaller elements: data acquisition or sensory input; abstract representation of the problem; hypothesis generation; deduction; and avoidance of bias. Rather than entering into a wordy explanation of these elements of CDR, we are going to examine four case illustrations to achieve clarity.

**Case 2: The importance of keen observation in data gathering**

A 34 year old woman underwent emergency abdominal surgery for acute abdominal pain 19 days ago in a district hospital that resulted in appendectomy. Four days later she has another procedure for omental patch repair of a perforated duodenal ulcer. She continues to be ill and is referred to a tertiary hospital purportedly for management of wound dehiscence and infection.

A year one resident who received the patient found her pulse to be 116 per minute, blood pressure 105/70 mm Hg, respiratory rate 30 per minute and temperature $38^0$ C. Her abdomen was distended but soft, with moderate tenderness in the right upper quadrant; a midline incisional wound was superficially dehisced but not grossly infected. On questioning the resident said, "she doesn't look that bad" and "her abdomen is soft." By contrast the expert immediately saw a woman in sepsis, potentially from a right sub-phrenic abscess due to a leak from delayed closure of a perforated duodenal ulcer which was missed in the first operation.

The resident was asked to observe the patient more closely, who was in fact anxious and not paying attention to her surroundings. He was asked to enquire about her gastrointestinal function: she confessed to have been vomiting following oral intake; he was asked to pay attention to her breathing: this was largely thoracic using her intercostal muscles; and he was asked to examine the right lung base, which showed poor air entry and dullness to percussion. There was clearly a difference in perception of the novice as compared with the expert. An oral contrast abdominal CT scan confirmed a large volume of fluid and air under the diaphragm on the right side and a duodenal leak of contrast.

In this case, the perception of the expert differed substantially from that of the year one resident; the difference was between "deep seeing" on the part of the expert as opposed to "superficial looking" by the resident. An effort should be made to facilitate the development of "deep seeing." It has been suggested by way of developing observation skills that students and junior trainees should be asked to pay attention to, observe carefully and describe what they see before interpreting information (Bleakley 2003).

The need to describe focuses attention; separation of observation from interpretation avoids bias. However, this advice is contrary to an expert's tacit use of prior knowledge and experience to detect subtle cues. Perhaps the implication is that we first need to carefully construct our mental knowledge structures through unbiased observation before we can use them to detect useful cues. The ability to discriminate based on visual and other cues in the judgment of illness falls in the realm of aesthetic sensibility (Bleakley 2003) which should receive attention during medical education beyond teaching history and physical examination skills in the conventional way.

**Case 3: The importance of abstract problem representation as a means of organising mental knowledge**

A 45 year old man from interior Sindh is known to have diabetes and is on oral hypoglycaemic medication. He also has liver cirrhosis and portal hypertension from Hepatitis C Virus (HCV) infection. After slipping on a wet surface and falling backwards four months ago he develops pain in the left groin spreading to the lower abdomen on the left side. Eventually he manifests a swelling in the left lower abdomen and fever for which he receives several courses of antibiotics. Initially after the fall he is able to walk with difficulty. However, two weeks prior to being seen in the clinic he could not even stand.

On examination he was found to be thin and pale and seemed to have lost weight. There was a tender large swelling extending from immediately above the left inguinal ligament to the level of the umbilicus; laterally it extended to the iliac crest, medially the border was ill defined. On a subsequent visit prior to admission he had developed a sinus from the swelling that was discharging frank pus. There were no bowel or bladder symptoms. An abstract representation of the problem was considered as follows:

> A middle aged man with multiple comorbidities, who following a relatively minor stretching injury in the left groin, gradually developed a large retroperitoneal pyogenic abscess in the left lower abdomen with loss of function in the left lower limb.

This enabled consideration of an acute inflammatory musculoskeletal problem as the pathophysiology with the following differential diagnoses: infected retroperitoneal haematoma, pyomyositis, spinal osteomyelitis and septic arthritis of the hip.

However, on further examination the spine appeared normal although its movements were slightly restricted. Rotational movements of the left hip joint were normal; pain was elicited on attempted flexion and hyperextension of the left hip. Review of a plain abdominal CT scan showed an abnormal left psoas muscle with fluid inside it communicating with a larger extra muscular “abscess” cavity. After a percutaneous drain was placed in the abscess cavity using ultrasound (US), he was much better and could stand and walk.

Thus pyomyositis involving the left psoas muscle was the definitive diagnosis. By this time a vivid narrative had emerged in the form of an illness script connecting predisposing conditions (context), pathophysiology and clinical consequences that was ready for storage in long term memory as well-organised knowledge. The script read as follows:

> Context: a middle aged man with multiple comorbidities sustains a relatively minor stretching injury in the left groin in the recent past;
>
> Pathophysiology: Pyomyositis of the left psoas muscle;
>
> Clinical consequences: fever and gradual development of a painful retroperitoneal swelling in the left lower abdomen that recently started discharging frank pus through a sinus; he has loss of weight bearing and mobility in the left lower limb.

If a similar case were to be encountered in the future, it is expected that recall of the illness script would greatly facilitate diagnosis (Bowen 2006).

### Cases 4 and 5: The intuitive pathway to a hypothesis and the folly of not checking for bias

### Case 4

An 81 year old man presents with insidious onset of diarrhoea, vomiting and right iliac fossa (RIF) pain over 12 days. On palpation there is a tender, 5 x 5 cm, ill-defined mass in the RIF; white blood cell (WBC) count is 22,000/ $mm^3$ and C Reactive Protein 312 mg/ L (0-5 mg/ L). The clinical diagnosis is an acute appendicular mass. A plain CT scan confirms a mass in the region of the appendix. Intravenous (IV) cephalosporin and metronidazole are started. Late that evening concerned relatives call the surgeon saying the patient is in “agony”. The surgeon concludes that conservative management is not going to work. A decision for exploratory laparotomy is taken at 3 a.m. The operative findings are an acutely inflamed, oedematous caecum with omental and ileal adhesions. The appendix is also inflamed; its base cannot be identified. There is no free fluid. A decision is taken to close the abdomen without doing an appendectomy and continue treatment with antibiotic and metronidazole.

On day eight postoperatively the patient develops bloody (maroon coloured) loose stools; he becomes hypotensive and his haemoglobin (Hb) drops to 8.0 g/ dl. He is transfused. By this time there are no abdominal signs; the mass has resolved. Flexible sigmoidoscopy is normal. The diagnosis of an acute appendicular mass is no longer tenable.

The patient continues to bleed and transfers to another hospital where he undergoes transcutaneous embolization of a bleeding vessel in the caecum; the revised diagnosis is amoebic caecitis/ typhlitis, belatedly confirmed on serology. The patient survives.

Had serious note been taken of the patient's age, insidious onset of illness with diarrhoea and endemicity of amoebiasis in the region, typhlitis due to *E. histolytica* might have been considered as a hypothesis leading to the obvious deduction that serology for Immunoglobulin M antibodies would be useful. This could have been a highly consequential example of hypothetico-deductive reasoning at work saving the patient unnecessary surgery and perhaps the complication of a lower intestinal bleed requiring transfusion and an additional intervention; not to mention prolonged hospitalisation and additional expense.

Instead, in this case, "similarity" to an acute appendicular mass was mistaken for the probability of its occurrence. At 81 years of age the base rate of acute appendicitis is low as compared to a younger person; there are other diagnoses to consider especially given the nature of the presentation. When perception of resemblance overrides consideration of probability, representativeness bias occurs (Kahneman 2011). Failure to keep intuitive reasoning (system 1) under check tends to occur when one is tired (the decision to operate was taken at 3 a.m.) or overwhelmed (the patient's family was expressing grave concern about his pain). To be fair an abdominal CT scan was done to corroborate the intuitive diagnosis. However, the scan simply showed a mass lesion in the region of the appendix which, lacking specificity, did little to change the preoperative diagnosis.

## Case 5

A 58 year old man, who is hypertensive, underwent a coronary artery bypass grafting two years ago. Presently on a beta blocker, antiplatelet aggregation medication, an antihypertensive and a statin, he is admitted for interval cholecystectomy 6 weeks after conservative management of acute cholecystitis. He is also HCV reactive and is classified as Child's A with respect to the functional state of his liver. Ultrasound shows a thick walled gall bladder with multiple stones; there is no comment about the common bile duct (CBD). A laparoscopic procedure is converted to an open procedure because of dense adhesions around the gall bladder. He is sent home on the fifth post-operative day after cholecystectomy. However, he is re-admitted on the tenth post-operative day with fever, pain and tenderness in the right upper quadrant of the abdomen. WBC is 26,000/ $mm^3$; liver function tests (LFTs) are mildly abnormal (Table 13.1). A plain abdominal CT scan shows a localised sub-hepatic collection, a right-sided pleural effusion and in retrospect a calcified opacity in the CBD region which was not reported. He is given IV antibiotic (Meropenem) and metronidazole; two days later (twelfth post-operative day) his sub-hepatic abscess is drained trans-cutaneously; pus grew E. coli (Escherichia Coli) sensitive to Meropenem.

**Table 13.1: Case 5 LFTs during the third admission**

| Serum levels | $11^{th}$ post-op day | $16^{th}$ post-op day | $21^{st}$ post-op day | $23^{rd}$ post-op day |
|---|---|---|---|---|
| Total bilirubin in mg/dl | 29 (0-17) | 15 | 10 | 13 |
| Direct in mg/dl | 28 (0-3.4) | 12 | 1 | 12 |
| Indirect in mg/dl | 1 | 3 | 9 | 1 |
| SGOT in Units/L | 28 (0 50) | 18 | 86 | 92 |
| SGPT in Units/L | 20 (0-45) | 12 | 39 | 59 |
| Alkaline phosphatase in Units/L | 190 (40-129) | 164 | 176 | 257 |

SGOT= Serum Glutamic–Oxaloacetic acid Transaminase
SGPT= Serum Glutamic–Pyruvic acid Transaminase

Fever and leukocytosis settle transiently, drainage stops and an ultrasound shows abscess resolution. However, five days later (seventeenth post-operative day) the patient's fever spikes again and he is short of breath. WBC count is 18,000/ $mm^3$; a chest x-ray reveals a sizeable right sided pleural effusion and a CT shows a small residual sub-hepatic fluid collection. The pleural effusion is drained under a water seal which results in full expansion of the lung. Antibiotics are changed to levofloxacin and amoxicillin – clavulanic acid. However, the patient continues to have fever and chills intermittently, right upper quadrant abdominal pain, and shortness of breath. He also has episodes of diarrhoea and develops ankle oedema. Repeat trans-cutaneous drainage of the sub-hepatic collection is done and he is discharged with the drain in situ on the twenty-seventh post-operative day after 24 hours of being afebrile. At follow up a week later he is found to be afebrile, although fluid continues to drain which is bile stained. A cystic duct stump leakage is suspected. Eventually the patient undergoes Endoscopic Retrograde Cholangio-Pancreatography (ERCP) at another hospital that shows multiple CBD stones which are retrieved via an endoscopic sphincterotomy leading to the patient's full recovery.

Had notice been taken of the abnormal liver tests especially the persistent mild increase in the level of serum alkaline phosphatase, and had the speck of calcification along the CBD on the CT scan been detected as a result of suspecting that the sub-hepatic abscess and the cystic duct leak were both ultimately due to partial obstruction of the common bile duct with stones, ERCP may have been considered earlier. This could have avoided recurrence of sub-hepatic abscess, a second transcutaneous drainage, pleural effusion, prolonged antibiotics and several days of hospitalisation with its attendant cost.

This case demonstrates "anchoring bias." The initial assessment was a sub-phrenic abscess following a difficult cholecystectomy; although the surgeon did consider a cystic duct leak when bile stained fluid was recovered from the drainage tube, he failed to go a step further to consider stones partially obstructing the CBD. This failure of adequate mental adjustment is due to "anchoring," a phenomenon whereby "different starting points yield different estimates, which are biased toward the initial values" (Kahneman 2011).

In summary, intuitive assessment of a clinical situation to arrive at a diagnostic hypothesis is an ability that experts usually use to their advantage; it facilitates elucidation of the relevant history and enables subtle observation. If a hypothesis is not immediately forthcoming, abstract problem representation could serve to jog the memory for past experience that bears resemblance to the situation at hand. Generally, one or more hypotheses may be considered at the outset but are narrowed down by deductive reasoning. Cause effect analysis based on conceptual knowledge of basic sciences enables deductive reasoning.[3] Likewise, probabilistic analysis can be used for deduction whereby a focused physical exam finding or a test result is used to upgrade an a priori probability of a hypothesis to an a posteriori probability based on knowledge of the accuracy of the exam or test (Doust 2009; Gill, Sabin and Schmid 2005).[4] Premature closure on a hypothesis is prone to error from bias as we have seen in cases 4 and 5. Of the different kinds of bias that exist, we have discussed two: representativeness and anchoring. It is necessary to be aware of the pitfall due to bias and the circumstances that lead to premature closure. A useful tactic to avoid error from bias is to regularly consider a differential diagnoses, albeit one that is stringent; each differential is ruled in or ruled out with proper justification.

The case illustrations have highlighted elements of clinical diagnostic reasoning that can be targeted for teaching-learning. Although we have used different cases to highlight different elements it is clearly also possible to highlight many elements in a single case. Next, we shall consider strategies that can be used to develop CDR ability.

## Teaching methods

As stated at the outset, CDR is a learned cognitive ability; therefore it can and must be taught (Pelaccia et al. 2011). The aim is to enable organisation of useful knowledge in long term memory based on experience and promote a balanced reasoning approach involving intuitive and analytic reasoning. As illustrated by the cases, the elements of diagnostic reasoning that require special attention are data acquisition and the power of observation; abstract representation of the problem and

---

[3] The acquisition of knowledge of basic sciences in a conceptual form rather than as factual information enables its application to clinical problem solving. Deep learning is required to develop concepts and practice is required to apply concepts at first to prototypical problems and later to atypical ones (Bowen 2006; Woods 2007).

[4] A broad understanding of Bayes theorem is important to figure out how a pre-test probability of a hypothesis is modified by the availability of a new test result provided we know the accuracy of the test (no test being perfect). If a pre-test probability of a condition (base rate) is very low then no matter that a highly sensitive test is positive it is more likely to be false positive (Doust 2009). The converse is also true; this is exemplified by the use of plain radiographs to diagnose a perforated abdominal viscus; if the clinical suspicion of free perforation is high then it is legitimate to interpret a negative x-ray as being false negative.

organisation of knowledge in long term memory; early hypothesis generation; deduction using cause effect and probabilistic analyses; and the avoidance of bias as a result of premature closure.

Furthermore, CDR is a task that is situated in the real world (Pelaccia et al., 2011). Therefore its learning requires interaction with the patient, the environment and the attending surgeon for feedback; even though simulation may provide useful initial preparation, the development of diagnostic reasoning ability is deeply dependent on clinical experience in authentic conditions of practice with graded responsibility for patient care.

Two modes of instruction are discussed: the time honoured case based discussion and direct observation of a student's or trainee's performance.

1. Case based discussion: this is the traditional mode, by means of which a student or resident presents a case in the clinic, at rounds or in a formal setting. To make it effective, the student's or resident's narrative is interrupted to enable intermediate reasoning. It is an opportunity to assess different aspects of diagnostic reasoning and provide feedback. A respectful atmosphere is maintained without diminishing the seriousness of the task to reach a sound provisional diagnosis. The teacher being in the dark about the final diagnosis is an advantage; reflection in light of any discrepancy with the final diagnoses contributes to learning (Kassirer 2010). The merit of this method is that it has found a niche in clinical practice, albeit one needing improvement. Its drawback is that it takes place after the patient encounter and so concentrates mainly on the analytic pathway to diagnosis (Pelaccia et al. 2011).
2. Direct observation: this is a time-intensive method that requires specific teacher training and is yet to find a durable place in clinical practice. Its advantage is that it takes place in real time in the workplace. As a result it enables different elements of CDR to be observed and assessed for providing timely feedback. In particular, it covers the learner's use of intuitive and analytic pathways and the interaction between them. In the case of an early learner simple questions act as prompts, e.g., the question, "what do you think is the likely pathophysiology?" within a few minutes of the patient encounter conveys the importance of arriving at a hypothesis by taking note of the patient's context and presenting clinical features. Asking for an abstract representation of the problem further helps to refine the hypothesis; asking "why do you think so?" sets in

motion a train of deductive reasoning based on an understanding of disease mechanisms, whereas "could it be something else?" stimulates a consideration of differential diagnoses with a view to avoid premature closure and error from bias. Direct observation provides the opportunity not only to assess the organisation of mental knowledge and the reasoning process but also learners' self-confidence in their knowledge and skills and their ability to deal with internal (e.g., lack of knowledge) and external (e.g., time constraint) pressures (Patel, Sandars and Carr 2015). Thus, direct observation assesses what a student or resident actually "does" in the real world.

Of course many other things contribute to teaching-learning: role modelling, organisation of learning experiences, establishment of a conducive learning environment, effective governance of the education programme and supportive institutional policies, to name a few.

## Conclusions

1. Physicians' clinical diagnostic reasoning ability has lasting value and is unlikely to be displaced by technological advances in investigation or progress in AI.
   a. By enabling selection of the right test and correct interpretation of the test result it improves diagnostic accuracy and patient safety; on a wider scale it promotes cost effective healthcare.
   b. The diagnostic approach of AI based on machine learning differs substantially from physicians' CDR; with the exception of certain targeted diagnostic tasks, e.g., medical image recognition, AI will serve to augment CDR not replace it.
2. Clinical diagnostic reasoning is a learned or acquired ability; therefore, it can and must be taught. It entails organising mental knowledge based on experience and relevant theory and adopting a balanced reasoning process that combines intuitive and analytic pathways.
   a. Intuition leads immediately to a hypothesis in familiar clinical situations; it denotes recognition of a pattern based on previous experience. Unfortunately it is prone to bias as it tends to use partial information to assess the clinical situation.
   b. Analytic reasoning requires conscious mental effort and is used to arrive at a hypothesis in an unfamiliar or complex clinical situation; it is used more often to accept or reject a hypothesis through cause effect or probabilistic analyses.

3. From the teaching learning perspective it is useful to consider elements of clinical diagnostic reasoning that can be emphasised at opportune times to the learner; for example:
    a. The power of keen observation to gather subtle, pertinent information;
    b. Abstract problem representation to jog memory for a similar experience in the past or to organise knowledge in the memory for future use;
    c. Early (intuitive) hypothesis generation taking note of the contextual and clinical features of the case;
    d. Deductive reasoning using cause-effect or probabilistic analysis to accept or reject the hypothesis and ask for additional relevant information;
    e. Avoidance of premature closure by being aware of bias and as a result of considering pertinent differential diagnoses.
4. Diagnostic reasoning is a real world task; therefore, teaching-learning must involve students and trainees in direct care of real patients with graded responsibilities in authentic practice conditions.
    a. The time honoured case based discussion can be improved for teaching learning by attention to certain details but suffers the inherent drawback of providing assessment after the event and so concentrating mainly on students and trainees' analytic reasoning skills.
    b. Direct observation of students and trainees enables a more comprehensive assessment of what they actually do in the workplace; both intuitive and analytic reasoning can be assessed. It also enables evaluation of students and trainees' abilities to reflect on their reasoning and regulate themselves; coaching and immediate feedback can be provided too.

## Bibliography

Barzilay, Regina, Garry Kasparov, Peter Norvig, Marcus du Sautoy et al. *New Scientist Essential Guide #2: Artificial Intelligence.* Edited by Richard Webb. London: New Scientist Ltd., 2020.

Bleakley Alan, Farrow Richard, Gould David and Marshall Robert. "Making sense of clinical reasoning: judgment and the evidence of the senses." *Medical Education* 37, no. 6 (June 2003): 544-552. DOI: doi.org/10.1046/j.1365-2923.2003.01542.x.

Bowen, Judith L. "Educational Strategies to Promote Clinical Diagnostic Reasoning." *New England Journal of Medicine* 355, no. 21 (November 2006): 2217-2225. DOI: 10.1056/NEJMra054782.

Broderson, John, Lisa M. Schwartz, Carl Heneghan, Jack William O'Sullivan, Jeffrey K. Aronson and Steven Woloshin. "Over diagnosis: what it is and what it isn't." *BMJ Evidence Based Medicine* 23, no. 1 (January 2018): 1-3. DOI: http://dx.doi.org/10.1136/ebmed-2017-110886.

Croskerry, Pat. "A universal model of diagnostic reasoning." *Academic Medicine: Journal of the Association of American Medical Colleges* 84, no. 8 (August 2009): 1022-1028. DOI: 10.1097/ACM.0b013e3181ace703.

Das, Jishnu, Liana Woskie, Ruma Rajbhandari, Kamran Abbasi and Ashish Jha. "Rethinking assumptions about delivery of health care: implications for universal health coverage." *BMJ* 361, no. 8154 (May 2018): 1- 5. DOI: https://doi.org/10.1136/bmj.k1716.

Doust, Jenny. "Using Probabilistic Reasoning." *BMJ* 339, no. b3823 (November 2009). DOI:10.1136/bmj.b3823.

Gill, Christopher, Lora Sabin and Christopher H. Schmid. "Why clinicians are natural Bayesians." *BMJ* 330, no. 7499 (May 2005): 1080-1083. DOI: 10.1136/bmj.330.7499.1080.

Graber, Mark, Ruthanna Gordan and Nancy Franklin. "Reducing diagnostic errors in medicine: what's the goal?" *Academic Medicine* 77, no. 10 (October 2002): 981 – 992. DOI: 10.1097/00001888-200210000-00009.

Jauhar, Sandeep. "The Demise of the Physical Exam." *New England Journal of Medicine* 354, no. 6 (February 2006): 548-551. DOI: 10.1056/NEJMp068013.

Kahneman, Daniel. *Thinking Fast and Slow*. USA: Farrar, Straus and Giroux, 2011.

Kassirer, Jerome. "Teaching Clinical Reasoning: Case Based and Coached." *Academic Medicine* 85, no. 7 (July 2010): 1118-1124. DOI: https://doi.org/10.1097/acm.0b013e3181d5dd0d.

Monteiro, Sandra and Geoffrey Norman. "Diagnostic Reasoning: Where We've Been, Where We're Going." *Teaching and Learning in Medicine* 25, no. S1 (November 2013): S26-S32. DOI: 10.1080/10401334.2013.842911.

Patel, Rakesh, John Sandars and Sue Carr. "Clinical diagnostic decision-making in real life contexts: a trans-theoretical approach for teaching: AMEE Guide No 95." *Medical Teacher* 37, no. 3 (March 2015): 211-227. DOI: https://doi.org/10.3109/0142159X.2014.975195.

Pearl, Judea and Dana Mackenzie. *The Book of Why: The New Science of Cause and Effect.* United Kingdom: Penguin Books Ltd, 2019.

Pelaccia, Thierry, Germain Forrestier and Cedric Wemmert. "Deconstructing the diagnostic reasoning of human versus artificial intelligence." *Canadian Medical Association Journal* 191, no. 48 (December 2019): 1332-1335. DOI: 10.1503/cmaj.190506.

Pelaccia, Thierry, Jacques Tardif, Triby Emmanuel and Bernard Charlin. "An analysis of clinical reasoning through a recent and comprehensive approach: The dual-process theory." *Medical Education Online* 16 (March 2011): 5890. DOI: 10.3402/ meo.v16i0.5890.

Rajkomar, Alvin, and Gurpreet Dhaliwal. "Improving diagnostic reasoning to improve patient safety." *The Permanente Journal* 15, no. 3 (Summer 2011): 68-73. DOI: 10.7812/tpp/11-098.

Rajkomar, Alvin, Jeffrey Dean and Isaac Kohane. "Machine Learning in Medicine." *New England Journal of Medicine* 380 (April 2019): 1347-1358. DOI: 10.1056/NEJMra1814259.

Woods, Nicole N. "Science is fundamental: the role of biomedical knowledge in clinical reasoning." *Medical Education* 41, no. 12 (November 2007): 1173-1177. DOI: https://doi.org/10.1111/j.1365-2923.2007.02911.x.

Wooldridge, Michael. *The Road to Conscious Machines: The Story of AI.* United Kingdom: Pelican, 2020.

# CHAPTER 14

# THE FUTURE OF SURGICAL TRAINING

AMIR SHARIFF, NADEEM SIDDIQUI
AND SABAH UDDIN SAQIB

With the highly tactile and visual specialty that surgery is and the continuing innovations that are taking place in the practice of surgery, it is no surprise that training the next generations of surgeons must continue to evolve. Previous chapters have described the changes in surgical education and brought us to where we stand today. This chapter will explore the horizons of surgical education particularly focusing on the role of social media and simulation.

## Social media in surgical training

Traditionally surgical education and training have been very swift to adopt innovations in teaching and learning methods. These newly evolved learning methods have shown promising results to meet the requirements of an ever-changing medical, scientific, and societal landscape. Social media (SM) is one of these strategies that has gained wide acceptance in surgical training in the last few years. There is evidence to suggest an increasing engagement with SM among surgeons and surgical trainees (Kilkenny, McDonald and Brady 2017). Institutions aiming for the provision of surgical care and training courses also use SM with its faculty, students and also for interacting with the community (Figure 14.1).

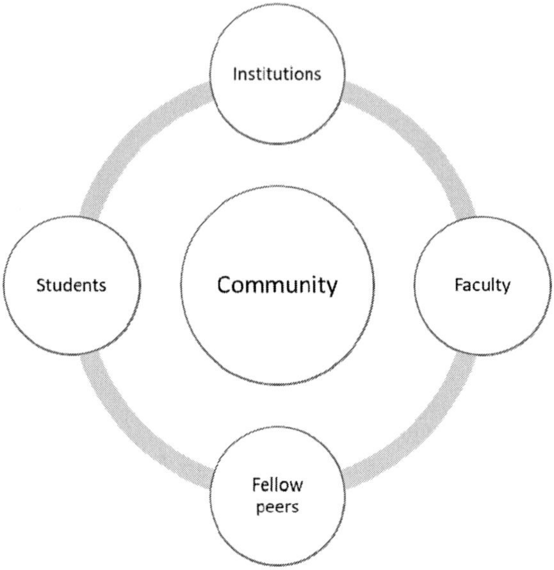


Figure 14.1: Different participants groups that use social media with the aim of interacting with each other or with the social community.

Hence, knowledge dissemination, surgical training, and patient interactions are a few fundamental aims of SM in surgical education and pedagogy.

SM incorporates a wide variety of platforms for education, training, and communication. Numerous sites ranging from social networking to blog share and video sharing have been developed, which have added a new dimension to learning and are gaining momentum in the surgical world. It behoves surgical educators to adapt to these new educational techniques and use them to meet the needs of the 21st-century learner (Evans and Schenarts 2016). Many social networking sites have been created for users to engage in either general (Facebook), professional (LinkedIn), medical (Doximity), or research (ResearchGate) interactions (Madanick 2015). In the following discussion, the role of the various SM tools in surgical training is described.

### *Blogs in surgical training*

A blog is an interactive (usually narrative text-based) website, managed by an individual, group, or organization with the opportunity to interact through comments that are regularly posted and shared (Ventola 2014).

Interacting through surgical blogs allows surgical trainees to keep abreast of the latest developments, innovations, and newer techniques of surgery. Surgeons from all around the world share their personal experiences, knowledge, and skills alongside new surgical procedures through blogs. Conventionally, it was surgical conferences and societies that were responsible for sharing such ideas and experiences. However, despite being low on the scale of evidence, blogs serve as an easily accessible alternative for knowledge sharing and in turn serve as an efficacious tool for surgical training. Surgical blog sites can take on various themes to better interact with their audience, which ranges from skilled surgeons and trainees to the general population. There are now numerous surgical blog websites that are popular among the surgical fraternity and provide the latest insights on current surgical practices. On the other hand, there are blogging sites which mainly concentrate on reviews about surgical products and equipment. Through these blogs young trainees aiming to become experts in their area of interest in surgery can receive mentorships and guidance from the experts which gives an added advantage of using blogs alongside training and education.

### *Twitter in surgical training*

With its short 140 characters message, Twitter is now serving as a very attractive microblog method for commodious and expressed communication. Due to its immediacy, surgeons have turned to Twitter to disseminate valuable information about surgery, including videos, journal articles, up-and-coming research, and events (Petrucci, Chand and Wexner 2017). Institutions responsible for surgical education and training run their Twitter accounts to give the latest updates regarding surgical diseases and available methods for the cure. Medical journals likewise share recent articles on Twitter promoting research in a fast and effective way. Surgical trainees can better connect with their peers and well known surgical specialists by following their Twitter handlers. Hashtag movements related to surgical topics promulgate information briskly all around the world. #SurgEd and #SurgTweeting are a few examples of very useful hashtags on topics related to surgical education and training. Journal clubs and grand rounds can be followed through their hashtags all over the world, hence making Twitter a very valuable SM tool for learning and sharing knowledge.

## *YouTube in surgical training*

With more than 1 billion users, YouTube is a valuable tool for surgeons that allows them to search a wide range of surgical videos. Surgical trainees are expected to be well prepared before undertaking an operation. The use of surgical video is emerging as a powerful tool to facilitate acquiring new surgical skills and accelerate learning new techniques. Real-time operative videos are now providing a very efficacious tool for surgical training and have been proven very effective in reducing harm to the patient. Most complications during surgery happen at the start of the learning curve of a surgeon. Studies have shown that video-enhanced learning is associated with the early attainment of surgical skills without increasing morbidity to the patient when compared with conventional methods of learning (Figure 14.2).

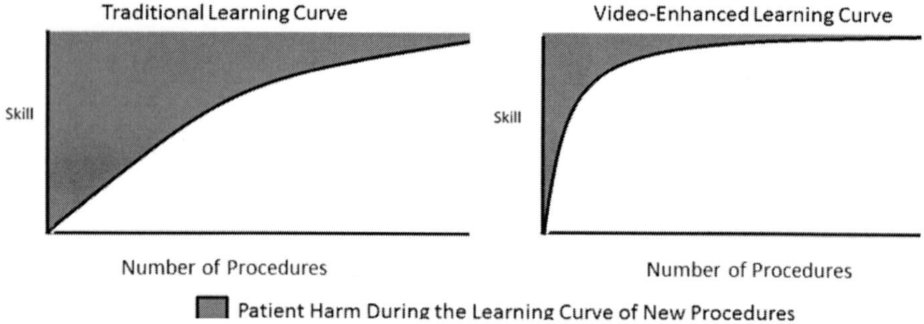


Figure 14.2: Reductions in patient harm while learning a new procedural skill.[1]

Video lectures like the Ackland anatomy series have helped surgical trainees become familiar with anatomy through human cadaveric dissection. Surgical educational websites such as giblib.com, webSurg, the International Hernia Collaboration, and others have gained significant appreciation within the surgical community. A survey by Rapp et al. evaluated surgical preparation methods of medical students, residents, and faculty and found that most respondents reported using videos as their preferred way of preparing for surgery with YouTube being the preferred source (Rapp et al. 2016).

[1] Ibrahim, A. M., O. A. Varban and J. B. Dimick. "Novel Uses of Video to Accelerate the Surgical Learning Curve." *J. Laparoendosc. Adv. Surg. Tech. A.* 26, no. 4 April 2016: 240-242. DOI:10.1089/lap.2016.0100.

### *Facebook in surgical training*

Closed SM groups over Facebook represent a novel paradigm in online learning and education. These groups are useful media and generate educational content helpful for surgical trainees. Various scientific groups and pages on Facebook post current information on core surgical topics and provide surgeons an opportunity to share their work with a diverse audience all over the world. Surgeons can share their work, deliver presentations and interact live with trainees over Facebook. Challenging cases can be shared with near immediate advice and feedback from surgeons from across the globe. Specific pages on Facebook also provide young trainees an opportunity to interact with their peers while preparing for different kinds of board exams. This category of social media is now playing a very vital role in continuing medical education. Institutes now run their Facebook accounts with the help of their active SM team to interact with the community and appreciate the work of their faculty and trainees. The Society of Gastrointestinal and Endoscopic Surgeons (SAGES) initiated eight closed Facebook groups in 2017, covering all of the society's surgical disciplines including the SAGES Master's Program Foregut Group, the SAGES Master's Program Colorectal Group, and The SAGES Master's Program Bariatric Group. These groups were inspired by and modelled after the success of The International Hernia Collaboration (IHC), one of the first examples of a closed Facebook group.

### *Mobile apps in surgical training*

With the ever-increasing use of smartphones, various apps have been launched to give quick and easy access to virtual learning, a novel method of surgical training. Educators are teaming with graphic designers and gaming experts to create apps aimed at teaching surgical trainees a variety of procedures. One example is the Touch Surgery app which is available in 226 countries with more than 1 million users who can practise more than 50 surgical procedures in more than 10 surgical specialties (Warshaw and Sarr 2011). Such mobile apps now provide an efficacious tool for surgical trainees to augment their knowledge and skills before they embark on independent practice.

## Social media as a new master trainer

Surgical education is increasingly supporting the idea of utilizing social media as a core component of training. Recent debates on work-life balance in surgical residencies have reduced hours spent in clinics, operation rooms, and clinical wards. Social media is giving a good option for trainees to enhance technical knowledge and augment their surgical skills by utilizing some part of their unoccupied time. The easy accessibility of the Internet in remote parts of the world provides them equal opportunities to remain updated with recent advances and novel procedures and surgical techniques. Through SM, trainees can receive immediate feedback on their clinical and research work by experts from all around the world. Such diverse feedback not only improves outcomes but also increases collaboration among surgeons and trainees in different parts of the world. Chand and Qureshi in their recent article described the importance of "surgical replay" (2014). This concept is derived from training sessions of professional athletes who use the video of their previous performance to improve their skills. Surgeons very often now record their videos of operating procedures which they share on various SM sites. These videos give them the ability to improvise their technical skills after retrospectively reviewing them. Moreover, their peers can also give feedback on operative videos which greatly helps in the acquisition of new techniques. Hence SM in the current period serves as a master trainer which is helping both surgeons and trainees in many different ways. To constructively incorporate SM sites in surgical training, educators must actively work to integrate them in the various teaching and training models of surgical residents.

## Perils of social media in surgical training

The evolution of SM in the last few years has not only changed the way information is shared but also raised many technical and ethical issues. In recent debates, the increasing use of SM in surgical education has been considered a threat to professionalism. Frequent posting of unprofessional online content by medical students and residents is an example of the questionable use of SM (Chretien et al. 2009). Sharing patient contents without informed consent on SM is a breach of patient confidentiality. Any such misconduct on part of professionals will inhibit the trust of the public in healthcare providers.

SM allows all facets of an individual's life to be shared with others easily. In this regard, the fine line between a surgeon's professional and personal life can be easily breached. One example of this newly available interaction occurs when a patient delivers a "friend request" to his or her physician. Inevitably, the physician is placed in an awkward position, as increasing social interaction after accepting the request can affect professional conduct and declining might negatively impact their interactions. To overcome this problem, common sense is a good guide for how to behave when using SM. Many hospitals and healthcare organizations have issued official SM guidelines that also act as the basis for legal action if violated.

## Simulation in surgical education

The role of simulation has gained tremendous popularity and acceptance in medical education, especially surgical training. Simulation has established its role for acquisition of procedural and technical skills in different surgical specialties. Currently more focus has been placed on the development and utilization of simulators for essential non-technical skills like communication, leadership, time, and team management. Simulation is also widely used as an effective tool for summative and formative assessment with the provision of providing real time constructive feedback in newer high fidelity simulators. This successful role of simulation in surgical training and assessment has led to its wider use in the process for certification and credentialing for different surgical skills and procedures.

Patient safety remains the most important factor in the conceptualization, development, integration and implementation of simulation in surgical training. Trainees can practise surgical skills in a non-pressured and controlled environment which not only ensures the safety and wellbeing of the patient but also addresses the ethical concerns related to the resident's hands-on training with real patients. Simulation training provides repeated attempts to master surgical skills in a simulation lab, ensuring achievement of competence in a particular skill before actually performing on real patients. Surgical training with simulation can lead to better patient outcomes and lower complication rates.

## Challenges related to simulation for surgical education

The concept of integration of simulation in surgical education and training sounds fascinating but comes with its own challenges. Institutions which excel in integration and implementation of simulation in surgical training have been able to navigate through these challenges with innovations to address the issues related to simulation implementation. Some of the major challenges related to surgical simulation include the following.

***Cost effectiveness:*** Development and implementation of simulation technology is not cost effective and remains one of the major concerns for institutions. This becomes particularly important for low- to middle-income countries.

***Hesitancy by surgical educators:*** Integration of simulation training in the surgical residency curriculum has faced general scepticism and reluctance by surgical faculty and supervisors. Factors contributing to this are an increased time commitment, the struggle to learn new simulation techniques to be effective teachers, inadequate financial compensation for the added responsibility, more vigorous and active involvements with trainees, and general inability to switch from traditional educational methods. Simulation is seen to be a rival and competitor of traditional training rather than complementary to it – the latter being its actual role in the training of surgical residents.

***Shortage of trained faculty:*** This is one of the major reasons for the underutilized role of simulation in surgical training. Presence of active, effective and certified faculty is of vital importance. Trained faculty not only helps in the implementation of simulation in a surgical training programme but also improves and innovates the existing system to make the simulation programme more productive and sustainable.

***Lack of standardized simulation curriculum:*** Most of the institutes utilizing simulation training for surgical residents have their own self-developed curriculum. These curricula are dependent on the experience of the faculty, the time available for residents, the time faculty members spend on simulation training and the availability of simulators in that institute. This can result in an ineffective use of simulators which does not address the need and learning objective of residents at that level of training. There is a desperate need for the development and implementation of high quality simulation curricula which has defined learning objectives and effective simulation tools to meet these objectives. There should be a regular evaluation process of this curriculum to identify gaps and effort should be made to address these gaps for improvement.

***Lack of coordinated research:*** The available literature on the use of simulation in different surgical specialities is present but quite sketchy and haphazard. Different types of simulators with invalidated assessment tools used for participants with varying degrees of experience are reported in a limited number of studies.

***Inadequate logistics and support staff:*** These are mandatory for the development and smooth functioning of simulation labs.

## Future of surgical simulation

Despite these challenges, the future of simulation seems to be promising in terms of further advancements and technological excellence. The very factors like patient safety, ethical concerns and transparency which initially introduced and advocated the role of simulation in surgical training, are pushing the industry and technology for more creativity in simulation. The new concept of using simulation technology not only for surgical training and assessment, but also for its role in better outcomes of surgical procedures has opened up the new arena for research and development of simulation technology. Here are some of the interesting and emerging concepts in simulation technology which can play fundamental roles in surgical education and training in the future.

***3-D virtual cadavers*:** There is a decline in the availability of human or animal cadavers because of ethical concerns. Simulation technology has responded to this challenge with the option of 3-D virtual cadavers. Students can view the virtual cadavers from different angles and can manipulate these cadavers with the help of virtual probes (Washmuth et al. 2020). Advancements in 3-D technology and having 3-D reconstructed images of virtual cadavers have given surgical students and teachers a new dimension of learning and teaching. Residents can practise multiple times on the same cadaver or multiple cadavers can be used at the same time by the group of students. This modality offers the advantage of performing a virtual dissection before the actual performance in real life and has shown to make a surgeon more time efficient. The learning curve is short for both teachers and students to learn this technology. One of the major drawbacks is the inability to feel the texture of different organs of the body. Continuous faculty involvement and training is also a challenge for effective implementation of this modality in surgical education.

***Virtual Library:*** Collection of virtual cadavers over a period of time can help in establishing a huge virtual cadaveric library. The main feature of this library is the presence of a large number of cadavers with similar a disease pathology but different anatomical variations. Students can learn to virtually dissect the tissues in many of the normal anatomic variants, anomalies and diseases of different organ systems in the body. This library will also help the students to virtually practise and dissect the tissue to achieve the necessary expertise before performing the operation on real patients. Addition of a patient's Computed Tomographic (CT) scan in the library can further help in the education of certain complex surgical diseases and operations of different anatomical varieties. The development of such effective libraries will need good collaboration between educational institutes at national and international levels.

***Virtual Patients:*** Virtual patients are interactive computer based simulators which are used in healthcare education, training and assessment. Virtual patients can be used in objective structured clinical examinations (OSCE) settings where artificially intelligent patients provide appropriate human, social, behavioural and cultural (HSBC) responses. Many of these virtual patients are able to respond with adequate verbal and nonverbal language like facial movements and emotional responses. Compared to real patients, they offer the advantage of being easily available on demand and modifiable; there's also a minimal chance of variance and subjective bias when assessing trainees. Studies have shown virtual patients to be more time and cost efficient. In a recent meta-analysis, virtual patients were found to be more effective for knowledge improvement and skills like clinical reasoning and teamwork (Kononowicz et al. 2019).

***Mannequins:*** Mannequins have been used in medical education since the 1970s, but with recent advancements in technology and software, they can now provide a very realistic educational experience with a high degree of verisimilitude. Mannequins with higher flexibility and fidelity, as well as real time feedback being provided during the encounter, have positively affected the educational experience of the trainee (Massoth et al. 2019). Improvements in tissue characteristics, the enhanced feel of the texture and bleeding from the tissues can help to teach procedural skills like chest tube placement, vascular anastomosis and endotracheal intubation more effectively.

***Virtual Reality (VR) simulators for pre-operative warm up:*** The concept of virtual holographic dissection has led to the concept of pre-operative warm up dissection on virtual reality simulators. This pre-op dissection has been found beneficial for decreasing operation time and results in fewer surgical errors. These effects are beneficial for both novices and experts. Doing 15 minutes of pre-op simulator warm up is associated with better motor and psychological performance and improved concentration in the operating room. This modality has been shown to improve psychomotor skills in laparoscopic cholecystectomy but due to very limited literature, improvement in all surgical parameters cannot be proved (Moldovanu et al. 2011). More research is needed to assess the actual benefit which pre-operative virtual warm ups can offer in different surgical specialities (Pike et al. 2017).

***In situ training:*** This is a blended mode of surgical training with the use of simulators in real clinical environments rather than practising on simulators in a simulation lab. This method of training is especially helpful in building team training, communication and professionalism among trainees. Compared to the very controlled and regulated conditions in the simulation lab, in situ training helps to identify gaps which are present in real life (presence of drugs or equipment in the right place, communications between different teams, adequate hand over for continuity of care etc.) and gives opportunities for improvement. Implementation of in situ training in surgery teams has been shown to improve communications, coordination and teamwork in trauma patients (Steinemann et al. 2011). Further research work is required to completely establish and integrate this modality in surgical training (Rosen et al. 2012).

***Tele simulation:*** This is a process in which telecommunication and simulation resources are utilized for the purposes of education, training and assessment of the learners at an offsite location. This modality helps in overcoming the geographical barriers for surgical education. In the absence of any simulation lab, smaller and less developed facilities can enjoy quality education and training, which is not only cost effective but also a great source for networking and collaboration among centres. Tele simulation has been successfully used in teaching basic laparoscopic skills (Henao et al. 2013; Okrainec, Henao and Azzie 2010), triage for trauma (McCoy et al. 2019) and simple high impact procedures like tube thoracostomies in critically ill patients (Jewer et al. 2019).

***Virtual environment:*** With the advancement and combination of tele-simulation technology and virtual reality simulators, came an immersive three dimensional virtual world called the "virtual environment" or "second life". The virtual environment has been shown to have very good acceptability by today's digitalized generation of students. This second life is particularly effective for teaching social and team networking skills which are essential for modern surgeons. A virtual hospital has been developed by Imperial College's Faculty of Medicine using second life, and provides a platform for e-learning activities with regard to the diagnosis and management of various diseases (Larvin 2009; Patel et al. 2013). Virtual environment technology has also been used in the military setting for soldiers suffering from post-traumatic stress disorders. Veterans can return virtually to their home environment during rehabilitation of their illness which has a positive influence on the overall outcome of the disease. One of the greatest benefits of second life is its accessibility at any time from any computer without the need of an educator. This modality has been used in general surgery procedures and in physician' responses to emergency or disaster preparation with good success (Cohen et al. 2013).

***Augmented reality:*** While virtual reality places subjects within an entirely simulated environment, augmented reality creates a "mixed reality environment" by superimposing digital information onto a real world image. Augmented reality devices require a display, a position tracking system and software to incorporate the data. Devices range from head mounted devices to smartphones. Intra-operatively, a head mounted device can potentially provide anatomic information as well as guidance on operative steps and instrument navigation. A systematic review evaluating augmented reality in surgical training concluded that this modality improved the trainees' competency and post-operative complication rates, however at the expense of a prolonged duration of surgery (Williams et al. 2020).

## Conclusion

As discussed above, the future of training in surgery is bright and exciting with numerous avenues and technologies that will be utilized in imparting the knowledge, skills and attitudes necessary to make a good clinician and surgeon. There will be challenges in incorporating these advances. Continual adaptation will become the mantra of surgical educators as our methodologies continue to change.

## Bibliography

Chand, M. and T. Qureshi. "Evolution in surgical training: what can we learn from professional coaches and elite athletes?" *J. R. Soc. Med.* 107, no. 7 (April 2014): 290–292. DOI: 10.1177/0141076814532395. PMID: 24781158.

Chretien, K. C., S. R. Greysen, J. P. Chretien and T. Kind. "Online Posting of Unprofessional Content by Medical Students." *JAMA* 302, no. 12 (September 2009): 1309-1315. DOI: 10.1001/jama.2009.1387. PMID: 19773566.

Cohen, D., N. Sevdalis, D. Taylor, K. Kerr, M. Heys, K. Willett, N. Batrick and A. Darzi. "Emergency preparedness in the 21st century: training and preparation modules in virtual environments." *Resuscitation* 84, no. 1 (January 2013): 78-84. DOI: 10.1016/j.resuscitation.2012.05.014. PMID: 22659598.

Evans, C. H. and K. D. Schenarts. "Evolving educational techniques in surgical training." *Surg. Clin. North Am.* 96, no. 1, (February 2016): 71–88. DOI: 10.1016/j.suc.2015.09.005. PMID: 26612021.

Henao, O., J. Escallón, J. Green, M. Farcas, J. M. Sierra, W. Sánchez and A. Okrainec. "Fundamentals of laparoscopic surgery in Colombia using telesimulation: an effective educational tool for distance learning." *Biomedica* 33, no. 1 (March 2013): 107-14. DOI: 10.1590/S0120-41572013000100013. PMID: 23715313.

Jewer, J., M. H. Parsons, C. Dunne, A. Smith and A. Dubrowski. "Evaluation of a Mobile Telesimulation Unit to Train Rural and on High-Acuity Remote Practitioners Low-Occurrence Procedures: Pilot Randomized Controlled Trial." *Journal of Medical Internet Research* 21, no. 8 (August 2019): e14587. DOI: 10.2196/14587. PMID: 31389340.

Kilkenny, J., J. J. McDonald and R. R. Brady. "Increased Engagement with Social Media in Colorectal Surgery." *Colorectal Dis.* 19, no. 6 (June 2017): 592-594. DOI: 10.1111/codi.13712. PMID: 28477367.

Kononowicz, A. A., L. A. Woodham, S. Edelbring, N. Stathakarou, D. Davies, N. Saxena, L. T. Car, J. Carlstedt-Duke, J. Car and N. Zary. "Virtual patient simulations in health professions education: systematic review and meta-analysis by the digital health education collaboration." *Journal of Medical Internet Research* 21, no. 7 (July 2019): e14676. DOI: 10.2196/14676. PMID: 31267981.

Larvin, M. "E-Learning in surgical education and training." *ANZ Journal of Surgery* 79, no. 3 (March 2009): 133-7. DOI: 10.1111/j.1445-2197.2008.04828.x. PMID: 19317777.

Madanick, R. D. "Education becomes social: the intersection of social media and medical education." *Gastroenterology* 149, no. 4 (October 2015): 844–847. DOI: 10.1053/j.gastro.2015.08.037. PMID: 26311278.

Massoth, C, H Röder, H Ohlenburg, M Hessler, A Zarbock, D M Pöpping and M Wenk. "High-fidelity is not superior to low-fidelity simulation but leads to overconfidence in medical students". *BMC Medical Education* 19, no. 1 (January 2019): 29. DOI: 10.1186/s12909-019-1464-7. PMID: 30665397

McCoy, C. E., R. Alrabah, W. Weichmann, M. I. Langdorf, C. Ricks, B. Chakravarthy, C. Anderson and S. Lotfipour. "Feasibility of telesimulation and Google glass for mass casualty triage education and training." *Western Journal of Emergency Medicine* 20, no. 3 (May 2019): 512. DOI: 10.5811/westjem.2019.3.40805. PMID: 31123554.

Moldovanu, R., E. Târcoveanu, G. Dimofte, C. Lupaşcu and C. Bradea. "Preoperative warm-up using a virtual reality simulator." *JSLS: Journal of the Society of Laparoendoscopic Surgeons* 15, no. 4 (October 2011): 533. DOI: 10.4293/108680811X13176785204409. PMID: 22643511.

Okrainec, A., O. Henao and G. Azzie. "Telesimulation: an effective method for teaching the fundamentals of laparoscopic surgery in resource-restricted countries." *Surgical endoscopy* 24, no. 2 (February 2010): 417-22. DOI: 10.1007/s00464-009-0572-6. PMID: 19565299.

Patel, V., R. Aggarwal, D. Cohen, D. Taylor and A. Darzi. "Implementation of an interactive virtual-world simulation for structured surgeon assessment of clinical scenarios." *Journal of the American College of Surgeons* 217, no. 2 (August 2013): 270-9. DOI: 10.1016/j.jamcollsurg.2013.03.023. PMID: 23870219.

Petrucci, A. M., M. Chand and S. D. Wexner. "Social Media: Changing the Paradigm for Surgical Education." *Clin. Colon Rectal Surg.* 30, no. 4 (September 2017): 244-251. DOI: 10.1055/s-0037-1604252. PMID: 28924397.

Pike, T. W., S. Pathak, F. Mushtaq, R. M. Wilkie, M. Mon-Williams and J. P. Lodge. "A systematic examination of preoperative surgery warm-up routines." *Surgical endoscopy* 31, no. 5 (May 2017): 2202-14. DOI: 10.1007/s00464-016-5218-x. PMID: 27633438.

Rapp, A. K., M. G. Healy, M. E. Charlton, J. N. Keith, M. E. Rosenbaum and M. R. Kapadia. "YouTube is the most frequently used educational video source for surgical preparation." *J. Surg. Educ.* 73, no. 6 (November-December 2016): 1072–1076. DOI: 10.1016/j.jsurg.2016.04.024. PMID: 27316383.

Rosen, M. A., E. A. Hunt, P. J. Pronovost, M. A. Federowicz and S. J. Weaver. "In situ simulation in continuing education for the health care professions: a systematic review." *Journal of Continuing Education in the Health Professions* 32, no. 4 (September 2012): 243-54. DOI: 10.1002/chp.21152. PMID: 23280527.

Steinemann, S., B. Berg, A. Skinner, A. DiTulio, K. Anzelon, K. Terada, C. Oliver, H. C. Ho and C. Speck. "In situ, multidisciplinary, simulation-based teamwork training improves early trauma care."

*Journal of Surgical Education* 68, no. 6 (November 2011): 472-7. DOI: 10.1016/j.jsurg.2011.05.009. PMID: 22000533.

Ventola, C. L. "Social media and health care professionals: benefits, risks, and best practices." *P&T* 39, no. 7 (July 2014): 491–520. DOI: PMID: 25083128. PMCID: PMC4103576.

Warshaw, A. L. and M. G. Sarr. "Social media in surgical education and practice." *Surgery* 150, no. 1 (July 2011): 1. DOI: 10.1016/j.surg.2011.05.021. PMID: 21683852.

Washmuth, N. B., T. Cahoon, K. Tuggle and R. N. Hunsinger. "Virtual Dissection: Alternative to cadaveric dissection for a pregnant nurse anaesthesia student." *Health Professions Education* 6, no. 2 (June 2020): 247-55. DOI: 10.1016/j.hpe.2019.11.001.

Williams, M. A., J. McVeigh, A. I. Handa and R. Lee. "Augmented reality in surgical training: a systematic review." *Postgraduate Medical Journal* 96, no. 1139 (September 2020): 537-542. DOI: 10.1136/postgradmedj-2020-137600. PMID: 32229513.

# CHAPTER 15

# QUALITY ASSURANCE IN ACADEMIC TRAINING: ESSENTIALS FOR THE PROGRAMMES AND THE FACULTY

QAMAR RIAZ
AND MUHAMMAD RIZWAN KHAN

## Abstract

Quality is a very subjective term and therefore may have different meanings for different stakeholders. There is a lot of debate in the literature about the acceptable definition of quality and the methods of quality assurance in academic training programmes, highlighting the fact that quality assurance is a complex process. Moreover, the quality assurance resources available for academic programmes may be completely different from the methods used for the academic faculty. This chapter aims to provide an overview of different methods available for quality assurance in academic training programmes. Since academic quality assurance is an evolving concept in developing countries, we shall recount the local perspective from Pakistan as well as the Aga Khan University to provide an insight to the readers on the current situation in the country and the opportunities available for further enhancement. Quality assurance and accreditation in the 21st century will require consensus on a set of "universal" attributes or standards of a quality educational experience, a focus on the learner rather than the institution, and a willingness to open up the entire process to a much broader group of stakeholders. The process may be evolving and not true science; but an investment in the quality assurance of academic programmes is a true investment into the future of communities.

# I. Introduction and background

## A. What is quality?

Quality is a very subjective term and therefore may have different meanings for different stakeholders in different contexts depending on the processes or outcomes under study (Vroeijenstijn 1995); hence a universal definition may be difficult to achieve. Quality is something that everyone likes to talk about and would feel when it is present, but the exact definition may be a challenge. Quality has been variously defined in the literature as having "added value," "fitness for purpose," being related to "end-user satisfaction," and "meeting desired outcomes" (Vroeijenstijn 1995).

## B. Quality assurance in academia

The concept of quality assurance (QA) initially emerged from industrial and commercial practice but has now been embedded into higher education and academia. Academic QA is a verification that a certain academic programme or activity has attained the desired level of quality and this quality or standard is likely to be sustained.

Ironically, measuring quality is as difficult as defining it, especially in an academic setting. It is a challenging process and cannot be accomplished unless there are well-defined outcomes and targeted areas of interest. The usual practice of identifying certain performance indicators and linking them with quality may not be the true representative of quality. This may also be called "quantification" of the quality data. There are several variables in academics that may be difficult to quantify and may be based on a subjective perception of the stakeholders. One common example used in the academic literature is how to assess the research output of a programme or university and—perhaps more importantly—the total number of publications, the rigorous methodology used, the citation index of the publications, and the impact of the publication on the health and life of the population, among other factors. The last of these may be difficult to measure but may be the most significant factor in assessing the impact and hence the quality of a publication. Similarly, when we look at the quality and outcome of academic programmes, the relevant question may be how to define the success of its graduates and how to measure it—is it the grades and pass rate of the students in the summative assessment, the professional competence of the trainees, or the fitness of the graduates to meet the needs of the society and the community? There are numerous such examples in the academic setting which emphasize the fact that assessment of the true essence of quality remains a challenge.

The quality assurance process in academia remains close to the assessment methods used in academia and must meet certain basic requirements including validity, reliability, and relevance. The key factor in quality assurance in academia and any parameters or indicators used for quality assurance must be relevant to the goals and objectives of the academic programme as well as its impact on the society. While quality assurance can be managed through the institutional monitoring system, the process demands transparency and dissemination of results to all the stakeholders.

Another important question is whether an assessment of quality is a one-time event or an ongoing process. Since academic processes are usually designed in a spiral fashion and the trainees move along the spiral over a period of time, it is quite clear that any quality improvement endeavour is usually a broad-based cyclical activity involving all the policies, standards, systems, and processes related to both quality management and quality control. Striving to achieve quality in educational institutions requires continuous review and revision of the curriculum, the teaching-learning methods, the assessment methods, and the overall student outcomes as a measure of the quality of the educational process experienced during each and every stage of a learner's professional development. In other words, quality assurance is a continual process, where data is collected to measure the quality of the educational programme and identify strengths and weaknesses to develop an improvement plan.

Although the academic programme and the supervising faculty are closely interlinked, the quality assurance processes for both these entities are distinctly different. The quality assurance indicators for the academic programme are usually related to the academic content of the programme, the teaching-learning environment of the programme as well as the ultimate student and programme outcomes, and all these factors are also influenced by the academic input of the supervising faculty. But the quality assurance for the supervising faculty is altogether different and may not have been adequately addressed in different academic centres across the world. Hence these two entities must be distinguished in academic literature and given due emphasis as separate entities.

In this chapter, we shall focus on quality assurance in academic training with a special focus on the training programmes in medicine and faculty development. In the end, the process adopted for the evaluation of the postgraduate programmes at the Aga Khan University, Karachi, shall be described to add a local perspective on the process of quality assurance.

## II. Quality assurance in academic medicine

Medical education broadly aims to train healthcare professionals in the knowledge, skills, and attitudes important for providing quality patient care. Any quality healthcare provider system relies predominantly on the quality of the medical education and its medical graduates (Karle 2006). Unfortunately, the literature is full of concerns about the quality of education and training of medical students and residents (Wilkes, Cassel and Klau 2018). The issue of quality and standardization of medical education and training was first raised by Abraham Flexner in his ground breaking report describing the condition of medical education in the United States (Ludmerer 2010). The proliferation of public and private medical schools (which may be of dubious quality) and postgraduate training programmes, as well as the international migration of trainees and practising physicians further elevated the concerns about the quality of medicine as an academic discipline (Sullivan and Mittman 2010). It was soon recognized that assuring quality in academic medicine is vital to maintaining or improving standards of healthcare delivery. As a result, in recent years, quality assurance has become an integral part of medical education globally to ensure scientific rigor and educational excellence in the preparation of physicians at all levels.

Any academic programme in medicine has several components that include the trainee students, the faculty, and the learning environment, and then there are many other stakeholders including the training institution, the regulatory bodies, and the community expectations. The students and trainees usually have a defined curriculum, set of learning objectives, and course of training leading to a distinct academic and professional achievement (Schiekirka et al. 2015). The academic performance of the students over the course is regularly monitored by using various formative and summative assessment methods by the supervising faculty and the certifying bodies (Gibson et al. 2008).

Quality assurance is a complex process and the institutions generally use two main approaches to address their quality assurance commitments. The first is to develop a mechanism of external evaluation or audit to validate that the institution or programme is complying with established standards (Hajifathali et al. 2006). The second strategy is for the institution to prepare a self-study or inquiry brief that provides an internal analysis of the strengths and weaknesses of the institution based on a set of standards provided by the quality assurance agency. Most of the academic programmes use these two methods in combination at various time intervals (Harvey 2002). Self-study will be used to focus attention on areas of improvement, while an audit verifies baseline compliance with standards. The major purpose of the two approaches remains the same and the whole idea is to identify the strengths and weaknesses of the current system with the development of a future plan which shall be validated again after its implementation. The decision about the method and type of evaluation is influenced by the goal of evaluation and definition of quality. The literature emphasizes internal evaluation as the first step, followed by external evaluation. In the case of external evaluation specifically, the terms of reference should be clear, and understood and interpreted by both the external review panel and the institute or programme to be reviewed in the same way (Stensaker 2003; Szanto 2005).

There are at least three well-defined approaches to monitoring the quality of academic training programmes (Joshi 2012):

A. Programme evaluation
B. Evaluation of the institutional learning environment
C. Accreditation – road to quality assurance

**A. Programme evaluation**

Evaluation refers to the process of determining the value of a programme or product, or efficiency in the case of a process (Cook 2010). In education, evaluation refers to the use of information to make a decision about the value or worth, effectiveness, and efficiency of an educational programme, irrespective of its scope and duration (Harvey 2002; Goldie 2006). Cronbach defined evaluation as "an examination conducted to assist in improving a program and other programs having the same general purpose." Some other terms used interchangeably are curriculum evaluation, outcomes evaluation, audit, benchmarking, and measurement against performance indicators, among others (Cook 2010).

Programme evaluation is a systematic method for collecting, analysing, and using the information to answer questions about projects, policies, and programmes, particularly about their effectiveness and efficiency (Goldstein 2010). It is the most fundamental pathway to quality assurance in medical education and training. ACGME defines programme evaluation as a "systematic collection and analysis of information related to the design, implementation, and outcomes of a program, for the purpose of monitoring and improving the quality and effectiveness of the program" (ACGME 2010a). In the context of medical education, evaluation can refer to several discrete processes ranging from overall evaluation of a training programme to evaluation of faculty teaching during a lecture, or workshop, or rotation within a training programme at undergraduate or postgraduate levels (Durning, Hemmer and Pangaro 2007).

Several models have been described in the literature for evaluating educational programmes; the ones most commonly used are (Frye and Hemmer 2012):

**1. Experimental/quasi-experimental evaluation approach**

This is one of the earliest models used to evaluate educational programmes. It depends on the assumption that a linear causal relationship exists between programme elements and desired programme outcomes (Kim and Steiner 2016). Since true experimental designs are not feasible and may not be ethical in an educational setting, evaluators most often use quasi-experimental designs. Additionally, these designs if used alone can provide information about the outcome of a standalone educational activity but have questionable validity and usefulness in the complex environment of an educational programme.

**2. Kirkpatrick's approach**

Kirkpatrick's model assesses four hierarchical "levels" of programme outcomes: (1) learner satisfaction or reaction to the programme; (2) measures of learning attributed to the programme (e.g., knowledge gained, skills improved, attitudes changed); (3) changes in learner behaviour in the context for which they are being trained; and (4) the programme's final results in its larger context (Kirkpatrick 1996). It has been extensively used worldwide for evaluating learner outcomes in training programmes (Smidt et al. 2009). While this model relies on linear causality too, the primary reason for its popularity is the clarity of its focus on programme outcomes and clear description of outcomes beyond simple learner satisfaction. This model however does not take into account intervening variables that may affect learning such as learner motivation, variable entry levels of knowledge and skills, relationships between important programme elements and the programme's context, and the effectiveness of the resources used (Holton 1996).

### 3. The logic model

The logic model, commonly used in the evaluation of medical education programmes, is grounded in the assumption that the relationships between the programme's educational methods and the desired outcomes are clearly understood (Balmer, Rama and Simpson 2019). It focuses on the four basic components of an educational programme, namely:

1) Inputs: these include facilities, faculty skills, faculty time, staff time, staff skills, educational technology, funds, and leadership support;

2) Activities: instructional and assessment strategies, innovations, or changes planned for the educational programme;

3) Outputs: an immediate result of activities that occurred in a programme such as the number of learners who attended a planned educational event, or characteristics of faculty recruited; and

4) Outcomes: includes short-term, medium-term, and longer-range changes (impact) as a result of the programme's activities.

### 4. The CIPP Model

The CIPP or the context/input/process/product model (Stufflebeam 2000) is similar to the logic model in terms of its components. However, as opposed to the logic model, which is most useful when used during the planning stage, CIPP model studies can be used both formatively (during the programme's processes) and summatively (retrospectively).

An individual model or a combination of them can be selected to plan evaluations for a specific educational programme. Depending on the model(s) selected, an evaluation may use a variety of assessments, tools, and sources including peer review, surveys of students, graduates and employers, patients, and faculty, and utilize both qualitative and quantitative indicators (Cook 2010).

A programme evaluation typically has one of these two purposes (Goldie 2006):

- Formative evaluation: it aims at the improvement of a programme, project, or activity, and is often undertaken during the course of the educational programme.

- Summative evaluation: it determines the overall value or worth of an educational programme for summative decision making, and is frequently conducted at the end of the programme.

The intensity of the programme evaluation process depends on the intent of the evaluation process. Similarly, the interest of the stakeholders is an important determinant of the overall outcome of the evaluation process. In any case, the evaluation process provides a great insight into the future roadmap for the programme. The process needs to be repeated at regular intervals to ensure that the recommendations coming out of the evaluation process are implemented and evaluated.

**B. Evaluation of the institutional learning environment**

The learning environment is a dynamic and complex structure comprised of the entire range of components and activities within which learning happens within a medical school (Soemantri, Herrera and Riquelme 2010). It includes the setting, learners, faculty, curriculum, teaching and learning methods, learning resources, physical infrastructure, monitoring and evaluation, and their interactions (Papp, Markkanen and Bonsdorff 2003). Genn defined the learning environment as "the curriculum's most significant manifestation and conceptualization, educational and organizational, which embraces everything that is happening in the medical school" (Genn 2001). 'Learning environment' is the umbrella term that can be applied to the whole spectrum of undergraduate, postgraduate, and graduate education in any discipline.

The clinical learning environment, the environment in which patient care is learned, has long been recognized as an essential component across the continuum of the health professions education (Spencer 2003; Weiss, Bagian and Nasca 2013). It is at the core of medical education as it is the avenue where learners at both undergraduate and postgraduate levels learn the essential skills of history taking, examination, decision making, interaction with patients and peers, empathy, and professionalism (Spencer 2003; Nasca, Weiss and Bagian 2014).

It is imperative to have an environment that ensures a high-quality educational experience in the clinical setting for medical professionals. Existing evidence supports a close relationship between a positive environment and achievement of learning outcomes indicating the quality of a programme and hence that of its graduates. The learning environment has been shown to directly affect performance – both at undergraduate and postgraduate levels – including factors such as clinical proficiency, attitudes, values, and behaviours. According to Genn, the "environment of the medical school is notable, not only because it derives from and is a manifestation of the curriculum, but because the environment is a determinant of the behaviour of the medical school's students and teachers" (Genn 2001). The learning environment has also been shown to affect resident wellness and mental health (Dolmans et al. 2008; Jennings and Slavin 2015). According to the UK Standing Committee on Postgraduate Medical Education, a working environment that is conducive to learning is critically important to successful training (Oxley, Medical et al. 1996; Standing Committee on Postgraduate Medical and Dental Education 1996). Learning environments not only determine the performance of their learners but also define the attitudes of the faculty (Hafler 2011). It is therefore important to have a periodic evaluation of a learning environment in order to identify any problems, and take timely measures to resolve them should any arise.

Measuring learners' perceptions is the most common method of evaluating a learning environment in healthcare education (Soemantri, Herrera et al. 2010); however, faculty perceptions of the learning and teaching environment are equally important. Roff and McAleer claimed that determining learners and faculty's perception of the factors that constitute the learning environment of any programme or institute can aid in a timely modification of these factors to enhance learning and ensure the attainment of learning objectives (Roff et al. 2001). Faculty viewpoints or perceptions about the educational environment are important not only for themselves but also for the learners and can contribute to improving the quality of the educational environment in any institution (Hoffman and Donaldson 2004). Thus, measuring learner and faculty perceptions about the learning environment and identifying factors that may deteriorate the learning are crucial to the development of safe health practitioners. This could facilitate the identification of areas requiring improvement so that resources could be directed to strengthen them; it could also reinforce areas that are functioning well, thus ensuring a learning experience that would offer the best possible learning outcomes (Till 2005; Cate, Snell and Carraccio 2010).

Various generic and specific instruments have been developed to measure learning environments as perceived by undergraduate and postgraduate medical, dental, or nursing students in different healthcare education settings (Whittle, Whelan and Murdoch-Eaton 2007). According to a review article, a total of 28 instruments were developed until 2012 to measure perceptions of learners in Medicine regarding their learning environment, of which 13 evaluated postgraduate only, 13 evaluated only undergraduate learning environments in hospitals or medical schools, and 2 were used for both undergraduate and postgraduate environments. Among the different instruments developed for measuring learning environments, the most commonly used instruments are the Dundee Ready Education Environment Measure (DREEM) (Roff et al. 1997), and Postgraduate Hospital Educational Environment Measure (PHEEM) (Clapham, Wall and Batchelor 2007). Other instruments have been developed for specific disciplines, settings and levels of education, such as: ACLEEM – the Ambulatory Care Learning Education Environment Measure (Riquelme et al. 2013); D-RECT – the Dutch Residency Educational Climate Test (Boor et al. 2011); ATEEM – the Anaesthetic Theatre Educational Environment Measure (Holt and Roff 2004); and UCLEEM – the Undergraduate Clinical Education Environment Measure (Strand et al. 2013).

It is essential that the instrument selected for evaluating the quality of the learning environment is valid, reliable, and can effectively and accurately measure the learning environment to inform decisions. While evaluating learning environments is important, it is vital to understand that using these instruments alone may not be the true reflection of the quality of the institute or programme under evaluation.

### C. Accreditation – the road to quality assurance

When the procedure, services, operations, and outcomes of an educational institute or programme are evaluated by an external body against pre-defined standards, the quality assessment process is termed accreditation. Accreditation is both a status and a process (Harvey 2004).

Accreditation has been defined as, "the process by which a designated authority (professionals, programme or institute/organization) reviews and evaluates an educational institution using a set of clearly defined standards and procedures, as having a particular status or being qualified to perform a particular activity" (Zanten, Boulet and Greaves 2012).

Medical education differs from other study programmes in terms of the restricted choice of courses and use of specific teaching strategies such as problem-based learning, clinical teaching, and interaction with real patients (Karle 2004). Yet, there is significant variation in the structure and quality of undergraduate and postgraduate medical education around the world (Karle 2004), and also differences in how organizations assess the quality of education. It is therefore generally recommended to use standards while accrediting educational programmes (Lilley and Harden 2003).

The purpose of developing these standards is to assist institutions, organizations, and national authorities in achieving and maintaining the quality of medical education (Davis and Ringsted 2006). While there may be global variation in accreditation standards, certain standards should be essential for determining quality (Abdalla 2012). The World Federation for Medical Education (WFME) recommendations stress that global standards should be modified or supplemented to suit local regional, national, and institutional needs, priorities, and contexts.

Accreditation may be of programmes or institutions. The purpose of institutional accreditation is to ensure that the institute meets the specified minimum (input) standards resulting in the achievement of a license to operate. It is usually based on an evaluation of whether the institution meets specified minimum (input) standards, such as staff qualifications, research activities, student intake, and learning resources. It might also be based on an estimation of the potential for the institution to produce graduates that meet explicit or implicit academic standards or professional competence. Programmes may be accredited for their academic standing; their ability to produce graduates with professional competence to practise is usually referred to as “professional accreditation”.

There are many accrediting bodies around the world working to ensure the quality assurance of undergraduate, graduate, and postgraduate medical programmes. In 2003, the WFME published the Trilogy of Global Standards for Quality Improvement for basic (undergraduate) medical education (BME) (World Federation for Medical Education 2003a), postgraduate medical education (PME) (World Federation for Medical Education 2003b), and continuing professional development of medical doctors (CPD) (World Federation for Medical Education 2003c). Then, in 2015 the WFME published recommendations on the use of the BME standards. The Accreditation Council for Graduate Medical Education (ACGME) and General Medical Council (GMC) are the accreditation bodies responsible for setting standards and accrediting the various postgraduate training programmes in the United States and the United Kingdom, respectively (General Medical Council 2021). Each postgraduate specialty programme may also have its specialty-based standards which are set by the respective colleges (Royal College of Physicians and Surgeons of Canada 2021).

The standards set by the international accrediting bodies may also be used to evaluate and accredit the programmes outside the primary country, which helps standardize the programmes across the world. The ACGME has an international arm called the Accreditation Council for Medical Graduates International (ACGME-I) which provides accreditation services to programmes outside the United States (ACGME International 2021). Moreover, each country may have its own standards for accreditation of training programmes, developed by its various national bodies and universities. The College of Physicians and Surgeons Pakistan (CPSP) is one such institution available in Pakistan, which is responsible for the standardization and accreditation of various postgraduate programmes in the country (College of Physicians and Surgeons Pakistan 2021).

## III. Quality assurance for the faculty

The faculty is the most important teaching and learning resource for the students, programmes, and the universities. Teachers not only have extensive subject-specific knowledge and skills, but they are also probably the most effective tool to transfer that knowledge directly to their learners. Faculty members are also responsible for the development of various programmes including the curricula, teaching-learning methods, and assessment strategies. Due to the very fact that they are responsible for the development of academic programmes, they are also the ones who take the credit for the success or responsibility for the failure of such programmes. Hence it is justifiable to say that the quality assurance of the programmes is directly based on the qualification, dedication, and quality assurance of its faculty members. Despite its huge significance, quality assurance for faculty remains a challenge for academic entities since it is a complicated process ranging from the recruitment of suitably qualified personnel to the continuous development of various attributes of these personnel, including their pedagogical, research, and related academic capacities (ENQA et al. 2015).

A number of approaches may be used for the quality assurance of the faculty members responsible for academic training and programmes, including:

A. Qualification and recruitment
B. Enhancement and appraisal of teaching capacities

C. Recertification and continuous faculty development

**A. Qualification and recruitment**

Institutions and organizations need to make a conscious effort to understand the essential purpose of recruitment of faculty in their programmes. Most of the clinical programmes in medicine are heavily biased towards clinical practice and providing essential patient care. The faculty being recruited for this purpose may be adequately qualified for the clinical needs of patient care, but may not have satisfactory skills as a teacher or mentor. It is commonly and erroneously thought that every qualified physician has the adequate attributes to qualify as a teacher and is able to transfer the knowledge and skills to the next generation, but this aspect should be given special consideration for the recruitment of faculty for academic programmes. The graduate of the clinical programmes may not have the required teaching, assessment, and management skills to reasonably address the teaching requirements of the programme. Special consideration should be given to the development of this aspect in the future faculty of academic programmes and a specific evaluation of this attribute needs to be done at the time of recruitment to match the needs of the programme with those of the faculty (Brennan and Shah 2000).

Another important consideration is the balance between the service and academic demands of the programme. Most academic activities in this day and age need some time for the proper assessment of trainees and the documentation of this assessment should make a meaningful conclusion about their progress. Any recruitment should have a built-in compensation for the academic contribution of the faculty otherwise it may result in disillusion and poor outcomes.

**B. Enhancement and appraisal of teaching capacities**

Faculty development is one of the most important factors that affects medical education. The faculty in academic programmes should be provided adequate resources to further enhance their teaching capabilities. Modern challenges such as limited working hours for the trainees and evolving teaching and learning methods including competency-based curricula may pose a serious challenge for the faculty of busy clinical programmes. Any change in curricula needs to have a special focus on faculty development to sustain and enhance the change, otherwise, it is doomed to fail without exception. The use of modern technology may also be a challenge for the older group of teachers including the use of e-learning methods, blended learning, and online assessments. Moreover, the assessment methods in academic training have been evolving over the years and there has been a lot more focus on workplace-based assessment methods, which may be a relatively new concept for some faculty members (Bettaz and Kamal 2019; Badran, Baydoun and Hillman 2019).

It is strongly recommended that all new faculty should be oriented to the academic needs of the programmes at the time of induction. They may also be given an essential refresher course to enhance their teaching-learning skills and to familiarize them with the recent changes in academic settings. The institutes should identify the development processes that have proven to be successful, and identify new needs to meet the demands of the evolving medical education – demands which may not be addressed by traditional methods. Also, the academic institutions need to develop an academic plan for the pedagogical development of their faculty on a regular basis.

The yearly appraisal reports should include evaluation of the faculty by the learners with special emphasis on formative feedback to the faculty on the positive and negative aspects. If serious deficiencies are identified in certain academic aspects, they should be addressed on a priority basis by providing opportunities for academic development. There is evolving evidence to suggest that faculty development and accreditation have largely been under-developed in countries like Pakistan (Arif et al. 2019).

**C. Recertification and continuous faculty development**

The concept of recertification for faculty is more closely related to the healthcare disciplines than any other specialized field. The purpose of recertification after a certain time is well developed in the United States as compared to other countries (American Board of Physician Specialties 2021; National Board for Professional Teaching Standards 2021). The process usually involves a summative assessment and the purpose of the periodic recertification is to ensure that the physicians have updated knowledge in their specialties and can offer the best possible care to their patients. The alternate approach used in this regard is to ensure that physicians should demonstrate that they have been involved in the process of continuous professional development for the minimum subscribed hours, resulting in the development of maintenance of certification programmes.

While such processes have been developed for physicians, no such requirements have been established for the quality assurance of the faculty of academic programmes. This may be a novel approach to address the quality assurance of teaching faculty with regards to their academic standards as teachers and needs to be explored further.

## IV. Quality assurance and accreditation in Pakistan

Pakistan is a developing country with huge healthcare needs and limited resources. The first private medical school in Pakistan opened in 1983. Between 1997 and 2005, the total number of medical schools doubled; currently there are 117 approved medical schools, 72 of which are private (Amin et al. 2010).

The Pakistan Medical Commission (PMC) is the sole authority for accrediting, regulating, and ensuring the quality of undergraduate medical and dental education in Pakistan (Pakistan Medical Commission 2021). The PMC uses standards or "regulations" to evaluate a medical college. Traditionally, the accreditation process in Pakistani medical colleges has focused predominantly on the evaluation of physical infrastructure and the number of faculty only, instead of educational processes and outcome measurements (Khan et al. 2020).

Accreditation of postgraduate programmes in Pakistan is mainly a function of the CPSP which was established in 1962 by a special act of the parliament of Pakistan. The CPSP offers accreditation and certification for various postgraduate training programmes in medicine, surgery, and dentistry. CPSP is currently the only postgraduate medical examination body in Pakistan and awards the membership degree in 22 programmes and fellowship degree in 73 specialties. The CPSP also offers sub-specialization in certain areas known as second fellowships.

The CPSP has devised a process for accreditation of various training programmes and training institutions across the country. The process involves an application for accreditation by the programme which includes basic data on the physical infrastructure, teaching-learning facilities, academic resources, and the supervising faculty. Once the data is reviewed, a physical visit of the site is made by the CPSP representatives to ensure compliance with the stipulated requirements. Once the accreditation status has been achieved, the programmes can enrol the trainees who must be registered with the CPSP and complete certain mandatory training and assessment requirements. The CPSP has also developed a framework for logbook and competencies for various levels of training, but compliance with these standards remains the responsibility of the individual supervising faculty already registered with the CPSP. After programme accreditation, there are no rigorous processes for ongoing monitoring and re-visits by the CPSP to ensure compliance with their requirements and this may result in serious deficiencies in the absence of strong internal institutional guidelines.

Accreditation fosters quality improvement, transparency, and above all, public trust (Davis and Ringsted 2006). The current model of accreditation is unable to meet the challenges faced by medical education, i.e., the global drive towards adopting outcomes-based curricula, and the integration of technology and e-learning. This requires redefining standards as measures of quality and embracing rigorous processes of evaluation and accreditation that are in line with the regional and global standards. It is important to substantiate medical education accreditation standards and provide evidence to validate the decisions made by the various accrediting agencies that utilize these standards. While national accreditation may be a legal requirement, internationally recognized accreditation has become the gold standard procedure of quality assurance in medical education (Sayek and Karle 2007; MacCarrick, Kelly and Conroy 2010). Pakistan should aim for evaluation and certification by the international accrediting agencies such as the WFME or ACGME. Studies have shown significant changes in the educational processes, administration, and implementation of the curriculum and monitoring of learning outcomes as a result of the accreditation process itself (Al Mohaimeed et al. 2012).

## V. Programme evaluation process for postgraduate programmes at the Aga Khan University

The Aga Khan University (AKU) was the first private medical university in Pakistan. It was established in 1983 with an international mandate and has campuses across 6 countries and 3 continents. The AKU campus on Stadium Road in Karachi is the largest campus of the university and consists of a Medical College, the School of Nursing and Midwifery, and a state of the art tertiary care University Hospital. An impact study conducted by the US-based Centennial Group International concluded that AKU has an annual economic impact of US$1 billion in Pakistan and supports 42,000 jobs per annum (The Aga Khan University 2017). Moreover, AKU was ranked among the top 100 universities for clinical medicine in the Shanghai Ranking of Academic Subjects 2019 released by the Academic Ranking of World Universities (The Aga Khan University 2019).

Apart from the flagship MBBS program, AKU offers numerous graduate and postgraduate programmes including a PhD programme in health sciences. Given the huge economic and academic impact of the university, AKU has established certain internal standards for quality assurance and standardization of its academic programmes. Postgraduate Medical Education (PGME) programmes at AKU were initiated in 1986 and the Department of PGME at AKU was established in 1995. PGME at AKU currently offers a total of 70 postgraduate programmes including a yearlong internship programme, 34 residency programmes, and 35 fellowship programmes. All of AKU's residency programmes and 17 fellowship programmes are currently accredited with the CPSP. The vision statement of AKU PGME states that "Postgraduate Medical Education at AKU strives to instil critical thinking and analysis into its graduates to promote evidence-based health care and research abiding by the principles of ethics and professionalism" (The Aga Khan University 2021). Each programme is carefully structured to produce skilled technologists and to facilitate a process of broad professional and personal development.

For the purpose of quality assurance, an internal process for the development and approval of new academic programmes has been devised for PGME at AKU. The programme proposal developed by the programme faculty is submitted to the PGME office after an internal faculty review. The submitted application is reviewed by the PGME sub-committee on programme review and then submitted for an independent external review by at least three faculty members including two subject experts and at least one expert in medical education. The feedback provided by the independent reviewers is collated by the PGME office and usually results in a significant revision of the programme proposal, leading to its academic enhancement. Once approved by the PGME office, the proposal is forwarded to the university leadership as well as the national accreditation bodies, as appropriate.

In addition to the programme approval and accreditation by CPSP, a process for regular evaluation of AKU's PGME programmes has also been developed. The internal review process conducted by the PGME office at AKU is quite extensive and a step-wise process. The first step consists of the completion of the Programme Information Form (PIF) by the programme director. The PIF form is quite a detailed review of the programme and its salient contents are listed in Figure 15-1.

**PGME Program Information Form (PIF)**

- Basic Program Information – program director / faculty
- Department Residency Committee – membership, meetings & minutes, agenda
- Candidate selection process, numbers & attrition
- Stated goals and objectives of the program
- Curriculum, Teaching learning & Scholarship
- Weekly academic schedule – didactic & clinical
- Working hours, on-call days & rotations
- Supervision and the learning environment
- Process of trainee assessment and feedback
- Process of summative assessment and promotion
- Compliance to quality processes of the institution
- Compliance to the requirements of the accreditation bodies
- Teaching and learning of the core competencies
- Adequacy of academic resources including library, internet and scholarly supervision
- Adequacy of training resources including patients, laboratory and technology
- Process of faculty evaluation & grievance
- Academic output of the program – presentations, publications and academic travels
- Academic success rate including pass rate for the exit examinations

Fig. 15-1: Salient features of the Programme Information Form.

This is followed by the nomination of the review committee consisting of the identified programme faculty and programme trainee representative, as well as at least one faculty member from another programme. The committee reviews the PIF form and the provided documentary evidence, which is then followed by meetings with the trainees, programme faculty, staff, and programme director. The review committee submits its report to the PGME office where a further evaluation of the programme is conducted and comparisons are made across the programme. The external review, on the other hand, reviews the programmes as well as the learning environment and resources offered by the institution for its academic programmes. Both the internal and external reviews compare the outcomes of the programmes with their stated goals and objectives, provide an overview of the overall impact of the programmes, and also identify their strengths, weaknesses, opportunities, and potential threats to them. Different evaluation templates have been used by the PGME office for the internal review of its programmes, but templates are usually based on the standards set by the ACGME. Recently, an extensive self-review of some of the university's PGME programmes was conducted in terms of the WFME's published standards for postgraduate programmes.

As noted from Figure 15-2, the PGME programmes have undergone several review processes conducted by the internal programme faculty as well as external faculty of international repute.

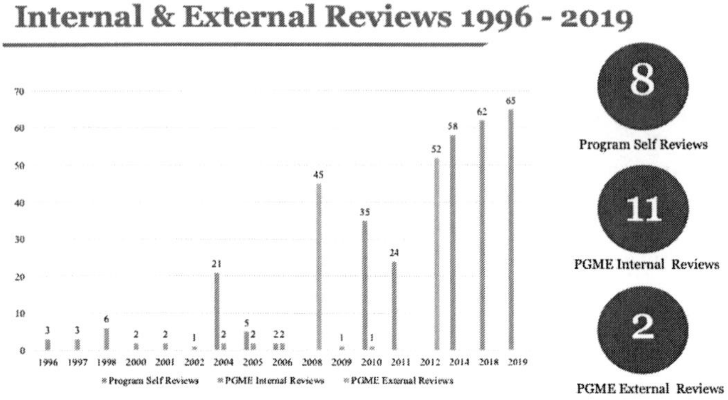


Fig. 15-1: Internal and external reviews of PGME programmes at AKU.

Such processes have helped our programmes to refine curricula, including their teaching-learning and assessment strategies. The outcomes of such reviews have also helped us in improving the quality of life of our trainees (and increasing their remuneration), impacting their mental wellbeing. Aga Khan University Hospital has been accredited with the Joint Commission International (JCI) since 2006 and was re-accredited as an academic medical centre in the year 2018. The annual review of PGME programmes is also a requirement of JCI and AKU has been in regular compliance in this regard.

Apart from internal and external evaluations, AKU has recently shifted its focus to the accreditation of its programmes by the international arm of ACGME. ACGME-I is a global accreditation body that verifies that medical education institutions, as well as their postgraduate programmes for residents and fellows, meet the highest academic standards. By improving the quality of teaching, learning, research, and professional practice, ACGME-I seeks to improve healthcare that ultimately benefits the public. This is an extensive, multi-step process, and involves multiple stakeholders including PGME trainees.

## VI. Conclusions

Medical education in the 21st century presents challenges to quality assurance that were unimaginable just a quarter of a century ago. Quality assurance and accreditation in the 21st century will require a consensus on the set of "universal" attributes or standards of a quality educational experience, a focus on the learner rather than the institution, and a willingness to open the entire process up to a much broader group of stakeholders. The process may be evolving and not a true science, but an investment in the quality assurance of academic programmes is a true investment into the future of communities.

## Bibliography

Abdalla, Mohamed Elhassan. *Accreditation in Medical Education: Concepts and Practice.* Jazan: Faculty of Medicine, Jazan University, 2012.

Accreditation Council for Graduate Medical Education. "About us." Accessed February 25, 2021. URL: https://www.acgme.org/About-Us/Overview.

ACGME International. ACGME-I Mission. Accessed February, 25, 2021. URL: https://www.acgme-i.org/.

Aga Khan University. About Postgraduate Medical Education at AKU. Accessed February, 02, 2021. URL: https://www.aku.edu/mcpk/pgme/Pages/vision.aspx.

Aga Khan University. "Shanghai Ranking: AKU ranks in the top 100 global universities". Accessed February 25, 2021. URL: https://www.aku.edu/news/Pages/News_Details.aspx?nid=NEWS-001884.

Aga Khan University. "AKU's Economic Impacts in Pakistan" 2017. Accessed February 02, 2021. URL: https://reports.aku.edu/PakistanImpactStudy/.

Al Mohaimeed, AbdulRahman, Farid Midhet, Issam Barrimah, and Mohamed Nour-El-Din Saleh. "Academic Accreditation Process: Experience of a Medical College in Saudi Arabia." *International journal of health sciences* 6, no. 1 (Jan 2012): 23. DOI: 10.12816/0005970.

American Board of Physician Specialties. "Physician Board Recertification Standards." Accessed February, 02, 2021. URL: https://www.abpsus.org/physician-board-recertification-standards/.

Amin, Zubair, William P. Burdick, Avinash Supe, and Tejinder Singh. "Relevance of the Flexner Report to Contemporary Medical Education in South Asia." *Academic Medicine* 85, no. 2 (February 2010): 333-39. DOI: 10.1097/ACM.0b013e3181c874cb.

Arif, Seema, Zunaira Liaqat, and Ayesha Afzal. "Quality Assurance & Accreditation of Teacher Education in Pakistan." *UMT Education Review* 2, no. 1 (2019): 01-21. DOI: https://doi.org/10.32350/uer.21.01.

Badran, Adnan, Elias Baydoun, and John R. Hillman. *Major Challenges Facing Higher Education in the Arab World: Quality Assurance and Relevance.* Switzerland: Springer, 2019.

Balmer, Dorene F., Jennifer A. Rama, and Deborah Simpson. "Program Evaluation Models: Evaluating Processes and Outcomes in Graduate Medical Education." *Journal of graduate medical education* 11, no. 1 (February 2019): 99-100. DOI: https://doi.org/10.4300/JGME-D-18-01084.1.

Bettaz, Mohamed, and Marwan Kamal. "On the Quality Assurance of Faculty Members." In *Major Challenges Facing Higher Education in the Arab World: Quality Assurance and Relevance*, 277-88: Switzerland: Springer, 2019.

Boor, Klarke, Cees Van Der Vleuten, Pim Teunissen, Albert Scherpbier, and Fedde Scheele. "Development and Analysis of D-Rect, an Instrument Measuring Residents' Learning Climate." *Medical teacher* 33, no. 10 (February 2011): 820-27. DOI: https://doi.org/10.3109/0142159X.2010.541533.

Brennan, John, and Tarla Shah. *Managing Quality in Higher Education: An International Perspective on Institutional Assessment and Change.* Buckingham, UK: Open University Press, 2000.

Cate, Olle ten, Linda Snell, and Carol Carraccio. "Medical Competence: The Interplay between Individual Ability and the Health Care Environment." *Medical teacher* 32, no. 8 (July 2010): 669-75. DOI: https://doi.org/10.3109/0142159X.2010.500897.

Clapham, Michael, David Wall, and Anna Batchelor. "Educational Environment in Intensive Care Medicine—Use of Postgraduate Hospital Educational Environment Measure (Pheem)." *Medical teacher* 29, no. 6 (Jul 2007): e184-e91. DOI: https://doi.org/10.1080/01421590701288580.

Cook, David A. "Twelve Tips for Evaluating Educational Programs." *Medical teacher* 32, no. 4 (March 2010): 296-301. DOI: https://doi.org/10.3109/01421590903480121.

College of Physicians and Surgeons Pakistan. About CPSP. Accessed February, 25, 2021. URL: https://www.cpsp.edu.pk/about-cpsp.php.

Davis, Deborah J., and Charlotte Ringsted. "Accreditation of Undergraduate and Graduate Medical Education: How Do the Standards Contribute to Quality?" *Advances in health sciences education* 11, no. 3 (August 2006): 305-13. DOI: 10.1007/s10459-005-8555-4.

Dolmans, D. H. J. M., I. H. A. P. Wolfhagen, Erik Heineman, and A. J. J. A. Scherpbier. "Factors Adversely Affecting Student Learning in the Clinical Learning Environment: A Student Perspective." *Education for Health* 21, no. 3 (February 2008): 32. URL: https://www.educationforhealth.net/text.asp?2008/21/3/32/101553.

Durning, Steven J., Paul Hemmer, and Louis N. Pangaro. "The Structure of Program Evaluation: An Approach for Evaluating a Course, Clerkship, or Components of a Residency or Fellowship Training Program." *Teaching and learning in medicine* 19, no. 3 (December 2007): 308-18. DOI: https://doi.org/10.1080/10401330701366796.

European Association for Quality Assurance in Higher Education (ENQA), European Students' Union (ESU), European University Association (EUA), European Association of Institutions in Higher Education (EURASHE), Education International (EI) and BUSINESSEUROPE. *Standards and Guidelines for Quality Assurance in the European Higher Education Area (ESG).* Brussels, Belgium: EURASHE, 2015.

Frye, Ann W., and Paul A. Hemmer. "Program Evaluation Models and Related Theories: Amee Guide No. 67." *Medical teacher* 34, no. 5 (April 2012): e288-e99. DOI: https://doi.org/10.3109/0142159X.2012.668637.

General Medical Council. Registration and licensing. Accessed February, 25, 2021. URL: https://www.gmc-uk.org/registration-and-licensing/.

Genn, J. M. "Amee Medical Education Guide No. 23 (Part 1): Curriculum, Environment, Climate, Quality and Change in Medical Education–a Unifying Perspective." *Medical teacher* 23, no. 4 (July 2001): 337-44. DOI: https://doi.org/10.1080/01421590120063330.

Gibson, Kathryn A., Patrick Boyle, Deborah A. Black, Margaret Cunningham, Michael C. Grimm, and H. Patrick McNeil. "Enhancing Evaluation in an Undergraduate Medical Education Program." *Academic Medicine* 83, no. 8 (August 2008): 787-93. DOI: 10.1097/ACM.0b013e31817eb8ab.

Goldie, John. "Amee Education Guide No. 29: Evaluating Educational Programmes." *Medical Teacher* 28, no. 3 (July 2006): 210-24. DOI: https://doi.org/10.1080/01421590500271282.

Goldstein, Naomi. "Chapter 2: What is program evaluation?" In *The Program Manager's Guide to Evaluation*, 6-10. Washington, DC: Office of Planning, Research and Evaluation, Administration Administration for Children and Families, 2010.

Hafler, Janet P., Allison R. Ownby, Britta M. Thompson, Carl E. Fasser, Kevin Grigsby, Paul Haidet, Marc J. Kahn, and Frederic W. Hafferty. "Decoding the Learning Environment of Medical Education: A Hidden Curriculum Perspective for Faculty Development." *Academic Medicine* 86, no. 4 (April 2011): 440-44. DOI: 10.1097/ACM.0b013e31820df8e2.

Hajifathali, A., M. Noori Avarzamani, A. M. Niaie and E. Negahban. "External Evaluation: A Requirement for Accountability and Responsiveness." *Journal of Medical Education* 8, no. 2 (September 2006): e105248. DOI: 10.22037/jme.v8i2.743.

Harvey, Lee. "Evaluation for What?" *Teaching in higher education* 7, no. 3 (August 2002): 245-63. DOI: https://doi.org/10.1080/13562510220144761.

Harvey, Lee. "Quality Assurance in Higher Education: Some International Trends." Paper presented at the *Higher Education Conference, Oslo*, 22-23 January *2002*. URL: https://www.qualityresearchinternational.com/Harvey%20papers/Harvey%202002%20Some%20International%20Trends,%20Oslo.pdf.

Harvey, Lee. "The Power of Accreditation: Views of Academics." *Journal of Higher Education Policy and Management* 26, no. 2 (January 2004): 207-23. DOI: https://doi.org/10.1080/1360080042000218267.

Hoffman, Kimberly G., and Joe F. Donaldson. "Contextual Tensions of the Clinical Environment and Their Influence on Teaching and Learning." *Medical education* 38, no. 4 (February 2004): 448-54. DOI: https://doi.org/10.1046/j.1365-2923.2004.01799.x.

Holt, M. C., and Sue Roff. "Development and Validation of the Anaesthetic Theatre Educational Environment Measure (Ateem)." *Medical teacher* 26, no. 6 (June 2004): 553-58. DOI: https://doi.org/10.1080/01421590410001711599.

Jennings, M. L., and Stuart J. Slavin. "Resident Wellness Matters: Optimizing Resident Education and Wellness through the Learning Environment." *Academic Medicine* 90, no. 9 (September 2015): 1246-50. DOI: 10.1097/ACM.0000000000000842.

Joshi, Medha A. "Quality Assurance in Medical Education." *Indian Journal of Pharmacology* 44, no. 3 (May-June 2012): 285. DOI: 10.4103/0253-7613.96295.

Karle, Hans. "Global Standards and Accreditation in Medical Education: A View from the Wfme." *Academic medicine* 81, no. 12 (December 2006): S43-S48. DOI: 10.1097/01.ACM.0000243383.71047.c4.

Karle, Hans. "International Trends in Medical Education: Diversification Contra Convergence." *Medical Teacher* 26, no. 3 (July 2004): 205-206. DOI: https://doi.org/10.1080/01421590410001667418.

Khan, Abdul Waheed, Ahsan Sethi, Gohar Wajid, and Raheela Yasmeen. "Challenges Towards Quality Assurance of Basic Medical Education in Pakistan." *Pakistan Journal Of Medical Sciences* 36, no. 2 (January-February 2020): 4. DOI: 10.12669/pjms.36.2.1319.

Kim, Yongnam, and Peter Steiner. "Quasi-Experimental Designs for Causal Inference." *Educational Psychologist* 51, no. 3-4 (September 2016): 395-405. DOI: https://doi.org/10.1080/00461520.2016.1207177.

Lilley, P. M., and R. M. Harden. "Standards and Medical Education." *Medical Teacher* 25, no. 4 (July 2003): 349-51. DOI: 10.1080/01421590310001595581.

Ludmerer, Kenneth M. "Commentary: Understanding the Flexner Report." *Academic Medicine* 85, no. 2 (February 2010): 193-96. DOI: 10.1097/ACM.0b013e3181c8f1e7.

MacCarrick, Geraldine, Cathal Kelly, and Ronan Conroy. "Preparing for an Institutional Self Review Using the Wfme Standards–an International Medical School Case Study." *Medical teacher* 32, no. 5 (April 2010): e227-e32. DOI: https://doi.org/10.3109/0142159X.2010.482396.

National Board for Professional Teaching Standards. Maintenance of Certification. Accessed February, 25, 2021. URL: https://www.nbpts.org/national-board-certification/maintenance-of-certification/.

Nasca, Thomas J., Kevin B. Weiss, and James P. Bagian. "Improving Clinical Learning Environments for Tomorrow's Physicians." *N. Engl. J. Med.* 370, no. 11 (March 2014): 991-93. DOI: 10.1056/NEJMp1314628.

Pakistan Medical Commission. Recognized Colleges & Qualifications. Accessed February, 25, 2021. URL: https://www.pmc.gov.pk/Colleges.

Papp, Inkeri, Marjatta Markkanen, and Mikaela von Bonsdorff. "Clinical Environment as a Learning Environment: Student Nurses' Perceptions Concerning Clinical Learning Experiences." *Nurse Education Today* 23, no. 4 (May 2003): 262-68. DOI: https://doi.org/10.1016/S0260-6917(02)00185-5.

Riquelme, Arnoldo, Oslando Padilla, Cristian Herrera, Trinidad Olivos, José Antonio Román, Alberto Sarfatis, Nancy Solís, et al. "Development of Acleem Questionnaire, an Instrument Measuring

Residents' Educational Environment in Postgraduate Ambulatory Setting." *Medical Teacher* 35, no. 1 (September 2013): e861-e66. DOI: https://doi.org/10.3109/0142159X.2012.714882.

Roff, S. U. E., Sean McAleer, Ronald M. Harden, Mona Al-Qahtani, Ashraf Uddin Ahmed, Horacio Deza, Guido Groenen, and Praorn Primparyon. "Development and Validation of the Dundee Ready Education Environment Measure (Dreem)." *Medical teacher* 19, no. 4 (July 1997): 295-99. DOI: https://doi.org/10.3109/01421599709034208.

Roff, Sue, Sean McAleer, O. S. Ifere, and Soumya Bhattacharya. "A Global Diagnostic Tool for Measuring Educational Environment: Comparing Nigeria and Nepal." *Medical Teacher* 23, no. 4 (July 2001): 378-82. DOI: https://doi.org/10.1080/01421590120043080.

Royal College of Physicians and Surgeons of Canada. General Standards of Accreditation for Residency Programs. Accessed February, 02, 2021. URL: https://www.royalcollege.ca/rcsite/documents/canera/general-standards-accreditation-for-residency-programs-e.

Sayek, Iskender, and Hans Karle. "Quality Assurance Standards Task Force Global Standards: Route for Accreditation in Medical Education in Europe." *Turkish Journal of Medical Sciences* 37, no. 5 (October 2007): 257. URL: https://journals.tubitak.gov.tr/medical/issues/sag-07-37-5/sag-37-5-1-0710-5.pdf.

Schiekirka, Sarah, Markus A. Feufel, Christoph Herrmann-Lingen, and Tobias Raupach. "Evaluation in Medical Education: A Topical Review of Target Parameters, Data Collection Tools and Confounding Factors." *GMS German Medical Science* 13, Doc 15 (September 2015). DOI: 10.3205/000219.

Smidt, Andy, Susan Balandin, Jeff Sigafoos, and Vicki A. Reed. "The Kirkpatrick Model: A Useful Tool for Evaluating Training Outcomes." *Journal of Intellectual and Developmental Disability* 34, no. 3 (September 2009): 266-74. DOI: https://doi.org/10.1080/13668250903093125.

Soemantri, Diantha, Cristian Herrera, and Arnoldo Riquelme. "Measuring the Educational Environment in Health Professions Studies: A Systematic Review." *Medical teacher* 32, no. 12 (November 2010): 947-52. DOI: https://doi.org/10.3109/01421591003686229.

Spencer, John. "Learning and Teaching in the Clinical Environment." *BMJ* 326, no. 7389 (March 2003): 591-94. DOI: https://doi.org/10.1136/bmj.326.7389.591.

Standing Committee on Postgraduate Medical and Dental Education. *Appraising Doctors and Dentists in Training: A Scopme Working Paper for Consultation*. London: SCOPME, 1996.

Stensaker, Bjørn. "Trance, Transparency and Transformation: The Impact of External Quality Monitoring on Higher Education." *Quality in higher education* 9, no. 2 (August 2003): 151-59. DOI: https://doi.org/10.1080/13538320308158.

Strand, Pia, Karolina Sjöborg, Renée Stalmeijer, Gitte Wichmann-Hansen, Ulf Jakobsson, and Gudrun Edgren. "Development and Psychometric Evaluation of the Undergraduate Clinical Education Environment Measure (Uceem)." *Medical Teacher* 35, no. 12 (September 2013): 1014-26. DOI: https://doi.org/10.3109/0142159X.2013.835389.

Stufflebeam, Daniel L. "The Cipp Model for Evaluation." In *Evaluation Models: Viewpoints on Educational and Human Services Evaluation*, 279-317. Dordrecht: Springer Netherlands, 2000.

Sullivan, Louis W., and Ilana Suez Mittman. "The State of Diversity in the Health Professions a Century after Flexner." *Academic Medicine* 85, no. 2 (February 2010): 246-53. DOI: 10.1097/ACM.0b013e3181c88145.

Szanto, Tibor R. "Evaluations of the Third Kind: External Evaluations of External Quality Assurance Agencies." *Quality in Higher Education* 11, no. 3 (January 2005): 183-93. DOI: https://doi.org/10.1080/13538320500329509.

Till, Hettie. "Climate Studies: Can Students' Perceptions of the Ideal Educational Environment Be of Use for Institutional Planning and Resource Utilization?" *Medical Teacher* 27, no. 4 (July 2005): 332-37. DOI: https://doi.org/10.1080/01421590400029723.

Vroeijenstijn, A. I. "Quality Assurance in Medical Education." *Academic Medicine: Journal of the Association of American Medical Colleges* 70, Suppl. 7 (July 1995): S59-67; discussion S68. DOI: 10.1097/00001888-199507000-00021.

Weiss, Kevin B., James P. Bagian, and Thomas J. Nasca. "The Clinical Learning Environment: The Foundation of Graduate Medical Education." *JAMA* 309, no. 16 (April 2013): 1687-88 DOI: 10.1001/jama.2013.1931.

Whittle, S. R., B. Whelan, and D. G. Murdoch-Eaton. "Dreem and Beyond; Studies of the Educational Environment as a Means for Its Enhancement." *Education for health* 20, no. 1 (April 2007): 7. URL: https://www.educationforhealth.net/text.asp?2007/20/1/7/101640.

Wilkes, Michael, Christine Cassel, and Marc Klau. "If We Keep Doing What We're Doing We'll Keep Getting What We're Getting: A Need

to Rethink 'Academic' Medicine." *Medical Teacher* 40, no. 4 (January 2018): 364-71. DOI: https://doi.org/10.1080/0142159X.2017.1417580.
World Federation for Medical Education. Basic Medical Education. WFME Global Standards for Quality Improvement. Copenhagen: WFME 2003. URL: http://www.wfme.org.
World Federation for Medical Education. Postgraduate Medical Education. WFME Global Standards for Quality Improvement. Copenhagen: WFME 2003. URL: http://www.wfme.org.
World Federation for Medical Education. Continuing Professional Development (CPD) of Medical Doctors. Global Standards for Quality Improvement. Copenhagen: WFME 2003. URL: http://www.wfme.org.
Zanten, Marta Van, John R. Boulet, and Ian Greaves. "The Importance of Medical Education Accreditation Standards." *Medical teacher* 34, no. 2 (January 2012): 136-45. DOI: https://doi.org/10.3109/0142159X.2012.643261.

# CHAPTER 16

# SIGNIFICANCE OF MULTI-DISCIPLINARY TEAM (MDT) TUMOR BOARDS IN SURGICAL ONCOLOGY PG TRAINING

AHMED NADEEM ABBASI
AND BILAL MAZHAR QURESHI

Medical education has evolved a long way from conventional apprenticeship training to modern day structured training and education programmes. While technology and innovation have enhanced medical and surgical practices for better patient care, there has been an increase in the utility of multidisciplinary team working and the acceptance of its utility for deciding standard treatment to cancer patients. The multidisciplinary team (MDT) tumour boards have been a venture not only for better patient care, but also an opportunity for postgraduate trainees to understand principles of decision making in oncology.

Site specific multidisciplinary tumour boards play a pivotal role in the provision of high-quality comprehensive cancer care. This dictum has been thoroughly validated via a number of studies conducted across the world. In our region, our team of cancer carers came forward and have tried to establish site specific MDTs in various institutes of the country and region. As expected, many hurdles of a varied nature were encountered by our team and we are still travellers on this journey which we have started on voluntary basis. Site specific teams conduct this activity and maintain the quality of these boards (Boniface et al. 2016).

Our multidisciplinary tumour boards are constantly evolving. Starting off with general tumour boards to the development of site specific tumour boards to the use of videoconferencing (Dickson-Witmer et al. 2008), the MDT tumour board process is continuously being refined to improve the contribution it provides to the cancer care process.

A positive change in clinical practice is being observed and documented across the globe. Although now well established in many parts of the world for decades, in Pakistan we are in the phase of establishment of this activity and published data are scarce (Lamb et al. 2011). Without much to go by, it may be safe to say that, generally, the incorporation of these meetings at hospitals providing cancer care is still a work in progress. The fresh talent entering the healthcare system from medical colleges provides an opportunity to improve this current state.

The scientific evidence shows that MDT tumour boards have been shown to alter management decisions (Wheless, McKinney, and Zanation 2010) and reduce costs (Look Hong et al. 2010). The success of MDT tumour boards depends on the active and efficient participation of clinicians and effective management by hospital administration to make them productive, taking into account the time and effort that is needed (Jalil et al. 2013). A study from the United Kingdom identified the participation of key members, provision of description of patient related factors, use of proformas or checklists and patient selection for discussion as important considerations for a successful MDT tumour board (Wright et al. 2009). Another study in Canada presented more administrative support, introduction of billing and videoconferencing as suggestions to improve meetings (Brar et al. 2014). Studies have also shown that identifying areas of weakness and subsequent measures of intervention can have a positive impact (Brar et al. 2014). Using the multidisciplinary model, the University of Colorado Hospital has been able to successfully establish multiple site specific clinics where patients have all their required tests, cases discussed and meet the specialists involved all within a period of one to two days (Abbasi 2011).

Centres around the world continue to improve the multidisciplinary process to gain more benefit from it and improve the standard of care for their cancer patients, though we continue to lag behind. We hope to see MDT tumour boards established in all institutes of Pakistan where cancer care is being provided (Kurpad et al. 2011).

Practice change requires the thorough critical appraisal of contemporary scientific evidence. We are living in an era of rapid technological advancement. Nowadays, offering best management to our cancer patients is still a complex challenge where all avenues of potential benefit must be fully assessed. MDT tumour boards provide one such avenue. They have been shown not only to alter disease management (Boniface et al. 2016), but also improve patient survival (Forrest et al. 2005). Not only being of benefit to the patient, they also provide experience to specialists on how to combine treatments along with being a valuable teaching tool for medical students and junior doctors alike (Abdulrahman 2011).

Across the world MDT tumour board meetings have been shown to yield clinically beneficial outcomes. A study conducted in the UK showed a three year survival jump from 58% to 66% in patients with Duke C stage colorectal cancer by introduction of the MDT (MacDermid et al. 2009) tumour board, while a study in Australia showed a mean improvement in survival in patients with inoperable non-small cell lung cancer from 205 days to 280 days, when comparing with cases discussed in an MDT tumour board meeting with those that were not (Bydder et al. 2009). Thus their benefit can be demonstrated regardless of place or specialty. These meetings are gradually being conducted by centres treating cancer patients in Pakistan and statistics released by the City Tumour Board (CTB) Karachi showed that of the 264 cases presented between March 2010 and March 2012, the initial treatment management plan was changed in 70% of them (Asghar et al. 2013; Fader et al. 1998). Along with improving decision making and outcomes, MDT tumour boards have shown to drastically decrease the cost of treatment. Establishment of the University of Michigan Multidisciplinary Melanoma Clinic (UM-MDMC) saved third party payers roughly $1600 per patient by improving the way resources were used (Fader et al. 1998). The reduced cost is of exceptional importance in places such as Pakistan where it is a major limiting factor in the delivery of effective treatment options.

Developing countries will not be able to attain the same high standards of comprehensive cancer care if they fail to establish site specific multidisciplinary teams in their countries. While advising our colleagues on the establishment of these multidisciplinary boards, we recommended the frequency of weekly boards with the full back up of a committee overseeing their quality standards and acting as a mechanism of robust monitoring. Introduction of quality indicators and full auditing is obviously not possible in non-mandatory processes; therefore, it is now high time to develop these site specific boards as a compulsory activity and essential component embedded in every cancer carer's job role and description.

Comprehensive cancer care and management require a well-planned strategy. At the planning stage, all areas of potential benefit are being explored by healthcare providers. Establishment of site specific MDT tumour boards is an important and integral component of a patient centred plan (Barry and Edgman-Levitan 2012) of service development worldwide (El Saghir et al. 2014) across all disciplines which are involved in oncological treatment (Abbasi et al. 2016; Schmieder, Keilholz, and Combs 2016) .

The dictum postulating that tumour boards save the lives of cancer patients is a validated narrative and we hope that site specific multidisciplinary tumour boards will be established in all healthcare facilities providing care to cancer patients. The importance of these meetings, of implementing clinical practice guidelines and developing cancer care clinical pathways, has already been established (Kostaras et al. 2012).

Cancers require multidisciplinary management; treatment of adenocarcinoma of the rectum, for instance, should include a sequential approach to the use of local radiotherapy, systemic chemotherapy, and complex surgery. Educational activities like continuous medical education (CME) enhance the agreement of specialists from various disciplines to adhere to evidence based standards of care. A formal approach of education to enhance the multidisciplinary approach has already been proven for improved patient care (Phang et al. 2011).

It is always useful to understand the effects and outcome of non-surgical treatment through multidisciplinary tumour board meetings. The knowledge gained through these forums can help comprehend the level of expertise required for other essential treatment modalities, the effect on the quality of life of patients and the usefulness of improving the treatment outcome (Bossi and Alfieri 2016). Advancements in each of these modalities has led to improved patient outcomes like quality of life, survival and reducing toxicity, besides going through a complex course of treatments. Nowadays, patient support groups are available which help the patient through a multidisciplinary supportive team. They have definitely helped in understanding and addressing the unmet needs of patients and further improving upon these areas (Nguyen and Ringash 2018).

Multidisciplinary and interdisciplinary education for the diverse management of cancer patients remains important for healthcare professionals (McAvoy, Fletcher, and Elwood 2007). These concepts are even being utilised for programmes like cancer prevention (Teegarden et al. 2011). This is now recognised as an essential component of the oncology curriculum in undergraduate programmes, and is incorporated formally through various means into the curriculum (Ha and Parakh 2018). Interdisciplinary learning has been recognised as an important method within various domains including case discussion, small group collaboration and hands on experience of dialogues between different specialties (Murgu et al. 2018). Multidisciplinary rounds have been utilised for education and understanding of decision making in other specialties of oncology resulting in the enhanced learning of junior doctors (Szumacher et al. 2003). The effectiveness of interdisciplinary learning has been determined successfully in different programmes. Learning from the thinking and decision making process of other specialties provides food for thought, builds up communication and understanding and at the same time generates new ideas (Brenner et al. 2014).

The modern approach of cancer management requires decisions pertaining to the diagnosis of malignancy, appropriate staging and pre-treatment work up, choosing and sequencing the essential treatment modality and devising a follow up strategy, all to be discussed and decided in a multidisciplinary forum. This provides an opportunity for cross-disciplinary training of the surgeons who are often at the forefront. This is being endorsed and adapted by authorities in Europe at large (Benstead et al. 2017).

Core training of a particular surgical specialty may not provide enough of an opportunity to a postgraduate doctor to enable him or her to achieve proficiency to manage cancer patients requiring a definite multidisciplinary approach. This includes malignancies like breast cancer, which is now considered as a systemic disease requiring simultaneous input from pathology, radiology, genetics, medical oncology and radiation oncology. This has been studied from an educational point of view by trainees and programmes and the need of exposure to multidisciplinary ventures have been emphasised (Park et al. 2020). The requirement of a multidisciplinary team approach and these meetings as part of surgical oncology training has been incorporated into various educational programmes endorsed by many national and international societies (Kolacinska 2017).

Reflective practice of learning has established its role in postgraduate medical education. Formal, didactic teaching methodology has often been criticised in recent times for its limitations and lack of interest-based acquisition of knowledge for adult postgraduate learners. Multidisciplinary meetings provide an opportunity for students to learn the strategy of incorporating the perspective of other specialties to decide on the management plan for the patient. Useful traits like self-directed learning, professional self-awareness, learning developed in context, multidisciplinary and multilevel collaboration become useful components of continuing professional development (Brigley et al. 1997).

Interaction with professionals from other disciplines helps build up personal and professional confidence, at the same time developing honesty and greater respect for others. Various educational interventions have been undertaken to study the effectiveness of inter-professional education in recent times. Education planners support and agree with interaction between different co-workers with the aim of producing cohesive multidisciplinary teams (Munro, Felton, and McIntosh 2002).

Multidisciplinary team meetings provide a unique learning opportunity for junior doctors and expose them to the management of a variety of cases in a limited timeframe. Certain rare cases which may by encountered only a couple of times during professional careers are seen by trainees of different disciplines in a multidisciplinary team. The usefulness of the meetings is not just limited to the knowledge of the entity being discussed in a particular meeting, but also elaborates the learners' way of thinking and ability to manage patients (Harrison 2016). The majority of clinicians accept their usefulness and feel more satisfied managing patients after discussions in tumour boards, recognising the impact for changing their practice based upon the evolving evidence in literature (Sarff et al. 2008).

The effectiveness of tumour boards has been appraised in the context of enhancing inter-professional education. MDTs not only contribute to the enhancement of learner proficiency but also help improve patient outcomes. These ventures have been associated with advanced clinical results and efforts towards better care delivery through newer systems (Edwards et al. 2019). These MDT tumour boards, in fact, create a welcoming environment with significant networking and mentoring opportunities (Kratzke 2018).

Limiting the working hours of surgery residents has been incorporated into many modern training programmes moving from an apprenticeship towards a more structured approach. Working in a multidisciplinary team and attendance at tumour boards provide concentrated learning through discussion of the management of a variety of cases within a short period of time (Sarff, Ellis, and Vetto 2009). Therefore, emphasising the formal inclusion of these meetings in the surgery education curriculum is mandated.

Many institutions award CME credit hours to the participants attending MDT tumour board meetings. This is recognition of tumour boards' validity as a forum for enhancing existing knowledge in addition to a clinician's time devoted to increase the quality of service provided. However, the provision of CME credit hours is not always taken up as an incentive to attend these meetings for clinicians who are already convinced of participating in multidisciplinary care of cancer patients. Individuals may not even endeavour to claim credit hours for tumour boards as their ultimate aim may be focused towards education and quality service for cancer patients (Forman and Haykus 1988).

Multidisciplinary tumour board meetings provide an opportunity for discussion of cases to reach a consensus towards a quality care plan for patients. They also help clinicians learn the decision-making process of other disciplines involved in management of patient and provide prospects for trainees to gain experiences beyond cases seen only as part of clinical service. All efforts should be directed towards enhancing the experience of trainees so they can be involved in the organisation and attendance of site specific tumour boards.

## Bibliography

Abbasi, A. N. "Cancer management is a multidisciplinary team work." *J. Coll. Physicians Surg. Pak.* 21, no. 5 (May 2011): 259-61. URL: https://www.researchgate.net/publication/51129881_Cancer_Management_is_a_Multidisciplinary_Team_Work.

Abbasi, A. N., M. U. Karim, N. Ali, A. Hafiz and B. M. Qureshi. "Multidisciplinary Team Tumour Boards are a Lifeline for Our Cancer Patients in Lower and Middle Income Countries." *Clin. Oncol. (R. Coll. Radiol.)* 28, no. 12 (December 2016): 799. DOI: https://doi.org/10.1016/j.clon.2016.07.003.

Abdulrahman, G. O., Jr. "The effect of multidisciplinary team care on cancer management." *Pan Afr. Med. J* 9, no. 1 (June 2011): 20. DOI: https://doi.org/10.4314/pamj.v9i1.71195.

Asghar, A. H., A. N. Abbasi, A. Jamal, G. Haider and S. Rizvi. "City tumour board Karachi: an innovative step in multidisciplinary consensus meeting and its two years audit." *J. Pak. Med. Assoc.* 63, no. 12 (December 2013): 1534-5. PMID: 24397101.

Barry, M. J. and S. Edgman-Levitan. "Shared decision making—pinnacle of patient-centered care." *N. Engl. J. Med.* 366, no. 9 (March 2012): 780-1. DOI: https://doi.org/10.1056/NEJMp1109283.

Benstead, K., N. S. Turhal, N. O'Higgins, L. Wyld, M. Czarnecka-Operacz, H. Gollnick, P. Naredi and J. G. Eriksen. "Multidisciplinary training of cancer specialists in Europe." *Eur. J. Cancer* 83, (September 2017): 1-8. DOI: https://doi.org/10.1016/j.ejca.2017.05.043.

Boniface, M. M., S. B. Wani, T. E. Schefter, P. J. Koo, C. Meguid, S. Leong, J. B. Kaplan, L. J. Wingrove and M. D. McCarter. "Multidisciplinary management for esophageal and gastric cancer." *Cancer Manag. Res.* 8, (April 2016): 39-44. DOI: https://doi.org/10.2147/cmar.s101169.

Bossi, P., and S. Alfieri. "The Benefit of a Multidisciplinary Approach to the Patient Treated with (Chemo) Radiation for Head and Neck Cancer." *Curr. Treat. Options Oncol.* 17, no. 10 (October 2016): 53. DOI: https://doi.org/10.1007/s11864-016-0431-3.

Brar, S. S., C. Provvidenza, A. Hunter, J. C. Victor, J. C. Irish, R. S. McLeod and F. C. Wright. "Improving multidisciplinary cancer conferences: a population-based intervention." *Ann. Surg. Oncol.* 21, no.1 (January 2014): 16-21. DOI: https://doi.org/10.1245/s10434-013-3296-8.

Brenner, D. J., M. Vazquez, M. Buonanno, S. A. Amundson, A. W. Bigelow, G. Garty, A. D. Harken, et al. "Integrated interdisciplinary training in the radiological sciences." *Br. J. Radiol.* 87, no. 1034 (February 2014): 20130779. DOI: https://doi.org/10.1259/bjr.20130779.

Brigley, S., Y. Young, P. Littlejohns and J. McEwen. "Continuing education for medical professionals: a reflective model." *Postgrad. Med. J* 73, no. 855 (January 1997): 23-6. DOI: https://doi.org/10.1136/pgmj.73.855.23.

Bydder, S., A. Nowak, K. Marion, M. Phillips and R. Atun. "The impact of case discussion at a multidisciplinary team meeting on the treatment and survival of patients with inoperable non-small cell lung cancer." *Intern. Med. J.* 39, no. 12 (December 2009): 838-41. DOI: https://doi.org/10.1111/j.1445-5994.2009.02019.x.

Dickson-Witmer, D., N. J. Petrelli, D. R. Witmer, M. England, G. Witkin, T Manzone, J Napoletano, P Strusowski, J Spellman and D. Smith. "A statewide community cancer center videoconferencing program." *Ann. Surg. Oncol.* 15, no. 11 (November 2008): 3058-64. DOI: https://doi.org/10.1245/s10434-008-0101-1.

Edwards, S. T., E. R. Hooker, R. Brienza, B. O'Brien, H. Kim, S. Gilman, N. Harada, et al. "Association of a Multisite Interprofessional

Education Initiative With Quality of Primary Care." *JAMA Netw. Open* 2, no. 11 (November 2019): e1915943. DOI: https://doi.org/10.1001/jamanetworkopen.2019.15943.

El Saghir, N. S., N. L. Keating, R. W. Carlson, K. E. Khoury and L. Fallowfield. "Tumor boards: optimizing the structure and improving efficiency of multidisciplinary management of patients with cancer worldwide." *Am. Soc. Clin. Oncol. Educ. Book 34*, no. 1 (2014): e461-6. DOI: https://doi.org/10.14694/EdBook_AM.2014.34.e461.

Fader, D. J., C. G. Wise, D. P. Normolle and T. M. Johnson. "The multidisciplinary melanoma clinic: a cost outcomes analysis of specialty care." *J. Am. Acad. Dermatol.* 38, no. 5 Pt 1 (May 1998): 742-51. DOI: https://doi.org/10.1016/s0190-9622(98)70203-8.

Forman, W. B., and W. Haykus. "Tumor conference: the role of continuing medical education." *J. Contin. Educ. Health Prof.* 8, no. 4 (January 1988): 267-70. DOI: https://doi.org/10.1002/chp.4750080404.

Forrest, L. M., D. C. McMillan, C. S. McArdle and D. J. Dunlop. "An evaluation of the impact of a multidisciplinary team, in a single centre, on treatment and survival in patients with inoperable non-small-cell lung cancer." *Br. J. Cancer* 93, no. 9 (October 2005): 977-8. DOI: https://doi.org/10.1038/sj.bjc.6602825.

Ha, F. J., and S. Parakh. "Novel Approaches To Undergraduate Oncology Education." *J. Cancer Educ.* 33, no. 3 (June 2018): 500-504. DOI: https://doi.org/10.1007/s13187-016-1109-z.

Harrison, A. "Learning from the multidisciplinary team." *Clin. Teach.* 13, no. 4 (June 2016): 303-4. DOI: https://doi.org/10.1111/tct.12427.

Jalil, R., M. Ahmed, J. S. Green and N. Sevdalis. "Factors that can make an impact on decision-making and decision implementation in cancer multidisciplinary teams: an interview study of the provider perspective." *Int. J. Surg.* 11, no. 5 (June 2013): 389-94. DOI: https://doi.org/10.1016/j.ijsu.2013.02.026.

Kolacinska, A. "How Can We Improve Education of Breast Surgeons Across Europe?" *Chirurgia (Bucur)* 112, no. 4 (July 2017): 365-366. DOI: https://doi.org/10.21614/chirurgia.112.4.365.

Kostaras, X., M. A. Shea-Budgell, E. Malcolm, J. C. Easaw, W. Roa and N. A. Hagen. "Is there a role for clinical practice guidelines in multidisciplinary tumor board meetings? A descriptive study of knowledge transfer between research and practice." *J. Cancer Educ.* 27, no. 1 (March 2012): 42-5. DOI: https://doi.org/10.1007/s13187-011-0263-6.

Kratzke, C. “Smart Choices for Cancer Education Professional Development: Your Voice and Visibility for Leadership.” *J. Cancer Educ.* 33, no. 5 (October 2018): 1148-1150. DOI: https://doi.org/10.1007/s13187-017-1174-y.

Kurpad, R., W. Kim, W. K. Rathmell, P. Godley, Y. Whang, J. Fielding, L. Smith, et al. “A multidisciplinary approach to the management of urologic malignancies: does it influence diagnostic and treatment decisions?” *Urol. Oncol.* 29, no. 4 (July 2011): 378-82. DOI: https://doi.org/10.1016/j.urolonc.2009.04.008.

Lamb, B. W., K. F. Brown, K. Nagpal, C. Vincent, J. S. Green and N. Sevdalis. “Quality of care management decisions by multidisciplinary cancer teams: a systematic review.” *Ann. Surg. Oncol.* 18, no. 8 (August 2011): 2116-25. DOI: https://doi.org/10.1245/s10434-011-1675-6.

Look Hong, N. J., A. R. Gagliardi, S. E. Bronskill, L. F. Paszat and F. C. Wright,. “Multidisciplinary cancer conferences: exploring obstacles and facilitators to their implementation.” *J. Oncol. Pract.* 6, no. 2 (March 2010): 61-8. DOI: https://doi.org/10.1200/jop.091085.

MacDermid, E., G. Hooton, M. MacDonald, G. McKay, D. Grose, N. Mohammed and C. Porteous. “Improving patient survival with the colorectal cancer multi-disciplinary team.” *Colorectal Dis* 11, no. 3 (March 2009): 291-5. DOI: https://doi.org/10.1111/j.1463-1318.2008.01580.x.

McAvoy, B. R., J. M. Fletcher and M. Elwood. “Cancer education and training in primary health care—a national audit of training providers.” *Aust. Fam. Physician* 36, no. 11 (November 2007): 973-6. DOI: https://search.informit.org/doi/10.3316/informit.356697636599877.

Munro, N., A. Felton and C. McIntosh. “Is multidisciplinary learning effective among those caring for people with diabetes?” *Diabet. Med.* 19, no. 10 (October 2002): 799-803. DOI: https://doi.org/10.1046/j.1464-5491.2002.00788.x.

Murgu, S., R. Rabito, G. Lasko, C. Jackson, M. Mino-Kenudson, D. S. Ettinger, S. S. Ramalingam and E. S. Edell. “Impact of a Non-small Cell Lung Cancer Educational Program for Interdisciplinary Teams.” *Chest* 153, no. 4 (April 2018): 876-887. DOI: https://doi.org/10.1016/j.chest.2017.11.032.

Nguyen, N. A., and J. Ringash. “Head and Neck Cancer Survivorship Care: A Review of the Current Guidelines and Remaining Unmet Needs.” *Curr. Treat. Options Oncol.* 19, no. 8 (August 2018): 44. DOI: https://doi.org/10.1007/s11864-018-0554-9.

Park, K. U., L. Selby, X. P. Chen, A. Cochran, A. Harzman, C. Shen and M. E. Gregory. "Development of Residents' Self-Efficacy in Multidisciplinary Management of Breast Cancer Survey." *J. Surg. Res.* 251, (July 2020): 275-280. DOI: https://doi.org/10.1016/j.jss.2020.02.014.

Phang, P. T., R. Woods, C. J. Brown, M. Raval, R. Cheifetz and H. Kennecke. "Effect of systematic education courses on rectal cancer treatments in a population." *Am. J. Surg.* 201, no. 5 (May 2011): 640-4. DOI: https://doi.org/10.1016/j.amjsurg.2011.01.008.

Sarff, M., M. C. Ellis and J. T. Vetto. "Case log review produces translational change in surgical oncology education." *J. Cancer Educ.* 24, no. 3 (September 2009): 176-9. DOI: https://doi.org/10.1080/08858190902876213.

Sarff, M., W. Rogers, C. Blanke and J. T. Vetto. "Evaluation of the tumor board as a Continuing Medical Education (CME) activity: is it useful?" *J. Cancer Educ.* 23, no. 1 (March 2008): 51-6. DOI: https://doi.org/10.1080/08858190701818226.

Schmieder, K., U. Keilholz and S. Combs. "The Interdisciplinary Management of Brain Metastases." *Dtsch Arztebl Int.* 113, no. 24 (June 2016): 415-21. DOI: https://doi.org/10.3238/arztebl.2016.0415.

Szumacher, E., E. Franssen, C. Hayter, C. Danjoux, E. Chow, L. Andersson, R. Wong and A. Loblaw. "Multidisciplinary radiation oncology palliative care rounds as a continuing educational activity implementing the rapid response radiotherapy program at the toronto sunnybrook regional cancer centre." *J. Cancer Educ.* 18, no. 2 (June 2003): 86-90. DOI: https://doi.org/10.1207/s15430154jce1802_10.

Teegarden, D., J. Y. Lee, O. Adedokun, A. Childress, L. C. Parker, W. Burgess, J. Nagel, et al. "Cancer prevention interdisciplinary education program at Purdue University: overview and preliminary results." *J. Cancer Educ.* 26, no. 4 (December 2011): 626-32. DOI: https://doi.org/10.1007/s13187-011-0232-0.

Wheless, S. A., K. A. McKinney and A. M. Zanation. "A prospective study of the clinical impact of a multidisciplinary head and neck tumor board." *Otolaryngol. Head Neck Surg.* 143, no. 5 (November 2010): 650-4. DOI: https://doi.org/10.1016/j.otohns.2010.07.020.

Wright, F. C., N. Lookhong, D. Urbach, D. Davis, R. S. McLeod and A. R. Gagliardi. "Multidisciplinary cancer conferences: identifying opportunities to promote implementation." *Ann. Surg. Oncol.* 16, no. 10 (October 2009): 2731-7. DOI: https://doi.org/10.1245/s10434-009-0639-6.

# CHAPTER 17

# BUILDING AN ACADEMIC MEDICAL PRACTICE

SHARMEEN AKRAM AND FARHAT ABBAS

At the outset we must define what we mean by **"academic medicine"** and **"academic medical practice."**

One of the accepted definitions of **academic medicine** is, *"The capacity of the healthcare system to think, study, research, discover, evaluate, teach, learn and improve."* **Academic medical practice** on the other hand can be defined as physicians practising at an academic medical centre, where education, research, and clinical care are combined to provide the best possible care, making the optimum use of current knowledge, technologies, resources and therapies that other community hospitals may not have available to them (Awasthi et al. 2005; Block, Sonnino and Bellini 2015; Weissberg et al. 2000).

This takes us to the interrelated components of academic medicine, which can be better understood as defined by Boyer (Glassick 2000), the related competencies or scholarship which ensure completion of the full circle of academic competency through:

- Discovery
- Teaching
- Integration
- Application

In other words, when professionals are engaged in the so called traditional "*tripartite mission*" of educating the next generation of professionals, discovering the causes of and cures for disease, integrating the emerging new knowledge for the development of new protocols for diagnosis and treatment, and applying these to patient care, the patients' treatment outcome is likely to be better than if this holistic approach was not employed. It also provides an opportunity for the physicians at academic medical centres to develop local, regional, national and international leadership in patient care, research and education, as the case may be, and hence professional recognition is a key reward that is enjoyed by physicians at academic centres.

## Challenges in academic medicine

While the above case seems very appealing, the real situation is quite complex and a lot has recently been written about the so called "instabilities in academic medicine," that has made the successful accomplishment of the so called "tripartite mission" by almost every single physician in the current era quite challenging. It is worth reviewing the salient observations as per the *Milbank Memorial Fund Report* (Awasthi et al. 2005). Some of the key highlights of the report include:

- Things are not right in academic medicine but there is little agreement on the exact nature of the problem
- Medical education does not prepare graduates for careers in modern medicine
- Pressure on health services means that academic medicine is often restricted
- Lack of mentoring and career paths being unclear
- Problems with career progression for women
- Many countries lack a well-resourced institution to speak for academic medicine
- Leadership has often been inadequate
- Academic medicine relates poorly to its stakeholders – patients, students, practitioners, policy makers, the public and media
- Lack of capacity for "translational research" or what brings innovation to the bedside
- Research is often not concerned with the biggest health problems – the 10:90 gap
- Simultaneous competency in practice, research and teaching is a challenge
- Fewer doctors want to pursue a career in research
- Academic medicine may entail financial disincentive
- Significant gap between evidence-based practice and what actually happens
- The gap between academics and practitioners is growing

In other words, there are numerous challenges that a physician aspiring to have a strong academic practice faces today and the breadth of the issues are well beyond the control of any one individual, institution or authority. In essence, it is the ever changing nature of societies, their expectations and the provision of resources and opportunities, that continues to shape and reshape the demands and expectations of professionals, including those of the academic physician. At the same time, science is progressing at a pace that has never been witnessed before, and emerging knowledge is associated with the need to acquire new understandings of various types, forcing the constant demand for physicians to upgrade their knowledge and skills. Furthermore, information overload and its easy accessibility to the wider community has made the general public and patient population much more aware about the nature of their ailments, diagnoses and treatment options; this puts an additional demand on physicians to be well versed in all aspects and to have greater communication and coordinating skills at work.

It is important for the academic physicians of today to better understand what is driving the so called current change or reforms in academic medicine, as opposed to the conventional practice models of yesterday. By having a better understanding of what is driving this change, academic physicians will be better prepared to respond to increasing expectations and align their professional practice with the reformed environment. Though not fully understood, as stated above, some of the key drivers of reform are described in the *Milbank Memorial Fund Report* (Awasthi et al. 2005), including:

- New developments in science and technology, especially genetics and information technology (IT)
- The rise of sophisticated consumers
- Globalization
- Socio-economic conditions
- Emergent diseases – COVID-19 being a case in point
- The increasing gap between rich and poor
- The ageing of society
- Increasing accountability of all institutions
- Managerialism
- Gap between what can be done and what can be afforded in healthcare
- The rise of self-care
- The rise of ethical issues
- The 24/7 society

But what do these factors mean to an aspiring physician, to a recent medical graduate, to a young specialist aspiring for a strong academic medical practice career? How too do they relate to senior physicians, teachers, educators, institutions, policy makers, and other leaders in terms of dealing effectively with changing times?

First and foremost, the academic medical practitioner must realise that the nature, shape, scope, expectations and practice of academic medicine will continue to evolve quite rapidly, and in order to meet the expectations of the various stakeholders and drivers of the reformed academic medicine he/she must remain a "lifelong learner." It will be crucial that beyond formal medical education, academic physicians must remain continuously engaged in the self-initiated and self-motivated pursuit of new knowledge and skills that will enhance their overall performance and disposition as academic medical practitioners. It will be prudent to continue to explore and understand the changing environment, emerging horizons and newer ways of doing their work more effectively, the so called "societal expectations." Based on them they must reshape their ongoing learning.

Secondly, the so called "boundaries of medical education" have become quite broad and also quite porous, and hence the initial education and subsequent continuous learning must include much broader and quite diverse curricula to address the emerging needs. This takes us to the educationists, academic leaders, policy makers, etc.

The International Campaign to Revitalise Academic Medicine (ICRAM) (Awasthi et al. 2005; Clark 2005) emphasises that academic medicine must:

- Improve relations with stakeholders
- Be more globally minded
- Focus on teamwork
- Become more skilful in managing operations
- Focus on lifelong teaching and learning
- Emphasise role models and mentorship
- Promote evidence-based medicine
- Offer learner-centred teaching
- Promote research combined with implementation and improvement

It is hence crucial that individuals, groups, educationists, institutions and policy makers must align the overall scope of learning in accordance with what is expected/required today from an academic medical practitioner.

Attention should be paid to some of the highlighted drivers of the changing environment and recommendations to address the emerging challenges must be openly embraced and adopted by individuals and communities within medical practice in order for reform to be successful.

## Paradigm changes in medical education

In order to better understand the changing nature of the role that is expected to be played by a recent medical graduate, one may interpret the paradigm shifts that have occurred in medical education to accommodate these broad and ever changing expectations. These changes reflect changing societal needs, healthcare needs, changes in the provision of healthcare, and developments in the field of education (CanMEDS 2000). The objective is to prepare individuals for the effective acquisition, integration and application of knowledge (independent professional functioning) in a defined area, primarily through the development of knowledge, skills, and attitudes (Bickel 1996; Maudsley 1999; The Medical School Objectives Writing Group 1999; The Royal College of Physicians and Surgeons of Canada 1996).

An individual aspiring for a strong academic medical practice ideally must have been moulded by a system that has adopted and implemented the required broad changes in medical education (as below) and the individual must have the realisation that a much broader and wider role is expected of them in the form of the academic medical practitioner—several attributes of which could be gleaned from so called the "terminal competencies" of a medical graduate of today and the life-long learner attitude that will assist them in an ever changing environment.

Tables 17-1 and 17-2 show some salient changes that have occurred in medical education in order to address the emerging needs (Abbas and Coburn 2012; Boelen and Woollard 2011; Papa and Harasym 1999; WHO 1995; South-Paul 2007).

**Table 17-1: The shifting paradigms of medical education (Abbas and Coburn 2012; Papa and Harasym 1999).**

| **Drivers of change in medical education** | **Paradigm changes in medical education** (driven by the needs) |
|---|---|
| Medical education should be designed to serve the needs of the population that is ultimately being served | ➤Societal needs concept |
| The societal needs are ever changing | ➤Educational programmes must be flexible |
| Widely diversified and increasing societal needs | ➤Broadening of education |
| Better understanding of principles of learning/acquisition of knowledge | ➤Curricular reforms |
| Desirable characteristics/attributes/competences of graduating students better defined | ➤Focused and refined educational strategies/assessment methodologies |
| Desirable characteristics of medical educators/teachers | ➤Redefined "role profile" of teachers; evidence-based medical education versus opinion-based |
| Integration and application of knowledge, problem solving, and skills development | ➤Refined assessment methodologies, outcome-based education, curricular mapping, skills labs, e-learning |
| Emergence of innovative learning technologies | ➤Integration of learning technologies with education – simulators, information and communication technologies (ICT), e-learning, etc. |

**Table 17-2: Shifting paradigms in medical education (South-Paul 2007).**

| **Traditional** (focused on) | **Revised paradigm** (focused on) |
|---|---|
| • The individual | ➤The community |
| • Cure of disease | ➤Preservation of health |
| • Episodic care | ➤Continuous care |
| • Physician provider | ➤Teams of providers |
| • Paternalism | ➤Partnership with patients |
| • Provider-centred | ➤Patient-family centred |
| • Anecdotal care | ➤Evidence-based medicine |
| • In-patient focused | ➤Ambulatory/home-centred |
| • Individual accountability | ➤System accountability |

It is crucial that academic medical practitioners understand these reforms and changes that have occurred. They must figure out any so called "gaps" in their education and training and must attempt to bridge them through additional learning; secondly, they must adapt to the revised form of medical practice, particularly at academic institutions where models of reformed medical practice could be developed for the collective benefit of the individuals, departments, and institution, as well the patient populations and communities receiving care.

The Lancet Commission on the Education of Health Professionals for the 21st Century used a global outlook with a multi-professional perspective and a system approach considering the connection between education and health systems (Frenk et al. 2010). The summary recommendations, as given in Table 17-3, attempt to describe a global strategy for post-secondary education in medicine, nursing and public health. The focus is to train competent educated, ethical and critical health professionals who to participate in patient-centred and population-centred health systems as members of locally responsive and globally connected teams.

**Table 17-3: Proposed reforms by The Lancet Commission on Education of Health Professionals for the 21st Century (Frenk et al. 2010).**

| |
|---|
| **Instructional reforms:** |
| 1. Adoption of competency-based curricula that are responsive to rapidly changing needs rather than being dominated by static coursework. |
| 2. Promotion of interprofessional and trans-professional education that break down professional silos while enhancing collaborative and non-hierarchical relationships in elective teams. |
| 3. Exploitation of the power of information technology (IT) through development of evidence, capacity for data collection and analysis, simulation and testing, distance learning, collaborative connectivity, and management of the increase in knowledge. |
| 4. Adaptation locally but harnessing of resources globally in a way that confers capacity to flexibly address local challenges while using global knowledge, experience, and shared resources, including faculty, curriculum, didactic materials, and students linked internationally through exchange programmes. |
| 5. Strengthening of educational resources, since faculty, syllabuses, didactic materials, and infrastructure are necessary instruments to achieve competencies. |
| 6. Promotion of a new professionalism that uses competencies as the objective criterion for the classification of health professionals, transforming present conventional silos. |

**Institutional reforms:**

7. Establishment of joint planning mechanisms in every country to engage key stakeholders, especially ministries of education and health, professional associations, and the academic community, to overcome fragmentation by assessment of national conditions, setting priorities, shaping policies, tracking change, and harmonising the supply and demand for health professionals to meet the health needs of the population.
8. Expansion from academic centres to academic systems, extending the traditional discovery-care-education continuum to the community setting.
9. Linking together through networks, alliances, and consortia between educational institutions worldwide and across to allied sectors such as governments, civil society organisations, business, and media.
10. Nurturing of a culture of critical inquiry as a central function of universities and other institutions of higher learning.

Medical competence could be defined as "the habitual and judicious use of communication, knowledge, technical skills, clinical reasoning, emotions, values and reflection in daily practice for the benefit of individuals and communities being served" (Norcini 1999). So careful reviews of the broad competencies that are expected from a medical practitioner, as defined by various systems, are summarized in Tables 17-4 and 17-5 as follows.

**Table 17-4: Outcomes and competencies for postgraduate medical education (Norcini 1999).**

| **Royal College of Physicians and Surgeon Canada (RCPSC)** | **Accreditation Council for Graduate Medical Education (ACGME & ABMS)** | **General Medical Council, UK (GMC)** | **College of Physicians and Surgeons, Pakistan (CPSP)** | **Aga Khan University, Pakistan (AKU)** |
|---|---|---|---|---|
| Medical expert | Medical knowledge | Good clinical care | Clinically competent | Medical expert |
| Communicator | Interpersonal and communication skills | Relationship with patient | Effective team member/leader | Communication & interpersonal skills |
| Collaborator | Systems-based practice | Working with colleagues | Evidence-based practice | Systems-based practice |
| Manager | Patient care | Maintaining good medical practice | Health promotion and prevention | Evidence & practice-based learning and improvement |
| Professional | Professionalism | Probity | | Professionalism |
| Scholar | -- | -- | Educator | Scholar |
| Health Advocate | Practice-based learning and improvement | Teaching, training, appraising and assessing | Research and publications | |

**Table 17-5: Competency common to all**

- Biomedical ethics
- Communication skills
- Teaching skills
- Quality assurance/improvement
- Research and critical appraisal
- Management skills
- Advocacy
- Collaboration

It is important that the medical education in the context of undergraduate, postgraduate and continuing education should be seen as a *true continuum* extending from school, college, medical school, postgraduate medical education and medical practice (Harden 2006). Hence, the skillsets required for successful academic practice, as defined above in various systems which are quite interrelated and complementary, are acquired through formal medical education in school, universities, teaching hospitals, etc., and are continuously added and upgraded through a lifelong learning habit, which is mostly voluntary (though at times required by the system), self-motivated, and self-directed. It is here that the role of "*mentors and role models*" is invaluable and of the utmost importance. Established systems to help and motivate academic faculty to engage in lifelong learning through continuing medical education (CME) and continuous professional development (CPD) will be mutually beneficial for the institution and the individual faculty.

## Challenges for academic medicine in the developing world: additional issues

Establishing an academic medical practice in the developing world poses both opportunities as well as particular challenges when compared with the developed world. Many of the particular challenges listed below in the developing world context, though not exclusive, could also act as potential opportunities (such as large populations, widened disease burden, etc.) as they provide a base for the broad exposure and diverse experience of the practitioner.

- Large populations
- Wide disease burden
- Socio-economic challenges
- Limitations of infrastructure, education, finance, and natural resources
- Challenges related to women professionals
- Social, cultural, linguistic, and religious variations
- Maintenance of balance amongst educational, research and service throughputs
- Technology, equipment and innovation
- Cost of quality healthcare with absence of third party payers

Given these specific challenges, which represent only a subset of what could be the real case in various environments, it is important that an academic practitioner in a developing world setting is particularly aware of these issues and is ready to surmount them as best as possible to help achieve his/her specific goals. This should be done while maintaining the objectives of providing the highest possible level of service in a given setting/country/region and keeping international standards as a reference and benchmark. It obviously requires thoughtful deliberations and support at all levels from policy makers, academic leadership and various stakeholders, and is usually steered by the academic professionals trying to establish high quality care at leading academic institutions/organisations. It is particularly important that the academic faculty must assume a leadership role in steering these discussions and presenting a compelling case for support from policy makers and organisational leaders. As is often the case, it is always the motivated healthcare professionals who act as "*agents for change*," providing local solutions to local problems and addressing the needs of their patient populations and the communities they serve. This is a very satisfying experience and surely provides a good sense of accomplishment.

***Challenges related to women professionals***

We must pay attention to the additional challenges faced by women professionals, particularly in the developing world setting. These are rather additional unique, gender-based challenges which make it even harder for women professionals to achieve academic and clinical practice excellence and acquire leadership roles. Ranging from maintenance of a balanced professional and family life to combining motherhood with work, gender equity issues include gender discrimination, compensation, career development challenges, ability to avail opportunities for continued professional development, and more dire issues such as sexual harassment at work and in communities where they serve and increased incidence of mental health problems. With an ever increasing number of female medical graduates it is crucial that the system must recognise and address the unique issues faced by female professionals and must create supportive structures and appropriate policies in this regard.

## Academic leadership support

It is important that the organisational leadership supports the development of high quality academic medical faculty through well designed and carefully selected policies and procedures that focus on some of the following key areas related to hiring, retention, development, career progression, compensation, and motivation/engagement. It is particularly important that the particular issues in health sciences institutions are addressed. The areas relate to:

- Conflicts in maintaining a balance between service and academic needs (organisational, departmental, individuals)
- Ensuring adequate resources (human, capital, physical, etc.) to subserve justified needs in an ever growing, technology-driven environment
- Maintenance and enhancement of quality of educational programmes, research engagements and responses to societal needs
- Enhanced support, recognition and reward for teaching and research contributions
- Maintaining adequate bottom–up, top–down communication
- A healthy and conducive environment for women professionals for work and development
- Adequate faculty and staff compensation/retention
- Providing medical education and continuous professional development programmes that are responsive to the needs of healthcare professionals and offer opportunities for ongoing intellectual stimulation and professional renewal
- Maintenance of a healthy, stimulating, challenging and supportive university environment, conducive to the integration and delivery of quality education, research and service

So in conclusion, academic medical practice could be an exciting career in the life of a healthcare professional. When personal and professional requirements are judiciously and carefully assessed and adopted, it can bring humongous rewards throughout the lifetime of an individual. It is however a demanding, challenging and laborious commitment—not just a career but a lifestyle, one that individuals commit to and that should be taken up after careful self-assessment and perhaps appropriate counselling. Individuals must feel that they possess the right credentials, personal and professional attributes, passion and commitment much required for them to excel in this field. It is advisable that individuals must fully understand the scope and breadth of the required engagements; must undertake the essential required training and education to help them excel in the various areas that they are expected to perform well in; must find a specific focus and niche for themselves, which will help them shine in a busy and competitive environment; must find some intellectually stimulating and motivating role models and mentors for themselves; must engage in reflective practice; and must be ready to become lifelong learners in the quest for new and emerging knowledge and skills, reformed methodologies for teaching and learning, research engagements, and high quality academic clinical practice. They must not only try to find conducive and appropriate environments where their professional expertise could be best utilised but more importantly, also try to become agents of change in bringing about the much desired transformational changes in their own local and regional settings to respond to overall societal needs.

In the end, it is crucial that they must enjoy and derive satisfaction from their journey of discovery and self-development, positively influencing lives through teaching and clinical practice, training others, being an agent of change and a catalyst for transformed environments, and leaving a legacy via all the lives they have positively touched and influenced in one way or another.

## Bibliography

Abbas, F., and M. Coburn. “Education and training of an academic urologic surgeon.” *In Urolithiasis: Basic Science and Clinical Practice*, J. Talati, H. G. Tiselius, D. M. Albala and Z. Ye (eds.), 1982. London: Springer Verlag, 2012.

Awasthi, S., J. Beardmore, J. Clark, P. Hadridge, H. Madani, A. Marusic, G. Purcell et al. “Five Futures for Academic Medicine.” PLoS Med 2, no. 7 (July 2005): e207. DOI: https://doi.org/10.1371/journal.pmed.0020207.

Bickel, J. “Proceedings of the AAMC Conference on Students’ and Residents’ Ethical and Professional Development”. *Academic Medicine* 71, no. 6 (June 1996): 622-3. DOI: 10.1097/00001888-199606000-00013.

Block, Steven M., Roberta E. Sonnino and Lisa Bellini. “Defining ‘Faculty’ in Academic Medicine - Responding to the Challenges of a Changing Environment.” *Academic Medicine* 90, no. 3 (March 2015): 279-282. DOI: https://doi.org/10.1097/acm.0000000000000575.

Boelen, Charles and Robert Woollard. “Social accountability: The extra leap to excellence for educational institutions.” *Medical Teacher* 33, no. 8 (July 2011): 614–619. DOI: https://doi.org/10.3109/0142159x.2011.590248.

CanMEDS 2000: Extract from the CanMEDS 2000 Project Societal Needs Working Group Report. *Med Teach* 22, no. 6 (2000): 549-54. DOI: 10.1080/01421590050175505.

Clark, J. "Five futures for academic medicine: the ICRAM scenarios." *BMJ* 331 (July 2005): 101-104. DOI: https://doi.org/10.1136/bmj.331.7508.101.

Frenk, Julio, Lincoln Chen, Zulfiqar A. Bhutta, Jordan Cohen, Nigel Crisp, Timothy Evans, Harvey Fineberg et al. "Health professionals for a new century: transforming education to strengthen health systems in an interdependent world." *Lancet* 376, no. 9756 (December 2010): 1923–1958. DOI: https://doi.org/10.1016/s0140-6736(10)61854-5.

Glassick, C. E. "Boyer's expanded definitions of scholarship, the standards for assessing scholarship, and the elusiveness of the scholarship of teaching." *Acad. Med.* 75, no. 9 (September 2000): 877-80. DOI: https://doi.org/10.1097/00001888-200009000-00007.

Harden, R. M. "Trends and the future of postgraduate medical education." *Emerg. Med. J.* 23, no. 10 (October 2006): 798-802. DOI: https://doi.org/10.1136/emj.2005.033738.

Maudsley, R. F. "Content in Context: Medical Education and Society's Needs." *Academic Medicine* 74, no. 2 (February 1999): 143-145. DOI: https://doi.org/10.1097/00001888-199902000-00013.

Norcini, J. "Standards and reliability in evaluation: when rules of thumb don't apply". *Acad. Med.* 74, no. 10 (October 1999): 1088-90. DOI: https://doi.org/10.1097/00001888-199910000-00010.

Papa, F. J., and P. H. Harasym. "Medical curriculum reform in North America, 1765 to the present: A cognitive science perspective." *Acad. Med.* 74, no. 2 (February 1999): 154–64. DOI: https://doi.org/10.1097/00001888-199902000-00015.

South-Paul, Jeannette E. *Proceedings of Advancing Diversity and Excellence in Science and Engineering*. Ann Arbor, Michigan: University of Michigan, 2007.

The Medical School Objectives Writing Group. "Learning Objectives for Medical Students Education – Guidelines for Medical Schools: Report 1 of the Medical School Objectives Project." *Academic Medicine* 74, no. 1 (January 1999): 13-18. DOI: 10.1097/00001888-199901000-00010.

The Royal College of Physicians and Surgeons of Canada. *Final Report of the Task Force to Review Fundamental Issues in Specialty Education (Maudsley Report)*. Ottawa: 1996.

Weissberg, P. L., R. Jones, I. Taylor and J. Moxham. "Clinical Academic Medicine - Academics should be rewarded appropriately." *BMJ* 321, no. 7256 (July 2000): 300-302. URL: https://www.jstor.org/stable/25225234.

World Health Organization. "Changing Medical Education and Medical Practice for All." Executive Board, 25 January 1995. URL: https://apps.who.int/iris/handle/10665/172313.

# CHAPTER 18

# CONCEPTUAL FRAMEWORKS FOR BROADER EDUCATION OF SURGICAL RESIDENTS

JAMSHEER JEHANGIR TALATI
AND MUHAMMAD RIZWAN KHAN

## Abstract

The improved and yet inadequate state of health and health service delivery in Pakistan, a lower-middle-income country, indicates that all is not well. Surgical care is generally delivered more iniquitously than its medical counterpart because of the increased resources required. It is plagued by waiting lists, overfilled hospitals, and inactive stratification of tasks between hospitals. Surgeons taught the principles of community health sciences, health systems, family practice, research, epidemiology and statistics in undergraduate years have little time to apply that very knowledge to the problems in health delivery, within the vortex of intense and important work which saves lives.

The accumulated burden of unmet need requires addressing through new approaches, at the levels of people, professions, policy and governance. Some deficiencies in the context of bio-medical management are easier to identify and address; but the complexity of the shortcomings resulting from interactions of disparate and complex societal behaviours with various political, legislative and governance structures adds a different and more difficult dimension to the task at hand. The coming quintiles of the $21^{st}$ century will usher in some predictable changes but will demand preparation for unexpected and unknowable possibilities. If the health of the nation must be improved, residents need to be prepared to correct current deficiencies and anticipate, tackle and shape change for the benefit and preservation of humans.

As surgical interventions are efficacious in preventing death, it is time to remodel surgical training, reshape it anew; to enrich it with the relevant cross-disciplinary territories of knowledge and the required attitudes and skills. To encourage change and validity, and maintain contemporaneity, special pedagogical interventions with artful mentorship (in which teacher and student co-explore new avenues of actions) may be required. It has been suggested that the medical humanities curriculum model will be inadequate for the task, though the anchoring to the humanities (so essential for an understanding of human nature, society, and the individual in society) must remain. The completion of a capstone project, to be completed by the final year, judged by a panel of citizens, professionals and government representative could be an essential requirement for graduation.

The success of any alteration to an intense surgical residency will depend upon how ably it aids attainment of surgical competences to the same or higher level as at present, in a shorter time so as to allow freeing up "space" for learning through newer avenues.

Specially trained to facilitate navigation through the turbulences of life and the corridors of power, such broadly educated surgeons would be invaluable to universities and medical colleges as teachers. Countries will benefit from the changes in policy, governance, and management for health that they will instigate; and from their progressive thinking on how to reduce the inequities in surgical care that are so rampant today.

A special additional degree might need to be bestowed by universities on such graduates.

## Acknowledgements

We would like to express our gratitude to Professor Mushtaq Ahmed, Vice Dean, Aga Khan University Medical College, for review of early drafts, and Professor Camer W. Vellani, Distinguished University Professor, Aga Khan University, for discussions on defining the raison d'être of the broad education of health professionals.

This work has been shaped by the intellectual input from communicating with numerous faculty and staff of the Aga Khan University, over time, and especially its Department of Surgery where many faculty have taken initiatives in building valued social capital. It also owes a debt to the intellectual powerhouse of the Department for Educational Development.

## Introduction

This chapter is written in the context of surgical healthcare in lower-middle-income countries (LMICs), where, despite the excellence, intensity, and breadth of many surgical education programmes (SEPs), all that is seen on the surgical scene is not well.

What is the state of provision of surgical health in LMICs? The following three scenarios give us a slit-lamp glimpse of the deficiencies and limitations of health systems in one LMIC, and the consequent inequities and deficiencies, in contexts of access to modern surgery. They open our conversation on the missing elements in surgeons' education and the need for a further broadening of surgical education.

1. Within the same country, women in rural areas do not have access to safe caesarean sections, whilst tertiary urban private hospitals monitor foetal heart rate and uterine contractions with cardiotocography, to predict foetal distress. This is an example of gross inequity.
2. An internal-migrant labourer with abdominal pain, neglected because he is a daily wage earner (without a minimum guaranteed income from the government), does not know where to go for treatment. Turned away from the first public hospital (which is overfull), a "general doctor" cursorily examines him sitting on a stool and prescribes antibiotics. The pain worsens. He cannot afford the PKR 40,000 [USD 250] demanded as admission fee by a good secondary care private hospital. Admission to another public hospital is arranged finally by commendation (*sifarish)*. A ruptured appendix is removed. Can that be a country's standard of care? *Why are our public hospitals overburdened? Should sifarish be replaced by a body of community health workers? Are the district hospitals performing their share of work, or are they restricted in their scope of function by interference and inadequate human and other resources? Are urban community health workers functional, serving as lay health advocates, and directing some of the workload to appropriate lower level facilities? Is sifarish our society's solution to the lack of able community health workers?*
3. An accident victim with a spinal fracture sustained on a highway (when his car overturned at night), had no emergency call centre where he could obtain advice on what to do. A trauma centre (40 miles south) lay underutilised, because COVID-19 had reduced road travel and consequently accidents. The nearby hospitals did

> not have a ventilator or 24-hour access to blood transfusion services. The victim recovered after treatment of the fracture and transient paraparesis because a co-traveller was a surgeon and took him to the tertiary care facility where he worked. *What is the strength of the supportive information and transport components of our health systems? What should be the involvement of surgeons in the construction of call centres, roads, cities, and transport-for-health, and the appropriate placement and access routes to surgical facilities?*

A wide range of deficiencies and the iniquitous distribution of services prevent the attainment of swift surgery-for-all even in cities. We teach safe optimal care but address the needs of only those who can reach us. Currently, we cannot institute optimal care for all, and it is likely that this is not only because of the costs of human, physical, instrument, implant and other resources, but because we fail to design and organise innovative approaches that focus on critical issues integrally impacting outcomes and lowering costs. The history of industrialisation gives us a tip.

Iron as a construction material remained inaccessible to small business ventures; until the cost of smelting iron ore was drastically cut by substituting coke for the original coal for smelting. The price came down so fast that the communities enjoyed much profit from increased trade, which necessitated a bridge across the river to transport the iron—the "Iron Bridge" (West Midlands History 2021), built of iron.

*Are surgeons trained to find and implement critical disruptive modifications in the detection-treatment-follow-up of patients with results as dramatic as that of coke?*

The three scenarios are but examples from the sea of ominously growing burdens for surgeons which have to be reduced before new trends and problems (consequent on our processioning into the second quintile of the 21$^{st}$ century) swamp us; or unimaginable unknowns surface from the murky future to annihilate humans. We advisedly use the word processioning, because despite our affluence and technology, humans as a species are not progressing with the passage of time.

If such scenarios represent the state of health despite the educational efforts of a growing number of medical/nursing colleges and surgical training programmes (in Pakistan), the answer to the question, "are our educational programmes fully functional?" is clearly a no!

Further, the situation is complicated by many less cut-and-dried crystal-clear problems, some of which are outlined below.

## 1.0 The overburdening of health systems by florid production of disease through fault lines plaguing society

The following scenarios demonstrate another subset of deficiencies, this time resulting from human behaviour and societal issues.

a. The principal of a medical college laments that he cannot find physicians for the associated teaching hospital though >300 students graduate each year (Dawn 2021). With mandated merit-based admissions, disregarding gender, most students are now women, who on graduation and marriage may not be allowed to work. Some women refuse to see male patients or work at night. And many women are discouraged from taking up surgery as a career—a problem not unique to LMICs, as it is also seen in the USA (Haskins 2019).
b. The relatives accompanying an aunt with a mutilating oral cancer for surgery and radiotherapy, come in blatantly chewing betel nut (*areca catechu*), the cause of the cancer in the aunt. Here, "society" has failed to act upon the advice of doctors, because of ingrained sociocultural habits.
c. Hepatitis is rampant and hepatic cancer prevalent because of reuse of injection needles; AIDS flourishes in an environment which negates the use of condoms; and in the midst of COVID-19, the universal gregariousness of humans drives mask-less people to bars in the West, and to closely packed eateries in the East.
d. A container which has not been locked to the transporter topples as the truck swerves on the road, crush-killing a family of five in the adjacent car.
e. The motorcycle serves as a family car for seven … all riding without helmets. Babies <2 years old are laid face down with legs straddled over the petrol tank, clasping nothing, whilst the young father nonchalantly swerves his motorcycle zigzagging through the motorised traffic. Daredevil riding at night across road intersections leads to amputated limbs.
f. Unscrupulous thieves (Jamsheer 1992) steal manhole covers, and men fall into sewers, during their journey home on foot, during torrential rains; urologists have to repair damaged urethrae.

g. The lust for money, fuelled by viewing fashionable lives on film on ubiquitously available fancy phones drives young men without education to break into houses at night and shoot or kill owners who do not cough up their wealth. Copying the styles of actors, they pose as relatives and slip past guards to execute patterns learnt from sectors with "justified" criminals.
h. Death waits in the shadows, whilst worn bus tires, useless brakes, unlicensed drivers, and long-haul night driving, meet the accident victim. At times the drivers' "charas" (created from fresh cannabis buds) intake drops the driver into error zones.
i. The tokka (an unguarded chaff cutter for fodder) in farming villages claims digits and forearms.
j. An industrialist throws pollutants into a stream that flows into the sea and mangrove forests, where fish swim and shrimp breed. Where is the Environmental Protection Agency (EPA)—shut-eyed and palm greased? Sleeping, ignorant or short staffed?
k. A youth in a mountainous territory aspires to become a forestry officer. Why? He smiles and says there are great opportunities for taking bribes (*rishwat*).
l. It is easy for even a fruit seller, with no education other than life, to make money, not pay tax, send earnings to a friend abroad, illegally, and then have it return, officially, to get 5% interest on the returned dollars, leading to a life of ease; and yet the grocer leaves discarded rotten fruit and banana peel strewn on the market floor, adjacent to his shop, to collect flies and generate disease, causing an elderly person to slip on the path. It leads to an operating room for hip fracture, and death. The prevalent model is making money, to own a smart phone, to enjoy life, with little thought of education and social responsibility.

## 2.0 Defining corrective measures: will broadening SEPs help?

In light of the above problems, how should SEPs be redesigned?

These problems (with us for three-quarters of a century), within the structure of organised civil societies, manifest across all societal and governmental sectors, and are propelled partly by the unique and universal failings of human nature. Even Volkswagen executives in greed for money shamed Germany by their polluting deceit.

Problems such as the inadequacy of beds and equipment can be resolved by attention to improved management, design planning and astute fiscal sense. But the correction of inadequate physicians requires a new vision of health professionals (HPs), and therefore surgeons' training that focuses on active engagement of all HPs in an understanding of how societies work, and the interactions of individuals in that society. And what better way than engaging with all tiers of society to work cooperatively at new approaches to reduce disease generation, and build social capital?

None of this indicates that social capital is missing. It is simply pointing out that despite Pakistan being an exemplar of philanthropy, giving more than USD two billion annually (~1% of GDP) (Amjad and Ali 2018); despite families helping each other as do villagers, despite the focus on philanthropic education and welfare organisations, all is not well on the health scene, and sadly is much worse when one focuses on surgical disease.

In an educational context, this set of societally generated health problems requires (in addition to the management-oriented and discipline-based approach that many of the health services organisational issues require), an imaginative approach that increases the effectiveness of surgeons in bringing about changes across society; and hence requires a new level of study and the valued interaction of the surgical resident (SR) with society and its governance structures.

The need for enhanced broader education is reinforced when we study the reality and urgency of preparing SRs to meet the challenges posed by human progression (or our processioning) through the next two quintiles of the 21$^{st}$ century, loaded as they will be with uncertainties; global, climate, economic power block changes; technological advancement and human enhancement; and much more (see Table 18.1).

**Table 18.1: Conditions, present and future, which suggest the need for a broader education than one confined to professional education and training.**

| | |
|---|---|
| a. | Uncertainty per se, and in the global environment, economic power blocs and views on majoritarianism |
| b. | The persistence and escalation of inequity |
| c. | Technological support, human enhancement, and helpful cyborgs |
| d. | Problems that arise from human nature and its cruelty, acquisitiveness, discrimination, tribalism, and intolerance; unbridled creativity; an inability to answer some questions despite the intellectual capacity to formulate them; and the ways in which patients will desire treatment |
| e. | Difficulties implementing mega-change in the environment of medicalisation of the normal with treatment, surveillance and detection drives |
| f. | Widespread lack of processes that build valued social capital |

All of this should set the conditions that drive the purpose of extending surgical training and education (see Table 18.2) and the attributes and characteristics that have to be developed in our future surgeons (see Table 18.3).

**Table 18.2: The purpose of extending surgical training and education.**

| | |
|---|---|
| 1. | Reduce the disease burden as well as the current inequity in the delivery of health services |
| 2. | Refine health systems to reduce the need for health professionals to interact with people |
| 3. | Understand human nature, death, the value of life and of the human after death |
| 4. | Understand and be prepared to respond agilely to change, the singularity and possibility of extinction |
| 5. | Increase effectiveness in producing change by linking the minds of people, experts, philosophers, bureaucrats, politicians, legislature, and executive arms of governance |
| 6. | Build social capital |

**Table 18.3: General attributes that could support effectiveness in the 21st century.**

1. Alert awareness of environment
2. Highly developed and organised sense of curiosity
3. Agility
4. Ethical probity
5. True tolerance, accepting the possibility that the other person's views might just also be correct
6. Capacity to build social capital
7. Equanimity, serenity and stamina
8. Development of rational and original thought
9. Ability to "recognise, adapt to and manage the change" and when necessary, to take the lead to bring about change (Christobal, Engel and Jamsheer 2009)
10. Ability to assess previous approaches to a problem, include multiple perspectives from societal members, attract expert contributions from other disciplines and professions, and work collaboratively on a project for local, regional or global development

We acknowledge and list the many examples of elements of broader education (BE) currently intertwined in SEPs (see *Supplementary material S1*) but as the list of what is not happening, and what is missing, grows, a greater clarity will emerge as to what needs to be done. A change in the directions indicated above is an imperative.

**Supplementary material S1**

**Elements of broader education that are present in current surgical residency programmes**

SEPs currently have significant components of BE imbedded throughout training. These vicariously influence the decisions of SRs, as they work in wards and operating rooms (ORs), and deal with life and death, people, and families. They learn as they juggle home, family and work responsibilities. Caring for patients itself provides a unique template for learning, inaccessible by those who do not interface with human suffering.

SRs learn the value of teamwork during cardiac resuscitation; mortality and morbidity conferences; rounding with nurses in ICUs, wards and ORs; and when serving during electives in hospitals with constrained resources. These provide what can be classed as in situ BE, albeit of a vicarious, opportunistic, and varied nature.

Even for university SRs, advantaged by exposure to a palette of opportunities (including seminars and webinars on science, culture, cities, psychology, ethics, health and environment by erudite speakers) and unique experiences—for example, that of providing services during the COVID-19 pandemic—the acquisition of special educational messages from the presentations remains variable, unless the message is underlined when stated. Certainly, their acquisition is not assessed.

When residents accompany faculty in national disaster teams, (say) post-earthquake, they have experienced the sway that each after-shock generates, as they sleep atop earthquake-proof buildings.[1] These ingrain in their minds the potential of architecture to mitigate casualties; a preventive measure that reduces the burden of trauma and need for operation. Similarly visiting flooded areas primes them to think of a future water world,[2] when rising seas from global warming inundate established towns. How will they manage operating under such circumstances? Where should the operating room be positioned in future coastal hospitals? The exposure to the management of supply lines, food sources, acquisition and management of donations under such difficult circumstances; the abandonment of sleep, a clean shave or a bath, all in the service to humanity; these are factors that temper SRs in ways not attainable otherwise.

But such opportunities, by nature, are not available to all in each calendar year. They arise from unpredicted calamities and depend on personal volunteerism. The resulting *experiences are not uniform*.

In contrast, there is constant exposure to role model faculty members who might additionally be supporting a charity (for instance Smile Train for cleft lips);[3] obtaining the country's President's cooperation for early cancer detection (Aga Khan University 2020); or directing the building of an emergency COVID-19 hospital to support governments efforts (Aga Khan University 2020), demonstrating exceptional ability to coordinate with the university, government, armed forces and society to achieve a desired result.

---

[1] Verbal report of residents who visited Islamabad after the earthquake.
[2] Refers to the film *Waterworld* (1995).
[3] The charity Smile Train helps children with cleft lips and palates: https://www.smiletrain.org/.

> Additionally, when SEPs have a built-in period of electives with financial support for travel, residents are exposed to different cultures. In LMICs, workloads are heavy and leave little time to absorb local culture or manage domestic affairs. Nevertheless, SRs across the world learn social cohesion during musical evenings—song, rhythm and pitch are imbedded in humans. But, perhaps we now need to create the space required to reflect on past cultures and view collectively and discuss with residents, a classical painting such as (say) the *Oath of the Horatii* (Louvre 2009) and nudge them to trace what the picture represents—which was one way of avoidance of all-out war. And that message is so important, because war is historically, the greatest contributor to the trauma operating load. From such paintings, faculty could encourage SRs to reflect on human nature and the value of building trust, cohesion and avoidance of conflict, and from there to move on to understanding the devastating effect of the plague (that era's COVID-19) on learning in the Dark Ages before the flourishing of art in the Renaissance.
>
> Today, most BE is opportunistically acquired. In the absence of dedicated time for reflection, and faculty-assisted, self-chosen readings, the depth of interaction of art and resident, or a real case and ethics, or the intricacies of a mortality discussion, are left unexplored.

This paper makes a case for creating a mandated curriculum for extended broader education *imbedded* as an integral component of surgical residency education. It suggests that development of a special social capital posited on trust between the government, surgeons and society be a major focus for the change.

### 2.1 Challenges to the focus on links with governance structures

A frequently mentioned objection to linking with governments is often voiced as follows:

> "What is the use of linking educational programmes with government officials when the political executive changes with each election and the bureaucracy changes with promotions and internal decisions?"

The reference to the creation of a link with society and its governance structures (each peculiar to the country) is not intended as a form of familiarity with *individuals* in government and politics (who will come and go). The interactions are needed for an understanding of the steps and structures of plans; the wording and presentation of thoughts and the pragmatisation (and perhaps downgrading) of original designs and plans; the establishment of written communication with government as a record for follow-up and improvement; the understanding of the country in the context of world hegemony; and the understanding of health systems in the contexts of complexity of staffing, monitoring and coordinating a beehive of disparate helping initiatives (such as TB control, AIDS programmes, lady health visitors, polio programmes, community health workers, getting a gamma knife into one public hospital, EPI, school nutrition, water, sewerage…and COVID-19). In other words, we must search for and find the essential elements that must be altered, that must be done, and done in a way that is successful, given the current milieu of finances, management expertise, individuals, family, society, community, and governance structures.

An understanding of how the elected legislature (with limited tenure which is dependent on re-election) functions in coherence with a staid, continuing well tooled bureaucracy might create a better understanding of cooperation. A study of the impediments that hinder political governments in effective governance, the peculiarities of interference by political rivals in specific contexts of the country, and the importance of popularity to the survival of governments, will trigger studies of how other disparate societies have used their constitution to meld people together. In this context, of note is the formulation of the United States of America's constitution, which was greatly influenced by France's. Watching politicians in action will show how structures of politics allow vibrant enlivenment of people's desires, despite the entrenched views of the people holding the knowledge of how the government actually runs. It can show how the military leader can turn into an astute statesmen like Julius Cesar, and then into a philosopher (as Cicero did during the Roman Empire); and how laws are processed into acts (so important when maximizing the use of our bodies as potential transplant material on death). Combinations of observations, readings and trial strategies will ultimately affect change.

It is appropriate that the SR should be initiated into the rights of progression to a healthy society; something which lies embedded in the political rights of people.

## 2.2 Personally directed growth of the resident

To have a greater lifelong impact, broader education programmes must mentor the personalised growth of each individual SR, in the directions of his/her own choice, within the contexts and frameworks of the curriculum.

## 3.0 Social capital as a common undercurrent: an overarching objective

The surgeon, being a highly educated individual in society, has a responsibility for effective contribution to the social capital of the country. In the contexts of this paper, we define social capital as the outcome of a concern for other citizens; the contribution to the capacity of a society to communicate their problems effectively for resolution at various levels of the strata of society, including governance; and citizens' willingness to identify and contribute towards problem resolution. High social capital would be attained when different levels of governance show awareness, concern and are effective in attempting to try and resolve problems in the communities they serve. Social capital has been enhanced in the past, at times, by facilitating commerce, simplifying languages and coinage (as the Qin [Chin] emperor did around 300 BC). Today it requires the search for a language of communication that captures the attention of those who govern, and an all-enveloping caring attitude within the nation. In the past, social cohesion and social capital were built on an unstated threat of war in case of non-compliance. In today's world the resident could learn to build social capital from the platform of a multi-dimensional society.

As contribution to social capital is evidence of an attitude, and as attitudes are dependent on thoughts, the broader education programmes should also attend to the **development and refinement of thought.**

## 4.0 Can BE be left to lifelong learning?

The lofty objectives mentioned above mandate a curriculum. The broadening of education cannot be left to student choice or emerge from self-chosen lifelong learning (LLL) alone. LLL is invaluable for guidance during interactions with society but it is autopoietic—self-generated and self-directed, informal and personally interpreted learning (Talati 2012). Very effective but mostly unplanned and acquired from the circumstances at hand (whether from experience, reading a book or observing behaviours), LLL has no proscribed course. It is opportunistic, not pre-planned. Effective BE requires well-defined goals, objectives, instructional and assessment strategy, and evaluation. Within the structured framework, BE courses need degrees of freedom during their execution, to flexibly accept student's autopoietic approaches and the winding alleyways their thought processes take. This is important as one of the aims of BE is to assist residents in developing their individuality. The curricular structure advantages the programme by providing frameworks for evaluation which allow one's demonstration of value to the society to which we are all accountable.

How then may all the desired objectives be packaged pragmatically into a curriculum that will interest and fascinate the busy resident, and build the required attributes? What subjects should be learnt? What triggers will excite and engage learners? How will the SR be propelled on a lifelong search for suitable collaborators with knowledge outside their own comfort zone? How will they link with society and government? Strategies will have to be carefully designed as surgical skill development will compete for time.

A hypothetical framework for evolving a curricular structure is conceptualised in Table 18.4.

**Table 18.4:** ***Towards defining a methodological process to initiate an extended programme of BE of surgical residents of value to LMICs: questions that assist the development of curricula.***

The below-mentioned framework of questions could be used when determining the specific contents of a surgical education's extension to expand the vision of its residents. The answers mentioned in the unshaded segments, might be far different from what faculty, societal participants and residents in a workshop on development of the BE curriculum might suggest.

| | |
|---|---|
| *Who are your students? What is their background, and knowledge of local customs and culture?* | |
| | |
| *What is your purpose in extending broader education?* | |
| | |
| *What will be the existing micro- and macro-environment during the era for which the resident is preparing for (up to 2040, and beyond)? (A situational and anticipation analysis)* | |
| | |
| *What are your goals?* | |
| | |
| *Towards defining narrower objectives on which to design overall strategy* | |
| | Develop conceptual knowledge across many disciplines |
| | Build social competence, character, agility, productive curiosity, serenity, stamina and ability to contribute to social capital |
| | Instil a firm grounding in the principles and practice of data analysis, statistics, epidemiology, health delivery, health systems and public health |
| | Other considerations |

| *Should strategy include any of the following?* | |
|---|---|
| | Multimodal learning including case based teaching; bringing the resident to think broadly on real life issues that require change; identifying gaps in knowledge (and addressing them) and gaining familiarity through interaction if possible, with (or through viewing the modes of function of) legislators, national and government leaders, Pakistan Medical Commission, Colleges of Physicians and Surgeons, business leaders, investors, entrepreneurs, venture capitalists, or others as per the case; reading widely; and experiencing the cultures and modes of reactions of people and populations<br>Triggering curiosity and developing residents' ability to find solutions, changing tracks as real-time scenarios change<br>Developing the art of choosing appropriate communication strategies and effective communication delivery<br>Providing opportunities for the real world experience of building social capital, demonstrating its achievement through a capstone project |
| *Would the following approach to pedagogy be valued?* | |
| | Encourage active learning, interactive discussions, action plans, and pursuit of the understanding of fundamental structures of other disciplines (for example: design, for planning, business administration [Lemon 2018], finance). A focus on territories of learning rather than on disciplines |
| | Degrees of freedom of speech and exploration unlimited, but conditional: confinement within accepted universal moral codes and limited to comments based on data or other evidence as justification for action |
| | Encouragement of new, awkward thought, if supported by careful continued dissection of issues arising therefrom, be they exploratory and without evidence, but always followed by close dissection and analysis of consequence |
| | Solutions searched for across disciplines with residents encouraged to contact others to understand their way of thinking |
| | Active sequenced creation of social capital culminating in an established initiation of a *capstone project*: a multidimensional, pragmatic, valued project, that provides a pathway for application of the accumulated intellect and already completed contributory practical experiences, with a broad societal benefit. Such projects would have to demonstrate the extent of bridges and trust built with residents, professionals, financiers, business and the wider citizenry, across the country/internationally and do so in ways that extend their plans into the corridors of the movers and shakers in society—judiciary, legislation, politics and government |

| | |
|---|---|
| *Should assessment include the following?* | |
| | Ideas put forth by the residents should be evaluated on three counts to note if there is: (i) a sequenced plan for the production of outcomes of value, (ii) a list of what the different sectors of society suggest, and (iii) a discussion of how to approach a diversity of views with the potential value/effects of building social capital for improved health.<br>In addition, formal structures of assessment for basic constructs of the different disciplines will need to be conducted through standard written tests and a viva. |
| *Would having predetermined anchors or foci as concentrations on which to peg various leaning experiences be valued?* | |
| | Major anchors (which multiple cases would repeatedly refer to) could be: cities, death, human nature; and art, literature and history (especially regarding the development of social capital and human endeavours) |
| | Repeated, informal social interaction and communication with people in power, as critical anchors for gaining insights into *how society functions* |
| | Ancillary material will be required: specially constructed cases, portions of books, and films; webinars, exhibitions, drama presentations, musical concerts, and critical published papers (for example, the Princeton paper comparing the Chin and Roman empires around 300BC) https://www.princeton.edu/~pswpc/pdfs/scheidel/041305.pdf |
| *What could serve as frameworks for developing a micro-strategy?* | |
| | Once the broad frameworks have been established, details of territories of learning can be set. They can be composed of combinations of disciplines—for example: design, mathematics, force field analysis, strategic planning, business, finance and markets. These can be done in combinations that allow the development of a grasp of their structural concepts). With the building of social competence, character, agility and productive curiosity, serenity, and the ability to contribute to social capital, management and analysis of data can be included in case discussions. If a case needs to be put to the assemblies, then a group of students could plan for lobbying that idea to the people who are the movers and shakers. A visit to assemblies in action would also give a taste of how processes move through legislative assemblies.<br>What should be the guiding principles to select different foci of different learning experiences? |

Once course content has been defined, we can move onto artful mentoring (see Table 18.5). A good sample case is: 'Why was Virchow not charged with sedition?' The assigned projects (for example a project to lower the case burden on the government's free hospitals) can be used to guide the SR to valued learning in preparation for interactions in the outer, real, weakly controlled, unsheltered world.

**Table 18.5: One possible framework for a sample case titled: "Why was Virchow not charged with sedition?"**

| THE CASE | **Why was Virchow not charged with sedition?** |
|---|---|
| Brief summary | (The summary is not shown to students)<br>Rudolf Virchow discovered in the 19th century that the insanitary conditions of a township were responsible for the start of a typhus epidemic. Instead of focusing on the social determinants of health alone, he wrapped it in with his political thinking and proposed that the citizens be given distinct independent citizenship. He deviated from a useful focus and was not able to ensure that the parliament of the time understood the value of social determinants of health. Till today, there is only lip service paid to the social and economic determinants of health.<br>A hypothetical way in which the learning from the case might unfold under the guidance of a superb teacher is outlined in this table. |
| Purpose of the case | Understanding different ways of presenting problems to a government for solution.<br>An initiation into the way in which politics and activism at times get mixed with decisions which governments should take on purely scientific or carefully reasoned grounds.<br>To appreciate Virchow's ability to spot the neglected state of society as a determinant of health.<br>To search as to why nearly two centuries elapsed (from Virchow's report) before the social, economic and environmental determinants of health were given importance.<br>To dissect Virchow's behaviour and politics; understand the vagaries of human nature; and explore the relationships of scientists with those in power. |
| Anchors | Human nature, politics, legislature, failure to develop social capital, social and economic determinants of health (SEDOH). (This is not the main case for increasing residents' understanding of SEDOH.) |

| | |
|---|---|
| Threads | The links (vehicles) that connect different elements in this "case": social capital, history, poverty, political neglect, root cause of illness, the essentiality of water in the link with health and municipal responsibilities for supply. (The latter could be linked to a case with Velasquez's painting of the water carrier of Seville, juxtaposed with a photograph of a Bhistee distributing water in a goat skin pouch, in Karachi, a city of 20 million, in 2020.) |
| Hidden generic objective | To search for and obtain facts and develop opinions only after researching the topic and dialoguing or debating with others. (This is common to all cases.) To define the building blocks that would help meaningful communication with those in government. To be able to defend one's views and respond to others' challenging one's view. |
| Target of inestimable value | This case is aimed at initiating understanding of the need to retain the relevant focus that a task demands and not deviate from that to include personal political agendas. The resident is also made aware of social determinants of health and the political processes for implementing change. |
| *Key resources include* | McNeely I. F., *"Medicine on a Grand Scale": Rudolf Virchow, Liberalism, and Public Health.* 2002. The Wellcome Trust Centre for the History of Medicine at University College London Occasional Publication, No. 1<br>https://core.ac.uk/download/pdf/36688109.pdf<br>(The same resource could also be used for a case specifically directed toward development of social capital, specifically concerning interaction with government and legislature.)<br>Glover J., *Man of Iron: Thomas Telford and the Building of Britain.* 2017. Bloomsbury.<br>Other books can be selected by faculty teaching the course. |
| *First session* | Discussions could begin by drawing attention to the fact that Virchow developed his views from close observation of the inhabitants of the village of Sohrau in Silesia (the students should find out where it is situated; currently it is in SE Poland), to which he was sent to report on the typhus epidemic in 1848.<br>Discussions could then be focused on recognition of talent, ability, competency and knowledge. Residents could be asked: Why was a pathologist chosen for this task? When you want a task done, is it competency you look for or a degree? Or a friend? Or a compliant subordinate who follows your orders?<br>Or do certain tasks just require a special skill or attribute? Was epidemiology a known specialty in 1848? How do disciplines emerge in universities? When did epidemiology become recognised? What was the role of the Broad Street Pump and why did the typhus epidemic and Virchow not launch a discipline? Who was the first chair of mathematics in the world? |

| | |
|---|---|
| | Did someone with a university degree invent the steam engine? Was choosing Virchow a correct decision? Discussions could be held around topics such as: What is more important: a university degree, competence, ability, agility? Social competence? A majority opinion? Polls?<br>A troubling question very pertinent to all of us because of some of the world happenings in January 2021 is the question of majority opinion and wisdom from a stable group in a country, company or hospital etc. When we refer to the value of the principle illustrated in Fariuddin Attar's congregation of the birds, should we also be cognisant of the problems that majoritarianism poses…especially if decisions are based on a mob? Why did Attar raise the spectre of wisdom and knowledge of the group being paramount?<br>Students could be challenged by the question: 'What recent occurrences around the globe are potential avenues for human collaboration?' and 'Are they an inevitable manifestation of the system of governance? Are they demonstrative of the multiple faces of majoritarianism?<br>If it is competency you are looking for, if a technician were to be converted to a cyborg, and could operate tremor free to perfectly anastomosise a vasculature of ~1mm diameter, and replace a severed digit, should the technologist-cyborg be allowed to do at least a part of the operation? Would you call him a surgeon? Would you take your friend or dependent to him or her for surgery? As the performing craftsman would have an intact brain, can the cyborg take over the entire process of diagnosis, empathic management, surgery and postop management?<br>What or who is a cyborg? How will you differentiate human enhancement from replacement of lost parts by technology?<br>What should be the limits of human enhancement? (This should link up with another case or seminar on human enhancement, surgeon and society.) |
| | Who was Britain's "first engineer" [answer Thomas Telford]? (Telford brought up by his mother, started life as a stonemason. He lived in an area where the shepherds wrote poetry in Latin. How do you explain the use of Latin in Britain? Did Telford have a degree in engineering?)<br>The famous "iron bridge" in Shropshire, Britain, was built because commerce had been facilitated by the development of a *cheaper process* for smelting iron. The community became rich and a bridge was required to assist the flow of goods.<br>Why then is Telford buried in Westminster Abbey and not the "architect" of the bridge in Shropshire? What does it take to get recognised? Is being recognised important? Is it dependent on "friends in high places"? Have you read *Laton McCartney's* |

| | |
|---|---|
| | *Friends in High Places: The Bechtel Story: The Most Secret Corporation and How It Engineered the World* (1989)?<br><br>The teacher could then move on to considerations of recognition for individuals' accomplishment, and why recognition matters. How often do we praise our children? How often do we praise our colleagues? How can we prevent praise becoming meaningless? Is a system of sending out accolades to colleagues important in times of unusual stress such as pandemics? |
| *Attention to critical change* | What is the critical change that Bismarck should have brought about to improve the health of the nation? Was what Bismarck did, regarding supporting the poor financially, effective? Did it improve the country's health? Was Virchow unable to move from the particular example to the greater good of the nation? Was Bismarck's decision correct? How was it different from Virchow's focus? How different is it from the roll out of Pakistan's Ehsaas programme in 2020? What is Sania Nishtar's role in this? Do you think that the ideas expressed in her book *Choked Pipes* (2010) set the processes in motion? Did learning about how to deal with global issues and her experience with the WHO help make her more effective than Virchow?<br>What was the critical change that allowed iron to be produced in large quantities at a lower cost, that ultimately led to economic success for a community, which then built the bridge to improve commerce? (The catalyst was the use of coke.[4])<br>Can you find a similar critical factor that will make surgery low cost? |
| Faculty teaching the course could pick up any of the following approaches to challenge residents. The curriculum will guide which topic will be taken up in which year of the residency. | |
| | Virchow noted the general debasement of the population, which had rendered it susceptible to epidemic onslaughts. He noted "the poverty, shabbiness of their living arrangements, their poor eating habits, and their utter lack of hygiene;" the "vermin" and lice, and stated that "the Silesian leaves it to celestial providence to free his body occasionally by a heavy shower of rain, from the crusts of dirt accumulated on it" [25]. (Appreciate the language!) This experience made him appreciate the social *and political* cause of disease. |

[4] When distilling bituminous coal in retorts to obtain gas for illumination, or by burning it in kilns or pits, the residue left behind is called coke, which is simply coal charcoal, and is nearly pure carbon.
https://www.scientificamerican.com/article/coke-and-coal/

| | |
|---|---|
| | What are the social and economic determinants of health; and what are the educational and environmental determinants? Can you prioritise the listings of social determinants (found on WHO websites)? Provide your reasons for choosing the first three highest impact factors.<br>(The same question can be asked in years 3 and 6, so that the residents can themselves gauge the degree of change in their opinions over time. This draws attention to the changing nature of opinions…) |
| | Students will be tasked: in year 1 of the residency, write down what you feel your involvement should be in approaching health through the lens of social, economic, educational, environmental determinants of health. |
| | Students' attention could be brought to the following: In 1848, the conscientious government sent Virchow to investigate an epidemic. Observations initiated some beneficial actions.<br>In your country, how can you increase the sensitivity of government to initiate data collection on important issues not yet on their radar? What are the recent examples where the government has used data? What is the degree of involvement of people-government interactions in decision-making on COVID-19 related issues in your country?<br>What is the one surgical disease in which *you* think ONE government action has the potential to bring about a lowering of either incidence, cost or mortality? (One of the acceptable answers might be: if the government would disseminate knowledge of problems that arise from consanguinity and baradari marriages, and institute genetic testing of relatives of children found to have genetically induced renal stones, it would go a long way in reducing the incidence of renal stones in children.) |
| | Virchow made the mistake of suggesting independence for the area in which the epidemic raged. Why did he mix a political statement with a health remedy? Was he right in so doing so? Why was he making a statement in favour of Poles? Was he Polish? (Students on searching Internet sources might find out that Virchow was born in a town which is now a part of Poland.)<br>Was Virchow a politician? An activist?<br>Should physicians be activists or should they try and have their voice heard by governments by other means?<br>What do you think was the state of social capital in Poland at the time of Virchow? Was the monarch dictatorial or the prime minister?<br>Students can be asked to find alternatives to social activism. The value of non-confrontational negotiations, conversations, debates, and dialogues can be discussed. Examples of neutral persons |

| | |
|---|---|
| | negotiating peace deals or division of countries can be searched for. How did they do it? (Example: Clinton from USA helped Ireland; Marker from Pakistan negotiated the East Timor deal.) |
| *Duration* | Sessions related to this case could run across the six years of residency, with faculty choosing increasingly complicated issues to unravel as the student grows in knowledge and confidence in being able to express views based on careful reading and thinking. |

A presentation of SR's interim views, to a critical audience which includes all strata of society (the local and wider community) and people in the corridors of power, would assist in honing the SR's thinking.

Assigned or self-chosen projects could be modified by faculty to require the building of relationships across professions, between ranks of citizens, communities, and the government. Projects (including a culminating capstone project) provide experience; they should be mentored to inculcate habits of identifying complementary strengths outside of surgical professions and to develop methods, based on trust and tolerance, of building lasting associations with many sectors of society. As these relationships remain and become wider points of contact for use in times of future distress (when a real-life problem seems insurmountable), SRs should be guided on retaining contacts developed during course work.

Including those in "governance structures" of society during evaluations allows SRs to review their strategy and the fragility of their own locus of control, and learn when it is necessary to deploy rational, reasoned control, aggressive insistence on truth, leadership skills, dialogue, diplomacy, tact or collaboration whilst "ceding territory."

Inter-sectorial, inter-professional teams built during assignments, which are inclusive of non-medical professionals and citizens, provide experiences of pathways to successes in real life in the spheres of work, play, performance and social usefulness, as they facilitate the internalisation of processes that determine project success, to the same extent as witnessed when an SR "automatically" dons gowns and gloves, without the need to think of the individual steps.

If such a process is developed by the curriculum it would admirably arm the SR to become a valued citizen contributor to social capital.

## 5.0 Defining anchors, foci, and pedagogical strategies which sweep across territories of required knowledge, unbound by traditional disciplinary limitations

To maintain an active interface between society and SRs; to bring in societal problems which bear on health; to bring attention to the social, economic, environmental, and educational determinants of health; and to eradicate the peculiar inaction of humans for the good of their fellows, three topics of study appear most useful: the city, human nature, and death. Using these three anchors several cases could be elaborated. Case based teaching would be advantageous as each case can be individually constructed for longitudinal study incorporating various sensory stimuli that necessitate a change in the course of action.

As much as a dissection of death, the vagaries of living humans' vacillating thought and the variegated aspects of human nature demand critical study. Death, dying and use of the self for others after death is often a taboo subject avoided but requires deep reflection.

The modern city (a black hole that generates illness as prolifically as it generates the trash and sewage under the weight of which it is collapsing), needs new design principles to be incorporated, to abolish its isolationism; its anonymity, frustrations and vandalization by skyscrapers; its partitioning of children from animals and farms; its contribution to global warming; its wastage of water in extravagant flushing systems; its propensity to show off with the tallest and the most extravagant; its facilitation of socially unchecked behaviours (for example cigarette smoking, betelnut chewing, drugs and drinking); the unnecessary long haul transport of its food chain, with the attendant diesel exhaust as food for the lungs and associated plastic packaging and salt that kills people; and the motorization of movement, the use of lifts, the impossibility of cycling anywhere…with the resultant promotion of auto-transport often with one occupant/car (in the absence of city transport), clogging of roads and coronary arteries, the diffusion of dioxin, and much more. The transformation of cities is a fitting anchor; a purpose around which to build part of the curriculum, with other possible anchors being human nature, death, pollution and non-communicable diseases.

### 5.1 Transmission of conceptual subject matter as territories of knowledge, such as pollution, energy and conservation; and not as disciplines such as design, architecture, law, governance, business and economics

If only one subject in BE were to be taught, philosophy (in the original sense of the word, the study seeking truth) would fit admirably.

But effective function in today's world requires knowledge of an extensive range of subjects. Gradual assimilation of a conceptual understanding of any discipline can be acquired during perusal of a personally chosen problem for in-depth study, for which more than one discipline will be seen to interact with the problem, creating *knowledge territories sans frontiers*. This territorial approach (in contrast to a discipline based one) could be supported by: (i) accessing Internet resources which engage foundational understanding from many disciplines, and allow growth at a pace commensurate with SRs' requirements and abilities, as is done at Khan's Academy (Khan Academy 2021); and (ii) reaching out to successful people in allied professions, the community, in business (Christobal, Engel and Jamsheer 2009) and government, to learn first-hand what does and does not work. An alternative to attaining deeper understanding is to appreciate a different approach and seek help and collaboration in writing and executing plans from subject experts.

Relevant territories could include: "Upstream factors that generate illness" (which include pollution, industry, poverty, consanguinity, use of plastics for storing water, or addictions to alcohol, tobacco, sugars, and hard drugs) (Singh et al. 2012); global warming; or say, the provision of water and its distribution to a city, a need noted from the times of the Roman Empire.

Essential territories would be the study of how societies function; the variations in individual behaviour within society; how valued social capital is developed and can be destroyed; and the function of surgeons within evolving contexts of war, disaster, and peace. History, art, literature and philosophy can be the vehicles for enhancing understanding, but need not be a prime focus for learning of or about these subjects.

The effects of war (the largest contributor to conditions requiring surgeons' attention) (Garnett 2015), through the eyes of suffering, deprived populations with their disease susceptibilities (and not the historical narration of war), must be understood. However, the naval battles of

World War II do additionally provide tales of drama, heroics, strategies and counterstrategies that make interesting reading.

Artfully developed cases that have engaging sensory triggers that raise residents' curiosity and which evolve through twists and turns that nudge the learner to deftly change their understanding of what is happening, renew a search in a different territory/discipline. It can lead to them time seeking different solutions and strategies (as knowledge of usefulness of another discipline emerges) or studying the manufacture of products by industry (requiring knowledge of entrepreneurship, finance, budgeting and planning), which will hopefully result in the SR internalising new and useful concepts for solving problems.

### 5.2 Case-based teaching, supplemented by projects, is aptly suited to shaping the SR's territorial approach to learning

BE should propel SRs onto the runway of development that converts them into sage advisors who examine all facets of a problem in detail. It allows them to give governments, legislators and politicians valued advice and an assurance of continued support based on facts and data. It is here that practical experiences (for example developing a capstone project) allow SRs to establish an evolving, working relationship with a government. For that to happen, the SR's informal interdisciplinary and inter-institutional networks and networking with communities, other professions, and people in diverse occupations—linked ultimately with presentations to society and government—can enlighten governments through the presentation of problems and ideas for solutions. Activism is not required in a country with high social capital and should be eschewed. The case-based teaching approach can prime the individual to identify which linkages will need to be developed.

Is such an approach pragmatic? All professions might not think so, especially not surgery. But if every project protects a freedom (as Churchill drew attention to during the bombing of London in WWII, when he stated that the citizens would be ready to "fight the Nazis, from street to street, house to house," to protect their freedom, if the courts were functioning [History Extra 2021]), society will remain grateful to the profession for moving the issue through the corridors of power and surgeon-citizens will blur the distinction between the governed and government in a rich elaboration of social capital. Citizens will drive the move to universalise the broader education of its professionals.

Professions would need to consider a major change which would enable them to extend their traditional responsibilities to include outward-looking, proactive, inter-professional and inter-sectoral collaboration. You may ask: "Just how realistic is it to expect all professions to adopt such wide-ranging commitments? We propose that professions would need to consider a major change which would enable them to extend their traditional responsibilities to include outward-looking, proactive, inter-professional and inter-sectoral collaboration.

## 6.0 How can a faculty friendly extended BE be developed?

A conceptually sound curriculum based on needs assessment can be drafted to define content and strategy. Easy to develop on paper, faculty engagement in its preparation might result in a more doable curriculum. Commencing from a series of questions posed to faculty in a workshop setting (according to the pattern listed in Table 18.4), a pragmatic model could evolve through workshops which drive participant enquiry to a realisation of its value. Once that is attained, implementation will be facilitated. The possible shaping of the programme by cultural influences and restrictions imposed because of potential difficulties in obtaining resources will have to be guarded against.

The construction of the curriculum is foundational but the executives who bring that curriculum to life are the faculty and other teachers; it is they who will play the critical role in developing the 21st century surgeon. It is critical that the pedagogical strategies in the curriculum be set and taught by a body of "teachers" cognisant of the 21st century trends shaping the future of learning (Thornton 2016).

## 7.0 Will a medical humanities curriculum suffice?

The humanities courses in the Faculty of Arts and Sciences are well developed and effective. Social competence is admirably developed in these undergraduate programmes. However, approaches seen in undergraduate liberal arts education where curricula are built on a deep thoughtful study of subjects and associated activities are not suitable for transplantation into SEPs. A medical humanities curriculum (MHC) which includes the study of humanities, social sciences and arts for undergraduate medical education is included by many medical schools to improve empathic treatment and to incorporate a broader look at patient care (Batistatou et al. 2010). But it is not broad enough. The task of BE is to enlarge the SR's mind beyond the delivery of patient care. An imaginative approach is required that *immediately captures and sustains* the SR's interest in exploring new details of what would be considered "irrelevant subject material" if taught by discipline.

The MHC could be used as an initial template, expanding learning by using paintings and artefacts to initiate learning if there is a link leading to a demonstrable relevance to influencing human behaviour and disease prevention or cure. For example, a newspaper photograph of a water carrying "Bhistee," distributing water on foot in a goatskin bag in 2020 in Karachi, side by side with Velasquez's picture of the water seller and dusty roads in early 17$^{th}$ century Seville, in an era where macadamisation of roads with tar was unknown. A picture of the flooding of the streets of Karachi with sewage, juxtaposed to an aqueduct carrying water to Rome, brings to attention the importance of water and effective sewerage systems, and can lead to discussions on the waste of water in modern water closets. These pictures provide sensory stimuli that trigger learning, and can be followed down alleyways of thought generated by the SR viewing the picture, or down through a plan developed by faculty.

A case could be developed around the quandary of a principal of a Medical College in Pakistan, who couldn't find doctors for night duty, as reported in the newspaper *Dawn* on January 24, 2021, despite graduating over 300 doctors a year. This is reportedly because most graduates are women, not allowed to work at night or work at all by their husbands. Such a case would lead to the discussion of social customs and a pragmatic solution to the problem.

All cases must be developed within the framework of a curriculum.

Whatever the curriculum, a content, placement, relevance, and pacing that comply with student requests (Shapiro et al. 2009) should be ensured, as advised by Shapiro in his critique of the medical humanities curriculum.

The development of the curriculum itself might be facilitated by following a structured framework moving sequentially from situational analyses (of the world and the surgeon's world), intended goals and objectives, overall strategy, and pedagogy, to cases which are linked to repetitive themes (which could be called anchors) with specific attention on the inclusion of specific triggers for discussion.

Curriculum development will need to be supported by a *corps* of effective teachers and case-developers.

# 8.0 Pragmatics

Such an approach must be presented in ways that do not allow it to appear difficult to introduce or implement.

In this era of online education, faculty will need to review educational research to (i) seek the latest methods to promote learning in the contexts of objectives, (ii) promote learning originating from cases stretching across different disciplines, and (iii) accommodate the individualistic requirements of a diverse student body. Strategy should encourage growth of student confidence and allow learning at a different pace (Arguel et al. 2016). Changes in educational design will have to be reiterative—changing and flexing as feedback from students indicates the need for changes in pace and direction or introducing new halt points (for detailed explanation of difficult to understand topics) and alternative strategies when blockades appear on the pathway to the completion of assigned tasks (Agostinho, Bennett and Lockyer 2016; Dawkins 2016).

In informal discussions, during the development of this paper, multiple questions were raised: how will curricular strategies promote the goal of connecting surgeons with communities, health delivery systems, and governance structures; and how will they promote the development of social capital? Is there any free time at all in residents' schedules, to fit these courses in?

A detailed explanation is given in Supplementary Material S2 below.

**Supplementary Material S2**

***How new BE programme strategies could engage communities, professions, government and legislature***

Involvement with the community could be made to grow out of a clinical encounter, a planned research project, or a visit to a field site of research conducted by community health departments (say, a survey of settled squatters' settlements to determine the nutritional status of the children there). Additional research projects could review the link between nutrition and poor social conditions, or child behaviour in hospital and response to surgery. They could define nutritional measures to be instituted in the community (for example would zinc deficiency delay wound healing?). The clinical encounter noted in a reflexive journal and discussed with a mentor could, for a urological resident be a renal stone in a child. Mentoring faculty, by gentle probing, will need to ask why the stone formed, whether there could be genetic cause for the stone, how the resident will determine if this is so, how every member of the family would need to be screened, how endogamy and consanguinity would need to be determined in this patient's cousins, and in their tribe; and what the conditions are of the tribe, how easy it would be to investigate them (are they in isolated mountainous regions where there are only mule and horse tracks, is the next community far away and at such altitudes that consanguinity persists?). The student-mentor team would work out educational materials for the community in *their* language, and, by year 6, assess the effectiveness of their residency regarding the attitudes to and incidence of consanguinity. This is but one example of defining opportunities in clinical care encounters, showing how we can enter into the lives of communities and provide educational support to change their behaviours to improve their health.

All residents could be asked to plot the trajectory of any of their ill relatives (who are not entitled to free treatment at the hospital where they work) from the time of their first symptoms to getting admitted for surgery. In COVID-19 times, how many times was the person asked to do a COVID test prior to admission? What was the cost? When returning home, was there support for physiotherapy, nursing, lab tests, telemedicine consultations or a sense of abandonment? Did the relative turn COVID positive after admission to the hospital or after discharge? When the inability to pay full fees was discussed, was an option of (say) using a cheaper implant raised? Did the person have to order something from abroad for treatment?

Of greater value would be the tracking by residents of care at a public hospital for a relative or a poor servant, then contrasting this with healthcare at his or her hospital. In following the journey through the hospital, the SR could identify what can be easily done to ameliorate some of the difficulties patients have to endure. This would identify the weak links in the excellent care delivered in the public sector.

Some general practitioners' (GPs) offices could be visited to see if all have a couch for the patient to be examined on, whether they have gloves and essential equipment, and whether the family physician/GPs have updated their certification.

A research project could evaluate what happens when there are no beds in a public hospital. Is there a link with other public hospitals? Does the government pay private hospitals to take on patients refused by public hospitals? Is there a data information centre available for people to find out where there are empty beds, and which public transport to take? How successful is the government-private partnership in hospital management?

A national disaster (at a simple level, torrential rains) is a firm testing and learning ground for residents. Alternatively, in a plane crash in which all victims were burnt, there is an opportunity to visit the morgue and witness its scenes of distraught relatives unable to find their dear ones; the anguish that relatives feel when they are told this burnt body is your relatives', when they cannot understand what DNA is and how it helps, or the possibility of an error given the technique used and the person performing the test. The magnitude of the grief, and measures to help relatives, can be viewed, and ideas formed challenging the patterns of grief counselling for different segments of the country's population. The same accident could be an opportunity for contacting the municipal or town council representative and reviewing what role they play, talking to them and if something more can be done, convincing them to do so; and if the councillors are obdurate, seeing if there is a social group of people living on the same street, to redress grievances, to link up with them…and ask if they could help their neighbours in distress.

Residents could be posed with problems in a hypothetical patient: for instance, noting difficulties in procuring a liver transplant, the risks involved and noting that the deceased donor's liver can be accessed without risk to the donor as in a living transplant. In this instance, how would they go about drafting and processing a law which promulgates that—as in Spain (wherein the body belongs to the State on death)—the State can claim a dead body for the benefit of society? What would be the cultural impediments? What would be necessary for a law to be passed? Who needs to be approached for moving the process through legislation into law? How many years would this take? What changes the mode of thinking of societies? What triggers could be used to enlighten societies to think out their problems rationally? Talks by lawyers, concerned citizens, transplant surgeons, legislators, and politicians would be enlightening.

As groups of individuals in the same year would have different problems, and as any presentation from these groups would be made to the group of students in any of the 6 years of residency, the fallout benefit from the study by a small group of SRs would positively impact all residents, as the attendees would include even those residents not in a special programme of BE.

Before institutional partnerships with the government develop, government officials could be invited as faculty to teach on courses or be part of workshops arranged for or by residents. Webinars by lawyers, judges, environmental protection agencies, tax officials, or budget specialists from government and civil society, could initiate SRs on the path to finding out how the country runs its legislature, courts, laws, police, and municipal governance, and what staff, equipment, and infrastructure is required to manage cities.

The panel of judges for the capstone oration could include government officials, informed of their role: critique of the project in ways that would assist the presenting SR would strengthen their approach to participation in the civic responsibility of contributing to social capital.

Briefly, the pedagogical strategies would increase and extend contact of SRs from individuals to families and communities. Research communities would be built in which team members included persons from civil society, government, industry, and professionals from other disciplines; SRs would be exposed to webinars from different sectors of society and government, and, for example, a non-accusatorial and cooperative approach to ensure environmental protection could be developed.

## 8.1 Creating time to avoid the extension of residency training by an extra year

Certainly, time will be required for residents to search, think, interact, rethink, and develop useful documents, videos, posters, speeches, and working papers, as well as perhaps undertake community service. Faculty will need time for case construction, which can be reduced by having a library of useful ideas, web links as references for listed topics they address, and options for their use, listed and stored in a library of learning objects and sensory triggers.

The arguments against the programme based on unavailability of time will become less aggressive once the value of the programme is realised. Graduands will be eagerly sought for, as Assistant Professors who change the way surgery is practised.

Initially however, a reorganisation of the SR's schedules and working at the hospital will be required. To allow time for learning without interfering with the provision of service, the six year programme could be split into two phases.

In Phase I, the first two years of SEPs, residents could receive intensive instruction in classroom, skill labs, and research settings as a thorough "*Preparation for service*," before immersion into difficult patient care. Phase I would also require mandatory attendance of surgical grand rounds; morbidity and mortality conferences; and most of the residents' core presentations. They would be fully participatory in a limited number of consulting, outpatient clinics, at fixed times that would not clash with learning sessions. Phase-I SRs would not be involved in ward or emergency care but would increase efficiency on wards and in operating rooms as they enter Phase II, "*Learning from practice*."

In Phase-2 (years 3-6), SRs would learn from full active participation in service, and will have been so admirably prepared that they will facilitate processes and reduce operating room time wastage, knowing exactly what to do for patients with changing vital parameters. They will be capable of performing (with appropriate supervision) circumcisions, cystolithotomies, ureteroscopies and simple radical nephrectomies, for instance, efficiently, in <1 year.

Another approach to universalisation and popularisation, would be to demonstrate the value of these courses by placing course material on the web and encouraging it to "go viral" across networks, world-wide, hopefully exciting the Bill Gates of our world to support it as he did Khan's Academy.

Whilst these changes are discussed in the context of the SR, these principles are applicable across all medical, nursing, and dental programmes. SRs would benefit if the same case is discussed in business, management, law and public administration schools, from which will emerge a host of new ways of looking at the world's problems in health.

Where will the teachers come from? The many faculty with hidden talents and accomplishments in developing social capital can be encouraged to become natural teachers and mentors for extended broader education (XBE). The willingness of faculty to explore the case with students will be an asset.

An alternative approach to XBE based on a case-study, whilst yielding rich dividends, requires complex, time-consuming organisation, mentorship and concentrated study. SEPs other than those in university settings, may find it too resource intensive and impracticable.

An alternative model could focus on building social capital, using a series of pre-recorded webinars presented by those in government, industry, law, and different professions, as well as community leaders, as it would be less intrusive on faculty or surgical training time. Selected Ted talks could be included. These sessions could be scheduled at designated times (just like mortality conferences, today) and reviewed by SRs at leisure, who would search the literature later to gain a better understanding. Such seminars could be buttressed by films and required reading of portions of novels, plays or publications in the lay press providing sensory stimuli for the SR's development within the framework of the curriculum.

Their written summary of what they learnt could form the basis of continual assessment and the practical execution of a project for improvement of social capital could be included in the final evaluation.

The course could limit its focus on a few major topics: (i) understanding how society works; (ii) human nature and society; (iii) factors in inequity; (iv) persuasive dialogue with the power structures of society; (v) the impact of early childhood development, of nutrition, social, environmental and economic determinants of health; and (vi) the fine differences between the desired progression of humans and perceived progress as we define it today, inappropriately, in the contexts of better life-styles, fixation on money, consumerism and consequent blatant pollution.

The alternative strategy is advantaged by the ease of spacing teaching sessions within the existing schedules. Thirty-six seminars (six per year) accompanied by discussion sessions, online tests, assignments, and a culminating capstone project, can be more readily achieved.

But SRs would miss the interaction-induced growth of knowledge, the practical networking, and the development of tolerance, trans-disciplinary friendships and behaviours that is so much the essence of enlightened undergraduate education seen in liberal arts colleges and which would be the central feature of full XBE. The alternate programme's graduands, will not be as well equipped to survive and morph as the world *and world of the surgeon* changes, though capable of effectively championing some projects leading to improved surgical health—for example, assuring wider access to surgery and planning delivery systems for surgery across populations. BE and its modified forms would make SRs effective in reaching out into the community and up towards government, convincing them of the need for action. They would influence policy through the channels that build social capital. And if these courses were online and held simultaneously across the country's universities and programmes there would be potential for a networked collaborative growth of empowered graduating surgeons.

It is worth going the extra mile as BE graduands will avidly be inducted into faculty ranks, where they will continue their influence by bringing to light the value of systems-thinking and of linking disease to living but refuse-drowned cities, to pollution, over-population, poor maternal and early childhood care and to the non-evolving nature of human nature—with its covetousness, avarice, tribal nature, powers of discrimination, and our sad evolution into a consumeristic, polluting society demanding instant gratification (Fromm 2001).

Above all they will contribute to social capital which will enhance processes and systems that contribute to autocorrecting and evolving systems of governance.

## 9.0 Conclusion

Intellectually-charged, reasoning, broadly educated surgeons contributing effectively to social capital can transform and enlighten the inter-relationships across strata of society and its governance structures, as they strive to improve surgical health. Extended BE has potentials for becoming a model for an enlightenment of the caring professions, perhaps, of Kantian proportions.

## Bibliography

Aga Khan University. "Breast cancer is one of Pakistan's deadliest diseases." Accessed February 10, 2021. URL: https://www.aku.edu/news/Pages/News_Details.aspx?nid=NEWS-002352.

Aga Khan University. "COVID-19: supporting the Sindh government's measures." Accessed February 10, 2021. URL: https://www.aku.edu/news/Pages/News_Details.aspx?nid=NEWS-002122.

Agostinho, Shirley, Sue Bennett and Lori Lockyer. "The design process of university teachers: A descriptive model." In *Show Me the Learning, Proceedings ASCILITE 2016 Adelaide,* edited by S. Barker, S. Dawson, A. Pardo and C. Colvin, 17-19. Adelaide: Proceedings ASCILITE 2016. URL: file:///C:/Users/sarfa/Downloads/Content_Strategy_A_Lesson_from_the_Indus.pdf.

Amjad, Shazia and Muhammad Ali. "Philanthropy in Pakistan: Why civil society organizations get bypassed in favour of donations to individuals." *Stanford Social Innovation Review*. Accessed February 14, 2021. URL: https://ssir.org/articles/entry/philanthropy_in_pakistan

Arguel, Amael, Jason M. Lodge, Mariya Pachman and Paula de Barba. "Confidence drives exploration strategies in interactive simulations." In Show *Me the Learning, Proceedings ASCILITE 2016 Adelaide,* edited by S Barker, S Dawson, A Pardo and C Colvin, 33-42. Adelaide: Proceedings ASCILITE 2016. URL: file:///C:/Users/sarfa/Downloads/Content_Strategy_A_Lesson_from_the_Indus.pdf.

Batistatou, A., E. A. Doulis, D. Tiniakos, A. Anogiannaki and K. Charalabopoulos. "The introduction of medical humanities in the undergraduate curriculum of Greek medical schools: challenge and necessity." *Hippokratia* 14, no. 4 (October 2010): 241-3. URL: https://www.ncbi.nlm.nih.gov/pmc/articles/PMC3031316/.

Christobal, Fortunato, Charles E. Engel and Talati Jamsheer. "Network: TUFH Position Paper - The Ultimate Challenge? Higher Education for Adapting to Change and Participating in Managing Change." *Education for Health* 22, no. 3 (November 2009): 419. URL: https://www.educationforhealth.net/text.asp?2009/22/3/419/101513.

Dawkins, Roger. "Content strategy: a lesson from the industry for university learning analytics." In *Show Me the Learning, Proceedings ASCILITE 2016 Adelaide,* edited by S Barker, S Dawson, A Pardo and C Colvin. Adelaide: Proceedings ASCILITE 2016. URL: file:///C:/Users/sarfa/Downloads/Content_Strategy_A_Lesson_from_the_Indus.pdf.

*Dawn*. "'Open merit policy has caused doctors' acute shortage at healthcare facilities." Accessed February 10, 2021. URL: https://www.dawn.com/news/1603189.

Fromm, Erich. *The Sane Society*. New York: Rinehart & Company, Inc., 1955.

Garnett, D. "The Surgeon's Role." A Reenactor's Site! Accessed January 18, 2021. URL: http://www.dagarnett.com/surgeon.htm.

History Extra. "Churchill's greatest speeches". Accessed February 10, 2021. URL: https://www.historyextra.com/period/second-world-war/churchills-greatest-speeches/.

Haskins, Julia. "Where are all the women in surgery?" AAMCNews. Accessed March 11, 2021. URL: https://www.aamc.org/news-insights/where-are-all-women-surgery

Khan Academy. "A personalized learning resource for all ages." Accessed January 18, 202. URL: https://www.khanacademy.org/about.

Lemon Jack D. "Perspectives: The MD/MBA: An emerging Dual Degree in Health Care". *The Journal of the Lancaster General Hospital* 13, no. 2 (Summer 2018): 52-55 URL: http://www.jlgh.org/Past-Issues/Volume-13-Issue-2/MD-MBA.aspx.

Lexico. "Meaning of singularity in English." Accessed February 15, 2021. URL: https://www.lexico.com/definition/singularity.

Louvre. “The Oath of the Horatii: Department of Paintings: French painting”. Accessed February 10, 2021 URL: https://www.louvre.fr/en/oeuvre-notices/oath-horatii#:~:text=Work%20The%20Oath%20of%20the%20Horatii&text=In%20the%207th%20century%20BC,family%20are%20prostrate%20with%20suffering

McNeely, Ian F. *“Medicine on a Grand Scale”: Rudolf Virchow, Liberalism, and Public Health.* London: The Wellcome Trust Centre, 2014. URL: https://core.ac.uk/download/pdf/36688109.pdf.

Office for National Statistics. “Social capital in the UK: 2020.” Accessed February 15, 2021. URL: https://www.ons.gov.uk/peoplepopulationandcommunity/wellbeing/bulletins/socialcapitalintheuk/2020.

Shapiro, Johanna, Jack Coulehan, Delese Wear and Martha Montello. “Medical Humanities and Their Discontents: Definitions, Critiques, and Implications.” *Academic Medicine* 84, no. 2 (February 2009): 192-198. DOI: 10.1097/ACM.0b013e3181938bca.

Singh, S, J McCool, J Weller J and A Woodward. "Medical Education in the 21st Century: Students Driving the Global Agenda." *Education Research International* 2012, Article ID 185904 (March 2012). DOI: https://doi.org/10.1155/2012/185904

Talati, Jamsheer, “Lower Urinary Tract Injuries”. *In Surgery for All. A View from the Developing World*, edited by M. Ahmed, R. J. W. Blanchard, B. Eklof, T. S. Harrison, F. Moazam, S. K. Suleman, J. Talati and S. Tibblin, 95. Lahore, Rawalpindi and Karachi: Ferozesons (Pvt) Ltd., 1992.

Talati, Jamsheer. “The training of a ‘stone doctor’.” *Arab Journal of Urology* 10, no. 3 (2012): 220-229. DOI: 10.1016/j.aju.2012.05.003.

Thornton, Linda F. “The Future of Learning Isn’t About ‘Knowing’.” Leading in Context. Accessed February 10, 2021. URL: https://leadingincontext.com/2016/02/10/the-future-of-learning-isnt-about-knowing/.

University of Minnesota Extension. “Community Social Capital Model.” Accessed December 9, 2020. URL: https://extension.umn.edu/leadership-approach-and-models/community-social-capital-model.

West Midlands History. “The story of the Iron Bridge – The birth of the bridge”. Accessed February 10, 2021. URL: https://historywm.com/films/the-story-of-the-iron-bridge-the-birth-of-the-bridge.

# CHAPTER 19

# COLLEGIALITY AND PROFESSIONALISM: SETTING STANDARDS AND VALUES IN AN ACADEMIC AND DIVERSE DEPARTMENT

SHAISTA MASOOD KHAN

## Introduction

Collegiality is defined as a behaviour that encompasses and facilitates a positive and productive work environment; the beneficiaries being faculty, trainees, and other members of a department, university, research or practice. Whilst engraved for centuries it has evolved from a simplistic order to a diverse set of principles attributable to behaviours. It imparts certain privileges as well as obligations bound by ethical links to protect those at a disadvantage—the most challenging component being its applicability and assessment.

## Historical development

The first known usage of the term in print was in 1874. Used by Cicero to describe a gathering of priests, the word collegium was later adopted by the Catholic Church to refer to a gathering of bishops (Mangiaridi and Pellagrina 1992). Historically identifiable collegial medical institutions first appear in the era of Hammurabi, the ruler of Babylon (Petro 1992). The ruler is best known for the development of a code of laws, known as the Code of Hammurabi, which was used to regulate Mesopotamian society; the extant portion of code establishes a fee schedule and sets standards by creating punishments for failures/complications:

> "If a physician heals the broken bone or diseased soft part of a man, the patient shall pay the physician five shekels in money." (Hammurabi's Code: # 221).

Hippocrates is well accredited for laying the foundation of modern medical collegiality, still applicable and valid after 2,400 years. Medical schools that developed in the Middle Ages in Salerno, Bologna, Padua, Montpellier, Bruges, and Paris represented the first institutionally based collegial groups within medicine. The first academic usage of collegiality referred to the community of scholars at Oxford University.

The Royal College of Physicians in England was started to bring together collegial groups of practitioners (Laws Jr 1992) and faculties of medicine were established on the continent to provide for collegial groups of individuals active in medical practice who had set standards and principles by which they formed their organizations.

## Understanding collegiality

A collegium refers to a group of individuals subscribing to a common idea and pursuing a common goal. This entails certain obligations and privileges. When this is applied to an academic group it refers to a group that focuses on knowledge, the common goal(s) being its preservation, validation, communication and extension. The venue required to achieve these goals is a university. The academic output of a university can be productive if the environment is conducive to freedom of inquiry. John Henry Cardinal Newman, a non-academic religious person stated perfectly that the "University is a place where ideas, not men rule." A new idea should be nurtured through a complete cycle of inception and validity, concluding with acceptance or rejection. An idea may be rated as "good" or "bad." Often bad ideas are a springboard for good ideas. But how these ideas are processed by the collegium is crucial.

When critiquing, the idea and not the person should be critiqued in order to sustain the lifecycle of an idea. As a member of a collegium, one should promote free expression, apply logic and encourage positive competition. The critique of a person is usually directed by emotions with ultimate secondary personal gains.

## Modern concepts of collegiality

Collegiality over time has evolved with concepts and understandings that have shifted with an applicability that is more diverse. Although the collegium is referred to as a "common group," there is an element of "elitism." This happens as standards are set and "the group" delineates.

Although the term elite has a negative connotation, it is a fundamental of the creation of these groups. Although containing people of differing ethnic, religious and socioeconomic backgrounds, these are specially created groups. Mangiardi and Pellegrino identify that the group enjoys certain privileges but also has certain obligations. Fundamental to the functionality of this group is autonomy and freedom. Max Weber assumes a different outlook. A German social scientist and one of the founders of modern sociology, Weber described the conflicts between professionalism, which is considered pro ethical, and bureaucracy which he considered pro materialist. He considers collegial structure integral to advanced specialization.

Malcolm Waters, in his review of Weber's analysis, refers to authority based on knowledge (the professional collegium) and authority based on power (the bureaucracy). Bureaucracy is represented by a monocratic organizational structure. The theoretical knowledge base of the profession ensures the availability of expertise. Weber did not consider collegial formation successful for social regularization. The advantage Weber attributes to bureaucracy may provide an understanding of approving and licensing bodies' implementation of external reviews, regulation and control over medical practice (Laws Jr 1992).

## Obligations and privileges

In an academic ethos, two key partners work towards achieving the common goals: the faculty and the university. Both are united by collective commitment to some idea, the pursuit of which entails certain privileges and imposes certain obligations (Mangiaridi and Pellagrina 1992). To achieve maximum academic output, a university should facilitate high individual efficiency. The obligations of the university are to preserve, validate and teach existing knowledge free of external influences, and to attain new knowledge through research.

(1) Academic freedom of expression, enquiry, free and open communication, honesty and fastidiousness in the reporting of research results are vital.
(2) The university has an obligation towards facilitating the duties and privileges of the collegial relationship. It should also provide an environment, both in monetary and practical terms, to ensure these activities can take place without external influences (Mangiaridi and Pellagrina 1992).

The faculty's obligation is to practise honesty and fidelity in its research ethics, inclusive of its ethical obligations to other colleagues. These obligations (duties) should evolve into virtues circumventing mutual respect that are not confined to colleagues but concern society as well. Civility of communication must be understood in terms of critiquing ideas. Often critiques get misdirected to individuals and not the idea behind the research. This begins a negative competition and can lead to the death of the idea, before it has completed its lifecycle.

## Faculty citizenship

With the evolving understanding of collegiality, the new notion of faculty citizenship should be discussed.

What is faculty citizenship? Faculty citizenship is a pattern of behaviours within a faculty that promotes the welfare of the department and as a consequence the university. It is more generic without linkage to any specific faculty role. It comprises two components: faculty engagement and collegiality.

Engagement is performance of the assigned responsibilities and willingness to participate in additional opportunities, perhaps more service related and more measurable in nature (Hammer et al. 2019). This engagement may manifest as positive or negative.

Collegiality includes interpersonal behaviours that promote a positive and productive work environment and culture, that ultimately benefit other faculty, students and trainees, as well as the department, school, university, discipline, and profession in which the faculty is engaged (Hammer et al. 2019). The emphasis is on "patterns" of behaviour and not a single event as anyone can have a "bad" day or a "good" day.

It therefore helps the university to establish citizenship expectations for its mission and reward individuals that go beyond the basic requirements (Hammer et al. 2019). But crucial to the success of citizenship behaviours is due appreciation of the university for these efforts, in doing so avoiding "citizenship fatigue."

## Inequalities of an academic medical collegium

The stakeholders of a medical collegium extend beyond faculty. Prime in the group are patients, students, residents and nurses. As referred to earlier, there is an element of elitism in this group that has, in an invisible manner, violated the intended egalitarianism. An unseen inequality in power has become the "norm" between physician, patients and trainees—not forgetting that a physician colleague frequently occupies the seat of a patient. The medical collegium stands apart with intense moral obligations. With the ultimate goal rooted in the practicality of conducting research that can be transferred to the bedside for patients' benefits, the ultimate goal is improved patient outcomes.

The academic collegium rests on attainment of knowledge. Knowledge is truth and purity. Acquisition of knowledge (by research) should be true and transmission of this knowledge (research results, teaching) should be sincere. While recurrent narratives of the personal experience of trainees are well known (Hall and Wong 2017; Nicholson 2012), lack of collegiality is also experienced in our nursing colleagues (Reiger 2001).

The inequalities occasionally politically exceed geographical boundaries (Mullan 2015). As responsible members of a collegium, we carry the responsibility to disengage healthcare related events from political sanctions. This imbalance between the physician and patient is on account of:

1. The vulnerability of the patient
2. The moral nature of medical decisions
3. The physician's monopoly on medical knowledge

The patient is dependent on the physician and is forced to seek advice from them as they are more empowered in terms of knowledge and skill. This can be readily exploited on monetary or emotional fronts.

Medical decisions and care are integral to accurate knowledge and skill. A physician's collegiality focuses on the patient's betterment and hence competencies are required to deliver good care. Perhaps, here is where Max Weber's preference for bureaucratic control may ensure through credentialing processes the issuance and renewal of licenses.

The physician's monopoly on medical knowledge by default empowers them in accrediting programmes, in being admitted to or ejected from the medical community. As stewards of this body of knowledge, physicians are obliged to preserve, validate, teach, and extend medical knowledge, ensuring also that it is available to those who are partners in this venture (Mangiaridi and Pellagrina 1992). Our trainees as students and residents should not be denied the correct transfer of knowledge and skill by adequate supervision, and formal and informal teaching. These needs manifest more under extenuating circumstances when the support required exceeds theoretical knowledge with mentoring (Reiger 2001).

## Collegial ethics

While collegiality is well understood in a multitude of ways, collegial ethics is perhaps a relatively new term which recognizes experiences that are not so new. This is with reference to faculty support. It is generally a straightforward answer when we ask ourselves how to treat our fellow faculty members. Applying the social norms with complete friendly and cordial support is the answer. But what about times when a faculty is in trouble?

While several of us may have experienced these, we are not experts in handling them. Often a young member of faculty faces the giants of the corridors of power as an infant, and is forced to comment/share personal views. The goal of collegial ethics is to actively support our colleagues and to develop the skills needed to do so (Kuhar and Cross 2013). If help is intended to be delivered it should be timely and appropriate in order to gain benefit.

It may not be easy to help a colleague. Sometimes we are not sure what the facts are, or sometimes we lack the structure to channel our involvement. We also know that taking a stand on a controversial issue can be perilous and hurt our career (Bird and Hoffman-Kim 1998). Therefore, we may perceive a danger to ourselves and decide to stay out of it. What have been the responses observed in such situations:

1. Avoid the mental efforts to judge and "blame" the accused or the victim.
2. Avoid taking sides and remain out of it by adopting a stance of "being fair."

Both of these stances actually skirt the issue rather than addressing and preparing our own take on it. But should we get involved in every event? Some such incidences may be totally personal affecting the accused/victim.

A good start would be to ask:

*What would be the impact on our colleagues, and our institutions?*

*When are the losses or gains great enough that we must step up?*

*How much should we contribute just because we are fellow human beings?*

A crime has to be differentiated from a wrongdoing. While the crime is not to be supported, a wrongdoing should not result in "ethical guilt," incurred from lack of support rendering an "ethical debt." Judgement when required should be inclusive of compassion and fairness. The key elements to address such events are:

**Using appropriate language and communication**

We have to be careful about how we talk about a given situation or colleagues (Kuhar 2011). Unfortunately, the language used in conversations about hurt or accused colleagues is often not helpful and is often more like judgmental "gossip" or posturing than a thoughtful discussion. Hurtful things may be done and said in a casual setting, without realizing their impact and influence on others.

Discussions in a larger faculty group may muster and increase the required support and also help in knowing the correct details of the events. This avoids "gossip" based on presumptions and assumptions. There are several additional factors to consider. There is, for instance, the golden rule which is found in all or most societies: "Help others as we would like to be helped" (Runes 1959). If we truly want to be fair to ourselves and our colleagues, we need to withhold stating false opinions and speak the truth. Agreeing to something you really do not believe in creates an internal dissonance, and the data may surprise you. Experimental studies have found that after you agree to something you really do not privately believe in, your private opinion changes to bring it more in line with what you have said (Gawronski and Strack 2004; Festinger and Carlsmith 1959).

**"Do no harm"—or "Minimize harm," applying the basics of the Hippocratic oath**

This could happen if incorrect information is disseminated with added personal remarks that are inappropriately articulated. If harm cannot be eliminated it should be minimized. One of the integral requirements therefore is "courage." This has been underestimated in supportive and ethical matters. Mark Twain said that "courage is resistance to fear, mastery of fear—not absence of fear" (in Cipriano and Buller 2012).

Overall we need to be aware of whether the things we say or do are destructive to others in some way or not. Choose the golden rule as a useful guideline, and the mandate of the Hippocratic Oath—first do no harm.

Careful selection of language incorporating a neutral and supportive approach when discussing the issue or talking to colleagues is vital. Over recent decades, there have been remarkable advances in ethics in related areas such as the protection of animal and human subjects in research. Ethical training in those areas required that we spend time with related precedents, cases, rules and guidelines. We regularly review those rules and guidelines and update ourselves (Grants & Funding: NIH Central Resource for Grants and Funding Information n.d.; Office of Laboratory Animal Welfare n.d.). This raises our awareness of ethical behaviour in research and encourages correct action.

While we have developed the necessary expertise to recognize ethical transgressions in research, there is perhaps a need to develop expertise to learn and practise collegial ethics. Omar Bradley, a highly successful World War II general, said that, "The world has achieved brilliance without wisdom, power without conscience. Ours is a world of nuclear giants and ethical infants" (Bradley 1967). Overall we need to be aware of whether the things we say or do are destructive to others in any way.

## Assessing collegiality

Whilst a comprehensive understanding of collegiality has evolved, one of the most challenging tasks is measuring it. Collegiality is incredibly difficult to measure. Assessing behaviours more often incriminates the subjectivity of the assessors. The fact is that collegiality has always been difficult to achieve. Partly for this reason, the maintenance of the collegial environment has not yet been made explicit in such documents as academic faculty bylaws, Board of Trustees resolutions, etc.

One should be wary of the potential negative consequences of such evaluations; wary of a real or perceived violation of the basic spirit of collegiality, of academic freedom, judgement of personality and the modifying process of promotion/tenure. Hence its exclusion as a separate measure in the promotion and tenure process has been suggested. Instead, it should be incorporated in the three major arenas of faculty's practice: teaching, research and service. The challenging questions relate to who measures it; which tools are used; and finally to its documentation.

It could be an essential response segment of evaluation forms by students and peers, but several self-evaluation proprietary questionnaires are available. The Atlas Self-Assessment Matrix (S-AM) or Collegiality Assessment Matrix (CAM) are two such examples (Cipriano and Buller 2012); a locally created checklist and rubric is another option. Easterling suggests some collegiality behaviours such as verbal and nonverbal signs of respect; civility in interactions with each other; self-motivated collaboration and cooperation on departmental, teaching and scholarly activities; and intentional, professional interactions between peers (Easterling 2011).

As referred to earlier, it is the "patterns of behaviour" that are to be used. Letters from others could also contribute in identifying patterns of behaviours. Finally the department chairs' evaluation of faculty citizenship behaviours would widen the catchment, making it more robust. However, one should be cautious of the easy documentation of "lack of collegiality" that would have a negative impact.

Once defined and operationalized, it should be decided if these assessments would be used across the board (annual performance etc.), or only for high stakes reviews such as promotion and tenure. These expectations should be measured as having been met, not met or having exceeded the expected performance levels. They should be used, for instance, in identifying components of professional development and the annual evaluation or recognition/award of high levels of collegiality. What has been lacking is giving due recognition and importance to collegiality in an academic unit. A separate award should be instituted for this attribute.

## Departmental implementation

The significance of collegiality remains undisputed. What is required is better presence and visibility in academic departments as a capacity and an attribute. Awareness amongst faculty can be enhanced by revisiting faculty citizenship, which is becoming extinct. Mandatory workshops to build the necessary knowledge and capacities should be conducted. Through assessment tools, patterns of behaviour can be identified. Besides offering support to correct any deficiency, a special award to acknowledge members with this quality can be added to the departmental appreciation armamentarium.

## Conclusion

Collegiality has historically evolved over centuries. An integral component of the social and academic setup, its understanding and applicability have transgressed from its initial group of bishops to employees in organizations and faculty in academia. Several facets have been consistent from the Codes of Hammurabi to the recent collegial ethics. Crucial to its survival is to be reminded that it refers to a collegium that is endowed with the freedom to work towards a mutual goal. Monotony without the dynamism to innovate and a sustained uniformity would assure its extinction; this is a journey that has already started. The privileges of a medical collegium—inclusive of the freedom to pursue medical knowledge, perform therapeutic interventions, and the freedom to engage in research and experimentation—are bound with obligations of sharing medical knowledge with colleagues and trainees through teaching. The moral covenant to patients, adherence to a medical code and the stewardship of knowledge are unavoidable obligations.

## Bibliography

Bird, S. J. and D. Hoffman-Kim. "Damned if you do, damned if you don't: The scientific community's responses to Whistleblowing." *Science and Engineering Ethics* 4 (March 1998): 3–6. DOI: https://doi.org/10.1007/s11948-998-0001-6.

Bradley, O. *Collected Writings, Vol 1*: Cosmological Economics, 1967.

Cipriano, R. E. and J. L. Buller. "Rating faculty collegiality." *Change* 44, no. 2 (March 2012): 45-48. URL: https://eric.ed.gov/?id=EJ960022.

Easterling W. V. "Collegiality: A singular concept?" *Indiana University-Purdue University Indianapolis (IUPUI) Scholar Works Repository*, Heading: Collegiality as behaviour (March 2011): 6. URL: https://scholarworks.iupui.edu/handle/1805/2539.

Festinger, L. and J. M. Carlsmith. "Cognitive consequences of forced compliance." *Journal of Abnormal and Social Psychology* 58, no. 2 (March 1959): 203–210. DOI: https://doi.org/10.1037/h0041593.

Gawronski, B. and F. Strack. "On the propositional nature of cognitive consistency: Dissonance changes explicit, but not implicit attitudes." *Journal of Experimental Social Psychology* 40, no. 4 (July 2004): 535–542. DOI: https://doi.org/10.1016/j.jesp.2003.10.005.

Grants & Funding: NIH Central Resource for Grants and Funding Information. "NIH regulations, policies and guidance: ethical guidelines and regulations." Accessed August 26, 2010. URL:

http://grants.nih.gov/grants/policy/hs/ethical_guidelines.htm
Hall, Justin N. and Shermon G. Wong. "A Call for Collegiality in Residency." *Journal of Graduate Medical Education* 9, no. 3 (June 2017): 401. DOI: https://doi.org/10.4300/JGME-D-16-00851.1.
Hammer, Dana P., Leigh Ann Bynum, Jean Carter, Nicholas E. Hagemeier, Daniel R. Kennedy, Parto Khansari, Pamela Stamm and Brian Crabtree. "Revisiting Faculty Citizenship." *American Journal of Pharmaceutical Education* 83, no. 4 (May 2019): 7378. DOI: https://doi.org/10.5688/ajpe7378.
Kuhar, M. J. "Collegial ethics: What why and how." *Drug and Alcohol Dependence* 119, no. 3 (December 2011): 235–238. DOI: doi.org/10.1016/j.drugalcdep.2011.10.015.
Kuhar, Michael J. and Dorthie Cross. "Collegial Ethics: Supporting Our Colleagues." *Sci. Eng. Ethics* 19, no. 3 (September 2013): 677–684. DOI: 10.1007/s11948-012-9364-9.
Laws Jr, Edward R. "The Advantages of Collegiality." *Bulletin of the New York Academy of Medicine* 68, no. 2 (March-April 1992): 297-302. URL: https://europepmc.org/backend/ptpmcrender.fcgi?accid=PMC1810159&blobtype=pdf.
Mangiaridi, J. R. and E. D. Pellagrino. "Collegiality: What is it?" *Bulletin of the New York Academy of Medicine* 68, no. 2 (March-April 1992): 292-6. URL: https://www.ncbi.nlm.nih.gov/pmc/articles/PMC1810187/
Mullan, Zoe. "Collegiality without borders." *The Lancet Global Health* Vol 3, no. 1 (January 2015): 1e1-e61 DOI: https://doi.org/10.1016/S2214-109X(14)70375-4.
Nicholson, Joshua M. "Collegiality and careerism trump critical questions and bold new ideas: a student's perspective and solution. The structure of scientific funding limits bold new ideas." *Virginia Polytechnic Institute and State University, Blacksburg, VA, USA Bioessays* 34, no. 6 (June 2012): 448–450. DOI: https://doi.org/10.1002/bies.201200001.
Office of Laboratory Animal Welfare. "PHS Policy on Humane care and use of laboratory animal models tutorial." Accessed August 25, 2010. URL: http://grants.nih.gov/grants/olaw/tutorial/index.htm.
Petro, Jane. "Collegiality in History." *Bulletin of the New York Academy of Medicine* 68, no. 2 (March 1992): 286-91. URL: https://www.ncbi.nlm.nih.gov/pmc/articles/PMC1810169/.
Reiger, Paula T. "Collegiality." *The Oncologist* 6, no. 1 (February 2001): 3. DOI: https://doi.org/10.1634/theoncologist.6-1-3.

Runes, D. D. *Pictorial history of philosophy.* New York: Philosophical Library, 1959.
Thinkexist Quotes. "Twain, M". Accessed on April 26, 2010. URL: http://thinkexist.com/quotations/courage/3.html.

# CHAPTER 20

# WORK-LIFE BALANCE AND BURNOUT IN A SURGICAL CAREER

RIDA MITHA
AND MUHAMMAD SHAHZAD SHAMIM

## Work-life balance: definition, traditional perspectives

Balance as defined by the Oxford English Dictionary is, "an equal distribution of [a] weight or amount." Whereas this definition may be literally accurate, another definition more relevant to sociology and more applicable to our specialty as doctors is, "stability of body or mind" (Guest 2002). By this standard, the term work-life balance (WLB) should be straight forward, as defined by Akhtar et al., as the management of the actual and desired proportion of one's work and private life (2020). Jones, Burke and Westman define it in other simpler words as, "the equilibrium between personal life and career work" (2013). However, both these definitions imply that the two aspects of life are separate, and we all know that for doctors, there is always an overlap between the two, sometimes impossible to demarcate. In fact, students for a long time were taught in medical schools to consider being a doctor, not as a career, but as a way of life. For this and several other reasons, it is perhaps appropriate to say that the correct definition of the phrase remains dynamic, and thus elusive, as it may vary according to professions, individuals, and also for each individual, according to their circumstances.

The concept of a WLB dates back to the Industrial Revolution in the late 1800s, when the working hours of women and children became restricted, eventually leading to a 44-hour work week law in 1938, to allow women to spend more time at home. However, this was not applicable for professionals such as doctors, who in those days were never really considered off work, or on leave (Raja and Stein 2014). In recent decades, as more data are emerging on the effects of long working hours on patient care, as well on the mental health of healthcare providers, a healthy WLB is gaining more popularity. A relatively specific Google search for, 'work-life balance for surgeons' reveals 1,850,000,000 results (as of February 2022).

Traditionally there are five main models used to describe the relationship between work and life outside work (O'Driscoll and Randall 1999; Zedeck and Mosier 1990).

1. The *segmentation model* hypothesizes that work and non-work are two distinct entities of life that are lived separately and have no influence on each other;
2. A *spillover model* hypothesizes that one world can influence the other in either a positive or negative way;
3. A *compensation model* proposes that what may be lacking in one area of life, can be made up in another;
4. An *instrumental model* whereby activities in one part of life can facilitate success in the other; and
5. The final model, a *conflict model*, which hypothesizes that with high levels of demand in all spheres of life, possibly some significant overload on an individual can occur.

The pressures of work have also been intensifying, so much so that in the UK even though the average number of hours worked has remained steady, the proportion of people working more than 48 hours in a week has increased (Guest 2002). This along with a higher proportion of women from all social classes engaged in paid employment has led to an increased interest in the conflict and spillover models of WLB. With the onset of longer work hours, more exhaustion and the growth of evening and weekend work, little scope is left for "quality" family or leisure time, further sparking interest in the need for WLB.

Furthermore, facilitated by new technology there is an increased scope for work from home, which further blurs the borders between work and home. This was particularly seen during the COVID-19 pandemic. On any normal day, people are border-crossers as they move between home and work. However, this border becomes increasingly permeable when work-from-home strategies are put into place, giving opportunity for spillover and conflict to occur between the two spheres of life.

So, are these borders desirable? And if so, then, under what circumstances (Clark 2002; Guest 2002)?

Each person's environment has some givens—things that are difficult to alter. But the environment also provides choices and opportunities, for each person to exercise a degree of autonomy. Some aspects of work/family border management may be within a person's control: the amount of flexibility in one's working schedule; the degree to which a person can work at home or carry out family responsibilities during work time; the management of responsibilities in each sphere; and the amount of spillover between work and home. However, of note is that some jobs and some families may limit an individual's freedom to manage borders by allowing little independence and flexibility, or setting up negative repercussions for the individual (Clark 2002).

## Work-life balance for doctors

Medicine is both a demanding and valued profession. Doctors are required to work long hours, make difficult decisions and cope with death and distress, all while maintaining compassion (Shanafelt et al. 2015). Doctors spend more than a decade in post-secondary education and overall work substantially more hours than the average employed individual. Therefore, it is no surprise that doctors often struggle to integrate their professional and personal lives. It is also not surprising that medical training is associated with significant mental health problems with a recent review concluding that lack of WLB, long hours, lack of job satisfaction, being a female medical professional and being younger in age are important predictors of burnout in doctors (Amoafo et al. 2015).

There have been numerous studies depicting the work-life imbalance that doctors and doctors-in-training face during the course of their careers. What is important to understand is that balance changes at different parts of one's career. In 2015, Nievas et al. (2015) described a resident's perspective of WLB, stating that overnight calls and weekend calls define and shape the lives of residents. Even with work hour regulations, their reduced duty hours were made up by working weekends; hence, family time was unlikely to be recovered. Days off included catching up on lost sleep, and regaining the strength to survive another day. The same paper also reflected on an attending physician's point of view regarding WLB. In their opinion, "considering work and life as two opposite forces is like dividing ourselves into two pieces that cannot coexist" (Nievas et al. 2015). It is better to accept the reality that work will absorb a large part of a doctor's life and spending time worrying about how much one has to work or how many overnight calls one has to do will only lead to further stress, while still having to do the same amount of work. It is not surprising that several studies demonstrate that depression, substance abuse, and suicide levels among medical students and doctors are two to six times the national averages (Cohen and Patten 2005; Dyrbye, Thomas and Shanafelt 2006).

In late 2015, with increasing concerns about the incidence of burnout and lack of WLB in doctors in the UK, a large study was conducted to assess the WLB of doctors in training in the UK, from the perspectives of trainees and trainers (Rich et al. 2016). 96 trainees and 41 trainers from London, Yorkshire and Humber, Kent, Surrey, Sussex, and Wales were interviewed over the course of the study. Five themes came to light illustrating key contributors to work-life imbalance.

1. Trainees felt they had to prioritize work over home life to cope with a difficult job while also completing their training requirements;
2. Frequent transitions at work and home could disrupt personal relationships;
3. Trainees felt they lacked time to cope with personal pressures outside of work which they perceived as significantly affecting their learning and performance;
4. Low morale and a feeling of exploitation was exacerbated by the proposed junior doctor contract; and
5. A greater negative impact was perceived in women due to structural barriers and discriminatory attitudes.

The study showed that along with long hours and the high volume of patients to care for, trainees were expected to work in their evenings and holidays to fulfil their training obligations, leaving little to no time for activities outside of work. As part of the NHS, trainees frequently changed workplaces, which could result in having to spend time away from family and friends, putting a huge strain on relationships. A trainer taking part in the study also stated that, "the geography and the lack of autonomy [are the biggest problem for trainees]. […] Having to move and not having control over where and when you move is difficult." On an extreme end of the spectrum, some trainees felt becoming a doctor was a dehumanizing experience going as far as to say, "you can't be a person and a doctor" (Rich et al. 2016).

The lack of WLB was felt to have a larger effect on the learning, performance and career progression of trainees with children (or who wanted children) and women in particular. Trainees described negative attitudes from seniors towards pregnancy, and towards women who wanted to work less than full time. A female surgery resident detailed, "I've had people say to me, so 'you're either a woman or a neurosurgeon, you can't be both [...] it made me lose the passion for my specialty and for my job'" (Rich et al. 2016).

In June 2011, a large national survey was conducted in the US to see the rates of burnout and satisfaction in terms of WLB amongst doctors across all specialties. A probability based sample of the general US population was also surveyed for comparison with doctors (Shanafelt et al. 2012). It was observed that doctors practising dermatology, general paediatrics and preventive medicine had the highest rated satisfaction of WLB, while doctors practising general surgery, general surgery subspecialties and obstetrics/gynaecology had the lowest rates.

The study (Shanafelt et al. 2012) also compared 6,179 non-retired doctors to 3,442 employed non-doctors. Doctors worked a median of 10 hours more per week compared to the population controls. 40.1% of doctors did not think their work schedule left enough time for personal or family life compared with 23.1% of controls ($P < .001$).

A follow-up study was done from August to October 2014 (Shanafelt et al. 2015), where US doctors and a probability-based sample of the general population were surveyed, similar to the survey done in 2011. When compared to 2011, the rates of satisfaction with WLB were lower in 2014 (40.9% vs. 48.5%; $P<.001$). Furthermore, satisfaction with WLB was lower in 2014 for all specialty disciplines with the exception of obstetrics and gynaecology and general surgery; 5,313 doctors were also compared with 5,392 employed, non-physician population control subjects. Doctors had a lower rate of satisfaction with WLB than the general US working population (36.0% vs. 61.3%; $P<.001$) and remained less likely to be satisfied with WLB compared with the population (odds ratio, 0.68; 95% CI, 0.62-0.75; $P<.001$).

Closer to home, a study conducted at the Aga Khan University Hospital between September and December in 2016 assessed satisfaction with work as well as the emotional and personal lives of residents in various medical and surgical specialties (Khan et al. 2020). A total of 275 residents were included in this study, with the subjects working a mean of 83.20±22.3

hours per week and spending 6.42±3.3 hours per week on academic activities. Only 13 subjects (4.7%) believed they had a WLB, 109 (39.6%) expressed moderate dissatisfaction with work-related factors, 119 (43.3%) were dissatisfied with life outside work, and 102 (37.1%) were dissatisfied with their health. 165 residents (60%) also believed their job had negatively affected their private lives.

When asked to suggest measures to improve WLB a hike in pay scale was suggested by 238 respondents (86.5%); 229 (83.3%) suggested a reduction in work hours; and 179 (61.8%) felt WLB monitoring by the Department of Postgraduate Medical Education (PGME) would be helpful.

## The Libby Zion Case (1984): a landmark case that brought doctors' working hours to light

Libby Zion was an 18-year old college student admitted to the New York City Hospital in 1984 with a fever and an earache. On admission her temperature was 103.5°F with no obvious aetiology. Seven hours later her axillary temperature was 107.8°F, after which she died (Bell 2016).

Upon admission she was looked after by an emergency room resident and an intern. No attending physician had seen Libby (Patel and Popp 2014). At the time, the same residents were covering dozens of other patients. The unexpected death left the family distraught and Libby's father requested an investigation into his daughter's death, due to which a grand jury investigation was convened.

This prompted a series of regional investigations that resulted in recommendations of profound changes in graduate medical education (Patel and Popp 2014). 18 months of deliberation by an appointed committee, including comments from all representatives of organized medicine such as the American College of Physicians, led to the enactment of "The 405 Regulations," also known as "The Libby Zion Regulations" or "The Bell Regulations." Findings by the committee emphasized the issue of supervision of young doctors by attending physicians. The recommendations also included limits on the hours worked by doctors, stating that, "Residents shall have a work week which will not exceed an average of 80 hours per week averaged over a 4-week period and should not be scheduled for more than 24 consecutive hours with one 24-hour period of non-working time per week hours" (Patel and Popp 2014).

The case led to widespread discussion on doctor burnout and the extreme fatigue faced by doctors. Several years had gone by before a general agreement was reached regarding the cause of Zion's death. Zion had taken a prescribed antidepressant, phenelzine, prior to her admission at the hospital. The combination of phenelzine with pethidine (given to her by the resident and intern) led to the development of serotonin syndrome, a condition leading to increased agitation. Her fever reached dangerous levels and she died soon after of cardiac arrest.

## Burnout

Professional burnout is a syndrome characterized by a loss of enthusiasm (emotional exhaustion), feelings of cynicism (depersonalization), and a low sense of personal accomplishment (Shanafelt et al. 2012). Findings of studies suggest that burnout may erode professionalism, influence quality of care, increase the risk of medical errors, and promote early retirement (Dyrbye et al. 2010; Shanafelt et al. 2010; Shanafelt et al. 2011; Wallace, Lemaire and Ghali 2009). Burnout also seems to have adverse personal consequences for physicians, including contributions to broken relationships, problematic alcohol use, and suicidal ideations (Shanafelt, Sloan and Habermann 2003; Shanafelt et al. 2012).

Shanafelt et al. also assessed rates of burnout amongst US doctors and compared them to a population based sample of the general US population in 2011 (2012), with a follow-up study in 2014 (Shanafelt et al. 2015) and reported extremely disturbing numbers. In 2011 (Shanafelt et al. 2012), they reported 37.9% of US doctors had high emotional exhaustion, 29.4% had high depersonalization, and 12.4% had a low sense of personal accomplishment. In total, 45.8% of doctors were considered to be experiencing at least 1 symptom of burnout based on a high emotional exhaustion score or a high depersonalization score. Emergency medicine, general internal medicine, neurology, and family medicine had the highest rates of burnout, whereas pathology, dermatology, general paediatrics, and preventive medicine had the lowest rates. Doctors were also at higher risk for emotional exhaustion (32.1% vs. 23.5%), depersonalization (19.4% vs. 15.0%), and overall burnout (37.9% vs. 27.8%) ($P<.001$ for all) relative to the population control. Characteristics associated with a lower overall risk for burnout were being older (OR for each year older, 0.99) and being married (OR vs. being single, 0.71) ($P<.001$ for both). Hours worked per week was also associated with a higher risk for burnout (OR, 1.02 for each additional hour; $P<.001$).

In their follow-up study in 2014 (Shanafelt et al. 2015), 46.9% of US doctors had high emotional exhaustion, 35.6% had high depersonalization, and 16.3% had a low sense of personal accomplishment. On aggregate, 54.4% of doctors had at least 1 symptom of burnout based on a high emotional exhaustion score and/or a high depersonalization score. When compared with 2011, rates of burnout among doctors were even higher (54.4% vs. 45.5%; P<.001). We must remember that these were the days before the Covid pandemic, and if the same study was to be conducted again, the numbers may have gone further up.

Doctors also had higher rates of emotional exhaustion (43.2% vs. 24.8%; P<.001), depersonalization (23.0% vs. 14.0%; P<.001), and overall burnout (48.8% vs. 28.4%; P<.001) compared to the general US population. After adjusting for age, sex, relationship status, and hours worked per week, doctors remained at increased risk for burnout compared with the population (odds ratio, 1.97; 95% CI, 1.80- 2.16; P<.001) (Shanafelt et al. 2015).

Keeton et al. (2007) assessed predictors of burnout in 935 practising doctors in the US who were not in residency training programmes. They found that measures of burnout (emotional resilience and personal accomplishment) were strongly associated with career satisfaction. The strongest predictor of burnout was control over schedule and hours worked. Control alone explained 30% of the variability in emotional resilience and 20% of variability in personal accomplishment. Total number of weekly hours worked was the second strongest modifiable predictor of emotional resilience and personal accomplishment. These findings are consistent with those of previous studies that also found control and hours worked correlated with career satisfaction and burnout (Richardsen and Burke 1991; Stoddard et al. 2001; Visser et al. 2003).

Roberts et al. (2014) also explored rates of burnout among doctors; 130 internal medicine hospitalists and 448 outpatient general internists were included in the analysis. They reported 52.3% of hospitalists and 54.5% of outpatient internists were affected by burnout (P=0.86). High scores on the emotional exhaustion subscale (43.8% vs. 48.1%, P 5 0.71) and on the depersonalization subscale (42.3% vs. 32.7%, P 5 0.17) were common. Hospitalists were more likely to score low on the personal accomplishment subscale (20.3% vs. 9.6%, P = 0.04) when compared to outpatient general internists.

## Burnout and WLB in surgeons

A career in surgery brings with it significant challenges that can lead to substantial personal distress for the individual surgeon and their family. Burnout among surgeons is increasing at an alarming rate with current reports exceeding 50% (Peckham 2016). A study of the graduates of a single academic medical centre suggested that approximately one third of US surgeons may experience burnout (Campbell et al. 2001).

Shanafelt et al. (2010) did one of the first studies on burnout in surgeons in 2009; 32% of the surgeons initially contacted responded to the survey of which 7,112 were fellows and 769 were associate fellows. Overall, 32% of participants reported high emotional exhaustion, 26% demonstrated high depersonalization, and 13% had a low sense of accomplishment. On aggregate, 40% of respondents had either a high emotional exhaustion score and/or a high depersonalization score and were considered burned out. Approximately 30% of the study participants screened positive for depression. High overall risk of burnout was associated with a younger age and having a spouse employed outside of home as a non-doctor healthcare professional (e.g., nurse, therapist, pharmacist, etc.). Having children was associated with a lower risk of burnout, especially if the youngest child was > age 21. Further characteristics associated with a high overall risk of burnout were specialization (with a higher risk among trauma surgeons, urologists, otolaryngologists, vascular surgeons, and general surgeons), being on call for a higher number of nights per week, increased work hours per week, a greater number of years in practice, and having compensation determined entirely by billing.

Balch et al. (2009) also presented alarming findings in their paper. They found that only 36% of surgeons felt their work schedule left enough time for personal and family life and only 51% would recommend their children pursue a career as a physician or surgeon. They also found a significantly higher rate of divorce among surgeons compared with their internal medicine colleagues. In addition, in a study of 1,118 married physicians, surgeons were found to have a divorce rate of 33% even after 30 years of marriage.

Another study done in 2001 by Campbell et al. (2001) also demonstrated the prevalence of burnout amongst surgeons. 582 actively practising surgeons were included in the study, and were evaluated with regard to 3 elements of burnout: emotional exhaustion, depersonalization and feeling of low personal accomplishment; 32% of surgeons scored high in emotional exhaustion, whereas, 13% scored high in depersonalization. Only 4% showed evidence of feelings of low personal accomplishment. Compared to general surgeons, orthopaedic surgeons were shown to have a significantly higher percentage of depersonalization ($P<0.5$). Other notable findings of the study included an inverse correlation between the number of weeks of vacation taken per year and emotional exhaustion ($P<0.05$), and that burnout was more evident in younger surgeons than older surgeons.

## Burnout – prevention

Burnout has many potential adverse consequences including medical errors, suicide, depression, and absenteeism (Dimou, Eckelbarger and Riall 2016). Healthcare organizations have an economic stake in doctors' well-being, as evidence shows doctors' well-being is related to patient satisfaction, a key outcome variable tracked by most organizations (Haas et al. 2000; Spickard Jr, Gabbe and Christensen 2002). The satisfaction of doctors will enhance recruitment and retention of existing staff, saving the cost of staff turnover (Buchbinder et al. 1999; Crouse 1995; Doan–Wiggins et al. 1995; Williams et al. 2010).

The best prevention, it seems, for doctors' burnout is to promote personal and professional well-being on all levels: physical, emotional, psychological, and spiritual (Spickard Jr, Gabbe and Christensen 2002). However, doctors' well-being requires a significant role to be played by healthcare organizations and doctors themselves. Spickard et al. (2002) made specific suggestions for healthcare organizations to promote doctors' well-being, including establishment of a doctors' health committee whose job it is to review corporate decisions and contracts for their impact on doctors' well-being; establishment of a mentor programme to guide junior doctors through their professional and personal lives; provision of confidential support groups; flexible scheduling to allow time off for critical family events such as births, deaths, graduations, caring for aging patients; and leaves of absence to pursue travel and vocational interests.

Doctors also have a role to play in their well-being. Weiner et al. studied the methods used by 130 primary care doctors to promote their own well-being. The 6 main practices found were spending time with family and friends, religious or spiritual activity, self-care, finding meaning in work, setting limits at work, and adopting healthy positive outlooks on life, such as focusing on success (Weiner et al. 2001).

A recent systematic review and meta-analysis evaluated the effectiveness of interventions to reduce burnout in doctors and whether different types of interventions (physician-directed or organization-directed interventions), doctors' characteristics (length of experience), and healthcare setting characteristics (primary or secondary care) were associated with improved effects (Panagioti et al. 2017). Twenty independent comparisons from nineteen studies were included in the meta-analysis (n=1550 physicians). Twelve studies focused on physician-directed interventions including mindfulness-based stress reduction techniques, educational interventions targeting doctors' self-confidence and communication skills, exercise or a combination of these approaches. Amongst the organization-directed interventions, 5 studies evaluated simple workload interventions that worked on rescheduling hourly shifts and reducing workload. Three studies tested more extensive organization-directed interventions incorporating discussion meetings to enhance teamwork and leadership, structural changes, and elements of physician interventions such as communication skills training and mindfulness (Panagioti et al. 2017).

Physician-directed interventions were associated with small significant reductions in burnout whereas organization-directed interventions were associated with medium significant reductions. The effects of organization-directed interventions were significantly larger than the effects of physician-directed interventions (Cohen Q=4.15, P=.04). Interventions in primary care settings were associated with small to medium reductions in burnout whereas interventions in secondary care settings were associated with small significant reductions in burnout. However, this difference remained non-significant (Q=0.51, P=.48) (Panagioti et al. 2017).

## Conclusion

Burnout and satisfaction with WLB remain critical problems amongst doctors across the globe today. The issues raised not only create personal and professional conflicts amongst doctors but have shown to have a significant impact on healthcare organizations and patient satisfaction. Given the extensive evidence that burnout among doctors has effects on quality of care, patient satisfaction, turnover, and patient safety, these findings have important implications for society at large (Shanafelt et al. 2015). This review demonstrates a need for evidence based interventions addressing the drivers of burnout among physicians. These interventions must address contributing factors in the practice environment rather than focusing exclusively on helping doctors care for themselves and training them to be more resilient.

## Bibliography

Amoafo, E., N. Hanbali, A. Patel and P. Singh. "What are the significant factors associated with burnout in doctors?" *Occupational medicine* 65, no. 2 (March 2015): 117-121. DOI: https://doi.org/10.1093/occmed/kqu144.

Balch, C. M., J. A. Freischlag and T. D. Shanafelt. "Stress and burnout among surgeons: understanding and managing the syndrome and avoiding the adverse consequences." *Archives of surgery* 144, no. 4 (April 2009): 371-376. DOI: https://doi.org/10.1001/archsurg.2008.575.

Bell, B. M. "Reconsideration of the New York State laws rationalizing the supervision and the working conditions of residents." *Einstein Journal of Biology and Medicine* 20, no. 1 (March 2016): 36-40. DOI: https://doi.org/10.23861/ejbm200320511.

Buchbinder, S. B., M. Wilson, C. F. Melick and N. R. Powe. "Estimates of costs of primary care physician turnover." *Am. J. Manag. Care* 5, no. 11 (Nov 1999): 1431-1438. PMID: 10662416.

Campbell Jr, D. A., S. S. Sonnad, F. E. Eckhauser, K. K. Campbell and L. J. Greenfield. "Burnout among American surgeons." *Surgery* 130, no. 4 (October 2001): 696-705. DOI: https://doi.org/10.1067/msy.2001.116676.

Clark, S. C. "Communicating across the work/home border." *Community, Work & Family* 5, no. 1 (April 2002): 23-48. DOI: https://doi.org/10.1080/13668800020006802.

Cohen, J. S. and S. Patten. "Well-being in residency training: a survey examining resident physician satisfaction both within and outside of residency training and mental health in Alberta." *BMC medical education* 5, no. 1 (December 2005): 1-11. DOI: https://doi.org/10.1186/1472-6920-5-21.

Crouse, B. J. "Recruitment and retention of family physicians." *Minnesota Medicine* 78, no. 10 (October 1995): 29-32.

Dimou, F. M., D. Eckelbarger and T. S. Riall. "Surgeon burnout: a systematic review." *Journal of the American College of Surgeons* 222, no. 6 (June 2016): 1230. DOI: https://doi.org/10.1016/j.jamcollsurg.2016.03.022.

Doan–Wiggins, L., L. Zun, M. A. Cooper, D. L. Meyers, E. H. Chen and F. T. W. T. Force. "Practice satisfaction, occupational stress, and attrition of emergency physicians." *Academic Emergency Medicine* 2, no. 6 (June 1995): 556-563. DOI: https://doi.org/10.1111/j.1553-2712.1995.tb03261.x.

Dyrbye, L. N., M. R. Thomas and T. D. Shanafelt. "Systematic review of depression, anxiety, and other indicators of psychological distress among US and Canadian medical students." *Academic medicine* 81, no. 4 (April 2006): 354-373. DOI: 10.1097/00001888-200604000-00009.

Dyrbye, L. N., M. R. Thomas, D. V. Power, S. Durning, C. Moutier, F. S. Massie Jr, W. Harper et al. "Burnout and serious thoughts of dropping out of medical school: a multi-institutional study." *Academic Medicine* 85, no. 1 (January 2010): 94-102. DOI: https://doi.org/10.1097/ACM.0b013e3181c46aad.

Guest, D. E. "Perspectives on the study of work-life balance." *Social Science Information* 41, no. 2 (June 2002): 255-279. DOI: https://doi.org/10.1177/0539018402041002005.

Haas, J. S., E. F. Cook, A. L. Puopolo, H. R. Burstin, P. D. Cleary and T. A. Brennan. "Is the professional satisfaction of general internists associated with patient satisfaction?" *Journal of general internal medicine* 15, no. 2 (February 2000): 122-128. DOI: https://doi.org/10.1046/j.1525-1497.2000.02219.x.

Jones, F., R. J. Burke and M. Westman (eds). *Work-life balance: A psychological perspective*. United Kingdom: Psychology Press, 2013.

Keeton, K., D. E. Fenner, T. R. Johnson and R. A. Hayward. "Predictors of physician career satisfaction, work–life balance, and burnout." *Obstetrics & Gynaecology* 109, no. 4 (April 2007): 949-955. DOI: https://doi.org/10.1097/01.AOG.0000258299.45979.37.

Khan, S. A., M. Waqas, M. Siddiqui, B. U. Ujjan, M. Khan, M. E. Bari and M. A. Azeem. "Work-life balance amongst residents in surgical and non-surgical specialties in a tertiary care hospital in Karachi." *JPMA. J. Pak. Med. Assoc 70* no. (2), 252–258. (February 2020): 252. DOI: https://doi.org/10.5455/JPMA.285942.

Nievas, I. F. Fernandez and D. Thaver. "Work–life balance: A different scale for doctors." *Frontiers in pediatrics* 3, (December 2015): 115. DOI: https://doi.org/10.3389/fped.2015.00115.

O'Driscoll, M. P. and D. M. Randall. "Perceived organisational support, satisfaction with rewards, and employee job involvement and organisational commitment." *Applied Psychology* 48, no. 2 (April 1999): 197-209. DOI: https://doi.org/10.1080/026999499377619.

Panagioti, M., E. Panagopoulou, P. Bower, G. Lewith, E. Kontopantelis, C. Chew-Graham, S. Dawson, H. v Marwijk, K. Geraghty and A.

Esmail. "Controlled interventions to reduce burnout in physicians: a systematic review and meta-analysis." *JAMA internal medicine* 177, no. 2 (February 2017): 195-205. DOI: https://doi.org/10.1001/jamainternmed.2016.7674.

Patel, N. and R. L. Popp. "Learning lessons: the Libby Zion case revisited." Journal of the American College of Cardiology. Elsevier USA. (December 2014). DOI: https://doi.org/10.1016/j.jacc.2014.11.007.

Raja, S. and S. L. Stein. "Work–life balance: History, costs, and budgeting for balance." *Clinics in colon and rectal surgery* 27, no. 2 (June 2014): 71. DOI: https://doi.org/10.1055/s-0034-1376172.

Peckham, C. "Medscape Lifestyle Report 2016: Bias and Burnout." Medscape. Accessed January, 2016. URL: http:// www.medscape.com/features/slideshow/lifestyle/2016/public/overview.

Rich, A., R. Viney, S. Needleman, A. Griffin and K. Woolf. "'You can't be a person and a doctor': the work–life balance of doctors in training—a qualitative study." *BMJ Open* 6, no. 12 (December 2016): e013897. DOI: https://doi.org/10.1136/bmjopen-2016-013897.

Richardsen, A. M. and R. J. Burke. "Occupational stress and job satisfaction among physicians: sex differences." *Social science & medicine* 33, no. 10 (January 1991): 1179-1187. DOI: https://doi.org/10.1016/0277-9536 (91)90234-4.

Roberts, D. L., T. D. Shanafelt, L. N. Dyrbye and C. P. West. "A national comparison of burnout and work-life balance among internal medicine hospitalists and outpatient general internists." *Journal of hospital medicine* 9, no. 3 (March 2014): 176-181. DOI: https://doi.org/10.1002/jhm.2146.

Shanafelt, T. D., J. A. Sloan and T. M. Habermann. "The well-being of physicians." *The American journal of medicine* 114, no. 6 (April 2003): 513-519. DOI: https://doi.org/10.1016/S0002-9343 (03)00117-7.

Shanafelt, T. D., C. M. Balch, G. Bechamps, T. Russell, L. Dyrbye, D. Satele, P. Collicott, P. J. Novotny, J. Sloan and J. Freischlag. "Burnout and medical errors among American surgeons." *Annals of surgery* 251, no. 6 (June 2010): 995-1000. DOI: https://doi.org/10.1097/SLA.0b013e3181bfdab3.

Shanafelt, T. D., C. M. Balch, L. Dyrbye, G. Bechamps, T. Russell, D. Satele, T. Rummans et al. "Special report: suicidal ideation among American surgeons." *Archives of surgery* 146, no. 1 (January 2011): 54-62. DOI: https://doi.org/10.1001/archsurg.2010.292.

Shanafelt, T. D., S. Boone, L. Tan, L. N. Dyrbye, W. Sotile, D. Satele, C. P. West, J. Sloan and M. R. Oreskovich. "Burnout and satisfaction with work-life balance among US physicians relative to the general US population." *Archives of internal medicine* 172, no. 18 (October 2012): 1377-1385. DOI: https://doi.org/10.1001/archinternmed.2012.3199.

Shanafelt, T. D., O. Hasan, L. N. Dyrbye, C. Sinsky, D. Satele, J. Sloan and C. P. West. "Changes in burnout and satisfaction with work-life balance in physicians and the general US working population between 2011 and 2014." *Mayo clinic proceedings* 90, no. 12 (December 2015): 1600-1613. DOI: https://doi.org/10.1016/j.mayocp.2015.08.023.

Spickard Jr, A., S. G. Gabbe and J. F. Christensen. "Mid-career burnout in generalist and specialist physicians." *JAMA* 288, no. 12 (September 2002): 1447-1450. DOI: https://doi.org/10.1001/jama.288.12.1447.

Stoddard, J. J., J. L. Hargraves, M. Reed and A. Vratil. "Managed care, professional autonomy, and income." *Journal of general internal medicine* 16, no. 10 (October 2001): 675-684. DOI: https://doi.org/10.1046/j.1525-1497.2001.01206.x.

Visser, M. R., E. M. Smets, F. J. Oort and H. C. De Haes. "Stress, satisfaction and burnout among Dutch medical specialists." *CMAJ* 168, no. 3 (February 2003): 271-275. PMCID: PMC140468.

Wallace, J. E., J. B. Lemaire and W. A. Ghali. "Physician wellness: a missing quality indicator." *The Lancet* 374, no. 9702 (November 2009): 1714-1721. DOI: https://doi.org/10.1016/S0140-6736(09)61424-0.

Weiner, E. L., G. R. Swain, B. Wolf and M. Gottlieb. "A qualitative study of physicians' own wellness-promotion practices." *Western Journal of Medicine* 174, no. 1 (January 2001): 19. DOI: https://doi.org/10.1136/ewjm.174.1.19.

Williams, E. S., T. R. Konrad, W. E. Scheckler, D. E. Pathman, M. Linzer, J. E. McMurray, M. Gerrity and M. Schwartz. "Understanding physicians' intentions to withdraw from practice: the role of job satisfaction, job stress, mental and physical health." *Health care management review* 35, no. 2 (April 2010): 105-115. DOI: https://doi.org/10.1097/01.HMR.0000304509.58297.6f.

Zedeck, S. and K. L. Mosier. "Work in the family and employing organization." *American psychologist* 45, no. 2 (February 1990): 240. DOI: https://doi.org/10.1037/0003-066X.45.2.240.

# CHAPTER 21

# MANAGING IN THE FACE OF SURGICAL COMPLICATIONS

ASAD JAMIL. RAJA

A simple definition of surgical complication is, “any deviation from the normal postoperative course” (Dindo, Demartines and Clavien 2004). A more comprehensive definition (of postoperative complication) is, “an undesirable, unintended event that would not have occurred had the operation gone as well as could be reasonably hoped” (Sokol and Wilson 2008).

More than 350 million surgeries are performed worldwide each year. Recent reports have revealed that adverse event rates for surgical conditions remain unacceptably high, despite multiple nationwide and global patient safety initiatives over the past two decades (Kim et al. 2015). Surgical complications are dreaded by surgeons because not only do they have diverse consequences for the patients and their families, but they also dispirit them personally. The technical and moral burden of adversities weighs heavily on them. Surgeons are also considered to be the most stoic and least likely to seek help. This makes matters worse, and the cumulative effect of such misadventures leaves them hesitant, dejected and may lead them into a spiral of making more errors. Burnout is also common in such situations (Greenberg 2020). Different patient safety checklists, timeouts and sign outs have made improvements in many system issues and have led to the reduction of human errors. Interestingly, adverse events resulting from surgical interventions are actually more frequently related to errors occurring before or after the procedure, than by technical surgical mistakes during the operation. These include (i) breakdown in communication within and amongst the surgical team, care providers, patients, and their families; (ii) delay in diagnosis or failure to diagnose; and (iii) delay in treatment or failure to treat (Griffen et al. 2007; Newman-Toker and Pronovost 2009).

In any early surgical career there are different sets of challenges, which are commonly related to experience, that contribute to complication rates. In later years, the potential for developing complications also increases as the spectrum, volume and complexity of work expands. One would expect that with experience these may reduce, but this is not always the case. Unfortunately, it has been observed that with time, factors like complacency, indifference, attitude and over delegation contribute to adverse outcomes even by experienced hands. It is evident that there is no age or stage at which a surgeon is exempt from surgical complications. It is the digression from the basic fundamental principles and teachings of surgery which has a bearing on the surgical outcomes.

Managing in the face of surgical complications sadly makes one wish that it had never happened. Reflecting on adverse outcomes, one needs to critically examine the common fallacies observed in the patient journey. There is no learning if one keeps repeating the same mistakes and expecting a different outcome. The surgical patient's journey starts much before the actual surgery and continues throughout the events during and after surgery. The desired attributes to nurture, which may help reduce adverse outcomes include: good communication skills; patient selection abilities; sound judgment; preparation and optimization; knowing one's limitations; willingness to seek help; anticipation and recognition of complications; and lastly reflection and self-improvement.

Regular audits, critical reviews and constant introspection of one's outcomes are necessary for learning, and they help build up to the ultimate goal of an uneventful patient recovery. This is crucial for development of a safe, astute and reflective surgeon: elements that are essential for both patient safety and for one's own well-being.

## By failing to prepare you are preparing to fail

Surgery is inherently invasive. It is a specialty where one first inflicts more insult and injury to the already sick, before making them better. Surgical trauma needs to be controlled and calculated with aims to minimize the insult. It must be well prepared, purposeful, timely, precise, performed with intent and well managed. Understanding this generic philosophy can help improve surgical outcomes.

Good communication and counselling with the patient and family are the best ways to inform, prepare, develop rapport and build trust. This helps them understand the goals of care, expected outcomes and any uncertainties in their minds. The discussions need to be coupled with integrity, sincerity and empathy. Appraisal of the patient's condition must happen as often as it is required. Keeping the patient and family on board throughout the journey is essential. Many problems, incidents and litigations that are cited are due to poor communication, lack of information and transparency. These interactions, if handled appropriately and honestly, are very helpful especially when things are not going well. Always pay attention to effective and regular communication with the patients and families.

Competence is fundamental to patient safety and to avoid surgical complications. Adequate preparations and patient optimization for elective surgery are the keys to success. Understandably, emergency surgery is associated with higher risks, for usually there is little or no time to optimize the patient, and there may be many unknowns which may adversely impact the outcomes. However, failure to investigate, prepare and optimize a patient for elective surgery is likely to cause harm to the patient, and is indefensible. In high risk elective patients, consider other lesser or low risk options or even doing nothing—a living problem is better than a dead solution (Raja 2017).

Surgical judgment is necessary for patient selection and timing for surgery. It is a complex ability which is acquired through constant reflection on past experiences and situations. It gives one an astute sense for avoiding trouble by knowing when or when not to operate. A well prepared patient and surgeon is necessary for a good outcome. Elective surgeries need to be done during working hours, especially major cases. These should start early on the list when the surgeon and the team are fresh; when colleagues' help is available if needed; and when all backup services and staff are available to support any eventuality. Besides, it is well known that fatigue and lack of sleep impair judgment, memory and reflexes which adversely impact patient outcomes (Nurok, Czeisler and Lehmann 2010; Rothschild et al. 2009).

Preoperative anaesthetic review and appropriate work up for all elective cases are mandatory. All necessary requirements for surgery must be prepared: special drugs; blood and blood products; instruments and equipment; and even prior case discussion with backup help should be prepared if necessary. Additional factors that should be considered include: appropriate positioning, securing the patient from risk of fall or injury, possibility of other harms from awkward positioning or energy devices. Clear communication between surgical and anaesthesia teams is necessary. Attention should also be given to special monitoring requirements along with staying alert to anticipated issues and events likely to stress or destabilize the patient's hemodynamic condition. Circulating staff should also be informed of the likely need of special medical surgical supplies beyond the routine.

During surgery follow the principle of doing it right and well, the first time around. This will minimize drastically the procedure related complications; for once these set in, it is difficult to rectify things. If one is not happy at any crucial and susceptible step, fix it or correct it there and then to your satisfaction. Speed is not a recommended trait as it is tantamount to being cavalier with someone else's life. However, one has to be deft to keep pace with things and move on. Prolonged surgery and anaesthesia also adversely impact the outcomes. The best way is to have a balance; to slow down at crucial, difficult and technically demanding steps and speed up at other times. Someone's life is dependent on every stitch one puts or every vital step one takes. No matter how many times it may have been done before, it still needs the same care and attention to detail every time it is done. Never be complacent.

Never underestimate the impact of surgical trauma to the body. Its effect on patient physiology, especially in the already sick, elderly and those with poor reserves is incredible. Avoid prolonging surgical trauma by defocusing during any procedure and unnecessarily adding procedures for benign incidental findings. Ensure having meticulous surgical technique, tissue handling and minimizing blood loss, and avoid hemodynamic instability, all of which have a bearing on the surgical outcomes.

A befitting quote by the writer Stephen King may help surgeons remain out of trouble: "There's no harm in hoping for the best as long as one is prepared for the worst" (King 1982).

## Asking for help – before it happens, after it happens

A good surgeon encompasses both surgical technique and the ability to recognize the limits of professional competence. Not overestimating the required abilities as a surgeon, and to possess the virtue of humility, i.e., what can broadly be defined as an awareness of one's strengths and especially, one's weaknesses. In cases deemed beyond one's expertise, the first premise is that they should be referred to another specialist colleague. Otherwise, one is likely to cause serious harm and adverse outcomes.

Facing diagnostic dilemmas and challenges in decision making are common in surgical practice. Delays and indecisiveness are likely to impact outcomes. They may result in failure to intervene, inappropriate deferment, or even choosing a wrong intervention. In such difficult cases, it is prudent to consult a colleague and get their opinion. A fresh and different perspective may assist in making a right and timely decision. Concurrence of another colleague is reassuring too, and helps boost one's confidence. This saves the patient from any harm and the surgeon from the fallouts of a complication. Asking for help is a strength, not a weakness. Seeking the help of peers in difficult cases should be part of a culture of any department and norm of good surgical practices.

During any surgical procedure, and even in the most experienced hands, there will be a situation where one is likely to need help. The help required may be as trivial as eyeballing something; to concur with a change of plans; or to seek actual physical assistance in the face of complexity or adversity. One needs to have insight and judgment to recognize the point where carrying on further would be harmful to the patient. The threshold to seek help should be very low. There must be no egos in seeking advice or help regardless of whether it is trivial or of major assistance in the procedure. Encountering complexity or an unfamiliar situation is well recognized in surgery. Nobody is safe from such surprises; it is how one deals with them that is important. It reflects the true character of a surgeon who puts patient welfare above all other egos. Such conduct and behaviour are also essential as a role model for young trainees. It is better to take this course instead of compromising patient safety and facing complications.

If appropriate help is not readily available and pursuing further is likely to cause harm, contemplate making a safe exit. Either, abandon or abbreviate the procedure, or palliate if necessary and come out. Save the patient by doing what is essential and minimally required. One can later revisit if necessary to rectify things or do a definitive procedure with experienced help and with a patient in a better physiological state. Damage control principles are based on the same philosophy. There is no point continuing to correct anatomy by fancy repairs or reconstructions and at the end of it all lose the patient to deranged physiology.

In summary, the hallmarks of a safe surgeon are knowing and working within one's limitations, and being ready to seek help at any stage of the surgical patient's journey. Senior colleagues must set examples by inviting their junior colleagues to give advice and opinions on a difficult case or help in a procedure. It breaks the myth that only juniors require help. It also gives juniors a quiet confidence that after all it is not a big deal to seek help. Such gestures need to be done regularly and formally even if there is dubious need. It serves the purpose of testing the water, setting an example and a culture of good surgical practices. These fundamentals will greatly help in reducing surgical complications.

## Anticipate and be proactive rather than reactive

Anticipation and a proactive approach are cardinal features of managing surgical patients, if one intends to reduce and detect surgical complications. A careful, detailed evaluation of every patient helps in anticipating any possible issues. Relevant monitoring and a care plan should be developed according to the individual needs and requirements of each patient. In the immediate phase of postoperative recovery, it is necessary to anticipate generic complications like inadequate reversal or hemodynamic instability. In addition, the type of procedure and the postoperative risk assessment dictate the need for close monitoring and further disposition of the patient. These decisions have a bearing on early detection of evolving problems especially in high risk patients. Failure to anticipate, detect and intervene may mean missing the opportunity to deal with complications in a timely fashion, and the opportunity to salvage the situation.

Unfortunately, despite critical monitoring and even getting enough warning signs (suggesting the patient is not doing well) most surgeons stay in denial. Deviation from a normal postoperative course, a cardinal sign in such situations, is usually ignored. They can respond by micromanaging every symptom and sign instead of stepping back and paying attention to the evolving global organ dysfunction. What it actually requires is to question the reasons for the patient's deviation from a normal postoperative course. The majority of patients in surgery never crash suddenly; there are always preceding tell-tale signs. Changes in physiological parameters occur long before clinically catastrophic deterioration (Brown et al. 2018).

Furthermore, in the face of deteriorating patient conditions, new explanations or new diagnoses are entertained. The obvious, and any problem related to the procedure, seems to become invisible. This results in unnecessary investigations and dubious interventions which are at times detrimental and responsible for further delays, especially when they add no value to the situation. The cost of being in denial is paid heavily by the patient and the healthcare resources. This is where, if doubt exists, an independent and experienced perspective on the patient's condition must be sought. This must be routine practice in such situations, for it is common and natural for primary attendings to sometimes lose the plot. It is better to seek timely help rather than lose everything.

The other common mistake observed when an intervention is eventually performed for a complication, is an attempt to belittle the problem. There is failure to do enough and what is necessary. This is again a reflection of the "denial" mindset. Instead of being aggressive, dubious and cosmetic interventions are done, or limited or inappropriate procedures are performed (through limited explorations). This is a disregard for the principles of surgery, a lack of appreciation of the patient's dire physiological state and the consequences of one's actions—particularly when this is the only opportunity to salvage the situation in such a critically ill patient. The second hit of surgical insult knocks out whatever remaining reserves there are in the patient. There may not be another opportunity. The patient is already in extremis, and it is now or never.

Surgery can be a very humbling experience, but never see it as any kind of humiliation in the face of adversity. Complications are no crime and are common; but remaining in denial and not offering timely or appropriate intervention, or seeking help when things are not going well are indefensible.

## Audit and reflection

Experiential learning in surgery can only be achieved through constant reflection on experiences, and reviews at Mortality and Morbidity Conferences (MMCs). MMCs remain a core audit activity within the departments of any academic medical centre. They are deeply rooted in the premise that we can learn from our mistakes, thereby improving the care we provide. These forums however have only variably matured in different departments and centres. Commitment to the aims of the meeting by all participants and the quality of their interactions play a crucial role in the effectiveness of an MMC. Good leadership is also necessary to create an enabling environment, where faculty can feel assured to self-report and have a frank discussion. Participants must be able to contribute towards a constructive and non-judgmental discussion. A climate of blame is unlikely to lead to open discussion and fruitful improvements.

The maintenance of a decorum and civility to the proceedings is essential. Colleagues need to be cautious in their remarks and choice of words when making their comments. They should be made with all humility, in a tone and demeanour that are sympathetic and supportive. A due acknowledgement of hindsight is helpful. Never press home or impose any views. An individual who is reeling with an adverse outcome needs some kind words to recover their morale. The schema is to push across the learning point; one just has to make it palatable. Sometimes sharing one's own similar misadventures and what one has learnt from them is very reassuring and a subtle message is conveyed. If the faculty is clearly reflecting and articulating the learning experience from the case, then there is no point to press further. The best thing to do for a faculty when faced with an adverse outcome is to sincerely reflect on the issue, and what they would do differently next time when faced with a similar situation. This would be enough to end the agony and discussion. There is no point being defensive. It leads one nowhere and reflects the inability to fulfil a moral obligation to minimize (as much as possible) the recurrence of similar complications.

At the end of the meeting the case summary should be given, including an analysis of the turning points that led to the adverse outcome. These should be categorized under the following headings: human factors, system factors, and patient factors. The conclusion of the discussion should answer the questions: "Was there a preventable harm? Did a safety incident occur that should trigger the formal duty of candour?" (The Royal College of Surgeons of England 2021). It's not easy but it is an important exercise for individual learning, reflection and improving systems. Sometimes, there may not be sufficient data or enough of a consensus to make any firm conclusions. In such cases decisions may be deferred and discussed again later with more and new information. It is however, essential and possible to wrap up the discussion in the majority of cases and make conclusions in order to put in the remedial processes to close the audit loop.

It is well known that healthcare providers may have a difficult time accepting their fallibility, acknowledging mistakes and disclosing errors. Fear of litigation, shame, blame, and concern about reputation, are just some of the barriers preventing physicians from being more candid about such events at any forum. While "duty of candour" expects proper complication/error, disclosure includes a timely explanation of what happened, who was involved, why the error occurred, and how it could be prevented in the future. The difficult challenge is to strike a balance between expectation and reality.

A way forward to allay the anxiety amongst surgeons about the consequences of surgical complications may help in finding the solution. It seems developing teams with good practices and support structures entrenched within the system may be helpful. A Royal College of Surgeons publication identifies a number of characteristics of such well-functioning teams (Royal College of Surgeons of England 2021). These allude to having several traits that a team shares to have a high degree of trust, where team members: admit mistakes and weaknesses; ask for help; accept questions and input about their area of responsibility; give one another the benefit of the doubt before arriving at a negative conclusion; take risks in offering and accepting feedback; and appreciate and tap into one another's skills and experiences. Also recommended are a code of conduct based on mutual respect and trust between participants; commitment to the task of an objective review of adverse outcomes; encouragement of contributions from all participants; constructive discussion and debate; valuing different opinions; and challenging those in the group who do not adhere to these principles.

Development of such teams within departments on the principles outlined will help allay some of the fears and disquiet associated with the discussion of surgical complications. Hopefully, this will help to some extent in dispelling feelings of shame, guilt and victimization. Being sensitive to the predicament of colleagues, sincere reassurance and extending support are the most valuable assets team members can offer. There has to be a realization that complications and medical errors afford the opportunity for individuals and institutions to be candid about their weaknesses while improving patient care processes.

Over and above the historical format of MMCs, a broader agenda has evolved in time of understanding medical errors, quality improvement initiatives and optimizing the duty-readiness and well-being of the healthcare provider. This has challenged the format and value of traditional models of MMC. As a result, some feel that the purpose of the MMC has become clouded and ill-defined: is it an educational conference that promotes mastery of clinical acumen, or is it a venue to drive quality improvement by addressing systems-based issues in delivering care? Or can it serve both purposes (Gregor and Taylor 2016)?

It is an interesting debate and one feels many times too that the regular MMC agenda seems to have been hijacked. However, realistically speaking, medical errors, quality and system issues were always embedded in MMC discussions. It is only that they have come to the fore now. It is very difficult to isolate or box them up in different compartments. They are linked and many times the issues are inseparable. Each element has its impact on the outcome and sometimes multiple elements are responsible. It helps dissect issues better, and apportion the responsibility appropriately where it lies. This then also helps in quality improvement initiatives and rectifying system errors. This may also help deflect sometimes the unnecessary pressure on the faculty with an adverse outcome, especially when the problem lies somewhere else.

## Second victim syndrome

Second victims are healthcare providers who are involved in an unanticipated adverse patient event. This may be a medical error or a complication or an injury which leaves them traumatized. Frequently, these individuals feel personally responsible for the patient outcome. Many feel as though they have failed the patient, second guessing their clinical skills and knowledge base (Scott et al. 2009; Wu 2000).

Medical errors and poor outcomes adversely impact the involved providers, especially surgeons, as well as the patients and their families. Unfortunately our current system does little to support these "second victims" who experience various degrees of emotional and psychological stress, including confusion, loss of confidence and debilitating anxiety. These factors contribute to the alarmingly high rates of professional "burnout," substance abuse, and suicide of healthcare providers, as well as increasing the likelihood of subsequent medical errors (Marmon and Heiss 2015).

Surgeons often bear the burden of their mistakes in isolation. They may struggle with guilt, shame and a crisis of confidence. It seems they are often unprepared to deal with the aftermath of surgical complications. Counterintuitively, they may shy away from transparency for fear of litigation and blame, despite evidence that patients cite poor communication and lack of transparency as primary drivers to file a lawsuit in the wake of any complication.

In addition to its direct emotional effect, complications can negatively impact a physician's performance. A survey reported that participants who were negatively affected by a complication reported difficulty concentrating, declining clinical judgment, loss of confidence, trouble sleeping and difficulty enjoying leisurely activities and daily life—symptoms that overlap with clinical signs of depression (Patel et al. 2010).

In a recent study, a cohort of academic surgeons in Boston were asked to describe their experiences with intraoperative adverse events and the emotional impact these events had on them. One surgeon stated, "We all hide our grief, suffer in silence. The pain can be close to debilitating." The responses of over 125 surgeons provide alarming insight into the distress faced by many colleagues when things go wrong. They replay and relive these moments, suffering quietly, wishing they had done better. In the absence of accepted rituals for helping colleagues to deal with difficult events, each of them is left to cope and heal alone (Pinto et al. 2013).

Mindful efforts to improve the healthcare culture and develop personal support systems can help surgeons become more resilient, provide higher quality patient care and have longer productive professional lives. Institutional support systems are necessary to assist "second victims" to recover from the impact of an adverse patient event.

Coping strategies for providers include discussing the event with others, seeking professional counselling, and implementing quality improvement projects. Physicians and healthcare organizations need to find adaptive ways to deal with complications that will benefit patients, providers, and their institutions (Han et al. 2017).

## Need for support

Surgeons live and act within a moral community. Although the clinical and technical features of their work are crucially important, so too are the more subtle moral dimensions. The overview of the ethics of surgical complications has been mostly about moral perception and its effects on individuals. Involvement in an adverse event, especially due to a medical error, can be devastating for physicians. The culture of medicine has high expectations and standards, where emotional reactions to adverse events are generally not acknowledged or openly discussed. This environment leaves physicians highly vulnerable. Common reactions of physicians involved in adverse events include sadness, shame, fear and isolation. Left unaddressed, these emotional reactions can be devastating—potentially leading to depression, anxiety, burnout and even suicide. Such fallout may negatively impact clinicians, teams, institutions and consequently, the quality of patient care (Helo and Moulton 2017).

There is enough evidence in the literature suggesting that this is a serious and a deep rooted problem. We cannot continue to ignore the cumulative impact of second victim phenomenon, as all of us are at risk. Many adopt coping mechanisms, some of which are healthy and good, but others are harmful and could put their careers and personal lives at risk (Hu et al. 2012). A concerted effort is required to better recognize the impact on the individual and identify colleagues who are in distress and struggling. This requires a culture that supports second victims as much as it promotes the safety of our patients.

It is a common observation and there is evidence to suggest that "second victims" most commonly turn to peers for help. Many centres have started peer support programmes that have been described as a means to support colleagues in times of need. Through these programmes, surgeons and trainees are identified by peers following major intraoperative or other catastrophic adverse events, and a confidential approach is taken to let them know they are not alone. A trained peer supporter (a surgeon) is immediately available to chat. It is observed that most of the surgeons accept the offer to speak with a peer supporter. Most report feeling relieved to have someone to speak to, and to know that others have been in their shoes. It seems a cultural shift where there is the collective sense that nobody should be left to struggle alone. It has been described as a shift in focus from failure and vulnerability to personal resiliency and a sense of rejuvenation (Shapiro and Galowitz 2016).

Many colleagues argue that it is imperative that healthcare institutions devote resources to programmes that support physician well-being and resilience. Recommended important components for the peer support conversation are: outreach call, invitation/opening, listening, reflecting, reframing, sense-making, coping, closing and resources/referrals. They argue that creating a peer support programme is one way forward, away from a culture of invulnerability, isolation and shame, and towards a culture that truly values a sense of shared organizational responsibility for clinician well-being and patient safety (Bohnen et al. 2019, Hecht et al. 2020).

## Conclusion

Surgery can be very unforgiving and errors in medicine are common due to the imperfection of human nature. The two combinations make nobody immune to surgical complications. The important thing is how one prevents them from happening; how one ensures early recognition and a chance to salvage things; what one does to handle things technically when complications happen; how one handles the patient, the family and the team; how one analyses, introspects, reflects, reports, shares and learns from the experience; how one manages oneself and one's conscience in the aftermath of everything; and lastly knowing if one needs help, and where this help and support available are.

Admittedly no surgeon would wish to never go through the above cycle, but unfortunately that is just wishful thinking. Therefore, it is better to be well prepared and have humility as a surgeon, knowing well how things can go wrong and it may be one's turn tomorrow to be in the dock. Be kind in comments and remarks, and support colleagues in learning from their adversities, helping them rehabilitate and build back their confidence. Rest assured that it may be sooner rather than later, when one may be seeking that same support and help. That is the nature of the beast called "surgery."

## Bibliography

Bohnen, Jordan D., Keith D. Lillemoe, Elizabeth A. Mort and Haytham M. A. Kaafarani. "When Things Go Wrong: The Surgeon as Second Victim." *Annals of Surgery* 269, no. 5 (May 2019): 808-809. DOI: 10.1097/SLA.0000000000003138.

Brown A., A. Ballal, M. Al-Haddad. "Recognition of the critically ill patient and escalation of therapy." *Fundamental Principles* 20, no. 1 (Dec 2018): 1-5 DOI: 10.1016/j.mpaic.2018.11.011.

Dindo, Daniel, Nicolas Demartines and Pierre-Alain Clavien. "Classification of surgical complications: a new proposal with evaluation in a cohort of 6336 patients and results of a survey." *Ann. Surg.* 240, no. 2 (August 2004): 205–213. DOI: 10.1097/01.sla.0000133083.54934.ae.

Greenberg, Jayson S., "A Call for Help—Reflections on Burnout, CABG Surgery, and the Super Bowl." *JAMA* 323, no. 4 (January 2020):311-312. DOI: 10.1001/jama.2019.22083.

Gregor, Alexander and David Taylor. "Morbidity and Mortality Conference: It's Purpose Reclaimed and Grounded in Theory." *Teaching and Learning in Medicine* 28, no. 4 (June 2016): 439-447. DOI: 10.1080/10401334.2016.1189335.

Griffen, F. Dean, Linda S. Stephens, James B. Alexander, H. Randolph Bailey, Scott E. Maizel, Beth Howell Sutton and Karen L. Posner. "The American College of Surgeons' closed claims study: new insights for improving care." *J. Am. Coll. Surg.* 204, no.4 (April 2007): 561-69. DOI: 10.1016/j.jamcollsurg.2007.01.013.

Han, Kelsey, Jordan D. Bohnen, Thomas Peponis, Myriam Martinez, Anirudh Nandan, Daniel D. Yeh, Jarone Lee, Marc Demoya, George Velmahos and Haytham M. A. Kaafarani. “The Surgeon as the Second Victim? Results of the Boston Intraoperative Adverse Events Surgeons’ Attitude (BISA) Study.” *J. Am. Coll. Surg.* 224, no. 6 (June 2017): 1048–1056. DOI: 10.1016/j.jamcollsurg.2016.12.039.

Hechi, Majed W. El, Jordan D. Bohnen, Maggie Westfal, Kelsey Han, Christy Cauley, Cameron Wright, John Schulz et al. “Design and Impact of a Novel Surgery-Specific Second Victim Peer Support Program”. *J. Am. Coll. Surg.* 230, no. 6 (June 2020): 926-933. DOI: 10.1016/j.jamcollsurg.2019.10.015.

Helo, Sevann and Carol-Anne E. Moulton. “Complications: acknowledging, managing, and coping with human error”. *Transl Androl Urol.* 6, no. 4 (August 2017): 773-782. DOI: 10.21037/tau.2017.06.28.

Hu, Yue-Yung, Megan L. Fix, Nathanael D. Hevelone, Stuart R. Lipsitz, Caprice C. Greenberg, Joel S. Weissman and Jo Shapiro. “Physicians' needs in coping with emotional stressors: the case for peer support.” *Archives of Surgery* 147, no. 3 (March 2012): 212–217. DOI: 10.1001/archsurg.2011.312.

Kim, Fernando J., Rodrigo Donalisio da Silva, Diedra Gustafson, Leticia Nogueira, Timothy Harlin and David L. Paul. “Current issues in patient safety in surgery: a review.” *BMC Patient Safety in Surgery* 9, Article number 26 (June 2015). DOI: https://doi.org/10.1186/s13037-015-0067-4.

King, Stephen. *Different Seasons*. Viking Press, Penguin Random House, New York: First Edition/First Printing 1982.

Marmon, Louis M. and Kurt Heiss, “Improving surgeon wellness: The second victim syndrome and quality of care.” *Seminars in Pediatric Surgery* 24, no. 6 (December 2015): 315-318. DOI: 10.1053/j.sempedsurg.2015.08.011.

Newman-Toker, David E. and Peter J. Pronovost. “Diagnostic errors-the next frontier for patient safety.” *JAMA* 301, no. 10 (March 2009): 1060-2. DOI: 10.1001/jama.2009.249.

Nurok, Michael, Charles A. Czeisler and Lisa Soleymani Lehmann. “Sleep deprivation, elective surgical procedures, and informed consent.” *N. Engl. J. Med.* 363, no. 27 (December 2010): 2577-2579. DOI: 10.1056/NEJMp1007901.

Patel, Amit M., Nichole K. Ingalls, M. Ashraf Mansour, Stanley Sherman, Alan T. Davis and Mathew H. Chung. “Collateral damage:

the effect of patient complications on the surgeon's psyche." *Surgery* 148, no. 4 (October 2010): 824-830. DOI: 10.1016/j.surg.2010.07.024.

Pinto, A., O. Faiz, C. Bicknell and C. Vincent. "Surgical complications and their implications for surgeons' well-being." *British Journal of Surgery* 100, no. 13 (December 2013): 1748-55. DOI: 10.1002/bjs.9308.

Raja, Asad J. *Being a Surgeon: The Ten Commandments*. Illinois, Chicago, North America: Trafford Publishing, 2017.

Rothschild, Jeffrey M., Carol A. Keohane, Selwyn Rogers, Roxane Gardner, Stuart R. Lipsitz, Claudia A. Salzberg, Tony Yu et al. "Risks of Complications by Attending Physicians after Performing Night time Procedures." *JAMA* 302, no. 14 (October 2009):1565-1572. DOI: 10.1001/jama.2009.1423.

Royal College of Surgeons of England. "Duty of Candour." Accessed February 7, 2021 https://www.rcseng.ac.uk/standards-and-research/standards-and-guidance/good-practice-guides/duty-of-candour.

Royal College of Surgeons of England. "The High Performing Surgical Team: A Guide to Best Practice." Accessed February 7, 2021 https://www.rcseng.ac.uk/standards-and-research/standards-and-guidance/good-practice-guides/hpst/.

Scott, S. D., L. E. Hirschinger, K. R. Cox, M. McCoig, J. Brandt and L. W. Hall. "The natural history of recovery for the healthcare provider 'second victim' after adverse patient events." *Qual. Saf. Health Care* 18, no. 5 (October 2009): 325-30. DOI: 10.1136/qshc.2009.032870.

Shapiro, Jo and Pamela Galowitz. "Peer Support for Clinicians: A Programmatic Approach." *Academic Medicine* 91, no. 9 (September 2016): 1200-1204. DOI: 10.1097/ACM.0000000000001297.

Sokol, Daniel K. and Wilson J. "What is a surgical complication?" *World Journal of Surgery* 32, no. 6 (June 2008): 942–944. DOI: 10.1007/s00268-008-9471-6.

Wu, Albert W. "Medical error: the second victim." *BMJ* 320 (March 2000): 726–727. DOI: 10.1136/bmj.320.7237.726.

# CHAPTER 22

# BEYOND THE KNIFE: CAREERS FOR SURGEONS OUTSIDE SURGERY

RASHID JOOMA AND HINA SATTAR

The making of a surgeon is demanding of time and effort and the traditional progression from medical school to residency training, followed by the challenges of establishing oneself in surgical practice, is a linear journey leaving little scope for personalisation. One's interests and creative instincts get squeezed out by the exigencies of the profession, particularly early in one's surgical career, and this one-dimensional trajectory may be a risk factor for disillusionment and burnout. However, surgeons are often creative and artistic by temperament and it is commonplace for them to seek leisure in photography, woodwork, painting and other such pursuits. But what of going beyond hobbies for leisure and investing effort and time in alternate career options to cultivate in tandem with the surgical work or even as a new occupation? Indeed, many of us are living in good health and vitality beyond Shakespeare's "threescore and ten." Should we be thinking about preparing the stage to take to following retirement from surgery?

We have identified and spoken to seven individuals who have distinguished themselves as surgeons but have also stepped beyond surgery to alternate occupations. These may have been to fulfil personal creative passions, to serve their profession or their communities, or just to allow alternate revenue streams. In all cases these surgeons are doing work which is fulfilling for themselves and impactful in a larger sense and we invite you to share in their journeys.

# Dr Akhtar Jamal Khan: the Surgeon and the Entrepreneur

*Dr Khan is a widely respected and popular ophthalmologist. Not only has he created his own branded facility, Akhtar Eye Hospital, he has also established a flourishing pharmaceutical manufacturing company.*

Dr Khan believes that leadership is not an acquired quality but is rather built around inborn traits of personality. Born under the sign of Leo, he always had the attributes to lead and bring about a change in the world. During his time in medical college, though never interested in political activities, he was however extremely social. Later, while working as a consultant in England, he desired to serve his country and began to think of returning to Pakistan to be able to give back to the community. On his return, he turned away from working in a government hospital and instead chose to practise in a private setting. When he was training, the foldable silicone intraocular lens—or IOL—had become widespread in ophthalmology and when he returned, he introduced the first IOL implant in a private hospital in Pakistan. The hospital also became very busy and was the first private hospital to offer a postgraduate programme.

When asked about his motivation to set up his own hospital, he told us that he was aware that the government hospitals in Pakistan would not fund new technology such as the IOL, and hence he decided to build a hospital that provided the latest trends in technologically advanced procedures. He further went on to say that in order to achieve something like this you need to have determination, funds and the willingness to take risks. In his opinion, to be an entrepreneur, it is important to respect and satisfy your client and have something that sets you apart. He added that there is a creative peak in the career of every doctor which usually declines after 10 to 12 years and the crest of this tide must be taken advantage of.

With regards to his entry into the pharmaceutical manufacturing industry, he advanced two reasons: firstly, it was a project for his retirement. Secondly, being familiar with the ophthalmic products on the market, he discerned that there was scope for improvement in the market. He initially commissioned a laboratory in his hospital to produce simple eye drops and gradually over the years expanded the manufacturing lines to ointments and steroids. At present, his company has a dedicated facility in Korangi which produces ointments, drops, injections and other general pharmaceutical products. When we inquired how much he relies on the other people in his company, he revealed that he is actively involved in the processes himself.

More recently he has entertained the idea of producing quality surgical sutures in Pakistan and his company is currently working on introducing machines to develop its own surgical needles which, he stated, is a complex procedure. Dr Khan never personally publicises his own products believing it would be unethical to do so. The company has a marketing team to promote its products.

All this he did while he simultaneously looked after his patients. Despite his busy schedule, he has still managed to achieve a perfect balance between his family and work life. He believes that you cannot sacrifice one for the other. He further added that relentlessly making money can be soul destroying and indeed, *"chasing money is the death of a society."*

Speaking about his approach to patients, he said that during his training in England, he had learnt that a doctor should always be respectful and empathetic towards his patients and show them kindness and generosity. He also believes in philanthropy and has been involved with several charitable organisations which have established charity hospitals. His first such project was a charity eye hospital at Nagan Chowrangi called Pakistan Eye Bank Society Hospital, which was established in 1984 in collaboration with a welfare organisation. His greatest accomplishment, and indeed biggest decision, was coming back to his country. He had earned a lot of respect and comfort working as a consultant in England, but he had made up his mind to return to his homeland where he had nothing but the resolution to serve his people.

When asked about the advice that he would give to an ophthalmic surgery resident and whether or not he would encourage them to explore other pathways, he stated that he would most certainly encourage them to do so. He personally believes that the more you use yourself mentally, the more you expand your vision.

## Dr Lubna Samad: the Surgeon and the Researcher

*Dr Samad is an alumnus of the Aga Khan University (AKU), who trained as a paediatric surgeon and has worked extensively on Global Surgery policy and implementation. She is currently working as a paediatric surgeon at the Indus Hospital and is Director of the Centre for Essential Surgical and Acute Care at Indus Health Network*

Dr Samad spoke of her experience of public health research in conjunction with her career as a surgeon. When asked why she did not follow the standard AKU model of seeking residency in the USA after graduation, she told us that before starting her medical education with AKU, she had studied briefly at Dow Medical College. That exposure combined with the fact that her parents, both physicians, had led fulfilling lives working in the public sector made her opt to pursue her training in Pakistan. She felt that she did not need a western buffer and was comfortable working in Pakistan. Initially she worked at a public hospital (National Institute of Child Health) as a surgical trainee, and then went to England to complete her surgical training. Later she moved to Gilgit where her husband was working on a project and there, she attached herself to the local district headquarter hospital on a voluntary basis for two years. This was a revelation, teaching her more about the reality of surgical care delivery in Pakistan than all the years before that.

*"Things you do not plan shape your destiny more than things you plan."*

During her stay in Gilgit, besides her surgical work, she got involved with a public health study looking at the problems concerning the unsafe use of injections. She had always been interested in public health and one of her biggest influences was the Community Health Sciences rotation at AKU Medical College. She immensely enjoyed the community outreach exposure the department afforded, and this exposed her to the basics of epidemiological research. Later on, she was able to integrate this new found interest with her surgical career.

Ten years ago, she took a short online course on public health and surgery offered by the University of British Columbia. Through this experience, she discovered that there were people who were not only talking and thinking like her about the interface between surgery and public health, but actually building it into a career trajectory. Her interest in research has been focused on surgical systems in the developing world rather than on individual surgical conditions. For instance, it is well established that plastibell circumcision is a very safe and standardised procedure, yet day in and day out children die or suffer from complications due to a botched circumcision because it has been poorly performed. Access to safe and timely surgical care is very important. Although the knowledge and resources exist, vast numbers of people are unable to access the care that they need. This health delivery gap—also called the "last mile" gap—needs to be the focus of research and intervention. This gap can only be bridged based on an understanding of the challenges faced by our own populations and by finding locally relevant solutions based on this evidence.

Around 2009, a team of public health experts and clinicians studied disease patterns in the Indus Hospital's catchment population. Dr Samad's particular interest was in the utilisation of surgical services. The core question was: "What prevents a person in need from availing surgical care?"

Besides the cost and the travel, there are many other social, cultural and geographical access barriers that influence this situation. This pushed her to keep collecting local evidence and data to support what works and what does not. She also pointed out that there is a lot of innovation required in ensuring uptake of surgical system changes, since strategies developed abroad or even in Islamabad may not work in some communities for a wide variety of reasons.

She believes that the five years in medical school should be structured to give young aspiring specialist surgeons and physicians a variety of options to combine a specialisation track with other fields. The world over we can see physicians combine their Doctor of Medicine (MD) with a Master of Business Administration (MBA) or Master of Public Health (MPH) for example. The ability to cross cut two or more specialties together helps design unique or niche areas that can be tailored to meet the needs of your country or to pursue specific personal interests. From Dr Samad's perspective, that is innovation itself. Having said that, there may be doctors who want to focus on their surgical field only and that is fine. It is just that it is important for young graduates and medical students to be aware of the options that exist and choose what works for them at an individual level when making career choices.

When asked if she would like to get a PhD (Doctor of Philosophy) or MBA degree, she laughed and said that she is considering starting a PhD when her youngest child goes to college. Age should not be a limiting factor to pursuing one's interests. However, for those graduates that are interested in global health careers from an early stage in their medical education and training, pursuing an MPH at an early stage can provide a lot of valuable insight and skills. This one-year programme can be pursued before the start of their residency programme, and can add value to residency applications. However, many programmes in the US allow residents to take a gap year or two in between their training for an MPH or a global surgery research fellowship.

Though she expressed her concern over the lack of a wider horizon that medical college students at AKU and elsewhere are exposed to, she recognises that even in the traditional clinical model from a generation ago in Pakistan, people have found different avenues and done phenomenal work. These are all diverse experiences towards something more than the boundaries of clinical medicine alone. The student graduating today has the opportunity of formalised training that gives them that jump start in their careers. For example, combining an MD/MBA for those interested in administrative health management or an MD/MPP (Masters in Public Policy) if they are involved in policy development are excellent options. The ability to link two interests early on in a career and use it as a launch pad to do a lot more or moving to it actually at a later stage but just keeping your options open throughout life is very important.

She further added that this process is not prescriptive. It is about your personal journey. Many people suffer the consequences of pursuing medicine because they have not seen enough. However, these are invested years and provide a platform from which to diversify experience. When asked if broadening your horizon makes you a better surgeon, she pointed out that if you look at the outcome of a perfectly executed surgical procedure with no complications and gauge your success on that alone then you have succeeded. In that case, all you need to know is surgical technique. Nevertheless, if you consider your success the rehabilitation of a patient back into the community or long term improvement in the quality of life of a patient then you begin looking at parameters that are not always in your control in the surgical theatre. In her opinion, your technical expertise is only one factor; it is critical to have a broader understanding of your patient as a person and of their life. Only then you can ensure that your surgical treatment is maximising their welfare.

In the end, she advised that career choices should never be imposed. You can only show young surgeons the variety of opportunities that they have and the different ways in which they can combine a financially solid career or income with doing so much more to diversify their own and their patient's experience. You can expose and educate them about the variety of options out there. You can open windows where you spark an interest and facilitate its pursuit. However, there is also a role for that technically perfect surgeon as well and that is a huge contribution in itself.

## Dr Shahid Shamim: the Surgeon and the Educationist

*Dr Shamim is a laparoscopic surgeon who is one of our pioneering medical educationists. In his career, the pendulum of his activity has swung away from the procedural to the educational.*

Dr Shamim told us that during his years at Dow Medical College, he was quite active in arranging annual events such as the sports week and was involved in various social welfare activities such as the Patients' Welfare Association. He immensely enjoyed enriching the experience of other students and always strove to make things better for fellow students through innovative and creative thinking. Initially, he had no intention of doing anything else after graduating other than being a qualified surgeon with a busy practice. However, during his residency at Liaquat National Hospital, he realised that he did not just want to be a surgeon but also wanted to be a trainer of young surgeons. Also, during the course of his residency, he was introduced to two disciplines that were new to him. One was Medical Ethics and the other, Education and Training. He heard and understood the word "ethics" for the first time during his residency and it fascinated him. He felt that somewhere in his subconscious mind, he was looking for this word.

After he had completed his residency and obtained fellowships from the Pakistan and Scotland Colleges, he joined the Surgery Faculty at Ziauddin University. Along with his general surgery practice and surgical teaching, he began teaching sessions on ethics at Ziauddin. To enhance his own understanding and improve the content of his ethics course, he did the diploma course in bioethics from the Centre of Bioethics at the Sindh Institute of Urology and Transplantation. At the same time, his interest in medical education was mentored by the late Professor Naeem Jafri who was the doyen of Medical Education as a discipline in Pakistan and established one of the earliest Departments of Medical Education of the country at Ziauddin University. Professor Jafri seems to have discerned educationist potential in Dr Shamim and would regularly make him read topical literature. They would then have in depth discussions about the topic in his office. He would make him attend faculty development sessions with basic sciences and clinical skills teachers. This experience fuelled his interest in medical education. When he was in the UK for surgical training he kept up his interest by getting involved in several medical education activities. Later, when he joined Dow University of Health Sciences (DUHS) he was encouraged by the Vice Chancellor to initiate a programme for medical education, though this initiative was handicapped by the absence of qualified faculty. However, with the collaboration of a medical educationist based in the Gulf, the foundation of the first Master's programme in Medical Education in Pakistan was established at DUHS and he himself enrolled and completed his Master's in the first batch in 2012. At this time, he was selected for secondment to a medical university hospital in Saudi Arabia. He was recruited as a surgeon but with his known interest and his new qualification he was assigned to the establishment of a department of medical education. This five year journey was very fulfilling for him and a great learning experience. He went to Saudi Arabia primarily as a general surgeon but returned as a medical educationist.

When asked about his opinion on the importance of an individual being qualified as a medical educationist in order to reform the undergraduate curriculum, he stated that we need to understand who is a medical educationist first. There is a difference between an educator and a medical educationist. Medical educationists do not deal with the content or the discipline being taught. They manoeuvre the process of education. The methodologies of the teaching process have not drastically changed over time; instead they have become more organised and teachable. The educationist's role is to ensure that everybody receives an equal standard of training from any trainer and that is why it needs to be structured. In conclusion, the role of a medical educationist in an undergraduate or postgraduate programme is not related to the content being taught, but primarily involves the process of training and how the education has to be delivered to the student. Dr Shamim agreed that surgical training is largely skill training which is best learned by attaching yourself to a more experienced person and his support system. The medical educationist optimises this specialist training by making it objective and reproducible.

The change in his profession began after doing about 17 years of hardcore surgery. He had achieved his personal satisfaction from surgery during these years. Now he is still doing surgeries, but he chooses his procedures and keeps things the way he desires. He believes that he has achieved his goals in surgery. He is doing a lot beyond teaching just one or a few surgeons. He is training several trainers who are further facilitating multiple trainees and that is the bigger picture he wanted to achieve. Surgical procedures like the appendectomy or even the esophagectomy are done by many surgeons. However, there are few who can train surgeons on how to teach surgery and to develop or improve surgical programmes. Dr Shamim has progressed above the trainer level and is pleased with what he has done so far. From his perspective, he is extremely satisfied with his work because there was a lot that had to be done in medical education as it was a virgin territory.

He suggested that getting the knowledge and skills of becoming a better educator is indeed required by every surgeon who wishes to train young surgeons. They may not have done a Master's but instead attended certificate courses or workshops because they wanted to learn about improving education. He further stated that he has seen that a lot of surgeons are now going after medical education often as a course but occasionally as a Master's candidate. A Master's in Medical Education may not help you in becoming a better surgeon nor help your patients directly. However, if you do pursue a Master's, your medical education skills should not be contained within the department of surgery but rather should benefit the trainees in other departments as well. By transferring your knowledge and skills to others, you may have a larger impact on the overall delivery of healthcare.

Young surgeons should, from their early days, consider having an alternate career or a retirement plan. This may involve management, education or any other field of interest. They should think about the career that they would choose if it was compulsory for a surgeon to have a career outside the operating room. Continuing work of the same nature and at the same place for the rest of your life has been an old tradition but if someone has the potential to do more, he/she definitely should: his or her talents should not be wasted in doing things that others can take up.

## Dr Nobhojit Roy: the Surgeon and the Public Health Practitioner

*Dr Roy trained as a trauma surgeon in Mumbai and holds an MPH from Johns Hopkins and a PhD from the Karolinska Institutet, Stockholm. He has served on the Lancet Commission for Global Surgery. He currently works as an advisor to an Indian State Health Department to improve rural medical services and access to surgery.*

Dr Roy led the life of a regular urban referral centre surgeon until his involvement with the work of the Lancet Commission on Global Surgery brought home to him the fact that a large measure of the surgical problems of the population were beyond the remedy of the knife. The top finding of the Commission was that 5 out of 7 billion people in the world are never going to see a surgeon. He realised that even with all his training and the surgical art that he possessed, most people are not going to see him or his skill. This was the turning point when he pivoted to public health. He spent five years working with the Indian Ministry of Health while practising surgery, trying to develop the national standard treatment guidelines in surgery. In 2017, he moved on full time to public health and left the operating theatre to go to poorer parts of India to figure out how surgery happens there if it happens at all. He is still doing that today.

He completed his medical education in Mumbai. When asked if he could recall being drawn into thinking about and assimilating social issues during his medical school or pre-medical years, he stated that he was very active in his medical school's social and political activity. He realised that students and doctors are largely isolated from the socioeconomic determinants of health and this impacts their work more than they realise. He was actively involved in social work in college and was someone who wanted to uplift the social circumstances of the indigent. For many, he believes, these sentiments start at an early age but on the flip side, a lot of people get completely disillusioned and move over to the other side. In his experience, a lot of such students started off as student leaders, being righteous, but somewhere along the line they just broke and became really big practitioners today, not wanting to look back at that life. In relation to this, he quoted a well-known Bengali saying, *"If you **have to** be a communist at 25 years, you **will be** a capitalist at the age of 45."*

Thus, maintaining that spirit of altruism is difficult but worthwhile.

Asked about his public health qualification, he told us that he did his MPH in the middle of his career (when it is very difficult to take a long break) but that his learning had helped him a lot. He realised that an MPH alone does not add much value to your surgical training but being cross-trained does give you the supplemental tools of a public health expert and allows you to understand both surgery and the epidemiology of the surgical burden of disease.

As a public health expert, he addressed questions that are beyond the scope of surgery because surgeons are only specialists in a silo of the health system. They only observe the world of surgery. Putting the patient at the centre as an individual who has a choice and fixed amount of money, and how a surgeon assists them with their choices, is the key issue. As he got older, he got better at trauma surgery and somewhere along the way he realised the futility of the endless broken bones and broken heads. He realised that there cannot be an upward graph of 1.25 million injuries/deaths every year in India due to trauma, while the rest of the world's injuries are on the downslide. We have to address prevention over post-crash surgical treatment.

Dr Roy moved out of the operating theatre to become the National Advisor of Public Health Planning and Evidence, at the think-tank of the Ministry of Health, New Delhi. He found that there was much different between the states of this large country. His state of focus was Bihar, a poorer region, and he later moved to advise this state's Department of Health. His first task at the Department of Health was to address the concern that not a single C-section was done in the government hospital in the district of Madhubani (just south of Nepal), an area with a population of 5.5 million people. Dr Roy reported that the C-section rate, based on epidemiological data, should be 13,500. While people can die of complex pathological conditions, it was unacceptable that a woman should die of a physiological condition—pregnancy. He felt that his whole life as a surgeon was not justified. Therefore, he spent many months in Madhubani trying to figure out the dynamics of surgery beyond the operating theatre. It was there that he realised that in Mumbai he believed that he was a super surgeon as he had the best residents, nurses and technicians around him in the hospital. They made him feel competent by being helpful and efficient. However, in the middle of the night in the resource-constrained setting of the district hospital the situation was quite different, particularly for a woman convulsing with eclampsia who needed her baby delivered immediately. More courage was required to operate in these limited surroundings. He appreciated that it is easier to sit in the posh Mumbai hospitals and judge that the Bihari surgeon in Bihar is unable to perform surgery. He realised that you need to be there to put yourself in their shoes to recognise the obstacles.

When asked about his opinion on bringing up his family in a rural area and not being able to send his children to the best schools, he gave the example of his mentor who moved from upstate New York and lived in a small tribal village in India. He admitted that he is not as resolute as his mentor, but there are others who are not willing to step out of their urban comfort zone. He stated that you do not have to give up everything and your child does not have to go to a tribal school for you to be able to do your two-bits for society. There is space for all types of commitment, even if someone does it only for a short period of time. He stated, *"One does not have to leave the comfort of their surroundings to be able to contribute in this interconnected world. If learning is not contextualised, then what good is it? Most surgeons working in Mumbai and Karachi are better suited to practise at Memorial Sloan Kettering or Columbia Hospital in New York than the forsaken places in the boondocks of our own countries."*

Elaborating further on material versus spiritual rewards, he stated that he is not competing with the middle-class symbols of wealth. The woman who died because she did not receive surgery is more important to him than the BMW he drove. He did surgery to save people's lives and if a life is lost, his status automobile was empty vanity. However, he added that you do not necessarily have to give up all the trappings of a comfortable existence.

Nonetheless, he believed that surgical practice in India is still largely urban based and there were very few role models of rural surgical practice. A typical surgical resident would learn procedures relating to the gallbladder, appendix and hernia while his rural surgery residents had the skills to do everything from urology to plastic surgery. He stated that if you are able to broaden your spectrum, you would be in the McDonald's model of high volumes and low profits. With this model, you would eventually buy your Mercedes Benz in seven years of practice and also before your urban counterpart, while addressing the unmet need in surgery. This will be the new model in surgery in the years to come, and centres like Aravind Eye Hospital and Narayan Hrudayalaya have been pioneering models to show the way.

## Dr Shahid Shafi: the Surgeon and the Community Politician

*An AKU alumnus, Dr Shafi trained and then practised as a trauma surgeon in Texas. He obtained an MPH and an MBA and became involved with local politics in his community. He was elected as a councillor in the City of Southlake, Texas, and served 2 terms. He is currently the CEO of The Aga Khan University (AKUH).*

Dr Shafi participated in US politics for nearly a decade, from 2009 until November 2020 when he finished his second term on the city council of his town. This was a voluntary, part time position, but he dedicated 20 to 30 hours a week to serving in that role. He viewed this as a community service and an area of policy-making at a local level. In his profession as a trauma surgeon, he had many interactions with policy-makers and legislators. These interactions concerned various policies related to public safety and funding for trauma centres and hospitals. Thus, after sitting on the asking side of the table for many years, he decided to run for an elected office. He decided to be on the other side of the table, making the decisions, instead of asking questions.

He gave credit to AKU for his interest in public health. As he went through the curriculum of Community Health Sciences at AKU, he began to appreciate the importance of a health systems approach to tackling health problems. This fuelled his interest in working for several months at USAID after graduating from AKU before he left for the US where he obtained a degree in public health (MPH). The purpose of doing so was to understand the larger picture of the health system.

When asked about finding the time from his surgical schedule for his political work, he said that the council work required a significant slice of his time. He had to adjust his practice and call schedule to accommodate the time needed for the city council. This required cooperative and supportive partners in practice who understood and supported his passion and interest and covered for him when he was not available. The city of Southlake had a population of 30,000 citizens and the city council was responsible for ensuring public safety, which included police, fire and emergency medical services. The council was also responsible for providing utilities, such as water, sewage, electricity and Internet as well as infrastructure facilities like streets, parks and recreation development programmes. They had a budget of about $100 million a year and a full-time staff of nearly 350 people. Managing these services required time, which came at the expense of his family and personal time. He added that, in order to do both community and professional work, he was blessed to have understanding and supportive partners, both in practice and at home.

Dr Shafi also felt that his clinical practice helped with his city council work because it helped him connect with his constituents. Several of his fellow physicians in the hospital and most of his patients also lived in the same city. Typically, it is very unusual for people in the medical field to be involved with elected office. He could not recall another doctor who was interested in running for office. Most of the elected officials he worked with came from other professions.

When asked if he was a role model on this journey, he said that he had mentored several people, who were inspired by his work, to run for office. From 2014 to early 2020, he conducted several workshops in Texas on how to run for an elected office. Through these workshops, he trained approximately 150 people on how to choose an office to run for, build a team, raise money, and use data to identify and manage the voters; find experts to help you run the campaign; and figure out the issues in a particular race and find solutions.

His experience in US politics has been extremely positive. The issue of being a Muslim, however, rankled a handful of people but it was never a hindrance. He found Americans to be open minded, accepting and welcoming of all immigrants.

When asked if being a surgeon prepared him to run for electoral office, he responded in the affirmative. He indicated that a lot of things that he did as a surgeon prepared him for complex leadership roles. First, surgeons are very hardworking; they know how to get up early and work until late and they do not leave the bedside until the work is done.

Secondly, surgeons are trained to pay attention to detail. For instance they know that leaving even a little bleeder somewhere can be disastrous so, *"we are used to dotting all the i's, crossing all the t's to make sure that the field is absolutely dry when we leave."* This attention to detail helped him in exercising due diligence in the political and the legislative process because there are a great many documents to be read and each word has a special meaning, so one has to be attentive to detail.

Thirdly, surgeons are used to working in teams of anaesthesiologists, nurses, technicians etc.; in short, with others, in and out of the operating room. A team approach is also critical to success in public policy. Thus, there are many attributes of a surgeon that prepare you well for a legislative career.

## Dr Salman Faridi: the Surgeon and the Writer

*Besides being a senior general surgeon in Karachi, Dr Faridi is known as a health presenter on television and regular contributor to newspapers and magazines. He is currently Medical Director of Liaquat National Hospital and Medical College.*

Dr Faridi told us that he had always been captivated by words, being fascinated by language and having a passion for writing and poetry. He actively participated in debates and "baet-bazi" during his days in school and this was not only in English but in Urdu as well. During his college days, he would make frequent contributions to the college magazine. Though he never wrote a daily diary, he made it a habit to write regular long letters to his children when they were studying abroad. He has always been someone who has tried to convey things from a public platform and was actively involved in debates and student affairs in college. He now writes poetry regularly and feels that writing helps an individual convey their thoughts, views and emotions about those things that impact them in one way or another.

For some time now, he has been writing a weekly sports column for a leading English newspaper. He occasionally also writes articles on history, current affairs and economics. He previously hosted a television talk show about medical issues where a panel of experts and himself would answer live questions from the audience. When asked how he motivated his children or the young medics around him to develop a facility for writing for work or pleasure, he replied that his children have always been avid readers and have been writing since their childhood. Out of the 7,000 books that his family owns, 1,500 belong to his children. In his opinion, the key to writing is three-fold. First is reading. Secondly, if you are a person who is concerned about the society around you and you feel the need to contribute to its betterment that is where the motivation comes from. It is not enough to go through a profession and earn a living. That is something you need for survival. You have to be able to make an effective contribution to bring about happiness in other people's lives. In order to do so, you have to be touched and moved by your surroundings and then react to them. Finally, the real motivation comes from your society, being aware of what is happening in it and wishing to respond to it in a positive way.

When asked why a young surgeon should devote their scarce time to the luxury of reading and writing for pleasure, he said he recognised that the instinct of self-survival is fundamental, superseding other competing interests, and everyone is concerned about having a secure future and establishing themselves in their profession. But he stressed that, for surgical practice, you needed a certain degree of hand-eye coordination, skill and finesse. But is that all there is to it? Or is there the purpose of alleviating pain and misery or bringing happiness? If that element is present, then how can someone stop at treating the disease and say, for example, that he has resolved his patient's blood pressure and send him home to the same conditions that led to the blood pressure problem in the first place. He advised that if you have to make an impact, you need to run that extra mile and do a little more.

> "*You have to be someone who is more than just a doctor. You have to be a healer and there is a lot of healing that needs to be done at the societal level.*"

He believes that whether it is writing or some other field of interest, it is about what priorities you assign to it in your set up and your life. If you feel that it is important to you and it matters, you will find the time for it. As far as professional excellence is concerned, there is no end to it. There are some doctors who will see 30 patients in a day and feel that is enough and there are others who will cater to 200 patients in a day and still feel the need to do more. From his standpoint, you have to create segments and categories in your life that may be different for each individual.

Dr Faridi shared a poem with us that he had written during the COVID-19 lockdown, titled **"This Too Shall Pass."**

This too shall pass
As seasons always pass
With time all things will pass
The grass will grow again
And scented blooms
Once more will dazzle and return
Rebounding from a lesson harshly learnt
And nature triumphant will seed again
New breeds of men
And life will re-emerge with different shades
Of altered notes and tempered tones
That peep beyond
This rancid sulfurous haze
The past will sleep
As pasts have always done
Resting in its own eternal pose
The grass will grow again
And cover all with silence and repose
Cover all the sadness and the pain
To lie in books
As tales and stories that remain
And some truths to heed
As narratives of bygone days and deeds
Derived from all the graves
Bearing mournful eerie witness
To this grim apocalyptic phase.

## Dr Abdul Bari Khan: Surgeon and Hospital Administrator

*Dr Khan transitioned from his career as cardiac surgeon at Karachi's Civil Hospital to Administrator of the Indus Hospital and more recently to full time Strategic Health Planner and Fundraiser.*

While a medical student at Dow Medical College, Dr Khan was moved by the plight of professional blood donors at Civil Hospital in Karachi and brought together fellow students to create the first voluntary blood bank. The Saddar bomb blast of 1987 was the city's first mass casualty event and he became involved with another student led project, the rebuilding of the casualty facility at Civil Hospital through private donation. After his graduation, he trained in Cardiac Surgery at the National Institute of Cardiovascular Diseases and in 2000 returned as faculty to establish the first cardiac surgery service at Civil Hospital. However, witnessing the poor conditions of public hospitals with long waits for patients, he resolved to build a hospital that could provide quality care free-of-cost. Thus, the vision of Indus Hospital was born and in 2007 it opened in Karachi's Korangi area. The hospital commenced operations with 150 beds and has grown to a 300 bed facility in just a few years, providing free care to all patients.

Speaking about his experience of hospital management, he said that from the beginning of his role as the Chief Executive Officer of Indus Hospital, he delegated tasks and institutionalised the governance functions of the hospital. Nonetheless, during the early days besides management, he was involved in activities such as donor mobilisation and fundraising. He created a hospital management board and registered it as a section 42 company. The board gradually evolved into a network. He has not performed surgeries since 2019. He realised that he could only do 10,000 to 15,000 surgeries in his professionally active life, however, if he developed an institution where 10 to 15 people are performing surgeries, he could increase it to 1.5 to 2 lacs.

When we inquired if he would advise young surgeons to get an MBA degree if they aspired to roles in management, he replied that he would definitely recommend getting a degree or doing a diploma course in hospital management. He believes that had he himself done so, it would have made the adjustment to his management role easier and improved his learning curve for management functions such as finance. A surgeon does not know the difference between credit or debit and these were the things which he has become familiar with only by a slow process of experiential learning while dealing with the business side of healthcare. Besides finance, managing procurement and inventory, along with cost-efficiency, were new subjects for him. While experience is invaluable in learning new skills, and even though his involvement with Civil Hospital welfare projects in his student days had exposed him to these aspects of management, he was certain that if he had the chance to do it all over again, he would definitely get a degree in health management.

When asked about human resource management and competency issues in the workplace, Dr Khan stressed that being a surgeon was a big advantage because you are trained to work in teams. As a manager, he had been doing this from the beginning with emphasis on building coherent teams and building their capacities. However, it also depends on the institution where you have the team building capacity. He strongly believed that efficient and responsible teams in healthcare need good role models and he has always tried to lead from the front. He said,

> *"There is a limit to how much you can do with money. For good outcomes in healthcare, you need to have competent human resources organised in strong teams."*

When asked about conflict resolution issues one faces as a manager, he stated that one has to first and foremost avoid conflicts by creating a collegial and respectful culture in one's institution. Try to make all employees feel valued and discourage degrading or humiliating behaviours by staff members. If conflicts do arise, these must be dealt expeditiously and fairly by enforcing a cooling off period and then addressing the personal grievances and animosities that are often at the root of conflict. If conflicts are dealt with fairly they will occur less often.

He advised aspiring young surgeons to have a big and clear vision. There are two prerequisites in order to do so; you need time and resources. He recommended utilising time wisely. The resources will gradually come with time. He believes that you should have faith in God and belief in yourself in order to succeed.

# CHAPTER 23

# SEEKING FULFILMENT IN THE WORLD OF MEDICINE AND BEYOND

IFTIKHAR SALAHUDDIN

*Honour the physician with the honour due him,*
*according to your need of him for the Lord created him.*
*The healing comes from the Most High and He*
*gave skill to men, that He might be glorified in their works.*
*The Bible: Ecclesiasticus. 38: 1-15*

Abu Ibn Sina (980 AD) known to the Latin West as Avicenna was undoubtedly the greatest physician-philosopher of $11^{th}$ century Persia. Among the many who still visit his mausoleum in Hamadan (Iran), some are convinced that even in death the physician can heal their maladies. William Osler (1849-1919), a celebrated Canadian physician, after visiting his grave, famously remarked, "the great Persian has still a large practice, as his tomb is much visited by pilgrims, among whom cures are said to be not uncommon." The devotion of the visitors to Avicenna's tomb is a measure of their veneration for him. For the many who seek a cure, their faith in the physician transcends even death—an affirmation of their belief that a physician is an intermediary between man and God.

Avicenna learned the art of healing, not formally, but by apprenticing himself to itinerant healers of maladies who wandered in and out of Afshona (Uzbekistan). After successfully treating the Sultan who suffered from a strange and stubborn illness, the young physician was allowed access to the coveted Samanid Library. That is where he taught himself the finer aspects of medicine and metaphysics. While on his way home, he would meet a local vegetable dealer from India, who was clever with numbers, and would unravel for him the mystery of arithmetical calculations and algebra. That was ten centuries ago. Today, the science of medicine is vast, complex and expanding astronomically. Consequently, the art of medicine has become as daunting as it is fascinating.

The decades-long professional journey of a surgeon (or a physician) traverses an unpredictable terrain: long easy stretches, sudden turns, low valleys and sheer mountains—all test the endurance and dedication of the doctor. Traveling on this challenging course, surgeons acquire unique experiences and perspectives that shape both their professional and personal lives. A surgeon in the spring of his career is energetic, ambitious and even daring. With time, the summer of middle age tempers the brashness of youth, taming it to a measured caution of maturity. As the professional journey continues into the autumn of his career, a sobering realization dawns that the heydays of profession are ebbing away, and the busy doctor will have to accept a different routine of living.

Likewise, after a fulfilling career of a half-century, the long and satisfying journey of my professional life has reached its logical destination, and it is time for introspection—to reflect on the road well-trodden. As the 19$^{th}$ century Swedish philosopher Soren Kierkegaard observed, "life can only be understood backwards but it must be lived forwards."

In a surgeon's career the phase of training is critical—a determinative period during which the resident is moulded and groomed in the crucible of the profession. A lapidary unwearyingly polishes and shapes a nugget till it becomes a sparkling gem. By the same analogy, in the shadow of a consummate surgeon, the assistant acquires seminal skills which define the craft of surgery; time and experience hone these talents to an artform. Then the residency is also the time when the young surgeon, inspired by worthy teachers, imbibes the virtues which personify a caring surgeon: truthfulness, personal integrity, compassion and humility with grace. When the well-groomed resident finally evolves into a dexterous surgeon, he is well advised to remember at every surgery the words of the American poet Emily Dickenson: "Surgeons must take heed when they pick the knife; underneath their fine incisions stirs sacred life."

Once the residency is completed, the enthusiastic surgeon steps into the real world of the medical profession, and is confronted with distinct choices: either pledge to the higher ideals of a sacred calling, or practise the art of healing to gain a livelihood. In a moral sense, the latter choice is in conflict with the spirit of the profession—indeed it diminishes the dedication inherent in the noble art.

Unfortunately, in the mores of our society, the fame of a doctor is often equated with financial status. For many in the profession, pecuniary gains become an all-consuming priority and to that end there develops an insatiable craving to increase patient load and working hours. It is not uncommon for surgeons to declaim their practice as "high volume-high revenue." The "want" to see more patients is at the expense of the precious time essential, not only for patient care but also for reassuring the distressed families about those dear to them. In the melee of a busy practice, it is easy to forget that "non-revenue" patients also deserve adequate time and humane attention.

On a personal note, very early during my practice, I was taught an eternal lesson in humility and patience. It was the end of a long and tiring day, and I was anxious to leave for a game of billiards when an old woman from a far-off destitute area (*katchi abaadi)* shuffled into my office to consult me for an ear problem that had been nagging her for some time.

It was getting late and rather callously remonstrated with her for not coming earlier in the afternoon. Her frail body and wrinkled face bespoke her suffering and penury. She steadied her stick on the wall, sat down slowly with a sigh and explained that she lived alone with a paraplegic daughter who has to be tied to the bed securely before she could safely lock the house behind her. She said, "Today, my daughter was very restless, and it took me long to tie her up. I am sorry." For a very long time, I sat still, looking down. My eyes welled up and I couldn't face the woman and looked up only when the tears of my remorse fell on the ground.

Francis W. Peabody (1881-1927), the celebrated teacher of the Harvard Medical School, who valued altruism on a par with the professional attributes of a doctor, remarked that one of the essential qualities of the clinician is interest in humanity, "For the secret of the care of the patient is in caring for the patient and the family." It is in the nature of the profession that a physician becomes an intimate witness of man—at his birth, during his illness and ultimately at his death. A sacred bond of trust grows between the patient and the caregiver. The distressed families often share with the doctor their gloomy stories of despair only to seek the doctor's understanding and compassion. There are myriad strands of personal events which weave through the lives of every family—both poor and wealthy. A caring physician, just by listening patiently can often soothe the anguish and pain of suffering; the balm of a few kind words is far more healing than a handful of pills or elixirs.

At times the narratives are personal and the family seeks advice trusting the doctor's integrity and better judgement. A 23-year-old girl consulted me for a mass in the parotid which I biopsied. A week later, I had the onerous responsibility of telling the mother that her daughter had a malignancy and the treatment would entail extensive surgery and prolonged after-care. First, there was silence, and then the distraught mother tearfully revealed that her daughter was to be married in a few days and that the bride-groom's family (*baraat)* was already in town. She was apprehensive that the in-laws might call off the marriage if they found out that the bride has health issues and the scar on her face would become a stigma. She wondered if she could postpone sharing the news with them until after the wedding. I advised an honest approach and offered to personally discuss the condition with the prospective in-laws. After an emotional discussion, the in-laws simply asked if the treatment could wait till after the wedding. In a very stirring manner, the mother-in-law-to-be emphatically stated that she had already accepted the bride to be her daughter and would gladly accompany her for the treatments. My heart felt warmed by the knowing that humaneness and traditional values are alive and well in our society.

Looking back in history, the celebrated Russian writer of the $19^{th}$ century, Anton Chekhov (1860-1904) has written hundreds of similar stories. He was a quintessential family doctor in a village outside Moscow. Despite his busy practice, he found time to write. His stories are unique, each reflecting the lives of his patients and cumulatively illustrating a vast canvas of Russian society replete with human emotions: suffering of the sick, the joyous celebration of a new baby and the grief at the burial of a near one.

Chekhov often visited his patients, most of whom were serfs and peasants mired in suffering, occasioned by penury and want. He portrays poignantly the anguish of the toiling classes beholden in servitude to the landowners. The rich wearied him with their wanton callousness; he writes fervidly about the epicurean society, the effete aristocrats and their pervasive debauchery. His stories vividly evoke the unjustness and inequities of Russian society at the time. In one of his many poignant stories, he describes the wretched life of a woodcutter suffering in his destitute cottage in the shadow of the plush *dacha* (country house) of the cruel headman. Chekhov, the village doctor, imbued with concern for the grim life of the peasants, undertook an arduous 2000-mile journey into the vast and bleak rural landscape of Siberia to document and narrate the squalid life of villagers in Russia's hinterland. His writings unfortunately had little effect on the apathetic and obtuse Czarist autocrats. His friends however were curious how he found time in his busy practice to write so profusely. Chekhov quipped, “Medicine is my lawfully wedded wife and literature is my mistress; when I get tired of one, I seek the other.”

To a young and prosperous surgeon, a busy practice and hectic times seem enduring if not eternal. Few have the wisdom to see beyond the present and prepare for the inevitable golden age when it would be time to get out of the fast lane and blend into a less frenetic path of life. It is a difficult transition for most doctors, who, throughout their career have travelled exclusively on the professional track, addicted to the heady life of a busy doctor but remaining blinkered to the exciting world beyond medicine. At the end of their busy professional life, many feel lost because beside their profession they have no other interests to fall back on. Even friendships nurtured in busy times become difficult to sustain in retirement. Consequently, after the hectic days of a glorious career the quiet days of retirement seem too long, lonely and purposeless.

But the period of retirement doesn’t have to be that way. Indeed, in western societies, retirement is often welcomed and even taken prematurely to enjoy much-anticipated travels to exotic destinations or to pursue interests and hobbies for which there never was ample time. A satisfying career is the culmination of many years of preparation; retirement too needs to be carefully planned and tailored—not at the end of the career but throughout the active life. Life is lived but once—a life that is beautiful, a precious gift that we are blessed with, and the world offers a rainbow of choices besides one’s profession.

To taste the flavours of the wondrous world, one must touch it in many places—but first “look in thine own self!” Man, rich or poor is a sum of innate talents, some of which are waiting to be realised. The legendary Italian sculptor of the Renaissance period, Michelangelo (1475-1504), remarked that his statues have always been always there, hidden in stone—he simply uncovered them with a chisel. By the same analogy, perhaps there is a painter in you, an artist, a writer or a poet just waiting to emerge. But if that concealed genius remains dormant and undiscovered, life will no doubt move on; would become merely routine and monotonous, not full, challenging or interesting.

Along the same vein, it is imperative to discover oneself but not wise to live only by one’s own experiences. Many who attained success and fame have left a bright trail in their wake; walking in their footsteps illumines the road ahead. In the words of Buddha, “to walk safely through the maze of human life one needs the light of wisdom and the guidance of the virtuous."

In the chronicles of physicians who transcended the frontiers of medicine to seek fulfillment beyond, there were some, who, while remaining devoted to their calling, also found joy in fine arts–literature, music and poetry.

In the fraternity of Chekhov, who concurrently practised his profession and indulged in his passion for writing, was the $19^{th}$ century legendary Austrian surgeon Theodore Billroth (1829-1894). He was born to a wealthy aristocratic family in northern Germany. About the same time in a nearby town Johann Brahms (1833-1897) was born into a family of a lower social order mired in poverty. The backgrounds of the two boys could not be more divergent or their careers more disparate. Billroth became a renowned surgeon and founded a school of surgery in Vienna. Brahms would become the greatest composer of symphonies after Beethoven, Mozart and Haydn. He lived in Vienna, the home of musical geniuses like Wagner, Strauss, Beethoven and Mahler. Brahms was celebrated in the city and his symphonies drew enormous crowds and rave reviews. Billroth, himself a gifted pianist, met the famous composer after a concert, and they become lifelong friends—a friendship which celebrated the union of art and science. Brahms recognized the brilliance of the surgeon's mind and was impressed by his uncanny musical skills. He discovered that the surgeon was also an accomplished composer of music, and he would ask him to review his manuscripts before they were performed at concerts. Brahms, a lonely musician, valued the warmth and extrovert personality of Billroth, and the surgeon, who witnessed suffering and death all day in his profession, relaxed in the company of the composer. Billroth would spend evenings playing the piano with Brahms, and they discussed music well into the night. For a concert in Vienna, Brahms composed musical scores to be played by both of them. After the performance, the two friends received a rapturous ovation from the audience. Aware of Billroth's fame in surgery, Brahms named the symphonies Billroth I and Billroth II. At the concert, critics were surprised that a surgeon could also be an accomplished musician. Billroth replied, "I have never known a great man in research who is essentially not an artist. Science and art spring from the same source."

Unfortunately, later in life the friendship faded and Brahms became more sloven in his appearance and often criticised Billroth unfairly. At the grand funeral of Billroth, who died at the age of 60 from cardiac failure, Brahms, who hated pomp and ceremony, observed the event from afar. Two years later, Brahms died of a gall bladder malignancy and was buried in the same cemetery where Billroth rested. Their graves are next to those of Schubert and Beethoven near Mozart's monument.

Another remarkable physician who is celebrated for his accomplishments beyond his profession was also from $19^{th}$ century Germany, Albert Schweitzer (1875-1965). During his student days, Schweitzer became an accomplished musician and frequently played the organ at music recitals, and yet still found time to earn a degree in philosophy and a doctorate in theology. He took up medicine, albeit late in life, "to devote himself unsparingly to the betterment of mankind's condition." After graduation, Doctor Schweitzer, a devout Christian, decided to go Africa to serve humanity. He settled in French Equatorial Africa (now Gabon) where he founded a hospital at Lambarene on the Ogooué River. Despite meagre funds and primitive equipment, he treated thousands of patients with leprosy and the feared sleeping sickness. Over the years Schweitzer added a leper colony to his hospital where 36 white physicians and nurses took care of hundreds of African patients with leprosy. Throughout his practice in Gabon, philosophy remained his passion and he wrote a book, *Kuturephilosophi* (Philosophy of Culture) which defined ethical principles of all living things and preached "reverence for life."

French colonialists ruled Gabon during the First World War, and France was at war with Germany. Dr Schweitzer and his wife were from Germany and were arrested and interned in a camp for two years; but that did not deter the missionary doctor from pursuing music and other scholarly interests throughout his prison term. He appeared on the front cover of *Time* magazine as the "Greatest man in the world" (July 1949). In 1952, Dr Schweitzer was awarded the Nobel Prize "for his altruism, reverence for life, [and] tireless humanitarian work which has helped in making the idea of brotherhood between men and nations a living one." The celebrated physician died in 1965 at his hospital in Gabon. His grave on the banks of the Ogooué River is marked by a cross which he had made himself.

In our own contemporary society there are admirable doctors who are internationally renowned scientists and also celebrated writers. For instance, Dr Azra Raza is an eminent oncologist in the United States whose abiding interest in Urdu poetry culminated in a book on the legendary poet Mirza Ghalib. She recites his poetry with as much grace and panache as she does discoursing the finer nuances of mutation and cell biology.

Looking back, Chekov, Billroth and Schweitzer all led enriched lives, committed to medicine and equally enthusiastic about the arts. They embodied an ideal harmony of profession and passion. But for many doctors, jaded with medicine, the profession lost its lustre, and they found more satisfaction and fulfillment in other callings. A new world beckoned them; they followed their heart and abandoned medicine altogether.

"I do not know a better training for a writer than to spend some years in the medical profession," remarked W. Somerset Maugham (1874-1965) the famous English novelist and playwright who graduated from St. Thomas's Hospital in London. In his new career, he achieved international renown for his plays, short stories and books. Several movies are based on his stories.

Another British doctor who gave up medicine after a long but failed spell of medical practice was Arthur Conan Doyle (1859-1930), a writer who mesmerised the world with his mystery stories. His fictionalised uncanny detective in the stories, Sherlock Holmes, became more famous than the real-life author himself; in fact, people believed that Sherlock Holmes actually resided at the detective's fictitious 221 Baker Street address and many Londoners came seeking him, hoping to consult the conjured sleuth. Sherlock Holmes was introduced in 1887 in the story *A Study in Scarlet*; the detective became so popular that when he dies in the story *The Final Problem* (1893), there were widespread protests in England. Women wore black capes and men sported black arm bands. After reading several editorials in newspapers Conan Doyle was obliged to resurrect Sherlock Holmes in *Adventures of the Empty House* (1894). In the literary world, the period of Sherlock Holmes' absence is referred to as "the Great Hiatus."

For physicians, giving up medicine to take up writing was not a drastic transition, but some doctors were attracted to politics and a few attained international attention. For example, George Clemenceau (1841-1929), Prime Minister of France during the First World War, is considered the architect of the Treaty of Versailles between Germany and Europe.

Some doctors with radical views, or those concerned about human rights and freedom, made bewildering choices which obliged them to abandon a noble and humane routine to take up arms in the cause of revolutionary movements. Sun Yat-sen (1866-1925), the father of modern China, was born in late-19th century China when the country was suffering under the Manchus of the last imperial Qing dynasty. He went to medical school in Hong Kong and later joined a hospital in Hawaii. The westernised leader who converted to the Christian faith returned to China to practise medicine in Guangzhou but was deeply troubled by the spreading anarchy in the country and the ineptness of the rule of the Manchus. Sun Yat-sen gave up medicine and joined a revolutionary movement, which in 1911 staged a violent rebellion against the effete Qing dynasty. After liberating ancient China, he established the Kuomintang party whose powerful revolutionaries Mao Ze Dong and Chiang Kai Shek both revered the doctor as the supreme leader who had given the freedom to China.

Sun Yat-sen changed the destiny of his own country, but among the physicians who influenced world events was William Jardine (1784-1843) the wily physician and intrepid trader from Scotland. He is recognised as the architect of the 1839 Opium War which the British forced on China. Jardine graduated from the University of Edinburgh's medical school, and after being admitted to the Royal College of Surgeons, he opted to join the East India Company as their ship doctor, setting sail for India. The Company permitted the doctor to trade in opium which was being smuggled on their ships to China. Within two decades, Jardine's company became the wealthiest and the most influential opium trading house in the east. The Chinese became weary of the widespread addiction of the population to opium and the sprouting of opium dens across the country. The Emperor even addressed a letter to the English King who did not even acknowledge it. British hypocrisy was on open display; indeed the use and sale of the contraband opium in their own country were punishable by death. In 1839, when the British refused to stop shipping opium to the Middle Kingdom, the Chinese commissioner Lin confiscated and destroyed 20,000 cases of opium which had just arrived from Calcutta. The British were livid, and found the insult intolerable. Jardine, who by then had become a member of the Parliament– backed by renegade British opium traders– persuaded Lord Palmerston, the Foreign Secretary, to use force against the "up-start and insolent" Chinese to open the opium trade. The Chinese lost the war and signed the humiliating Nanking Treaty ceding their territory of Hong Kong to England. *Jardine and Matheson* is today a major trading house in Hong Kong.

In the world of revolutionary warfare, few can match the charisma and popularity of Che Guevara (1928-1967), the Latin American doctor, who has been venerated around the world, especially by millions of restless youths for emancipating the poor of Latin America and Africa. A physician from the University of Buenos Aires, he befriended Fidel Castro and joined the armed guerrilla movement against the oppressive Baptista government. After hiding as a fugitive for decades he was ultimately assassinated by the CIA deep in the jungles of Bolivia.

In the annals of doctors who chose a different calling over the medical profession, there were none more daring and adventurous than the physicians who gave up a modest life tending to the sick and set out to explore the so-called Dark Continent. In the process they discovered lands not then mapped; some explorers who were imbued also with missionary zeal spread God's word in the deepest recesses in the heart of darkness. There were many such dedicated physician-explorers: Surgeon Mungo Park (1771-1806), a graduate of the University of Edinburgh in Scotland, discovered and mapped the River Niger in the late 18th century. He returned to the river in 1805 and was killed, mistaken for a local rebel from a Muslim tribe.

Not to be forgotten in the annals of history—and amongst its noblest personae—was the Scottish missionary who was the most admirable British hero of the Victorian era. As a medical doctor he cared for his parishioners for many years, but eventually heeded to a higher calling-spreading the Lord's name in Africa. He lived over 30 years in Africa, mapping almost a third of the vast continent, and even after discovering the Victoria Falls, he continued his quest for the origin of the River Nile. While in Africa he witnessed the abhorrent practice of the slave trade, and used his enormous influence in England to raise his voice against the outrageous sin of human trade. When he went missing for several years, the British hired a swashbuckling renegade to search for him in the wilds of Africa. Henry Morton Stanley, a journalist, is recognised for greeting the missing explorer with the famous words, "Dr Livingston, I presume?" Dr Livingston died while praying in his cottage in the wilds of East Africa (1873). His African assistants cut open his chest to retrieve the heart which loved Africa and buried it in the soil. That is where the doctor wanted it to be. His frail and emaciated body was brought back to London by his two faithful assistants and interred in Westminster Abbey among the hallowed heroes of the British Empire.

Physicians and surgeons are uniquely blessed to witness humanity in its innumerable expressions; indeed the medical profession opens a wide window to civilisation. It allows doctors a vantage position to gaze at the world from a holistic perspective and at the same time seek avenues to a fulfilling existence. Man is as free as his dreams. Fear of the unknown shackles only the weak, but the strong take the high road beyond the horizon.

To quote Rumi, “Every mortal will taste death but only some will taste life. Death holds no terror for the one who can see beyond this life’s short and fitful span; the knocks of the rocks, the churning ocean’s swell do not affect the pearl inside the shell.”

# CHAPTER 24

# SURGEONS AND EMOTIONAL INTELLIGENCE

SYED MUHAMMAD NAZIM

## Introduction

Healthcare systems are not run by individuals but by teams. Surgeons are the leaders in a healthcare team and are expected to successfully manage both themselves and the rest of the team to accomplish the tasks (Gawande 2010; McKinley 2014). There is a growing demand from surgeons to not only demonstrate clinical and technical mastery but also possess strong personal and social qualities which would impact not only their well-being but the patient-doctor relationship and team dynamics as well (Lin, Kannappan and Lau 2013).

Surgical education and training are inherently stressful and the ability to effectively handle this stress is an essential component of surgical competence (Flin, O'Connor and Crichton 2008; Shapiro, Shapiro and Schwartz 2000). Surgical residency programmes aim to identify individuals who are not only sound academics but who also possess the intrapersonal and interpersonal qualities enabling them to thrive in an emotionally, socially, and physically challenging work environment for prolonged periods (Provenzano et al. 2021).

Emotional intelligence (EI) has emerged as a construct and a successful leadership skillset in recent years, particularly in business literature. Due to its role in the social relationship, it can thus be linked to favourable outcomes in fields of healthcare and healthcare education as well (Provenzano et al. 2021).

## Emotional intelligence

Intelligence as a concept can be described in many ways. Two traditional classifications include:

a) Verbal and propositional and
b) perceptual and organizational areas.

A third intelligence that was sought by investigators for decades includes one which accounts for individual differences in intelligence (Mayer, Salovey and Caruso 2008). Since emotions convey valuable information regarding individuals and their relationship with others, the effective understanding and management of emotions is considered a type of intelligence (Johnson 2015). In other words, emotion and intellect combine to form emotional intelligence.

The concept of EI was popularized and received significant attention with the publication of the American psychologist Daniel Goleman's book *Emotional Intelligence: Why it Can Matter More Than IQ for Character, Health and Lifelong Achievement* (Goleman 1995).

Emotional intelligence describes a wide variety of non-cognitive qualifications and competencies helping individuals manage emotional and environmental stressors as well as their ability to navigate relationships with others (Brannick et al. 2009).

EI was defined by Salovey and Mayer (1990) as,

> The subset of social intelligence that involves the ability to monitor one's own and others feelings and emotions, to discriminate among them, and to use this information to guide one's thinking and actions.

## Emotions and the brain

EI represents "the ability of the higher brain centres to monitor and direct more primitive emotional signals from phylogenetically older brain structures, such as the amygdala, in such a way that they are used constructively by the individual, rather than destructively" (Humphrey et al. 2007).

The amygdala, a primitive structure of the limbic system mediating basic and self-centred impulses, is controlled by higher cortical structures of the brain such as the frontal lobes. The way we react to a situation is a habit or automatic reflex and hence this response is an "act" before we have time to "think."

Individuals with a higher level of EI are not only able to identify their emotional states and those of others but could control them using the higher cortex. Thus EI teaches individuals to shift from self-gratification seeking behaviours to gratification received by emotional needs in the self and others (Johnson 2015).

## Emotional intelligence models and key elements

There is no uniformly accepted model of EI; however, three major models are most commonly referred to. These are:

- Salovey and Mayer (1990)
- Goleman (1995) and
- The Bar-On Model of Emotional-Social Intelligence (2006)

The common thread in all these models is defining the importance of emotional awareness and its impact on relationships with other individuals (Jensen et al. 2008).

Goleman defines EI as a group of five key elements: (1) self-awareness, (2) self-regulation, (3) motivation, (4) empathy, and (5) social skills (Fig. 24-1).

These skillsets enable the best leaders to maximize not only their performance but that of their followers as well (Salovey and Mayer 1990).

The first two, self-awareness and self-regulation, are skills that are inwardly focused, while the last two have to do with how we relate to others. The third skill, motivation, acts as a bridge between the others as it incorporates both what motivates the individual and provides an understanding of what motivates others (Endean 2018).

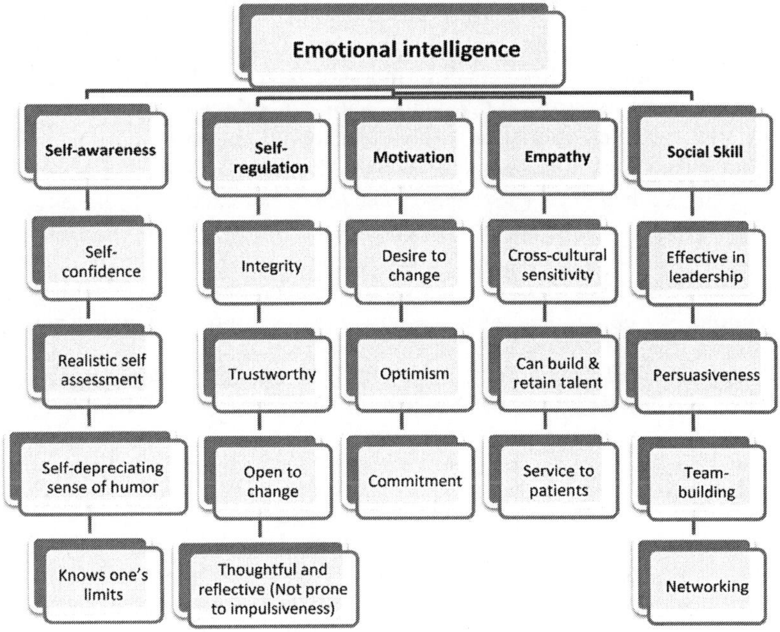


Fig. 24-1: Key elements of emotional intelligence

## 1. Self-awareness

Goleman described self-awareness as "knowing one's strengths, weaknesses, drives, values and one's impact on others" (Goleman 1995). An individual's self-image is either better or worse than how others view him. Self-aware individuals often have a humble sense of humour, know their limitations and seek help when needed. An example includes a "good" resident who knows his/ her limitations but also knows what he /she is capable of doing.

Various strategies are described to improve self-awareness including keeping a journal to write down one's thoughts and self-reflection about strong emotions such as anger.

## 2. Self-regulation

Goleman defined this skill as, "handling our emotions so that they facilitate rather than interfere with the task at hand; being conscientious and delaying gratification to pursue goals; [and] recovering well from emotional distress" (1998). It is the ability to control one's emotions and impulses, especially when they are negative; or in other words, the ability to think before acting or reacting. Individuals with self-regulation have a high degree of integrity. Individuals, who regulate themselves effectively, do not make an emotional or rushed decision and never compromise their values. They are the opposite of the "hothead." This is one of the important skills that surgeons need to develop. For example in instances of uncontrolled bleeding during surgery, the ability to control emotions and frustrations and to focus and address the problem results in a better outcome than a surgeon who loses his temper and expresses his / her emotions by yelling, placing blames on others and throwing an instrument.

To improve self-regulation abilities, it is suggested that the individual knows his "values" and "code of ethics," holds himself accountable, and practises being calm.

**3. Motivation**

Individuals with a strong motivation love challenges, look for ways to do things more efficiently, and are proud of a job that is done well. They are committed, open to change, and are optimistic. A motivated surgeon would encounter a challenging case and constantly look for ways to do it better by embracing change, new technologies, and adapting better skills.

**4. Empathy**

Empathy is being considerate of another person's viewpoint or feelings and having the ability to accept and understand a different point of view. Having empathy is critical to managing a successful team or organization. Through this ability, good relationships can be built with patients and other members of the team.

**5. Social Skills**

Goleman has defined this skill as, "handling emotions in relationships well and accurately reading social situations and networks; interacting smoothly; [and] using these skills to persuade and lead, negotiate and settle disputes, for cooperation and teamwork" (1998).

Social skills, like empathy, have to do with one's ability to interact with others. They entail having the ability to manage relationships to move in a certain direction. It involves team building and persuasiveness. Individuals with good social skills are great communicators and can manage change and resolve conflicts.

## EI and "success"

Goleman, in his famous book, claims that only 20% of a person's success can be attributed to IQ. This claim prompted many researchers to explore other factors that contribute the other 80% to a person's success. A person with high emotional intelligence not only contributes better towards academic success but is also said to function better under stress and as a team player, thus contributing to an organization's productivity (Mohzan, Hassan and Halil 2013).

## Conceptual model of EI: ability or trait?

EI is a multi-dimensional construct comprising cognitive and affective domains (Cherry et al. 2014). There is a debate in psychology literature whether EI is an ability, a personality trait, or a mixture of both.

The ability definition describes EI as, "the ability to monitor one's own and others' feelings and emotions, to discriminate among them, and to use this information to guide one's thinking and actions" (Salovey and Mayer 1990).

Trait theorists define EI as, "a constellation of emotion-related self-perceptions and dispositions, assessed through self-report" (Petrides and Furnham 2003).

Mixed model theories define EI as, "an array of non-cognitive capabilities, competencies, and skills" (Bar-On 2006).

Many EI related behaviours do not fall under a single competency but are widely applicable across competencies. The traditional intelligence quotient (IQ) is regarded as relatively static; however, EI is considered fluid and teachable to individuals across various age groups and can be measured using validated instruments (Bar-On 2006).

Proponents of different models of EI affirm however that EI can be taught, learned, and developed (Petrides 2012; Salovey and Sluyter 1997) through continual active training, learning, feedback, and practice throughout all ages (Goleman 1998).

## How is EI measured?

Several assessment tools have been developed and validated to measure EI in the literature (Consortium for Research on Emotional Intelligence in Organizations 2021). Due to the unresolved disagreement about the nature of EI as a construct, there are multiple different and conflicting approaches to the assessment of EI. The trait and mixed-models take into account the inherent subjectivity of emotional experiences belonging to the domain of personality (Davey 2005) and thus advocate the use of self-report as their measurement appliance.

Examples include:

- Emotional Quotient Inventory (EQ-i) (Bar-On 1997)
- Emotional Competence Inventory (ECI) (Boyatzis, Goleman and Rhee 2004)
- Emotional Intelligence Scale (EIS) (Schutte et al. 1998)
- Trait Emotional Intelligence Questionnaire (TEIQue) (Petrides and Furnham 2003)

The ability model views EI as a skill or competence that can be measured using objective performance testing. The Mayer-Salovey-Caruso Emotional Intelligence test (MSCEIT), for example, tries to capture ability EI through a series of problem-solving items and is scored by consensus or by expert opinion (Johnson 2015).

**Trait Emotional Intelligence Questionnaire (TEIQue)**

This questionnaire is based on the trait conceptualization of EI. It is a psychometrically validated 153-item self-assessment tool for EI, developed and scored by Dr K. V. Petrides's group at London Psychometric Laboratory, University College London (Petrides and Furnham 2003; Petrides, Pita and Kokkinaki 2007). Each item on the TEIQue is a statement answered on a 7-point Likert scale, depending on how strongly the respondent agrees or disagrees with a particular statement; (1 = completely disagree; 7 = completely agree). The items yield fifteen independent facet scores which then cluster into four broader factor scores for well-being, self-control, emotionality, and sociability (Table 24-1).

**Table 24-1: TEIQUE domains, facets and factor descriptions**

| Factor/Facet | High scorers perceive themselves as |
|---|---|
| **Well-being factor** | Possessing a generalized sense of well-being; feeling positive, happy and fulfilled |
| **Happiness** | Cheerful and satisfied with their lives |
| **Optimism** | Confident and likely to "look on the bright side" of life |
| **Self-esteem** | Successful and self-confident |
| **Sociability factor** | Excelling at social interaction and relationship building; able to exert influence in social settings |
| **Social awarenessAssertiveness** | Accomplished networkers with superior social skills |
| | Forthright, frank, and willing to stand up for their rights |
| **Emotional management** | Capable of influencing other people's feelings |
| **Emotionality factor** | Capable of perceiving and expressing emotions, and using these qualities to develop and sustain close relationships with others |
| **Relationships** | Capable of maintaining fulfilling personal relationships |
| **Emotional perception** | Insightful and clear about their own and other people's feelings |
| **Emotional expression** | Capable of communicating of their feelings to others |
| **Empathy** | Capable of taking in someone else's perspective |
| **Self-control factor** | Possessing a healthy degree of control over their urges and desires, also good at coping with external pressures and stress |
| **Impulse control** | Reflective and less likely to give in to their urges |
| **Emotion regulation** | Capable of controlling their emotions |
| **Stress management** | Capable of withstanding pressure and regulating stress |
| **Adaptability** | Flexible and willing to adapt to new conditions |
| **Self-motivation** | Driven and unlikely to give up in the face of adversity |

The items also generate a single global score. The TEIQue version 1.50 questionnaire takes approximately 15 to 25 minutes to complete and is available at http://www.psychometriclab.com. TEIQue has been tested across a variety of cultures and languages with high reliability (Cronbach-α for overall EI score of 0.92). It suffers, however, from its sole reliance on self-report and no objective metrics are available.

There is a short form (TEIQue-SF) available comprising 30-self-report items with a seven-point Likert scale rating. These item ratings are summed to give a global trait EI score ranging from 30-210.

**Mayer-Salovey-Caruso Emotional Intelligence Test (MSCEIT)**

The MSCEIT is an ability-based instrument developed to capture emotional intelligence objectively (Mayer, Caruso and Salovey 1999). It measures how well people perform emotional tasks and solve problems involving emotional situations (Mayer, Salovey and Caruso 2002). The MSCEIT version 2.0 yields a profile of scores describing the individual's ability to perceive, use and manage emotions. It was developed by the University of New Hampshire and Yale University. It is a validated instrument and has shown good evidence for face, content, and predictive validity (Doherty, Cronin and Offiah 2013).

It has been tested in a wide variety of settings such as research, corporate, education, and clinical fields (Mayer, Salovey and Caruso 2002). The MSCEIT assesses a respondent's level of correctness based on a normative sample of 5,000 people (2002). It has a total EI score and four branch scores: perceiving emotions, using emotions, understanding emotions, and emotional management (Table 24-2).

**Table 24-2: Subscales of MSCEIT V 2.0**

| Areas | Ability | Question types | How the ability may be used | Test sections |
|---|---|---|---|---|
| **Experiential** | **Perceiving Emotions** | Identifying emotions in faces, landscapes and designs | "Read" people's moods for feedback | Faces, picture |
| | **Using Emotions** | How moods impact thinking; relating feelings to thoughts | Creating the right feeling to assist in problem solving, communicating a vision, or leading people | Facilitation, sensations |
| **Strategic** | **Understanding Emotions** | Multiple choice emotion vocabulary questions | Being able to predict how people will emotionally react | Changes, blends |
| | **Managing Emotions** | Indicating effectiveness of various solutions to problems | Integrating emotion and thought to make effective decisions | Emotion management, emotional relationships |

Scores are positioned on a normal curve with an average score of 100, standard deviation (SD) of 15, and a maximum score of 145 (2002).

The measure comprises 141 test items and takes approximately 30 to 45 minutes to complete. Both a paper and pen version and online administration are available at www.mhsassessments.com. The test presents a series of photos and pictures in some subscales and the respondents are asked to identify the emotions portrayed. In other subscales, the respondents are asked to choose the most appropriate strategy to solve an inter-personal situation.

MSCEIT attempts to objectify experiences and situations that are emotion-laden and inherently subjective; it also uses expert and consensus scoring to determine the correct responses. This can lead to potential problems as individual differences in the way people perceive emotional information cannot be easily deemed "erroneous" by either an "expert" or a "panel of judges."

**The Bar-On Emotional Quotient Inventory (EQ-i):**

This inventory was created based on the Bar-On model which describes EI as, "an array of interrelated emotional and social competencies, skills and behaviours that impact intelligent behaviour."

It is a well-validated EI-measurement instrument (Bar-On 2006). The EQ-i is an online 133-item self-assessment instrument that uses a 5-point response set (ranging from "Not true of me" to "True of me"). It takes approximately 30-40 minutes to complete. It measures EI on five composite scale scores (intrapersonal, interpersonal, stress management, adaptability, and general mood) and fifteen content subscale scores (Table 24-3).

**Table 24-3: Subscales of Bar-On EQ-i**

| **Component** | |
|---|---|
| **1. Intrapersonal** | **Assessment of inner self** |
| Self-regard | The ability to respect and accept oneself as basically good. It is associated with feelings of security, inner strength and self-confidence |
| Emotional self-awareness | The ability to recognize one's feelings and emotions, to differentiate between them and to know what caused them |
| Assertiveness | The ability to express feelings, beliefs and thoughts. To defend one's rights in a non-destructive manner |
| Independence | The ability to be self-directed and self-controlled in one's thinking/actions, and to be free of emotional dependency |
| Self-actualization | The ability to realize one's potential capacities and affiliate them with feelings of self-satisfaction |

| | |
|---|---|
| **2. Interpersonal** | **Assesses interpersonal capacity and functioning** |
| Empathy | The ability to be aware of, understand and to appreciate the feelings of others |
| Social responsibility | The ability to act as a cooperative, contributing and constructive member of one's social group, even when one may not benefit personally |
| Interpersonal relations | This ability to establish and maintain mutually satisfying relationships that are characterized by intimacy |
| **3. Stress management** | **Assesses the ability to withstand stress** |
| Stress tolerance | The ability to withstand adverse events and stressful situations. This is similar to the concept of "ego strength" and "positive coping" |
| Impulse control | The ability to resist or delay an impulse, drive or temptation to act |
| **4. Adaptability** | **Assesses the ability to cope with environmental demands** |
| Reality testing | The ability to assess the correspondence between what is experienced and what objectively exists |
| Flexibility | The ability to adjust one's emotions, thoughts and behaviour to changing situations and conditions |
| Problem-solving | The ability to identify and define problems as well as to generate and implement potentially effective solutions |
| **5. General mood** | **Assesses one's general feeling of contentment** |
| Optimism | The ability to look at the brighter side of life and to maintain a positive attitude, even in the face of adversity |
| Happiness | Happiness combines self-satisfaction, general contentment and the ability to enjoy life |

Like MSCEIT, EQ-i scores have a mean of 100 and an SD of 15. The EQ-i is regarded as the most widely validated and used instrument and is available in 29 languages (Bar-On 2006; Jensen et al. 2008). It has shown excellent reliability (internal consistency) of 0.97 (Bar-On 2004).

This instrument has been used to examine patient satisfaction (Bar-On 1997), changes in residents' and medical students' EI over time (Bar-On 1997), and personal awareness of the emotional skills and competencies necessary to cope with the demands of a stressful operating theatre (OT) environment (1997).

A major criticism of EQ-i is the self-reported nature of the questions and critics have speculated that respondents may choose "socially desirable" choices rather than being truthful in their answers (Brackett and Mayer 2003; Conte 2005; Lewis, Rees, Hudson and Bleakley 2005).

### EQ-360

This inventory is a form of EQ-i which is distributed to six different raters who know the subject well. For use with surgical trainees, this instrument could potentially be distributed to attending physicians, fellow residents, interns, medical students, patients, nurses, families & friends, and other raters who may know the individual well. The addition of the EQ-360 to the individual's EQ-i profile may provide a more complete evaluation of an individual's EI (Jensen et al. 2008).

## Which measure of EI to use?

The self-report measures are criticized on the ground of the problem of social desirability bias and the potential for faking. There is also the added drawback that individuals are poor at "self" estimating their various intellectual abilities (Johnson 2015).

Combining "self-reporting" with assessment by co-workers (360° assessment) (Boyatzis and Goleman 1999) can counteract the potential for response biases. In 360° assessment, the external feedback by the people who work alongside surgeons generates a more complete evaluation and is therefore helpful for evaluating all areas of EI including self-awareness (McLeod and Sonnenberg 2017).

## Emotional intelligence in medicine and surgery

*"Medicine is not only a science but also the art of letting our own individuality interact with the individuality of the patient."*
Dr Albert Schweitzer (1875-1965) (Cherniss et al. 1998)

Emotional intelligence is a psychological "construct" made up of personal-emotional-social components of general intelligence (Arora et al. 2010). Although it has demonstrated worth in the business community, it is still a nascent field of research in the healthcare industry.

Healthcare is a complex field involving challenging diagnosis and treatment, a background of patient and family anxiety, and financial and regularity complexities (Fernandez et al. 2012). Several of the non-technical "soft" skillsets such as teamwork, leadership, communication, and decision-making skills are shown to correlate with EI (Talarico et al. 2013; Taylor, Farver and Stoller 2011).

Emotional intelligence is an essential part of a surgeon's repertoire. Skills in EI help surgeons understand, engage and motivate their team. They also enable productive interpersonal interactions, improved communication, constructive conflict resolutions, and dealing with complex problems (Fernandez et al. 2012). With the increasing complexity of surgical care, multi-disciplinary care, and the rising frequency of patient care transfers, these skills are even more important than ever before (Jensen et al. 2008).

In a busy day to day surgical practice, EI is important for the careful management of emotions. Taking an example, good emotional understanding involves listening to a frustrated patient or colleague's angry outburst without taking it personally, or trying to focus on what is best for the patient rather than "who is right" (Arora et al. 2010).

Within a multi-disciplinary team, today's surgeon is required to develop critical self-awareness skills to understand his strengths, weaknesses, needs, and desires. It is also important for him to recognize the effect of his behaviour on others within a team (Sharp, Bourke and Rickard 2020). Self-regulation and impulse control allows a surgeon to control his emotions and to think before he acts (Goleman 1995). Intrinsic motivation is associated with his passion for surgery, perseverance, and what he desires to achieve (Sharp, Bourke and Rickard 2020). Interaction with colleagues and patients allows the surgeon to place himself in the shoes of others. He gains the ability to realize the feelings of others and to demonstrate respect and value for others. This empathetic behaviour promotes great trust between him, his colleagues, and his patient to achieve a common team goal. This can be exemplified by an OT environment where effective communication and teamwork lead toward the best patient outcome by minimizing errors. Situational awareness in the OT could reduce the negative emotions of stress and anger and thus prevent bullying behaviours (Meires 2018).

There has been a recent interest in surgical literature in correlating EI with team leadership and communication (Barie 2005; Gewertz 2006). Research has also demonstrated that EI has a potential role in clinical outcomes, particularly by positively correlating with an improved doctor-patient relationship, patients' satisfaction, and trust (Weng et al. 2008; Weng et al. 2011).

## Surgical personality

There are many stereotypes associated with the characteristics comprising a "surgical personality". Surgeons are known to be "domineering, arrogant, aggressive, full of energy and mainly concerned with their prestige" (Bruhn and Oscar 1964). Because of these stereotyped characteristics that surgeons are thought to have, it is hypothesized that they possess poor EI (Stobbs and Ward 2014). It is also perceived by other medical disciplines and the general public that surgeons excel at the operating and technical side of their career but lack interpersonal skills (Stobbs and Ward 2014).

Surgeons, whether trainees or fully qualified, are subjected to a vast array of stressful situations (Al-Hamdan et al. 2017). Their expectations of a career in surgery often fall short due to multiple other factors like malpractice expenses, changes in reimbursement rates, and the rising demands for "clinical volumes" (Gewertz 2006).

There is a need for urgent action to improve the workplace environment for surgeons. Dr Lorna Bourke, Principal Lecturer in Psychology at Liverpool Hope University has expressed this as follows (Evans 2009):

> *Emotional Intelligence should be an explicit part of on-going contemporary surgical training and education. Surgeons are committed, resilient, driven individuals who are being lost to the profession while at their peak. For a surgeon, a "bad day at the office" would be a typical person's worst nightmare. Yet they often regulate their emotions by putting up a barrier without processing it properly, which can create real problems. We need a system where surgeons are given regular Emotional Intelligence testing and training, and strategies put in place to help them where they can talk about what they've been through, without them feeling as if they need to mask it.*

## Surgeons' responses to stress

The relationship between stress level and performance is complex. Stress could be detrimental or may be conducive to better performance (Wemm and Wulfert 2017). Surgeons' responses to stress are influenced by intrinsic characteristics such as their personalities and/or emotional intelligence. During surgical challenges, certain personality traits put surgeons at higher risk of experiencing stress whereas others confer upon them the ability to cope better with stress (Hassan et al. 2006; Schuetz et al. 2008).

Studies have shown that individuals with higher EI scores show greater self-efficacy in coping with stress and are likely to view a stressful task as a challenge rather than a threat as compared to individuals with low EI scores (Arora et al. 2011; Mikolajczak and Luminet 2008).

Acute stress is a particular problem in the OT where there are numerous stressors including distractions, interruptions, equipment failures, and technical complications (Arora et al. 2010; Sevdalis et al. 2008). Poor stress management skills compromise OT performances. A systematic review identified that stress can impair both psychomotor and teamwork skills in novice surgeons with clear repercussions not only on their training but on a patient's safety as well (Arora et al. 2009).

EI skills can also play an important role in perioperative care to facilitate interaction with interdisciplinary teams (e.g. effective exchange of information with anaesthetists) and in the resolution of conflicts. Identifying the individuals with poor stress management skills is important as these are often confined to the "hidden curriculum" and are not overtly taught (Arora et al. 2010). Arora et al. (2011) showed that training needs concerning managing stressors also differ and thus interventions need to be tailored to better equip trainees with the skills they need to cope.

## EI and medical students

EI is shown to be associated with the academic performance of medical students (Chew, Zain and Hassan 2013; Miri et al. 2013) and with the amount of stress affecting their lives (Birks, McKendree and Watt 2009). Students with low emotional intelligence have a risk of disturbed sleep habits and a chance of being indulged in health-damaging behaviour in response to stressors. Emotionally intelligent students however are more likely to manage stress using social support (Pau et al. 2004).

Various methods are used to assess the EI among medical students. These include behavioural interviews and multiple mini-interviews assessing a range of soft skills such as critical thinking, decision-making, and communication skills (Borges et al. 2009).

Doherty et al. (2013) analysed EI data using self-reported EQ-i and ability MSCEIT in graduate entry medical students who completed 8 sessions of personal and professional development (PPD) over a period of two years. They found that females scored higher compared to males and high self-reported EI was found to be associated with good performance on several bio-medical knowledge-based assessments. They concluded that the concept of EI assessment can be included in personal and professional development (PPD) courses within a medical curriculum.

Another area that has been explored by researchers is the role of problem-based learning (PBL) in the development of affective domains including an individual's personality and EI. PBL places students in situations where interpersonal skills are important and by using this method, students can begin to understand the characteristics of their own EI (Wood 2003).

The association of EI with the choice of a clinical specialty is another area of interest. Different medical specialties are sometimes thought to attract specific personality stereotypes. A primary care doctor is regarded as one who is more empathetic, patient-centred, socially conscious, and "connected," compared to a distant and cold but technically skilled surgeon (Borges et al. 2009). Borges et al. (2009) examined EI and specialty choice among year 1, year 3, and year 4 medical students. They found no significant difference in EI between students entering primary care versus non-primary care specialties and concluded that EI is not an effective predictor of even the broadest of specialty choice classification.

## EI in surgical education

The current literature surrounding EI in surgery is minimal and of a low impact. The areas covered include mainly: needs assessments to include opportunities for the improvement of surgical education (Erdman et al. 2017); measuring EI to assess residents' performance including their EI scores and comparison with the national average (Cofer et al. 2018); recognizing the risk of burnout (Lindeman et al. 2017); and EI based intervention (Erdman et al. 2017).

### EI and ACGME core competencies

The Accreditation Council for Graduate Medical Education (ACGME) established the following six core competencies for resident education:

- Patient care
- Medical knowledge
- Practice-based learning and improvement
- Interpersonal and communication skills
- Professionalism
- Systems-based practice (Webb, Young and Baumer 2010)

EI is related to a number of the core competencies that modern medical curricula seek to deliver (Arora et al. 2010). Arora et al. reportedly first published work linking EI to ACGME's core competencies. They performed a literature review to examine EI traits and relate them to the six competencies and found a strong correlation with patient care, professionalism, interpersonal skills and communications skills (2010).

### Empathy

Empathy is an emotional skill in healthcare. Studies have demonstrated that empathy deteriorates in surgical students and trainees over the course of their training and work (Hojat et al. 2004; Shapiro 2011). The possible mediating factors could be personality, sleep deprivation, stress, depression, and burnout. There is a rising need to incorporate the development of EI into medical training (Arora et al. 2010; Taylor, Farver and Stoller 2011; Webb, Young and Baumer 2010). Medical educators have a responsibility to provide training to the students to develop their ability to better withstand the emotional responses to stressors.

## EI, burnout and job satisfaction

Burnout in medicine is defined as a "state of mental and physical exhaustion caused by [a doctor's] professional life" (Lee, Medford and Halim 2015). Burnout may be related to personal characteristics, EI, or work experiences (Lindeman et al. 2017). Compared to the general population, physicians have higher rates of burnout; among physicians of all specialties, surgeons have the highest level of burnout, with an estimated incidence of around 40% (Shanafelt et al. 2009).

The Royal College of Surgeons (RCS) report has mentioned:

> *"Surgeons who are burnt out can begin to treat others as if they were impersonal objects, not caring about colleagues or work, becoming callous and blaming others."* (Dean 2020)

Surgical residency programmes are long and challenging with high attrition rates (Sullivan et al. 2013). The trainees experience high levels of physical and mental exhaustion and emotional detachment (McManus, Keeling and Paice 2004). Among general surgery residents, up to 69% experience at least one symptom of burnout (Elmore et al. 2016).

Burnout has been shown to negatively affect job performance. It is a major contributor to poor mental health (Cofer et al. 2018), clinician "depersonalization" and medical errors (Lee, Medford and Halim 2015) leading to a significant decline in productivity, decrements in clinical decision-making, and even potential thoughts of self-harm and suicidal ideation (Maslach, Schaufeli and Leiter 2001; Peterson et al. 2008). Emotional intelligence was found to have a negative relationship with neurosis and depression and a positive relationship with extroversion, acceptability, openness to new experiences, life satisfaction, and cognitive skill (Jacobs et al. 2008).

In a longitudinal cohort study involving residents of two general surgery programmes (Lindeman et al. 2017), authors observed severe burnout in 51% of residents with higher burnout scores observed in the female gender and during the beginning and end of the academic year. They observed that higher levels of EI appeared to be protective against burnout.

In another study, 73 general surgery residents participated in a survey. EI scores correlated positively with psychological wellbeing and inversely with depression and burnout parameters (Lin et al. 2016).

For surgical residents, work performance is formally assessed using faculty evaluations. In a study conducted at the University of Alabama, the authors (Hollis et al. 2017) evaluated the trait EI in general surgery residents and job satisfaction score and their relationship with measures of work performance, i.e., United States Medical License Exam (USMLE) scores, American Board of Surgery In-Training Examination (ABSITE) percentile, or faculty evaluations based on ACGME surgical milestone scores. They found a significant correlation between job satisfaction and EI. Individuals with low scores on EI, especially self-control, showed more burnout. There was however no association between residents' EI and surgical milestones or ABSITE scores.

The authors recommended the development of programmes to capture key factors associated with burnout and directed interventions to enhance EI among residents. They also recommended the recognition and management of emotions through trained faculty mentorship and coaching programmes. A systematic review regarding burnout interventions showed that a combination of person-directed and organization-directed interventions were more beneficial than one intervention alone (Awa, Plaumann and Walter 2010).

## EI and demographic characteristics

Most of the available literature describes higher scores of surgical residents compared to the general population in the domain of EI. Jensen et al. (2008) and Dugan et al. (2014) both reported surgical residents scores to be highest in stress management and lowest in interpersonal skills as measured by the Bar-On EQ-i. However, these low scores were still above the national average. Concerning the effect of age and experience on EI, there were inconsistencies in the literature. Jensen et al. (2008) found no significant difference across postgraduate training years among surgical residents across different age groups. Two studies found a positive correlation between EI and age or clinical experience among doctors and proposed that EI increases as one progresses through his career (Weng 2008; Weng et al. 2008). The life experiences of people increase with their age and as they mature, they become more sensitive to their feelings and the feelings of others (Lin, Kannappan and Lau 2013; Weng et al. 2008; Weng 2008).

With regards to gender, less variation was found between surgical residents compared to residents of other specialties, and specific traits of EI did not reveal a significant difference between male and female surgical residents in global EI scores (McKinley et al. 2014). Male surgical residents scored higher in stress management and emotion management while female surgical residents scored higher in impulse control and relationships (2014).

Although each surgical resident has his or her own particular development needs, the programme directors should select the areas which demonstrate low scores, especially attention to impulse control in male residents and stress management in females.

## EI in surgery: patient outcome and surgeon performance

Although EI of surgery residents is linked with burnout and job satisfaction, little is known in the literature regarding the relationship between EI and surgeons' performance in terms of patients' satisfaction and patients' outcomes. Compared to their medical counterparts, traditionally, surgeons are regarded as placing less emphasis on patient autonomy and provision of care (Weng et al. 2011). Poor application of EI in healthcare settings is believed to negatively impact quality of care, creativity, commitment, teamwork and safety and thus will harm an organization's reputation (Pfifferling 2008; Porath and Pearson 2010).

EI training may improve clinical diagnostic and prognostic abilities and the doctor-patient relationship (Pagnini, Manzoni and Castelnuovo 2009). A high level of EI can improve operating room performance due to situational awareness, communication, decision making, and leadership and teamwork skills.

Multiple factors are associated with patient satisfaction including a surgeon's behaviour (Wagner et al. 2002). Emotionally intelligent doctors are better able to perceive not only the needs of the patient but also can address any issues if they arise.

Dugan et al. (2014) have shown an increase in patient satisfaction scores after training of EI in doctors compared to previous satisfaction scores.

Although no specific articles have reviewed the effect of EI on patient safety, it can be hypothesized that surgeons with greater EI are safer, recognize their limitations due to self-awareness, and have greater communication and social skills.

Mustian et al. (2018) performed a retrospective cohort study to link the EI of general surgery residents with post-operative complications. They used TEIQue-SF to measure total EI and its various domains. For outcome measures, the record of post-operative complications was gathered from Quality Improvement in Training Initiative (QITI) reports. They found no significant correlation between EI and complication rates.

A large majority of complaints of healthcare professionals are linked with poor communication. An elevated level of EI can eliminate the communication barrier and, similarly, the ability to understand a patient's emotional state will help a surgeon better communicate and hence results in a satisfied patient (Doherty, O'Keefe and Traynor 2011; Kim and Lee 2016).

A key report from the Royal College of Surgeons states that

> "*Patient safety is at the centre of care provided by all clinicians and is enhanced by effective leadership and team working by all clinical staff*" (Dean 2020).

Ambady et al. (2002) showed a link between a surgeon's communication style in the outpatient clinic setting and number of lawsuits filed against them; they found that those who communicate poorly with a higher level of dominance had higher malpractice claims.

## EI in surgical education

From the limited available literature, evidence suggests that modern-day surgeons do have equal/better EI capabilities compared to other specialties (Stobbs and Ward 2014).

Arora et al. (2010) did a systematic review to explore the evidence on EI and modern doctor training. Their review included sixteen studies out of which four studies focused on undergraduates, one on medical school applicants and eleven on postgraduate trainees. Out of these eleven studies, six examined surgical, radiology, and other specialty residents, with the other five comprised of doctors and other members of the multi-disciplinary team. Nine different assessment tools were identified in those studies. Higher EI was reported to contribute to the doctor-patient relationship (three studies), communication skills (six studies), increased empathy (five studies), and stress management, leadership, & organizational commitment (three studies). They found that these attributes align with contemporary medical education, which aims to train physicians who possess not only the expert knowledge and skills but also the abilities to demonstrate competence in non-cognitive characteristics.

Another review was done by Provenzano et al. (2021) based on a Medline search which identified seven articles relating to "surgery" and "emotional intelligence." They found that integration of EI principles is a growing trend within surgical education. They found certain notable trends: 1) EI is partially inborn but proven to be learned; 2) surgical residents have a higher EI than the national average; and 3) educational shifts are needed to improve outcomes for the surgeon, patient, health network, and community at large.

In another meta-analysis Emilia et al. (2020) examined the current trends in the assessment of EI in the surgical education curriculum. They concluded that EI is a modifiable non-cognitive attribute enabling surgical residents to effectively recognize and manage emotion. It thus contributes to the ability to cope with stressors throughout their residency.

## EI among surgical residents

The surgical residency, compared to other medical specialties is a lengthy, comprehensive, and demanding endeavour that taxes the residents physically, mentally, socially, and emotionally (Lin et al. 2016). Despite this, "surgery culture" celebrates dedication to work at the cost of residents' personal needs and well-being, for instance by discouraging showing weakness or by keeping emotions and personal problems from interfering with the work (Mayer and Salovey 1997).

Lin et al. (2013) studied the applicants for the post of a general surgery residency programme at Stanford University, California. Applicants completed a TEIQue and a short survey in addition to the standard interview. They found that traditional faculty interviews do no adequately capture the EI trait of candidates and hence residency programmes should incorporate questions to reveal EI traits in applicants.

An EI training programme for ENT (otolaryngology) residents comprising a one-day seminar, simulation, and faculty mentoring showed higher EI scores and higher measures of patient satisfaction (Dugan et al. 2014).

In a study, Jensen et al. (2008) assessed the educational needs of general surgery residents concerning leadership, communication, and emotional intelligence measures using the Bar-On EQ-i. Residents scored strongly on EI self-assessment and EQ-i. The authors also identified that surgical residents scored higher than the norm for stress tolerance even though the "norm" for surgeons is likely to be higher than the general population. They concluded that EI-based interventions have the potential to impact two of the six ACGME core competencies (interpersonal communication and professionalism) and that enhancing leadership skills could indirectly impact third competency (system-based practice).

Stenton et al. (2011) compared EI between surgeons and psychiatrists using the Bar-On EQ-i tool and found no difference concerning the total EI scores of the two specialties, though surgeons scored higher in the subcategories of stress tolerance, self-regard, and optimism, while psychiatrists scored higher in empathy, impulse control, self-awareness, and social responsibility.

The authors thought that this was due to the intrinsic difference in the jobs of surgeons and psychiatrists. Being "thinkers and feelers," much of a psychiatrist's work is dealing with emotional problems for which emotional self-awareness and impulse control are important. Surgeons on the other hand, being "doers" had higher scores in self-regard and stress tolerance.

In a descriptive, cross sectional study, Chan et al. (2014) analysed EI among orthopaedic residents at a single institution using the MSCEIT. They found an overall low EI score and residents had difficulty in all four branches of MSCEIT, i.e., perceiving emotions, facilitating thought, understanding emotions, and emotional management. Their result indicated that higher mean total EI scores were found among junior residents, Caucasian residents and those younger than 30. They recommended dedicated EI education, training, and testing to optimize residents' competency in non-cognitive skills.

Ravikumar et al. (2017) conducted a cross-sectional study from two postgraduate training institutes in Delhi to measure EI using Schutte's self-report emotional intelligence test. It included residents from both medical (54%) and surgical (46%) specialties and the majority (72.5%) of doctors worked between 48 to 96 hours with 11.5% working more than 96 hours per week.

They found that 17.5% of participants reported "significant stress" in their lives and mostly reported it due to work or academia. The mean EI scores were not different for gender, marital status, and specialty or postgraduation years. However, the authors identified that the workload of the residents affected their emotional intelligence scores. The EI scores tended to decrease with an increase in the number of working hours per week. Similarly, lower EI scores were observed in residents who had night duty hours or emergency duty.

In another study, McKinley et al. (2015) aimed to describe the EI of residents across the specialties of surgery, pathology, and paediatrics from academic medical centres. They found a global EI level similar to that of the general population but residents scored higher in self-esteem, empathy, impulse control, self-motivation, and emotional management. They identified distinct areas of strengths and opportunities for EI development among the surgery, paediatrics, and pathology residents and concluded that residents from different specialties would benefit from targeted educational interventions emphasizing the different aspects of EI.

## EI teaching and development programmes

*"Old habits are hard to break."*

EI cannot be learned or modified in the way we typically learn about diseases or acquire surgical skills. When learning cognitive or technical skills, an error could be corrected by simply learning the facts or sharpening a psychometric skill such as doing wound dressing or suturing (Fernandez et al. 2012). A certain level of EI is inborn, but with persistence, practice, and feedback from colleagues and coaches, one can improve EI skills (Erdman et al. 2017).

The teaching and learning of EI involve personal skill acquisition and collaborative efforts by the surgeons, trainers, and administration (Humphrey et al. 2007; Zeidner, Roberts and Matthews 2002). Personal insight is important and efforts are directed towards modification of behaviours and minimization of poor personal interactions. Motivated learners can undertake self-study to gain these skills but this process is greatly facilitated by the presence of role models and mentors (Gewertz 2006).

The teaching of EI should be in an environment where students feel supported (Humphrey et al. 2007) and programmes should be well structured with explicit objectives and a clear purpose.

At the organizational level, experts have described a 4-phase model to enhance EI (Cherniss et al. 1998):

- First, both organizations and individuals must undergo preparation for change;
- Second, training should be undertaken to help people change the way they view the world and its emotional and social demands;
- Third, skills must be transferred effectively to the workplace environment; and
- Fourth, evaluations of how the skills have been applied and maintained should be carried out.

For self-improvement in EI, the first step is to recognize which areas in EI need improvement. It can be difficult to objectively see our words; to analyze our actions and attitudes that affect others. As surgeons are typically in charge and are the leaders of a team, they need to actively seek feedback with the genuine desire to hear and change (Goleman, Boyatzis and McKee 2001).

Sometimes feedback can feel far more painful and be perceived as personal rather than about behaviour. Creating a learning environment that is safe, non-judgmental, and conducive to self-insight is crucial.

The next step is to develop strategies to change negative habits. This strategy includes activation of the pre-frontal cortex to focus the brain on what is about to happen. It is helpful to think ahead about a situation (reflection before action) and think through a plan on various responses to that specific situation. Other strategies include keeping a journal about one's behaviour, volunteering as a coach, and meeting different individuals to know them better. The final step is constant practice and repetition to change the habit or response.

Administrative support is required to develop the conceptual framework and once it is in place, small- or large-group discussions and interactive activities can facilitate synthesis and application of teaching EI (Roth et al. 2019). Interactive scenarios and role-playing are some of the best teaching and learning strategies and could be supplemented by series of lectures, workshops, seminars, and community service experiences, amongst other things (Gewertz 2006; Glymph et al. 2015).

The residents must see EI as an integral part of their programme and not something to be developed entirely in a separate environment of workshops or seminars which are only complimentary. EI training should be holistic, inter-disciplinary and provide an opportunity for education and leadership development through practical and applied preparation (Johnson 2015).

A study from the otolaryngology programme showed that implementing faculty mentorship and simulations with a focus on recognition, understanding, and emotion management could not only increase the level of EI among residents but also lead to improved patient satisfaction (Dugan et al. 2014). Webb et al. (2010) attempted to measure the effect of formal EI coaching in residents with the use of training sessions. This intervention was unsuccessful due to lack of residents' protected time and hence authors emphasized the importance of designing and implementing programmes in a way that ensures the full participation of residents.

## Conclusion

There has been a realization of the importance of EI by the surgical community in both patient care and surgeon well-being. Surgeons face various factors daily which affect EI such as long working hours, lack of sleep, problems with interpersonal relationships and poor job satisfaction. EI should be more formally assessed and interventions should be designed and implemented to improve EI among surgeons to reduce stress and burnout, increase positive emotions, and improve leadership skills, interpersonal skills, and patient trust and outcomes.

## Bibliography

Al-Hamdan, Zaid, Islam Ali Oweidat, Ibrahim Al-Faouri and Estelle Codier. "Correlating emotional intelligence and job performance among Jordanian hospitals' registered nurses." *Nursing Forum* 52, no. 1 (January 2017):12-20. DOI: 10.1111/nuf.12160.

Ambady, Nalini, Debi Laplante, Thai Nguyen, Robert Rosenthal, Nigel Chaumeton and Wendy Levinson. "Surgeons' tone of voice: a clue to malpractice history." *Surgery* 132, no. 1 (July 2002): 5-9. DOI: 10.1067/msy.2002.124733.

Arora, Sonal, Hutan Ashrafian, Rachel Davis, Thanos Athanasiou, Ara Darzi and Nick Sevdalis. "Emotional intelligence in medicine: a systematic review through the context of the ACGME competencies." *Medical Education* 44, no. 8, (August 2010): 749-64. DOI: 10.1111/j.1365-2923.2010.03709.x.

Arora, Sonal, Louise Hull, Nick Sevdalis, Tanya Tierney, Debra Nestel, Maria Woloshynowyc, Ara Darzi and Roger Kneebone. "Factors compromising safety: Stressful events in the operating room." *American Journal of Surgery* 199, no. 1 (January 2010): 60-5. DOI: 10.1016/j.amjsurg.2009.07.036.

Arora, Sonal, Nick Sevdalis, Debra Nestel, Maria Woloshynowych, Ara Darzi and Roger Kneebone. "The impact of stress on surgical performance: A systematic review of the literature." *Surgery* 147, no. 3 (March 2009): 318-30. DOI: 10.1016/j.surg.2009.10.007.

Arora, Sonal, Stephanie Russ, K. V. Petrides, Pramudith Sirimanna, Rajesh Aggarwal, Ara Darz and Nick Sevdalis. "Emotional intelligence and stress in medical students performing surgical tasks." *Academic Medicine* 86, no. 10 (October 2011): 1311-7. DOI: 10.1097/ACM.0b013e31822bd7aa.

Awa, Wendy, Martina Plaumann and Ulla Walter. "Burnout prevention: a review of intervention programs." *Patient Education and Counselling* 78, no. 2 (February 2010): 184-90. DOI: 10.1016/j.pec.2009.04.008.

Bar-On, Reuven. *Bar-On Emotional Quotient Inventory (EQ-i): Technical manual.* Toronto: Multi-Health Systems Inc., 1997.

Bar-On, Reuven. "The Bar-On Emotional Quotient Inventory (EQ-i): rationale, description, and summary of psychometric properties". In *The Measurement of Emotional Intelligence: Common Ground and Controversy*, 115-45. New York: Nova Science Publishers, 2004.

Bar-On, Reuven. "The Bar-On model of emotional-social intelligence (ESI)." *Psicothema* 18 (January 2006): 13-25. URL: https://pubmed.ncbi.nlm.nih.gov/17295953/.

Barie, Philip. "Leading and managing in unmanageable times." *The Journal of Trauma* 59, no. 4 (October 2005): 803–14. DOI: 10.1097/01.ta.0000187809.46099.83.

Birks, Yvonne, Jean McKendree and Ian Watt. "Emotional intelligence and perceived stress in healthcare students: a multiinstitutional, multi-professional survey." *BMC Medical Education* 17, no. 9 (September 2009): 61. DOI: 10.1186/1472-6920-9-61.

Borges, Nicole, Terry Stratton, Peggy Wagner and Carol Elam. "Emotional intelligence and medical specialty choice: findings from three empirical studies." *Medical Education* 43, no. 6 (June 2009): 565-72. DOI: 10.1111/j.1365-2923.2009.03371.x.

Boyatzis, Richard, Daniel Goleman and Kenneth Rhee. "Clustering competence in emotional intelligence". In *The handbook of emotional intelligence: Theory development, and assessment, and application at home, school, and in the workplace*, 343-362. San Francisco: Jossey-Bass, 2004.

Boyatzis, Richard and Daniel Goleman. *Emotional competence inventory*. Bastion: Hay Group, 1999.

Brackett, Mark and John Mayer. "Convergent, discriminant, and incremental validity of competing measures of emotional intelligence." *Personality and Social Psychology Bulletin* 29, no. 9 (September 2003): 1147– 60. DOI: 10.1177/0146167203254596.

Brannick, Michael, Monika Wahi, Melissa Arce, Hazel-Anne Johnson, Stanley Nazian and Steven Goldin. "Comparison of trait and ability measures of emotional intelligence in medical students." *Medical*

*Education* 43, no. 11 (November 2009): 1062-8. DOI: 10.1111/j.1365-2923.2009.03430.x.

Bruhn, John, and Parsons Oscar. "Medical student attitudes toward four medical specialties." *Journal of Medical Education* 39, no. 39 (January 1964): 40–49. URL: https://pubmed.ncbi.nlm.nih.gov/14102917/.

Chan, Kevin, Brad Petrisor and Mohit Bhandari. "Emotional intelligence in orthopedic surgery residents." *Canadian Journal of Surgery* 57, no. 2 (April 2014): 89-93. DOI: 10.1503/cjs.022512.

Cherry, Gemma, Ian Fletcher, Helen O'Sullivan and Tim Dornan. "Emotional intelligence in medical education: a critical review." *Medical Education* 48, no. 5 (May 2014): 468-78. DOI: 10.1111/medu.12406.

Cherniss, Cary, Daniel Goleman, Robert Emmerling, Kimberly Cowan, and Mitchel Adler. "Bringing Emotional Intelligence to the Workplace: A Technical Report issued by the Consortium for Research on Emotional Intelligence in Organizations." Consortium for Research on Emotional Intelligence in Organizations. Accessed January 21, 2021. URL: http://www.eiconsortium.org/pdf/technical_report.pdf.

Chew, Boon, Azhar Zain and Faezah Hassan. "Emotional intelligence and academic performance in first and final year medical students: a cross-sectional study." *BMC Medical Education* 27, no. 13 (March 2013): 44. DOI: 10.1186/1472-6920-13-44.

Cofer, Kevin, Robert Hollis, Lauren Goss, Melanie Morris, John Porterfield and Daniel Chu. "Burnout is Associated with Emotional Intelligence but not Traditional Job Performance Measurements in Surgical Residents." *Journal of Surgical Education* 75, no. 5 (September-October 2018): 1171-1179. DOI: 10.1016/j.jsurg.2018.01.021.

Consortium for Research on Emotional Intelligence in Organizations. "Emotional Intelligence Measures." Accessed January 21, 2021. URL: www. eiconsortium.org/measures/measures.html.

Conte, Jeffrey M. "A review and critique of emotional intelligence measures." *Journal of Organizational Behavior* 26, no. 4 (June 2005): 433– 440. DOI: https://doi.org/10.1002/job.319.

Davey, Graham. *The Encyclopedic Dictionary of Psychology*. London: Oxford University Press, 2005: 306-307.

Dean, Erin. "Surgeons and mental health support." *Bulletin of Royal College of Surgeons of England* 102, no. 6 (September 2020): 240-243. DOI: doi.org/10.1308/rcsbull.2020.169.

Doherty, Eva, Dara O'Keeffe and Oscar Traynor. "Developing a human factors and patient factors safety programme at the Royal College of

Surgeons in Ireland." *Surgeon* 9, no. Suppl 1 (February 2011): S38-9. DOI: 10.1016/j.surge.2010.11.003.

Doherty, Eva, Patricia Cronin and Gozie Offiah. "Emotional intelligence assessment in a graduate entry medical school curriculum." *BMC Medical Education* 7, no. 13 (March 2013). DOI: 10.1186/1472-6920-13-38.

Dugan, James, Robert Weatherly, Douglas A. Girod, Carolyn Barber and Terry Tsue. "A longitudinal study of emotional intelligence training for otolaryngology residents and faculty." *JAMA Otolaryngology-Head & Neck Surgery* 140, no. 8 (August 2014): 720-6. DOI: 10.1001/jamaoto.2014.1169.

Elmore, Leisha , Donna Jeffee, Linda Jin, Michael Awad and Isaiah R. Turnbull. "National Survey of Burnout among US General Surgery Residents." *Journal of American College of Surgeons* 223, no. 3 (September 2016): 440-51. DOI: 10.1016/j.jamcollsurg.2016.05.014.

Endean, Eric. "Emotional intelligence and the vascular surgeon." *Journal of Vascular Surgery* 68, no. 2 (August 2018): 317-324. DOI: 10.1016/j.jvs.2018.03.420.

Erdman, Mary, Alisha Bonaroti, Gina Provenzano , Rachel Appelbaum and Marybeth Browne. "Street Smarts and a Scalpel: Emotional Intelligence in Surgical Education." *Journal of Surgical Education* 74, no. 2 (March-April 2017): 277-285. DOI: 10.1016/j.jsurg.2016.09.004.

Evans, Phillip. "Is there a link between problem-based learning and emotional intelligence?" *Kathmandu University Medical Journal* 7, no. 25 (January-March 2009): 4-7. DOI: 10.3126/kumj.v7i1.1756.

Fernandez, Claudia, Herbert Peterson, Shelly Holmstrőm and AnnaMarie Connolly. *Developing Emotional Intelligence for Healthcare Leaders, Emotional Intelligence - New Perspectives and Applications.* Accessed January 18, 2021. URL: https://www.intechopen.com/books/emotional-intelligence-new-perspectives-and-applications/developing-emotional-intelligence-for-healthcare-leaders.

Flin, Rhona, Paul O'Connor and Margaret Crichton. *Safety at the shard end: A guide to non-technical skills*. Surrey, England: Ashgate, 2008.

Gawande, Atul. "Health care needs a new kind of hero. Interview by Gardiner Morse." *Harvard Business Review* 88, no. 4 (April 2010): 60-61. URL: https://hbr.org/2010/04/health-care-needs-a-new-kind-of-hero.

Gewertz, Bruce. "Emotional intelligence: impact on leadership capabilities." *Archives of Surgery* 141, no. 8 (August 2006) : 812-4. DOI: 10.1001/archsurg.141.8.812.

Glymph, Derrick, Maria Olenick, Salvatore Barbera, Ellen Brown, Lauren Prestianni and Crystal Miller. "Healthcare Utilizing Deliberate Discussion Linking Events (HUDDLE): a systematic review." *AANA journal* 83, no. 3 (June 2015) :183–188. URL: https://pubmed.ncbi.nlm.nih.gov/26137759/.

Goleman, Daniel. *Emotional intelligence: Why it can matter more than IQ for character, health and lifelong achievement.* New York: Bantam Books, 1995.

Goleman, Daniel. *Working with emotional intelligence.* London: Bloomsbury publishing, 1998.

Goleman, Daniel. "What makes a leader?" *Harvard Business Review* 76, no. 6 (November- December 1998): 93-102. URL: https://hbr.org/2004/01/what-makes-a-leader.

Goleman, Daniel, Richard Boyatzis and Annie McKee. "Primal leadership. The hidden driver of great performance." Harvard Business review 79, no. 11 (December 2001): 42-51. URL: https://hbr.org/2001/12/primal-leadership-the-hidden-driver-of-great-performance.

Hassan, Iyad, Paul Weyers, Katja Maschuw, B. Dick, B. Gerdes, M. Rothmund and A. Zielke. "Negative stress-coping strategies among novices in surgery correlate with poor virtual laparoscopic performance." *The British Journal of Surgery* 93, no. 12 (December 2006): 1554 – 1559. DOI: 10.1002/bjs.5544.

Hojat, Mohammadreza, Salvatore Mangione, Thomas Nasca, Susan Rattner, James Erdmann, Joseph Gonnella and Mike Magee. "An empirical study of decline in empathy in medical school." *Medical Education* 38, no. 9 (September 2004): 934-41. DOI: 10.1111/j.1365-2929.2004.01911.x.

Hollis, Robert, Lauren Theiss, Allison Gullick , Joshua Richman , Melanie Morris , Jayleen Grams , John Porterfield and Daniel Chu. "Emotional intelligence in surgery is associated with resident job satisfaction." *The Journal of Surgical Research* 209, no. 1 (March 2017): 178-183. DOI: 10.1016/j.jss.2016.10.015.

Humphrey, Neil, Andrew Curran, Elisabeth Morris, Peter Farrell and Kevin Woods. "Emotional Intelligence and Education: A critical review." *Educational Psychology* 27, no. 2 (April 2007): 235-54. DOI: 10.1080/01443410601066735.

Jacobs, Madeline, Joseph Snow, Marilla Geraci, Meena Vythilingam, R. J. R. Blair, Dennis Charney, Daniel Pine and Karina Blair. "Association between level of emotional intelligence and severity of anxiety in generalized social phobia." *Journal of Anxiety Disorder* 22, no. 8 (December 2008): 1487–1495. DOI: 10.1016/j.janxdis.2008.03.003.

Jensen, Aaron, Andrew Wright, Avalon Lance, Kurt O'Brien, Charles Pratt, Dimitri Anastakis, Carlos Pellegrini and Karen Horvath. "The emotional intelligence of surgical residents: a descriptive study." *American Journal of Surgery* 195, no. 1 (January 2008): 5-10. DOI: 10.1016/j.amjsurg.2007.08.049.

Johnson, Debbi. "Emotional intelligence as a crucial component to medical education." *International Journal of Medical Education* 6, no. 6 (December 2015): 179-83. DOI: 10.5116/ijme.5654.3044.

Lee, Yeong, A Medford and A Halim. "Burnout in Physicians (Review)". *The Journal of Royal College of Physicians of Edinburg* 45, no. 2 (June 2015): 104-7. DOI: 10.4997/JRCPE.2015.203.

Kim, Bogyun and Jia Lee. "Relationships between personal traits, emotional intelligence, internal marketing, service management and customer orientation in Korean outpatient department nurses." *Asian nursing research* 10, no. 1 (March 2016): 18-24. DOI: 10.1016/j.anr.2015.10.005.

Lewis, Natalie, Charlotte Rees, Nicky Hudson and Alan Bleakley. "Emotional intelligence medical education: measuring the unmeasurable?" *Advances in Health Science Education: Theory & Practice* 10, no. 4 (November 2005): 339–55. DOI: 10.1007/s10459-005-4861-0.

Lin, Dana, Arthy Kannappan and James N Lau. "The assessment of emotional intelligence among candidates interviewing for general surgery residency." *Journal of Surgical Education* 70, no 4 (Jul-Aug 2013): 514-21. DOI: 10.1016/j.jsurg.2013.03.010.

Lin, Dana, Cara Liebert , Jennifer Tran, James N. Lau and Arghavan Salles. "Emotional intelligence as a predictor of resident well-being." *Journal of American College of Surgeons* 223, no. 2 (August 2016): 352-8. DOI: 10.1016/j.jamcollsurg.2016.04.044.

Lindeman, Brenessa, Emil Petrusa, Sophia McKinley, Daniel Hashimoto, Denise Gee , Douglas Smink, John Mullen and Roy Phitayakorn. "Association of burnout with emotional intelligence and personality in surgical residents: Can we predict who is at risk?" *Journal of Surgical Education* 74, no. 6 (November-December 2017): e22-e30. DOI: 10.1016/j.jsurg.2017.11.001.

Maslach, Christina, Wilmar Schaufeli, and Michael Leiter. "Job burnout." *Annual Review of Psychology* 52 (February 2001): 397-422. DOI: 10.1146/annurev.psych.52.1.397.

Mayer, J. and Peter Salovey. *What is emotional intelligence?* New York: Basic Books, 1997.

Mayer, John, David Caruso and Peter Salovey. "Emotional intelligence meets traditional standards for an intelligence." *Intelligence* 27, no. 4 (December 1999): 267–98. DOI: https://dx.doi.org/10.1016/S0160-2896(99)00016-1.

Mayer, John, Peter Salovey and David Caruso. *Mayer-Salovey-Caruso Emotional Intelligence Test (MSCEIT).* Toronto: Multi-Health Systems Publishers Inc., 2002.

Mayer, John, Peter Salovey and David Caruso. "Emotional intelligence: new ability or eclectic traits?" *The American Psychologist* 63, no. 6 (September 2008): 503-17. DOI: 10.1037/0003-066X.63.6.503.

McKinley, Sophia. The Emotional Intelligence of Resident Physicians. Doctoral dissertation, Cambridge. Harvard Medical School, 2014. URL: http://nrs.harvard.edu/urn-3:HUL.InstRepos:12407610.

McKinley, Sophia, Emil Petrusa, Carina Dijk, John Mullen, Douglas Smink, Shannon Scott-Vernaglia, Tara Kent, Stephen Black-Schaffer and Roy Phitayakorn. "A multi-institutional study of the emotional intelligence of resident physicians." *American Journal of Surgery* 209, no. 1 (January 2015): 26-33. DOI: 10.1016/j.amjsurg.2014.09.015.

McKinley, Sophia, Emil Petrusa, Carina Dijk, John Mullen, Douglas Smink, Shannon Scott-Vernaglia, Tara Kent, Stephen Black-Schaffer and Roy Phitayakorn. "Are there gender differences in the emotional intelligence of resident physicians?" *Journal of Surgical Education* 71, no. 6 (November-December 2014): 33-40. DOI: 10.1016/j.jsurg.2014.05.003.

McLeod, Scott and Lyn Sonnenberg. "The emotional intelligence of pediatric residents – a descriptive cross-sectional study." *Canadian Medical Education* Journal 24, no. 8 (February 2017): 44-51. URL: https://www.ncbi.nlm.nih.gov/pmc/articles/PMC5344067/.

McManus, I. C., A. Keeling and E. Paice. "Stress, burnout and doctors' attitudes to work are determined by personality and learning style: a twelve year longitudinal study of UK medical graduates." *BMC Medicine* 18, no. 2 (August 2004): 29. DOI: 10.1186/1741-7015-2-29.

Meires, Jan. "The Essentials: Using Emotional Intelligence to Curtail Bullying In the Workplace." *Urologic Nursing* 38, no. 3 (May/June 2018): 150-153. DOI:10.7257/1053-816X.2018.38.3.150.

Mikolajczak, Moïra and Olivier Luminet. "Trait emotional intelligence and the cognitive appraisal of stressful events: An exploratory study." *Personality & Individual Differences* 44, no. 7 (May 2008): 1445–1453. DOI: https://doi.org/10.1016/j.paid.2007.12.012.

Miri, Mohammad, Tayyebe Kermani, Hoda Khoshbakht and Mitra Moodi. "The relationship between emotional intelligence and academic stress in students of medical sciences." *Journal of Education & Health Promotion* 31, no. 2 (July 2013): 40. DOI: 10.4103/2277-9531.115836.

Mohzan, Maizatul, Norhaslinda Hassan and Norhafizah Abd Halil. "The influence of emotional intelligence on academic achievement." *Procedia-Social and Behavioral Sciences* 90 (October 2013): 303–312. DOI:10.1016/j.sbspro.2013.07.095.

Mustian, Margaux, Samantha Baker, Lauren Goss, Joshua Richman, Daniel Chu, Melanie Morri and Brenessa Lindeman. "Does the Influence of Emotional Intelligence in Surgical Residents Extend to Patient Outcomes?" Journal of the American College of Surgeons 227, no. 4S2 (October 2018): e203. DOI: 10.1016/j.jamcollsurg.2018.08.549.

Pagnini, Francesco, Gian Manzoni and Gianluca Castelnuovo. "Emotional intelligence training and evaluation in physicians." *JAMA* 301, no. 6 (February 2009): 600. DOI: 10.1001/jama.2009.81.

Pau A. K., R. Croucher, R. Sohanpal, V. Muirhead and K. Seymour. "Emotional intelligence and stress coping in dental undergraduates-a qualitative study." *British Dental Journal* 197, no. 4 (August 2004): 205-9. DOI: 10.1038/sj.bdj.4811573.

Pfifferling, John-Henry. "Physicians' "disruptive" behavior: consequences for medical quality and safety." *American Journal of Medical Quality* 23, no. 3 (May/June 2008): 165-7. DOI: 10.1177/1062860608315338.

Peterson, Ulla, Evangelia Demerouti, Gunnar Bergström, Mats Samuelsson, Marie Asberg and Ake Nygren. "Burnout and physical and mental health among Swedish healthcare workers." *Journal of Advanced Nursing* 62, no. 1 (April 2008): 84-95. DOI: 10.1111/j.1365-2648.2007.04580.x.

Petrides, Konstantinos. *Technical Manual for the Trait Emotional Intelligence Questionnaire (TEIQue)*, 1st edition, 5th printing. London: London Psychometric Laboratory, 2012.

Petrides, Konstantinos and Adrian Furnham: "Trait emotional intelligence: behavioral validation in Two studies of emotion recognition and reactivity to mood induction." *European Journal of Personality* 17, no. 1 (January-February 2003): 39–57. DOI: https://doi.org/10.1002/per.466.

Petrides, Konstantinos, Ria Pita and Flora Kokkinaki. "The location of trait emotional intelligence in personality factor space." *British Journal of Psychology* 98, no. 2 (May 2007): 273–89. DOI:

10.1348/000712606X120618.
Porath, Christine and Christine Pearson. "The Cost of Bad Behavior." *Organizational Dynamics* 39, no. 1 (January-March 2010) : 64–71. DOI:10.1016/j.orgdyn.2009.10.006.
Provenzano, G. R. Appelbaum, A. Bonaroti, M. Erdman and M. Browne. "Systematic review of emotional intelligence in Surgical education." 11th Annual Academic Surgical Congress. Poster presentation. Accessed January 21, 2021. URL: http://academicsurgicalcongress.org.
Ravikumar, Rajkrishna, O. P. Rajoura, Rahul Sharma and Manjeet Bhatia. "A study of emotional intelligence among postgraduate medical students in Delhi." *Cureus* 9, no. 1. (January 2017): e989. DOI: 10.7759/cureus.989.
Roth, Christine, Karen Eldin , Vijayalakshmi Padmanabhan and Ellen Friedman. "Twelve tips for the introduction of emotional intelligence in medical education." *Med Teach.* 41, no. 7 (July 2019): 746-749. DOI: 10.1080/0142159X.2018.1481499.
Salovey, Peter and John Mayer. "Emotional intelligence." *Imagination, Cognition and Personality* 9, no. 3 (March 1990): 185-211. DOI:10.2190/DUGG-P24E-52WK-6CDG.
Salovey, Peter and David Sluyter. *Emotional Development and Emotional Intelligence: Educational Implications*, 1st edition. New York: Basic Books, 1997.
Schutte, Nicola, John Malouff, Lena Hall, Donald Haggerty, Joan Cooper, Charles Golden and Liane Dornheim. "Development and validation of a measure of emotional intelligence." *Personality and Individual Differences* 25, no. 2 (August 1998): 167–177. DOI: https://doi.org/10.1016/S0191-8869(98)00001-4.
Schuetz, M., I. Gockel, J. Beard, P. Hakman, F. Dunschede, S. Moenk, W. Heinrichs and Th. Junginger. "Three different types of surgeon-specific stress reactions identified by laparoscopic simulation in a virtual scenario." *Surgical Endoscopy* 22, no. 5. (May 2008): 1263-7. DOI: 10.1007/s00464-007-9605-1.
Scutari, Emilia, Jeremy Egan and Michael Markiewicz. "Emotional Intelligence in Surgical Residencies: An Overview". University at Buffalo, School of Dental Medicine. Accessed December 26, 2020. URL: https://smbsweb.med.buffalo.edu/COS/abstractsubmission/abstracts/151226_Scutari_Emilia.pdf.
Sevdalis, Nick, Damien Forrest, Shabnam Undre, Ara Darzi and Charles Vincent. "Annoyances, disruptions, and interruptions in surgery: The

Disruptions in Surgery Index (DiSI)." *World Journal of Surgery* 32, no. 8 (August 2008): 1643-50. DOI: 10.1007/s00268-008-9624-7.

Shanafelt, Tait, Charles Balch, Gerald Bechamps, Thomas Russell, Lotte Dyrbye, Daniel Satele, Paul Collicott, Paul Novotny, Jeff Sloan and Julie Freischlag. "Burnout and career satisfaction among American surgeons." *Annals of Surgery* 250, no. 3 (September 2009): 463-71.DOI: 10.1097/SLA.0b013e3181ac4dfd.

Shapiro, Johanna. "Perspective: does medical education promote professional alexithymia? A call for attending to the emotions of patients and self in medical training." *Academic Medicine* 86, no. 3 (March 2011): 326-32. DOI: 10.1097/ACM.0b013e3182088833.

Shapiro, Shauna L., Daniel E. Shapiro and Gary E. Schwartz. "Stress management in medical education: A review of the literature." *Academic Medicine* 75, no. 7 (July 2000): 748–759. DOI: 10.1097/00001888-200007000-00023.

Sharp, Gary, Lorna Bourke and Matthew Rickard. "Review of emotional intelligence in health care: an introduction to emotional intelligence for surgeons." *ANZ Journal of Surgery* 90, no. 4 (April 2020): 433-440. DOI: 10.1111/ans.15671.

Stanton, Clive, Faisil Sethi, Oliver Dale, Michael Phelan, James Laban and Joseph Eliahoo. "Comparison of emotional intelligence between psychiatrists and surgeons." *Psychiatrist* 35 , no. 4 ( April 2011): 124 - 9. DOI: doi.org/10.1192/pb.bp.110.029959.

Stobbs, Nicola and Elizabeth Ward, "Do modern-day surgeons break the stereotype and show emotional intelligence in their leadership?" *Annals of Royal College of Surgeons England* 96, no. 8 (September 2014): e5-e8. DOI: https://doi.org/10.1308/147363514X14042954768592.

Sullivan, Michael, Heather Yeo, Sanziana Roman, Maria Ciarleglio, Xiangyu Cong, Richard Bell Jr and Julie Sosa. "Surgical residency and attrition: defining the individual and programmatic factors predictive of trainee losses." *Journal of American College of Surgeons* 216, no. 3. (March 2013): 461-71. DOI: 10.1016/j.jamcollsurg.2012.11.005.

Talarico, Joseph, Albert Varon, Shawn Banks, Jeffrey Berger, Evan Pivalizza, Glorimar Medina-Rivera, Jyotsna Rimal, et al. "Emotional intelligence and the relationship to resident performance: a multi-institutional study." *Journal of Clinical Anesthesia* 25, no. 3 (May 2013): 181–7. DOI: 10.1016/j.jclinane.2012.08.002.

Taylor, Christine, Carol Farver and James Stoller. "Perspective: Can emotional intelligence training serve as an alternative approach to teaching professionalism to residents?" *Academic Medicine* 86, no. 12 (December 2011): 1551–4. DOI: 10.1097/ACM.0b013e318235aa76.

Wagner, Peggy, Ginger Moseley, Michael Grant, Johnathan Gore and Christopher Owens. "Physicians' emotional intelligence and patient satisfaction." *Family Medicine* 34, no. 10 (November-December 2002): 750-4. URL: https://fammedarchives.blob.core.windows.net/imagesandpdfs/pdfs/FamilyMedicineVol34Issue10Wagner750.pdf.

Webb, Anita, Richard Young and Joane Baumer. "Emotional Intelligence and the ACGME Competencies." *Journal of Graduate Medical Education* 2, no. 4 (December 2010): 508-12. DOI: 10.4300/JGME-D-10-00080.1.

Wemm, Stephanie and Edelgard Wulfert. "Effects of Acute Stress on Decision Making." *Applied Psychophysioly & Biofeedback* 42, no. 1. (March 2017): 1-12. DOI: 10.1007/s10484-016-9347-8.

Weng, Hui-Ching. "Does the physician's emotional intelligence matter? Impacts of the physician's emotional intelligence on trust, patient–physician relationship, and satisfaction." *Health Care Management Review* 33, no. 4 (October-December 2008): 280-8. DOI: 10.1097/01.HCM.0000318765.52148.b3.

Weng, Hui-Ching, Hung-Chi Chen, Han-Jung Chen, Kang Lu and Shin-Yuan Hung. "Doctors' emotional intelligence and the patient-doctor relationship." *Medical Education* 42, no. 7 (July 2008) : 703-11.DOI: 10.1111/j.1365-2923.2008.03039.x.

Weng, Hui-Ching, James Steed, Shang-Won Yu, Yi-Ten Liu, Chia-Chang Hsu, Tsan-Jung Yu and Wency Chen. "The effect of surgeon empathy and emotional intelligence on patient satisfaction." Advances in Health Science Education: Theory & Practice 16, no. 5 (December 2011) :591-600. DOI: 10.1007/s10459-011-9278-3.

Weng, Hui-Ching, Yaw-Sen Chen, Chia-Shiang Lin, Yuan-Kun Tu, Hsi-Hsun Lin and Shang-Won Yu. "Specialty differences in the association between health care climate and patient trust." *Medical Education* 45, no. 9 (September 2011): 905-12. DOI: 10.1111/j.1365-2923.2011.03984.x.

Wood, Diana. "ABC of learning and teaching medicine: problem-based learning." *British Medical Journal* 326, No. 7384 (February 2003): 328–330. DOI: 10.1136/bmj.326.7384.328.

Zeidner, Moshe, Richard Roberts and Gerald Matthews. "Can Emotional Intelligence Be Schooled? A Critical Review." *Educational Psychologist* 37, no. 4 (June 2002): 215-31. DOI: https://doi.org/10.1207/S15326985EP3704_2.

# CHAPTER 25

# BIOETHICS - THE ELEPHANT IN THE (OPERATING) ROOM

AAMIR M JAFAREY

*"The practice of medicine is an art, not a trade; a calling, not a business; a calling in which your heart will be exercised equally with your head."*
*—William Osler*

Good residency programmes strive to produce well rounded, humane, and compassionate practitioners of the arts and sciences of healthcare. In this chapter, I will make a case for moving beyond the paradigm of limiting resident training to the acquisition of technical skills (in which they use only their heads), and moving towards a more holistic education where they learn also to use their hearts. I will emphasize an approach that goes beyond treating disease, and attempts to understand the illness and the patient as a whole. Describing the spectrum of the humanities, I will highlight the connection between them and the field of medicine, underlining the relevance of humanities in the instruction of medical trainees, not only to enhance their own sensibilities as medical practitioners but also to enrich their personal lives.

Describing how bioethics provides a natural bridge between the perceived fluidity of the humanities and the apparent concreteness of the medical sciences, I will use this chapter to emphasize the need for formalizing bioethics content within essential educational strategies for our trainees.

After presenting a broad situational analysis of bioethics in Pakistan, I will describe how we can use what we already have to ensure bioethics and humanities are seamlessly integrated into postgraduate educational curricula, without causing disruptions or being a burden on the trainees.

I will end by underlining the importance of addressing the needs of the elephant already in the room. I will make a case for providing formal institutional patronage for bioethics so that it develops as an academic discipline in its own right, embedded within medical institutions. The utility of bioethics is well beyond that of a regulatory instrument, or an exhibit to be showcased in medical symposia; it is a means of preparing the virtuous physician.

## Creating a messiah: much more than technical competency

*"Life is short*
*And the art long*
*The occasion instant*
*Experiment perilous*
*Decisions difficult"*
*—Hippocrates "Aphorisms"*

All residency training in general, but especially surgical residency training was classically modelled as an extended apprenticeship. You learnt from your master, acquiring not only clinical and diagnostic skills but also the mannerisms in which the skills were applied. This is not surprising, since surgical residency traces its roots to William Halstead who in 1889 initiated the first formal residency training programme in the USA, at Johns Hopkins Hospital. Halstead's all-male trainees, committed to bachelorhood as a prerequisite, had a 24/7 workweek with no breaks; graduation happened, if ever, only when the master felt a trainee was ready to practise independently.

Over the years, training programmes have, of course, undergone radical changes with humane hours, formal training structure, and objective assessment criteria being brought in (Sealy 1999). Modern residency programmes now aspire to much more than recreating the mentee in the image of her mentor.

From the apprenticeship, the trajectory of modern residency programmes has shifted towards providing a more holistic education. In addition to producing good professionals, programmes now desire to instil professionalism in their graduates. Professionalism encompasses, in addition to a technical skillset, an infusion of the highest moral and ethical values like trustworthiness, conscientiousness, empathy, compassion, respect, and so forth in the practitioner (Kirk 2007). Modern residency programmes boast graduates who display sound medical as well as ethical judgment.[1]

Residency programmes are well-positioned in equipping their residents with the latest diagnostic and treatment skills. Managing a patient, however, is not limited to only prescribing medicines, performing interventions, or excising tumours. Care for the patient oftentimes requires healing the patient as one treats the disease. Healing involves the spoken word, mannerisms, facial expressions, gestures, all constituting an array of attributes that an exposure to the humanities brings forth. It requires empathy and developing a connection between the healer and the one being healed. To heal, you need more than a scalpel and a pill.

Our therapeutic approaches are, perhaps out of necessity, reductionistic, deconstructing the patient into a set of neatly aligned, scientifically explainable, facts. Our focus is finding a diagnosis, identifying the diseases, the pathology. However, only when we reconstruct the patient and look beyond quantifiable data do we begin to see his illness, which constitutes not only the disease but the actual entirety of his affliction. It is only through this totality that we grasp the actual root cause of his fears and concerns, which obviously impact how his disease plays out. Only after acknowledging the patient's own microcosm of realities, his lived experiences, his sufferings, do we truly begin to appreciate what ails him. Remedying his ailment comes after understanding not only the disease but the illness too, which is oftentimes much broader than the diagnosis. As Sir William Osler famously said, "The good physician treats the disease; the great physician treats the patient who has the disease." A patient must be understood as much more than the numbers and images that can come to represent him in his hospital bed.

Illnesses induce vulnerabilities or enhance already existing ones, not only for the patients but also for their families. Recognizing these vulnerabilities is essential in dealing with patients and their illnesses, and it is these "softer" skills that guide the resident through these times. For the most

---

[1] As an example, the University of Arkansas for Medical Sciences. "Program Objectives, 2021". Accessed February 4, 2021. URL:
https://surgery.uams.edu/education/residencies-and-fellowships/general-surgery-residencies-and-fellowships/program-objectives/).
McGill University. "Program Goals and Objectives". Accessed February 4, 2021. URL:
https://www.mcgill.ca/generalsurgery/current-residents/program-goals-objectives

part, our residency training programmes leave the acquisition of these skills to the trainees themselves.

Take the case of a 77 year old adamantly refusing to undergo a curative resection of a colonic tumour. He will be regarded by the medical team as making an unreasonable, and entirely illogical decision. With the family members pushing the surgeons to go ahead and operate, energies are spent in balancing the principle of beneficence with the rights of the patient to make autonomous decisions for himself. The problem often lies beyond these prima facie principles, which disregard context.

Residency training programmes in Pakistan generally do not involve inculcating the art of meaningful and empathetic communication in our residents, our interactions with the patient generally being limited to whatever transpires during business rounds. Conversations with family members are also quite often either brief encounters in overcrowded hospital corridors, or attempts at rapidly fending off verbal volleys by irate relatives.

While there is no denying the fact that residents are overworked and have little time for anything more than patient management, good and effective communication, done humanely and empathetically, is very much a part of healthcare, and what makes medicine an art. A two-minute interlude, taking a chair and sitting by the bedside, and just gently talking with the patient is something never taught. Even a brief conversation asking him about his fears may go a long way in helping develop an understanding about his reasons for being so obstinate, and perhaps help him resolve his apprehensions. But our residents, generally lacking any meaningful training in communication skills, understandably feel more comfortable in incising their patients' belly rather than talking to him about his fears. Residency training prepared them well for the former, but not for the latter.

## The humanities: broadening the gaze

*"Wherever the art of medicine is loved, there is also a love of humanity."*
*—Hippocrates*

I have discussed above the perceived necessity of deconstructing the patient to arrive at a workable solution, and have advocated the need to reconstruct him in order to see the whole picture. Moving from identifying a patient as "bed 24-B, male, right inguinal hernia," to remembering his name and acknowledging an identity beyond the pathology that represents him is an important step in this reconstruction. Humanizing the patient requires going significantly beyond "married, with two children," and getting to know what these individuals actually mean in his life. Humanizing requires acknowledging the person's religious, spiritual, and social identities; since all of these aspects not only play out in how he lives his life but also affect how his affliction plays out in him. While the disease can be seen under a microscope, grasping the illness requires one to step back, and take in the entire canvas that represents the patients' life, vivid colours, blemishes, and all.

In order to grasp these details, the trainee has to be acquainted with the skills to not only understand the image on an MRI or PET scan, but also to begin appreciating the fine strokes of a Sadequain and a Van Gogh, the subtle nuances in verses by Ghalib and Shakespeare, the beat of Abida Parveen's rendition of a Sufi *kalam* and the rhythms of a Beethoven symphony.

Our education system in Pakistan is formulated in such a fashion that most students planning on opting for a career in the medical professions would have been, tenth grade onwards, entirely divorced from anything remotely related to the wide spectrum of the humanities. It is not surprising that even seasoned faculty involved in educating residents often find it difficult to describe what comes under the umbrella of the humanities, let alone discover and exploit a connection between the humanities and the medical training they impart.

Within the ambit of the humanities are included diverse areas of learning with culture as a common thread. This includes history, literature, languages, arts (including performing arts), philosophy, religious studies, anthropology, sociology and much more. The nature of the humanities is such that even a sprinkling of these influences, strategically designed and placed within the routine training of the residents, has the potential of igniting the required sparks. They do not have to add to the burden on the residents; they will actually help in unburdening some of the conflicts our residents quietly grapple with.

A well-tailored exposure to the humanities has a dual utility. Finer sensibilities, nurtured by an exposure to art, literature and philosophy, carry an intrinsic value for the trainees. These will help nurture an aesthetic discrimination within the individual, helping him develop an appreciation of artistic works, and appreciate life itself. As the French philosopher Vladimir Jankélévitch famously said, “It is possible to live without philosophy, without music, without joy, and without love, just not as well.”

In addition to this intrinsic value of a holistic education involving the humanities, there is also an instrumental value for trainees. An appreciation of these softer sensibilities inculcates tolerance, a trait so often needed in dealing with patients and their families. Exposure to art and literature helps in developing an appreciation of the unobvious, the view from the other side. It promotes social cohesion by nurturing an ability to appreciate a position other than the one immediately obvious to them. This aids decision-making, especially on contentious ethical issues. These sensibilities foster critical thinking, and thinking outside the box, a useful trait especially in the medical fields where innovation is a constant reality.

The connection between culture, the humanities, the arts, and the medical sciences is well established. Bioethics forms the perfect connection between the perceived abstractness of the humanities and the apparent concreteness of medical practice. The conceptualization of contemporary bioethics is difficult without considering its deep-rooted connections with the humanities. The values that bioethics draws upon, like empathy, respect for the person, justice, and many others, are deeply embedded in concepts borrowed from philosophy, theology, culture, sociology, history, and so on, all found within the umbrella of the humanities. The fact that there are centres and institutes devoted to exploring and developing this connection across the world is testament to the natural connection between biosciences, bioethics, culture, and the humanities. Just to mention a few, Durham University established its Centre for the Arts and Humanities in Health and Medicine in the 1990s, which has now become the Institute of Medical Humanities; Hong Kong University has the Centre of Humanities and Medicine; Johns Hopkins University has its Centre of Medical Humanities and Social Medicine, and closer to home, we have had the Centre of Biomedical Ethics and Culture (CBEC), at SIUT in Karachi since 2005.

## Bioethics finds a foothold

*"The beginning is the most important part of the work."*
*—Plato*

Over the past four decades, bioethics has increasingly been recognized for its utility as a regulatory instrument, both in human subject research governance, as well as in clinical care. With funding and the publication of research contingent on ethical review, ethical review committees[2] are now the norm across the world, regarded as an essential component of the research structure of any institution worth its name. Hospital ethics committees (HECs) mandated to provide consultations to deal with the ethical dilemmas arising during the provision of healthcare are also making a gradual appearance, if only to meet accreditation requirements of international agencies like Joint Commission International (JCI).[3]

Bioethics has also gained ground in medical and nursing curricula, and in the past three decades, programmes across the world have included it as a mandatory subject to be taught and examined (Nicolaides 2014; Okoye, Nwachukwu and Maduka-Okafor 2017). The World Medical Association has endorsed its formal inclusion in the medical curricula as an essential subject (World Medical Association 2017). There is however no consensus on how best to teach it, and several methodologies are still being tested for its seamless integration into medical curricula. There is certainly no "one size fits all" aspect of bioethics being taught or examined (Ghias et al. 2011; Greenberg 2016; Shamim et al. 2021; Willard 2015).

In Pakistan, bioethics made landfall in the mid 1980s at the Aga Khan University (AKU), with the subject being introduced informally into undergraduate medical education. Professor Jack Bryant introduced it into the coursework for medical students rotating through the community health sciences (Jafarey 2003; Moazam and Jafarey 2005). From this initial foothold, bioethics has gradually made formal space for itself in the various curricula being offered at this university. This came long before the national medical and nursing governing bodies made any

---

[2] Ethical review committees are also known as institutional review boards, research ethics committees, institutional ethics review committees, and several other similar terms.

[3] Three hospitals in Pakistan have JCI accreditation, and all have HECs structured along formal parameters. Other hospitals in Pakistan also have ethics committees, often providing an ethical review for research and ethics consultation in addition to playing policy advisory roles as well.

recommendations for its formal inclusion in these curricula. Now defunct, the Pakistan Medical and Dental Council (PMDC), in its recommendations, stopped short of making it mandatory to include bioethics in curricula.[4] Even though bioethics education has been embraced by medical curricula the world over as an integral part of education, apart from a few notable exceptions, graduates from a vast majority of Pakistani medical and dental institutions are still largely ignorant of the value of this burgeoning field. Hence it is even more important for residency programmes to step in and fill this void. Perhaps with the dissolution of the PMDC and the recent creation of the Pakistan Medical Commission (PMC), bioethics may get the space it requires in undergraduate curricula.

While bioethics still struggles to make academic space for itself in educational institutions in Pakistan, it has found some recognition at the governmental level. The National Bioethics Committee (NBC) was formally established in 2004 under the then Federal Ministry of Health.[5] The NBC has two subcommittees, the Healthcare Ethics Committee (HCEC) and the Research Ethics Committee (REC). The HCEC is mandated to take on ethical challenges at a national level regarding clinical ethics and has produced guidance, including ethical guidelines for pharmaceutical industry-physician interactions (National Bioethics Committee, Pakistan 2011). In 2017, after two years of deliberations, this committee has also developed a bioethics curriculum and a teaching handbook to help introduce bioethics formally in the medical and dental undergraduate curricula, thereby addressing a major gap that existed, and, in doing so, taking bioethics forward in the country (National Bioethics Committee, Pakistan 2018). Despite several attempts to engage with the PMDC regarding adoption of this curriculum, no progress was made, with the result that this document now resides only on various websites, with no evidence of it being utilized by medical teaching institutions.

The national REC has however demonstrated consistent contribution in the area of its mandate of providing timely ethical review. It has also

---

[4] The PMDC Code of Ethics under, "The Teaching of Medical Ethics" (section 8.2): "All the medical and dental colleges running MBBS and BDS, College of Physician and Surgeons of Pakistan, and Universities running the Postgraduate Medical Courses in Pakistan are advised to incorporate medical ethics into their curriculum". By an act of parliament in 2019, the PMDC stood dissolved and was replaced by the Pakistan Medical Commission.

[5] With the $18^{th}$ constitutional amendment, the health sector has been devolved to the provinces and the federal Ministry of Health dissolved. The NBC is now under the federal Ministry of National Health Services, Regulation, and Coordination.

demonstrated an ability to respond to newer challenges, such as the requirements for a rapid turnaround review process for COVID-19 related projects (National Bioethics Committee, Pakistan 2020).

In addition to finding a utility in Pakistan as a regulatory instrument, bioethics has also become a fad. It is unusual for a medical symposium or conference to be held without a customary "invited talk" on bioethics, before moving on to business matters. Its significance as a value in itself however still seems elusive.

## Bioethics and residency training

*Medicine, the most humane of sciences, the most empiric of arts, and the most scientific of humanities."*
*—Edmund Pellegrino*

Just as residents require structured technical training, they also require formal education in bioethics to be able to utilize it optimally in patient care and beyond. While acknowledging that surgeons were slower in embracing bioethics than their colleagues in other medical specialties, it has been rightly observed that due to increasing economic and technological challenges, basic grounding in bioethics for surgeons has become imperative (Tung and Organ 2000).

While at the turn of the twenty first century only a handful of US-based surgical residency programmes offered formal bioethics education for their trainees, in the next few years this drastically changed, and by 2009, practically all US surgical training programmes were offering bioethics education in one form or another (Helft, Eckles and Torbeck 2009).

The trajectory in Pakistan has been quite different. Despite its importance in healthcare, there is no structured methodology in place for imparting these skills to our trainees. There is also no evidence of any formal effort to include bioethics education in postgraduate residency training through official directives from the nation's postgraduate medical training regulatory authority, the College of Physicians and Surgeons of Pakistan (CPSP).

CPSP regulates all aspects of postgraduate medical training, and has put in place a variety of mandatory workshops, both for its trainees and training supervisors. Bioethics is not included for either category. In order to obtain a postgraduate qualification, each trainee must undertake original research on human subjects. This in itself would necessitate the requirement for at least an introduction to research ethics. However, CPSP does not consider it necessary to include this education formally into its repertoire of mandatory workshops. Instead, it relies on the trainee to provide an ethical clearance letter from their intuitional ethics committee to accompany their submission to the college.

This policy has a two-fold detrimental effect. With no central registration or accreditation of ethical review committees (ERCs) in the country, there is a huge variation in the quality of ethical review from institution to institution, which obviously is then reflected in the kind of research that is done by the trainees. Also, a unique opportunity to impart training in research ethics to CPSP registered trainees is lost—one which many postgraduate qualified fellows will never have in their careers in future.

In addition to an introduction to research ethics, trainees also need exposure to clinical ethics. While residents may be involved in sporadic research activities, linked to their dissertation or beyond, they are all involved in providing various aspects of healthcare throughout their careers. Their exposure to ethical dilemmas in their work is inevitable, yet they have practically no education in how to identify them when they arise, nor deal with them effectively when they do (DuBois et al. 2019). In fact, our doctors probably cause more harm with unethical medical practices than they do with unethical research.

Even for the few Pakistani medical graduates who are introduced to bioethics education during their medical schooling, the dilemmas they grapple with at that level are mostly theoretical, and not a lived reality for them. Residency, an entirely hands on experience, is different. The apprehensions in watching a patient worsen, the interactions with distraught family members as it happens, agonizing over having to shift patients out because there are no beds, obtaining consent for mutilating but life saving surgeries; these are all very real problems medical trainees face on a daily basis. Nothing in their residency training systematically prepares them to negotiate these situations; they handle them on little more than gut instinct. A new inductee may be struck by the inherent dishonesty of being instructed by his chief resident to procure wound dressing materials for a poor patient, using the name and account of another patient whose bills are being paid by an employer or insurer. But "Robin Hooding" is soon internalized, justified by expediency, with no possibility of any moral debate on it.

The first informal exposure to bioethics at AKU can be credited to Professor Farhat Moazam, at that time Chair of the Department of Surgery. In 1992, she introduced a series of short workshops for her residents, initially using the Four Principles approach, as advocated by Tom Beauchamp and Jim Childress in their book *Principles of Biomedical Ethics,* as a tool for residents to grapple with ethical dilemmas (Beauchamp and Childress 2001).[6] In 2002, for a brief period, residents in the Department of Surgery at AKU were fortunate to get some exposure to a formal bioethics curriculum designed especially for them. Professor Asad Raja, soon after his return to AKU after completing his Master's in Bioethics from the University of Toronto, launched this curriculum for surgery residents.[7] While the initiative did not last long, to the best of my knowledge it is the only example of a locally developed and formally written down bioethics curriculum meant for residents. This curriculum, using cases, aimed at teasing out ethical issues that residents face in real life while dispensing healthcare. The cases were contextual to the lived realities of the trainees and therefore were perceived as real issues rather that some esoteric, foreign notions that the already overworked residents were being asked to tax their minds with. Unfortunately, apart from personal archives, this document is not accessible for use.

The Postgraduate Medical Education Department of AKU offers some formal exposure to bioethics for residents. All residents at this university are currently required to attend two mandatory clinical ethics sessions in years two and four of their training.[8] Residents have recently also been asked to maintain an "ethics diary," recording ethical challenges from their

[6] I was a resident at that time and took part in at least two such workshops. The Four Principles approach was later abandoned as an approach in these workshops, since without taking into consideration sociocultural aspects it became difficult to accept any resolution. Professor Moazam later took a sabbatical in 2000 to pursue a Master's in Bioethics from the University of Virginia, the first one to do so from Pakistan, and later left the university to pursue a PhD in religious studies with a focus on bioethics, from the same university.

[7] Prof. Raja, then Associate Professor in the Department of Surgery at AKU Karachi, had obtained a fellowship to pursue a Master's in Bioethics from the Joint Centre of Bioethics, University of Toronto, Canada. He later became the PI of two successful grants, a planning grant and then a training grant from Fogarty International Centre of the US National Institutes of Health to initiate a Master's programme in Bioethics at AKU.

[8] In these two, three-hour sessions areas that are covered include principles of biomedical ethics, ethical decision making, privacy and confidentiality, medical errors, truth-telling, professionalism, and conflicts of interest.

second year onwards, so that they can be discussed in the final session in their second encounter.

Additionally, residents are also offered a certificate course in research ethics. However, since there is no mandatory requirement by the CPSP, it can safely be said that AKU sessions for residents are an exception rather than a rule in Pakistan.

## Bioethics: from the esoteric to the relevant

*Tum āsmāñ kī bulandī se jald lauT aanā*
*hameñ zamīñ ke masā.il pe baat karnī hai*
*—Shayar Jamali*

(Please do return soon from your flight in the skies
we have to tackle the challenges on the ground[9])

Bioethics has often been criticized as esoteric, alien and impractical, and best left to armchair physicians, the wannabe philosophers. Those in the trenches don't have time for it.

It is in fact those in the trenches who need to be armed with it the most, since they are the ones encountering ethical dilemmas on the go, and have no inkling as to how to deal with them other than by unconsidered gut instinct. For bioethics to work, it has to be indigenized; imported moral thought does not work. The successful use of technology, as in the optimal utilization of our imported PET scanners, cyber knives and robotics, largely depends upon following scientific parameters and adherence to globally uniform checklists and guidelines, whereas the application of bioethics requires local relevance within the context in which it is being applied.

Bioethics also shares its space with several other areas, some well developed like religion, law, and philosophy, while others are more diffuse, such as culture. Each of these, in their own way, play out differently within various contexts. This is why principles of ethics cannot just be taken from one place and applied elsewhere; the fit has to be just right.

Within the Pakistani context, for instance, it is often impossible to make ethical decisions without negotiating the "religious question," an aspect

---

[9] Author's translation.

that is entirely missing from mainstream contemporary bioethics discourse. In fact, *Principles of Biomedical Ethics*, first published in 1979 and now in its eighth edition, is considered the bible of contemporary bioethics (Beauchamp and Childress 2001). This text, however, does not factor in religion or culture within its analytical framework which is why it was abandoned as a favoured ethical tool during the initial informal sessions initiated for surgery residents, mentioned above (Roqué-Sánchez and Macpherson 2018). It is ironic, that in the few places where bioethics is taught in Pakistan, the four principles advocated in this book—respect for autonomy, beneficence, non-maleficence and justice—are utilized blindly, and without contextualizing, in attempting to resolve ethical dilemmas that are steeped in cultural nuances. This is perhaps one of the reasons for the prevailing perception of the foreignness of bioethics. In our context, an ethic that does not address religion and culture will fail to be relevant.

Take the example of termination of pregnancy. This question will play out very differently in different countries and cultures. Whereas in the US the debate will be around pro-life and pro-choice arguments, in Pakistan the discussion will immediately boil down to, "What does Islam say about it?" Following this will emerge the question of what position Pakistani law takes on it (Moazam 2012).

Since practically all obstetrics and gynaecology residency graduates will, at one time or another encounter this ethical question, it is imperative that their training includes not only the medical aspects of abortion, but also the ethical aspects, which will be informed by religious and legal debates. Misconceptions abound, and our practitioners do not realize the space available to them to deal with such situations, ethically, legally, and within dictates of religious rulings. Neither should the personal biases of the trainer mould the thought process of the residents, and only a structured curriculum taking this into account will guard against this. The prevailing ignorance around such matters is unconscionable and can only be addressed by strengthening training programmes to include such education as well.

Another deeply contentious area is that of brain death. This is a medical diagnosis, based on medical criteria, yet because of its nature, it impacts lives so profoundly that it almost always results in controversy. While our residents may be well trained to diagnose and declare brain death, they are entirely unequipped in dealing with what lies beyond this declaration. Dealing with the devastated family of a young motorcycle accident victim, full of life one day, on a ventilator the next, and meeting brain death criteria, requires not only a great deal of compassion, empathy, and patience, it also requires well-honed communication skills. In addition to all this, the resident must also have a thorough grounding in the religious and legal questions that arise immediately regarding the declaration of death based on neurological criteria (Moazam 2006).

Closely connected with brain death is the issue of deceased organ donation which is permissible under the organ transplantation law of Pakistan, even though its elaboration in law leaves much to be desired (Punjab laws, Government of Pakistan 2010). Additionally, there are several Islamic rulings from various jurisprudences in support of deceased organ donation for the sake of saving another person's life (Moazam 2011). Several Muslim majority countries have well established deceased organ donor programmes. For example, Iran and Saudi Arabia, both countries with strict enforcement of sharia law as per their own jurisprudential traditions have well established deceased organ donor programmes. However, this area always generates passionate opinions when the possibility of organ donation is brought up with the family. This is the critical time when the resident, who is going to be at the forefront, must have a clear understanding of the legal, religious and sociocultural aspects, and should be able to confidently address all concerns raised by the distraught family (Moazam, Jafarey and Shirazi 2014). If he succeeds in facilitating organ donation from the deceased, he will have helped multiple patients struggling at the fringes of existence regain meaningful extension of their lives. This negotiation requires sensitivity, care, and kindness, in addition to sound medical, legal and ethical knowledge.

## Bioethics: strategic dealienation

*"When you want wisdom and insight as badly as you want to breathe, it is then you shall have it."*
*—Socrates*

To be effective, ethics training requires a well-designed plan with clear and achievable objectives integrated into the wider curriculum. There can be no "textbook approach" for ethical dilemmas, and unlike medicine or otolaryngology, there can be no textbooks prescribed for ethics. Ethical dilemmas and how they are handled are very contextual and situation centred.

Pakistan is fortunate to already have a framework for a curriculum for undergraduate medical and dental students, and also one for surgical residents (the HCEC undergraduate curriculum and the AKU ethics curriculum for residents that I alluded to above). Both, unfortunately, are gathering cyber-dust. They can however be customized to suit the varying priorities of different fields, both in and outside of healthcare.

A perceived challenge in this formal inclusion of ethics and humanities in training curricula is the paucity of appropriately skilled instructors. But while you need an accredited instructor to train future surgeons, internists, anaesthesiologists and so on, incorporating a structured ethics curriculum in various residency programmes at this initial stage does not require a bioethicist armed with a degree. It requires willing faculty with an interest in bioethics to take it forward, given they are provided the space and freedom to do so.

An important step, therefore, is to train existing departmental faculty into bioethics leaders in addition to their assigned roles. This does not necessarily require a postgraduate qualification in bioethics, although that would help. Relevant short courses, workshops, and some self-directed learning by earmarked faculty can go a long way in creating enough understanding of the concepts that need to be transmitted down.

Perhaps the greatest challenge for finding a home for bioethics in the lives of residents is in making space for it. Bioethics, as an ad-on will only increase the burden that residents already carry on their shoulders. A stand-alone classroom session on bioethics will accomplish nothing more than some shut-eye for weary trainees.

A strategy that has worked well at the undergraduate level has been that of seamless integration of bioethics within purely "medical" topics being taught. Ward rounds present a natural integration point. First initiated by Sir Osler, ward rounds are the standard, time tested method of bedside clinical teaching. Being the greatest proponent for bedside teaching, he used to lead ward rounds in an octagonal-shaped rotunda, hence the title which has stuck over time (Sugg 1995).

Ward rounds have an undeniable similarity with the classical Socratic method, which alludes to philosophical discussions employing an open, two-way discourse where the teacher involves the students into a discussion in order to arrive at a conclusion, or just as happily, no conclusion at all. While ward rounds may not be discussing the meaning of life or the merits of pleasure over pain, they do engage the learners and the teacher in a two-way dialogue, fitting the ethos of the Socratic method. This moving class draws into discussion various aspects of patient management and can easily provide an opportunity to bring in various ethical aspects concerning the management of the particular patient as well.

For instance, a discussion on informed consent can be built into evening rounds. While going through the preoperative workup of a woman scheduled for a modified radical mastectomy for breast cancer the next morning, instead of just asking whether the consent was "done" and moving on, the team leader could initiate a discussion on the moral and legal aspects of consent. The discussion could bring in ethical and cultural values that come into play, and so on. Like so often happens, it may turn out that the husband had actually signed the consent form instead of the the patient herself, which could then open up the way to discuss social and cultural nuances that impact the process of obtaining consent in our country. Similarly, a structured bioethics curriculum could have topics of privacy and confidentiality built into ward rounds, which provide numerous opportunities to discuss these areas in clinical care, otherwise generally ignored and assumed to be known.

Case discussions generally work better than lectures in engaging residents. Actual cases seen in the wards which have raised ethical dilemmas can easily be introduced during the already scheduled core curriculum sessions and morning meetings and used to supplement the clinical discussions without seeming alien. For instance, an active case where a father is adamantly refusing corrective cardiac surgery on his new-born baby, saying that if God wants the baby to live, she will live even without the surgery. Such a case opens up an opportunity to not only discuss the limits of what physicians can do to cope with the inevitable frustrations while facing such challenges but also to discuss the wider questions of health systems, social services, and the responsibility of the institution and the state. Many of these are resolved questions in the developed nations, but we still need to look at them within the framework of our own economic and social realities.

Journal clubs can also be an excellent forum to bring in bioethics. During my second year of residency, I was introduced to bioethics through a case in the ward and a journal club discussion that followed.

The case was that of a baby suffering from an irreversible liver condition. The only way of saving her from certain death was the remote possibility of a liver transplant, a service not available in Pakistan at that time and prohibitively expensive abroad, even if an arrangement could be made.

Our bedside discussion on the medical options and the probability ended, but the team's moral discomfort remained. Our discussion continued in the corridor on whether we even ought to tell the parents that their baby had a remote possibility of surviving if she received a portion of a liver from one of her parents, or just tell them that nothing could be done. Opening up the practically impossible possibility of a liver transplant somewhere abroad would burden them with guilt at not being able to do anything, or perhaps lead them to sell all their possessions, borrow money and try, and fail.

As the discussion continued in the privacy of the seminar room, one view was that it was their right to know, while the other view was that it was unfair and unkind to burden them with this information. The journal club the following week was focused on exploring the ethical questions rather than just looking at the surgical aspects. This was an excellent example of integrating actual clinical care with an exploration of the ethical questions that surrounded it.

Grand rounds are generally an established feature in residency programmes. Residents can be asked to research the ethical aspects of patient care and bring them up as presentations during designated grand rounds. This way an already existing space and forum can be utilized to introduce structured bioethics components into the educational stream. Residents could also be encouraged and trained to include ethical challenges in each presentation they make, devoting perhaps two slides of their entire presentation to ethics. This will help them think "bioethically" even as they explore purely clinical topics.

Bringing in humanities exposure can be done in subtle, innovative ways without also causing major disruptions in schedules. Departments organize annual events, often with music or a *mehfil e ghazal*. During these gatherings, an informal reading of an excerpt from the powerful autobiographical account *When Breath Becomes Air* by Paul Kalanithi, himself a surgeon who succumbed to cancer, can be stimulating and help residents and faculty alike see the view from the other side. Similarly, a reading of an excerpt from Azra Raza's *The First Cell*, which is an excellent example of a perfect blending of the starkness of oncology with the fuzziness of human lives and richness of literature, can be an eye-opener for the residents.

A brief guest lecture exploring fairness and justice, using various modalities including pictures, paintings, and short literary excerpts can be tied in with actual global health issues, providing the residents with a rare opportunity to look at real-life problems through different lenses. Film viewing, in addition to providing entertainment and relaxation can also be used most effectively as a medium to make people think. For instance, feature films like *The Constant Gardner* or *Side Effect* can help explore the pharma industry and its influence on medical practice, or *Guzarish* and *The Sea Within* could be used to explore difficult end of life scenarios that are never discussed with residents.

Even changing gear briefly at the end of a core curriculum session on say, management of biliary sepsis, and displaying an image of the famous nineteenth century painting *The Doctor* by Luke Fildes, asking residents to think for a few minutes and comparing how healthcare has changed, may help them reflect on medicine not only as a profession but perhaps as a calling.

There are excellent resources easily available that compile a variety of such literary excerpts and other materials, which if used appropriately, systematically, and strategically, can make bioethics and humanities an interesting part of the residency experience.[10] However, one-off events, though good for breaking the monotony, are not very useful as far as providing structured education is concerned.

## Owning Bioethics

*Nahi Hai Na-Umeed "Iqbal" Apni Kasht-e-Wiran Se,*
*Zara Num Ho To, Ye Mitti Bohat Zarkhaiz Hai Saqi*
*—Allama Iqbal*

(Of these barren fields, Iqbal shall not despair;
A little rain, and this soil will yield rich harvests, oh Saqi![11])

Bioethics also needs to be recognized and developed as an academic discipline in its own right. That can only happen through locally developed academic programmes in bioethics, offering higher levels of learning to prepare the future leadership in this field. In 2008, AKU, through a grant brought in by its faculty, had an opportunity to start offering a Master's

---

[10] There are several excellent resources available such as *Medicine in Art (A Guide to Imagery)*, 1st Edition, by Giorgio Bordin and Laura Polo D'Ambrosio; *The Literary Companion to Medicine: An Anthology of Prose and Poetry* by Richard Gordon; and *The Moral of the Story: An Anthology of Ethics Through Literature* by Peter Singer and Renata Singer, just to mention three.

[11] Author's translation.

programme in Bioethics.[12] Unfortunately, the university did not step in with its own support when funding from the US National Institute of Health (NIH) ended, and the programme died. This reflected a lack of institutional support for bioethics as an academic discipline.

We cannot rely on external support to address our own issues for long. At this time, only one institution has funded, through its own resources, a formal bioethics-related academic entity. The Centre of Biomedical Ethics and Culture (CBEC), at the Sindh Institute of Urology and Transplantation (SIUT) in Karachi, established in 2005, offers structured university-level education through a postgraduate diploma as well as a Master's programme in Bioethics. Both courses are free of charge.[13]

Bioethics in Pakistan has largely been an orphan field, surviving for the most part on voluntary support from individuals. As I stressed above, institutional interests have largely been limited to tapping into its normative value as a utility for setting up ERCs and to a much lesser extent HECs, and to a sprinkling of ethics lectures to garnish annual symposia and conferences; bioethics is there more of a fashion statement rather than a value in itself.

In order to have a meaningful presence in educational programmes as well as in regulatory processes, the trans-disciplinary field of bioethics requires recognition in its own right.

AKU provides an excellent case study of an institution utilizing bioethics, without institutionalizing it. Bioethics has thrived at this institution, mainly driven by a handful of faculty having a personal interest in it. In the early 2000s, several faculty members, who we can rightly call trailblazers, invested their time and effort in bioethics. Putting their careers on hold, they went abroad to pursue formal bioethics education, proceeding on their own steam, or after winning external fellowships, and with no institutional support other than getting a leave of absence (Jafarey

[12] Prof. Asad Raja was the PI of the grant but when he left for AKU Nairobi, the lead was taken over by Prof. Aasim Ahmad.

[13] In January 2021, the Department of Bioethics at Shalimar Medical and Dental College (SMDC), Lahore, a private sector institution, has called for applications for its newly launched postgraduate diploma in Healthcare Ethics and Professionalism. The programme commenced in April 2021 with a maximum of 15 students.

2014).[14] Bioethics is now well integrated into various educational curricula, thanks mainly to the personal commitments of these faculty members and others who did not pursue formal bioethics education themselves. This was the first institution to initiate formal ERC and HEC as well as formally introduce bioethics within educational streams. The first workshops in research ethics and clinical ethics in Pakistan were held at AKU.

The Bioethics Group (BG) at AKU was initiated over two decades ago in 1997 as an informal interest group in bioethics (Jafarey 2002; Zaman 2018).[15] Over the years, the BG has provided not only the inspiration, but also the human and intellectual resources for the various academic ventures undertaken at the university, including conducting regular campus-wide ethics grand rounds and workshops. It continues to provide the nidus for seeding and germinating bioethics initiatives across the university. Despite this, the BG is yet to be provided with a formal institutional mandate for its work. From the mid-1980s up to the turn of the century, AKU was the only institution in the county with any recognition for bioethics. Yet to date, it has no formal administrative structure at this university, such as a department or centre of bioethics.

Systems cannot be sustainable if left to run on a volunteer basis. In order to grow and become self-sustaining, bioethics requires, like any other field worth developing, formal recognition and tangible institutional support. Bioethics curricula need to be designed by people who know the business, and integration should be done by field experts so that bioethics and the humanities become fundamental parts of various educational and training programmes. This requires staff, resources, and finances, which universities will have to commit if they want to take bioethics seriously.

---

[14] Professor Farhat Moazam, Founding Chair of the Department of Surgery, was the first person to opt for formal education in bioethics. She took a sabbatical from AKU in 2000 to pursue a Master's degree in Bioethics from the University of Virginia. Later she left the university to pursue a PhD in religious studies with a focus on bioethics, and came back to initiate the Centre of Biomedical Ethics and Culture (CBEC) at SIUT as its founding Chair.

[15] Professor Farhat Moazam initiated this informal group, its first meeting taking place in June 1997 with the support of the Dean of Health Sciences, Dr John Dirks. Members included faculty from different university departments, all with a shared interest in bioethics. Gradually, the group began to be looked upon as an informal institutional resource, even conducting the first ethics consultation at the hospital. At that time the group used to meet once every two weeks, over lunch which was budgeted through the Dean's office. I was invited to become a member in 2000.

A budgeted department, appropriately staffed, is the only way bioethics can have a meaningful presence in a variety of diverse departments and programmes, and in various institutional regulatory processes. People have to be employed and paid to do bioethics, like they are for seeing patients, performing procedures, or developing and modifying medical curricula. Faculty in such departments do not have to be bioethicists; they can be faculty with a formal interest in bioethics, having intersectional appointments with other primary departments. The departmental commitment formalizes their contributions, which need to be acknowledged appropriately.

The discipline of medical education, now an essential department in every medical teaching institution, in its initial years, was also seen similarly floating unmoored. It has gained recognition as an independent and essential department only in recent years. Bioethics needs to follow this trajectory.

The utility of bioethics ought not to be merely limited to providing an ethical review of research and consultations for difficult decisions, but in fact ought to be part of the training of virtuous physicians and researchers, who can then internalize the values instilled in them through systematic pedagogical efforts. Whether it is our undergraduate students or those enrolled in our postgraduate training programmes, their conduct and their skills reflect the education they receive.

Bioethics has arrived in Pakistan; the elephant is very much in the room. However, much like Kavaan, the world's loneliest elephant, bioethics remain chained to a post, as an exhibit (Khan 2020). Reducing bioethics to a mere utility for regulatory needs, or as a window dressing for appearance's sake, will be a disappointing reflection of extreme academic myopia. Given the intellectual space and institutional support, bioethics has the potential to do much more, not only as a service for the institution, but also to impact lives, the reverberations of which will travel far and wide.

## Bibliography

Beauchamp, Tom L, and James F. Childress. *Principles of Biomedical Ethics*. USA: Oxford University Press, October 2002. DOI: http://dx.doi.org/10.1136/jme.28.5.332-a.

DuBois, James M., Emily E. Anderson, John T. Chibnall, Jessica Mozersky, and Heidi A. Walsh. "Serious ethical violations in medicine: A statistical and ethical analysis of 280 cases in the United States from 2008–2016." *The American Journal of Bioethics* 19, no. 1 (January 2019): 16-34. DOI: https://doi.org/10.1080/15265161.2018.1544305.

Ghias, Kulsoom, Syeda Kauser Ali, Kausar S. Khan, Robyna Khan, Murad M. Khan, Arshi Farooqui, and Parvez Nayani. "How we developed a bioethics theme in an undergraduate medical curriculum." *Medical Teacher* 33, no. 12 (January 2012): 974-977. DOI: https://doi.org/10.3109/0142159X.2011.588890.

Greenberg, Rebecca A., Celine Kim, Helen Stolte, Jonathan Hellmann, Randi Zlotnik Shaul, Rahim Valani, and Dennis Scolnik. "Developing a bioethics curriculum for medical students from divergent geo-political regions." *BMC Medical Education* 16, no. 1 (July 2016): 1-6. DOI: https://doi.org/10.1186/s12909-016-0711-4.

Helft, Paul R., Rachael E. Eckles, and Laura Torbeck. "Ethics education in surgical residency programs: a review of the literature." *Journal of Surgical Education* 66, no. 1 (February 2009): 35-42. DOI: https://doi.org/10.1016/j.jsurg.2008.10.001.

Jafarey, Aamir M. "The bioethics group of the Aga Khan University, Karachi." *Issues in Medical Ethics* 10, no. 1 (January to March 2002): 163-164. DOI: https://ecommons.aku.edu/pakistan_fhs_mc_surg_surg/746.

Jafarey, Aamir M. "Bioethics and medical education." *The Journal of the Pakistan Medical Association* 53, no. 6 (June 2003): 209-210. DOI: https://www.jpma.org.pk/article-details/160.

Jafarey, Aamir Mustafa, Saima Pervaiz Iqbal, and Mariam Hassan. "Ethical review in Pakistan: the credibility gap." *The Journal of the Pakistan Medical Association* 62, no. 12 (December 2012): 1354-1357. DOI: https://jpma.org.pk/article-details/3877?article_id=3877.

Jafarey, Aamir M. "A degree in bioethics: an" introspective" analysis from Pakistan." *Indian Journal of Medical Ethics* 11, no. 2 (November 2016): 93-99. DOI: https://doi.org/10.20529/ijme.2014.024.

Khan, M. Ilyas. "Kaavan, the world's loneliest elephant, is finally going free." BBC News. Accessed February 13, 2021. URL: https://www.bbc.com/news/world-asia-55060433.

Kirk, Lynne M. "Professionalism in medicine: definitions and considerations for teaching." In *Baylor University Medical Centre Proceedings* 20, no. 1 (November 2017): 13-16. DOI: https://doi.org/10.1080/08998280.2007.11928225.

Moazam, Farhat, and Aamir M. Jafarey. "Pakistan and biomedical ethics: Report from a Muslim country." *Cambridge Quarterly of Healthcare Ethics* 14, no. 3 (June 2005): 249. DOI: https://doi.org/10.1017/S0963180105050346.

Moazam, Farhat. "Ethical and Social Dimensions of Brain Death." *Pakistan Journal of Neurological Science* 1, no. 1 (April – June, 2006): 39–41.

Moazam, Farhat. "Sharia law and organ transplantation: through the lens of Muslim jurists." *Asian Bioethics Review* 3, no. 4 (December 2011): 316-332. URL: https://muse.jhu.edu/article/461974.

Moazam, Farhat, Aamir M. Jafarey and Bushra Shirazi. "To donate a kidney: public perspectives from Pakistan." *Bioethics* 28, no. 2 (Dec 2014) 76-83. DOI: 10.1111/bioe.12010.

Moazam, Farhat. "'Doing Bioethics' in Pakistan." Bioethics Forum Essay of *The Hastings Center*, New York. Accessed February 13, 2021. URL: https://www.thehastingscenter.org/doing-bioethics-in-pakistan/.

National Bioethics Committee, Pakistan. "Guidelines for healthcare professionals' interaction with pharmaceutical trade and industry." Accessed February 13, 2021. URL: http://nbcpakistan.org.pk/assets/ppi_guidelines_may_2011-1--final-copy-on-pmrc-wbesite.pdf.

National Bioethics Committee, Pakistan. "Research ethics - Guidance document to help researcher fill the ERC application form." Accessed February 13, 2021. URL: http://nbcpakistan.org.pk/assets/nbc-erc-guidance-sheet-(2015).pdf.

National Bioethics Committee, Pakistan "Guidelines and teachers handbook for introducing bioethics to medical and dental students." Accessed February 13, 2021. URL: http://nbcpakistan.org.pk/assets/may-16-bioethics-facilitator-book---may-16%2c-2017.pdf.

National Bioethics Committee, Pakistan. "COVID-19 Emergency Response": Ethical Review of Health Research in Pakistan." National Bioethics Committee-Research Ethics Committee, TORs version 1.2. Accessed February 13, 2021. URL: http://nbcpakistan.org.pk/assets/rec-1.2-tors.pdf.

Nicolaides, A. "The critical role of ethics training in medical education." *African Journal of Hospitality, Tourism and Leisure* 3, no. 1 (May 2016): 1-12. DOI: http://hdl.handle.net/10500/20272.

Okoye, Onochie, Daniel Nwachukwu, and Ferdinand C. Maduka-Okafor. "Must we remain blind to undergraduate medical ethics education in Africa? A cross-sectional study of Nigerian medical students." *BMC Medical Ethics* 18, no. 1 (December 2017): 1-8. DOI: https://doi.org/10.1186/s12910-017-0229-2.

Punjab laws, Government of Pakistan. "The Transplantation of Human Organs and Tissues Act 2010." (Act V I of 2010). Accessed February 13, 2021. URL: http://punjablaws.gov.pk/laws/2428a.html.

Roqué-Sánchez, María Victoria, and Ignacio Macpherson. "Análisis de la ética de principios, 40 años después." *Revista Bioética* 26, no. 2 (June 2018): 189-197. DOI: https://doi.org/10.1590/1983-80422018262239.

Sealy, Will C. "Halsted is dead: time for change in graduate surgical education." *Current Surgery* 56, no. 1-2 (January-February 1999): 34-39. DOI: https://doi.org/10.1016/S0149-7944(99)00005-7.

Shamim, Muhammad Shahid, Adrienne Torda, Lubna A. Baig, Nadeem Zubairi, and Chinthaka Balasooriya. "Systematic development and refinement of a contextually relevant strategy for undergraduate medical ethics education: a qualitative study." *BMC Medical Education* 21, no. 1 (January 2021): 1-12. DOI: https://doi.org/10.1186/s12909-020-02425-6.

Sugg, Diana. "Show-and-tell for doctors making the rounds: In a tradition that began at Hopkins Hospital, doctors learn from patients and each other." *The Baltimore Sun*. Accessed February 13, 2021. URL: https://www.baltimoresun.com/news/bs-xpm-1995-09-23-1995266001-story.html.

Tung, Thomas, and Claude H. Organ. "Ethics in surgery: historical perspective." *Archives of Surgery* 135, no. 1 (January 2000): 10-13. DOI: https://doi.org/10.1001/archsurg.135.1.10.

Willard, Julian. "Structuring bioethics education: The question, the disciplines, and the integrative challenge." *Ethics and Social Welfare* 9, no. 3 (April 2015): 280-296. DOI: https://doi.org/10.1080/17496535.2015.1005555.

World Medical Association. "WMA resolution on the inclusion of medical ethics and human rights in the curriculum of medical schools world-wide." Accessed February 13, 2021. URL: https://www.wma.net/policies-post/wma-resolution-on-the-inclusion-of-medical-ethics-and-human-rights-in-the-curriculum-of-medical-schools-world-wide/.

Zaman, Riffat M. "AKU Bioethics Group: Fountainhead for Bioethics in Pakistan." *Bioethics Links* 14, no. 1 (June 2018): 1-2. DOI: http://www.siut.org/bioethics/AKU%20Bioethics%20Group%20Fountainhead%20for%20Bioethics%20in%20Pakistan.pdf.

# CHAPTER 26

# JOURNEY BEYOND IMPACT: MEASURING THE CONTRIBUTIONS OF SURGICAL GRADUATES OF THE AGA KHAN UNIVERSITY HOSPITAL

ARIF ALI, MASOOD UMER
AND GULZAR S. LAKHANI

## Introduction

Large tertiary teaching hospitals have traditionally been the setting for the major portion of the education of medical students and resident physicians. The experience of college education helps students to become potential influencers in a number of areas across the societal spectrum. Such growth can manifest itself in various arenas, be they intellectual, academic, social, emotional, or behavioural. One of higher medical education's fundamental and earliest objective has always been that a candidate should be a functioning and aware citizen (Brubacher and Rudy 1982). Colleges and universities have the societal responsibility to help their students and "improve their performance in citizenship," along with furthering their "cognitive learning" and "affective development," in order to form a "comprehensive personality" (Bowen 1977; Boyer 1987).

Since the founding of colleges and tertiary teaching hospitals, there has been a strong link between higher education and serving the greater society. Over the history of higher education, public service and social responsibility have been defined in many ways. The tradition of social responsibility, regardless of its operationalization, remains a central principle in the history of higher medical education (Kohlberg 1969; Kohlberg, 2016).

A genuine altruistic interpretation of contributing to society has become increasingly visible in recent decades. The strengthening of the linkages between education and service, and involvement of students at all levels has led to college-educated citizens becoming more involved with community service (Kohlberg, 2016).

It is safe to say that in a hospital with students on the wards, the patients are more carefully looked after and their diseases are more fully studied, with the aim of providing the most comprehensive and best possible care (Haesler 1993; Osler 1903).

In the USA in the 1990s, the Higher Education Research Institute at UCLA completed a national study of the effects of President Bill Clinton's Learn and Serve America Higher Education Program. The activity was organized by the Corporation for National Service, a body designed to facilitate the development of volunteer service programmes for college students. This longitudinal multi-institutional study allowed for evaluation of effects of service participation after examining students' precollege propensity to engage in service. Findings suggested that service participation is positively associated with a number of short-term cognitive and affective outcomes during undergraduate years (Astin and Sax 1998).

Generally though, there are few surveys reported in the literature regarding alumni contribution to society. The University of Washington conducted a survey of alumni containing seven items relating to contribution to society, service-related activities and citizenship (Korn 1999). While most studies of the long-term impact of college usually focus on whether college attendance or degree attainment make a difference (Pascarella and Terenzini 1991), few studies have been carried out to assess the long-term impact of particular college experiences such as community service and contribution. In Pakistan there has been scarce data collected regarding the roles of university alumni and their contributions at both national and international levels.

Alumni surveys need to be beneficial and meaningful. Surveys should be focused on engendering results that can impact policy making and improvement in education styles at the parent institution. The literature indicates that three such types of surveys exist (Cabrera, Weerts and Zulick 2005; Gore 2018; Pace 1979).

The first one is the alumni outcomes approach. This was the dominant approach of surveys in the USA from 1930 to 1970. With this approach, a variety of questions are asked regarding the level alumni have reached so far and the skills and status they have acquired after graduation. They are also asked about their job satisfaction levels (Pace 1979). Engagement in civic and political activities and tolerance for diversity are other secondary domains in this survey method. The benchmark in the outcomes approach to alumni assessment is represented by a yearly survey of the National Association of Colleges and Employers (NACE). NACE membership includes over eighteen hundred colleges and universities and more than nineteen hundred employer organizations. The 2002 NACE report reflected recent graduate data regarding earnings by majors, job, salary, and benefits expectations, as well as difficulties encountered in the job search according to different majors (Nagle and Bohovich 2002). The NACE survey assesses the impact of college by asking respondents whether college education was a worthwhile investment and the extent to which the college-based career service was helpful in finding a job. Bok and Bowen's book, *The Shape of the River* (1998), is also a good example of this. The book assesses and studies the impact of the primary institution on the alumni joining social activities like clubs, charities or professional organizations.

Other examples of alumni surveys include the American College Testing's Outcomes Survey and the State University of New York's Alumni Outcomes Survey. Both surveys measure faculty and campus experience. They help institutions improve their college experience (Kinnick 1985; Mentkowski 1998; Tremblay, Lalancette and Roseveare 2012).

Next is the competencies approach survey. This came after 1980 and in it alumni are assessed on their competencies of self-learning, interpersonal skills, vocational skills and critical thinking. Engagement of the alumnus with the primary institute, and his links to teaching and learning are also assessed. Students attain a lot of competencies after their graduation, which may or may not be linked to their primary courses in the index institution. The competency survey assesses whether competencies were obtained in the primary institute or thereafter (Pascarella and Terenzini 1991). Basically the few questions asked during this survey method are: what should be the focus of the institution on teaching a particular set of competencies? How much engagement should the institution have with the student to impact their future life? And how do the alumni apply those skills in later life to capitalize on the basic competencies learned? In the west, big public universities are frequently asked by lawmakers about their productivity. These surveys can help them provide data on the usefulness of their programmes. Their engagement with their alumni and the competencies produced by their organizations can bring about the change and impact their alumni are trying to establish in the community at large.

The third concept is that of the alumni giving back to the host institution. This may be in terms of money, time or knowledge. Primary institutions are becoming increasingly aware of the need to compile their alumni database and remain engaged with them. This helps them further their educational programmes. Another objective of these alumni surveys is to identify alumni who are the most financially or politically able to help an institution achieves its goals.

To conclude, there are many internal and external demands for assessment, accountability, and market-driven research in higher education (Dellow and Romano 2002). This is especially true for public and community colleges in the west where legislators and taxpayers have a strong voice in ensuring that postsecondary education yields economic and social benefits for the states and communities in which it is based. Outside the university, legislators, trustees, and the general public have increased their demands on higher education institutions to be more accountable, efficient, and aligned with public needs. Institutional leaders must consider how alumni research can be used to inform these key audiences about important issues of institutional quality and the overall impact that colleges and universities have on society.

We propose that data collection strategies should follow these stages of student development from early college decisions to student engagement, to alumni outcomes, to alumni giving. This approach would allow universities to form strong conclusions about the links between college experiences and student and alumni outcomes at critical stages of development. In addition, this approach would simplify data collection, reduce the length of the survey, and minimize measurement errors.

The Aga Khan University was founded in 1985, starting its Bachelor of Medicine, Bachelor of Surgery (MBBS) programme in 1988. By 2020, its postgraduate residency programmes had completed 25 years of PGME. Over the years it has graduated hundreds of students both in MBBS and residency programmes, contributing to society at both national and international levels.

The 2016 Alumni Survey represented the first ever comprehensive survey of AKU alumni from programmes in Afghanistan, Kenya, Pakistan, Tanzania, Uganda and the United Kingdom (UK) (Aga Khan University

Alumni Affairs 2017). It was also the first survey undertaken since 2007, which was limited to alumni from Pakistan (PK).

The survey not only probed attitudes, experiences and feelings towards the alma mater, but also served as a vehicle to gather demographic and career-related information, including further education and training, as well as various degrees of accomplishments and leadership roles. The overall response rate for the survey was the total number of respondents' actual degrees and diplomas conferred, including dual credentials (n = 3,571) divided by the number of total alumni (n = 13,066), which yielded a response rate of 27%.

Out of 1,372 total responses from medical college PK alumni, 710 or 52% were received from alumni living overseas, and when breaking down the number of overseas alumni with respect to individual programmes, for both graduate and postgraduate alumni who completed their programs in 2013 or earlier, 34% to 44% of the responses were from alumni based overseas. Also unsurprisingly, 84% of overseas MBBS responses from 2013 and earlier were from alumni based in the US.

*Net Promoter Score:* An increasing number of professionals in the area of marketing prefer the Net Promoter Score (NPS) as a more precise gauge of customer loyalty than simple satisfaction levels. The idea was first introduced by Frederick F. Reichheld in the *Harvard Business Review* in 2003, and later in his book, *The Ultimate Question* in 2006. Since then it has become the gold standard for many in terms of gauging the quality of customer relations. NPS can range from -100 to +100 and is arrived at using an 11-point scale, which is divided into three categories, namely: a. Promoters (9-10), b. Passives (7-8), and c. Detractors (0-6).

In 2011, San Diego State University (SDSU) conducted a study of 19 other North American public universities' undergraduate programmes, which included Binghamton University, McGill University, New Jersey Institute of Technology, Penn State University, Queen's University, Rutgers University, Ryerson University, Simon Fraser University, Trent University, University of British Columbia, University of California Berkeley, University of Maine, University of Michigan (Ann Arbor), University of Michigan (Flint), University of Minnesota, University of South Florida, University of Toronto, University of Virginia and University of Washington-Bothell. It was determined that the NPS of these universities ranged from +9 to +65, whereas SDSU's own alumni NPS came out at +23. In contrast, AKU's overall alumni NPS, derived from the question discussed earlier in this section "Would you recommend your AKU programme to others?" was calculated at 64.5. This was the same as the highest NPS amongst the 19 universities in the SDSU study cited above. While AKU programmes' NPS were impressive, both collectively and individually, there were a few that still managed to stand out. From programmes in Pakistan, Medical Education (Med) scored highest at 72 followed by nursing programmes and MBBS, each of which ranged in the 60s.

A survey was conducted and a questionnaire sent to all alumni of AKU to tell us about their current appointment, and their academic and clinical contributions at national and international levels. We also inquired about the volunteer and philanthropic work they have done over the years and any other work which has contributed in some way to the society at large.

## Methods

To assess the impact of alumni contribution to society, data were drawn from a survey which was conducted several months ago. A questionnaire was sent via email and alumni were asked to complete the survey questionnaire. Information regarding two distinct groups of alumni were analysed for this report: alumni who graduated from the MBBS programme and the alumni of postgraduate programmes who graduated from the postgraduate residency or fellowship programmes. They were analysed in two different cohorts.

## Results

### Basic Information

There was a total of 233 respondents. This included graduates from MBBS, residencies and fellowship programmes. Some participants were alumni from both undergraduate and postgraduate studies.

Table 26.1: Total number of study participants

| Groups | MBBS | Residency | MBBS + Residency |
|---|---|---|---|
| Total number of participants | 50 | 166 | 17 |

Among the MBBS graduates, most of the alumni perused their postgraduate studies in the US and are working there at different institutions in varied capacities—many of them in leadership positions such as researchers, clinicians and administrators. Two of the medical college alumni have joined our university, one as Dean of the Medical College and another as Chief Executive Officer of the hospital.

Forty eight participants stated that they are working for the government in key positions across all provinces of Pakistan and are trying to contribute to society by upgrading health facilities and services in their set ups. The majority of the faculty of our institute are also the graduates of the MBBS or residency programmes and they have also been actively involved in philanthropic and volunteer work.

### Number of publications

Regarding academic contribution, the number of publications in research and medical sciences by our alumni is tremendous. Some of them even have 150 to 200 publications in indexed journals (see below chart.)

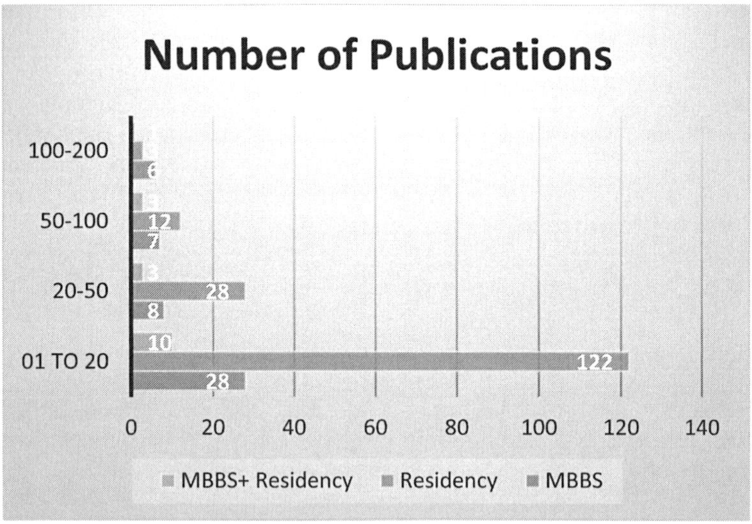


Figure 26.1: Number of publications in research and medical sciences by AKU alumni. *See centrefold for this image in colour.*

### Number of book chapters

Alumni academic contributions are not only limited to writing research papers. Many of them are the authors of book chapters in their respective areas of expertise and several of them have also actively participated in unique areas like Bioethics. One of the alumni is the pioneer of the first centre of biomedical ethics and culture in Pakistan and the chairperson of that centre is also a faculty member associated with AKU.

Seventy of the alumni among the 233 respondents are the authors of book chapters. Nine are authors of 5-10 book chapters and six are authors of more than ten book chapters, which is also a significant academic contribution (see chart overleaf).

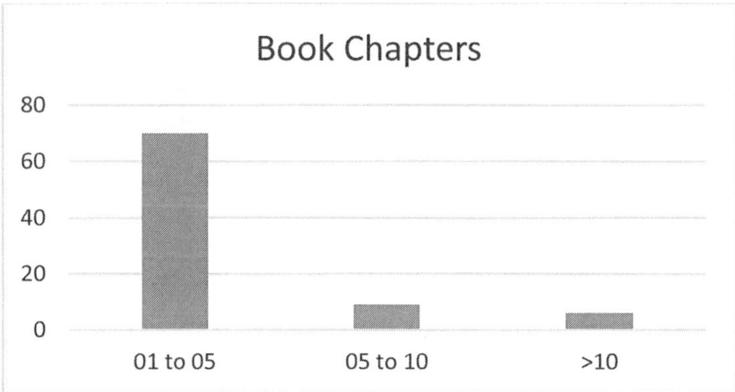


Figure 26.2: Number of book chapters

## Discussion

Medicine is unique among the professions in that medical school requires physicians to participate in extensive periods of applied clinical training at both the undergraduate and postgraduate level. A primary goal of the university is to have students and alumni participate in a sustained manner and contribute to their communities and societies. AKU has a deep commitment to promoting its past and current students to contribute to society and be good citizens. The purpose of this report was to examine how many alumni are contributing to society and in what ways. Responses to four specific questions regarding alumni's service-related behaviours provide information relevant to how well the AKUH is meeting this portion of its mission.

Many of the respondents declared their involvement in philanthropic activities and work during national calamities or disasters. The AKUH team was among the first teams of healthcare workers arriving in Azad

Kashmir to help in relief activities in 2005 when Pakistan was hit by a massive earthquake in that area, and they continued their services until the people affected were rehabilitated.

During unfortunate bomb blasts in different regions of Pakistan, the AKU/AKUH and its staff members always volunteered to help and were among the front runners in rescue and services.

Last year, was a great example during the Covid crisis. Our alumni were asked by the government to establish a Covid Isolation Centre on an urgent basis, which was successfully done within a week and it greatly covered the needs of the people of Karachi despite such a critical situation. The alumni from the medical college who currently hold leadership positions have been involved as infectious disease experts in the national and provincial Covid task forces, and have also worked with the government in providing tele-ICU services to various government and non-government hospitals, providing Covid treatment across the country.

The benefits to the community of institutional training programmes can also be quantified in economic terms, for instance when graduates start their practice in their local underdeveloped areas and try to implement the practices and set up healthcare facilities at primary, secondary and tertiary level centres. Their clinical research and scholarly activities also play a pivotal role in providing long term benefits to society, in terms of preventive care and finding new solutions or treatments for diseases. This also must be acknowledged and should be promoted by academic institutions.

The results from this examination of how AKU alumni demonstrate their worth and act as good citizens through their contribution to society are significantly positive. The analyses for this assessment show that AKUH alumni are good citizens, in that they contribute to the society via donating both time and money to philanthropic activities and organizations and/or events, along with their expertise. Over 50 percent of AKU alumni stated that they spend some amount of time in philanthropic activities, including tutoring/teaching, religious activities, medical/health causes, recreational activities, counselling/mentoring, school alumni programmes, and campaign/political causes, as well as public safety activities.

One study regarding the economic impacts of AKU, done in 2018, showed that AKU created an impact of Rs 103 billion ($1 billion) in one year. This was through high-quality education that increases alumni incomes, outstanding healthcare that keeps people healthy and productive, and its operations, which support businesses and jobs.

11,000 students have graduated from AKU in Pakistan, and an estimated 60% live in Pakistan. Alumni earn more over their careers because of the knowledge and skills they develop at AKU; they then create jobs as entrepreneurs and send money home from abroad. When calculating alumni income gains, only alumni living in Pakistan were counted. Alumni income gains were Rs 4.52 billion ($44 million), alumni start-ups generated Rs 2.2 billion ($22 million) and alumni remittances up to Rs 1.85 billion ($18 million). 5,260 jobs were created through our alumni.

## Conclusion

The benefits to the community and overall society of the training programmes of teaching hospitals extend far beyond their walls. By providing services to individuals and the community at large these programmes contribute in a very positive way and have a large outreach. Important aspect of planning, resource allocation, innovation and quality standards within the institution, are the main factors that may be contributors in providing long term benefits to society.

As per AKU's mission, the university is committed to the development of human capacities through the discovery and dissemination of knowledge and the application of service. From the results of this survey, it is clear that the AKU is fulfilling its mission by its current students and alumni who are experts in their area of work and through various modalities contribute to their community and overall society.

## Bibliography

Aga Khan University Alumni Affairs. "Alumni Survey Report: 2016." *AKU-NAMA*. Book 14 (2017): 01-23. URL: https://ecommons.aku.edu/alumni_survey/1/.

Aga Khan University. "The Aga Khan University's economic impact in Pakistan". AKU- Economic impact study (April 2018): (01-14). URL: https://www.akdn.org/publication/aku-economic-impact-study.

Astin, A. W. and L. J. Sax. "How undergraduates are affected by service participation." *Journal of College Student Development* 39, no. 3 (May/June 1998): 251-263. URL:

https://digitalcommons.unomaha.edu/cgi/viewcontent.cgi?article=1012&context=slcehighered.

Bowen, H. *Investment in Learning: The Individual and Social Value of American Higher Education*. San Francisco: Jossey-Bass, 1977.

Bowen, William G., and Derek Bok. *The Shape of the River. Long-Term Consequences of Considering Race in College and University Admissions*. New Jersey: Princeton University Press, 1998.

Boyer, E. *College: The Undergraduate Experience in America*. New York: Harper and Ro, 1987.

Brubacher, John S., and Willis Rudy. *Higher Education in Transition: A History of American Colleges*. USA: Row Publishers, 1982.

Cabrera, A. F., David J. Weerts and B. J. Zulick, "Making an impact with alumni surveys." *Special Issue: Enhancing Alumni Research: European and American Perspectives* 2005, no. 126 (Summer 2005): 5-17. DOI: https://doi.org/10.1002/ir.144.

Dellow, Donald A., and Richard M. Romano. "Measuring Outcomes: Is the First-time, Full-time Cohort Appropriate for the Community College?" *Community College Review* 30 no. 2 (Fall 2002): 42-54. DOI: 10.1177/009155210203000203.

Gore, Paul. *New Directions for Institutional Research.* USA: Jossey-Bass, 2018.

Haesler, W. K. "Why we should care about medical education." *HMO Magazine* 34, no. 1 (May 1993): 19–23.

Kinnick, M. K. "Increasing the use of student outcomes information, new directions for institutional research". *New Directions for Institutional Research* 1985, no. 47 (September 1985): 93-109. DOI: https://doi.org/10.1002/ir.37019854709.

Kohlberg, L. "Stage and Sequence: The Cognitive-Development Approach to Socialization." In *Handbook of Socialization Theory and Research*, edited by D. A. Goslin, 347-480. Chicago: Rand McNally, 1969.

Kohlberg, L. "Stages of Moral Development." In *Moral Education*, edited by C. Beck, B. Crittenden, and E. Sullivan, 23-92. Toronto: University of Toronto Press, 2016.

Korn, Jessica S. "Contribution to Society among Graduates of the University of Washington." *Office of Educational Assessment OEA report 99-10 (*May 1999): 01-25. URL: http://depts.washington.edu/assessmt/pdfs/reports/OEAReport9910.pdf.

Mentkowski, M. "Higher education assessment and national goals for education: Issues, assumptions, and principles." In *How students learn: Reforming schools through learner-centered education,* edited by N.

M. Lambert and B. L. McCombs, 269–310. American Psychological Association, 1998.

Nagle, Rhea A., and Jerry Bohovich. “A Report on NACE's 2002 Graduating Student & Alumni Survey—How College Job Seekers View Their Prospects.” *Journal of Career Planning & Employment* 62, no. 3 (Spring 2002): 28-34. URL: https://eric.ed.gov/?id=EJ646815.

Osler, W. *On the need of a radical reform in our methods of teaching senior students*. 1903.

Pace, C. Robert. *Measuring outcomes of college: Fifty years of findings and recommendations for the future*. USA: Jossey-Bass, 1979.

Pascarella, E. T., and P. T. Terenzini. *How college affects students*. San Francisco: Jossey-Bass, 1991.

Tremblay, Karine, Diane Lalancette and Deborah Roseveare. “Assessment of Higher education learning outcomes.” *AHELO Feasibility Study Report* 1 (April 2012): 141-172. URL: https://www.oecd.org/education/skills-beyond-school/AHELOFSReportVolume1.pdf.

# CHAPTER 27

# HOW TO SURVIVE AND EXCEL IN SURGERY RESIDENCY: WHAT MAKES A SURGERY RESIDENT OUTSTANDING?

SYED ATHER ENAM, SAQIB KAMRAN BAKHSHI AND AHSAN ALI KHAN

*Disclaimer: Any resemblance of the resident's name at the beginning of the article to anyone is purely coincidental.*

It is 6:30 in the morning. While most of the city is still asleep, Amna, a surgery resident, is on her way to the hospital. She joins the morning ward round, which starts at 7am, and an hour later, she is in the seminar room to give an academic presentation in the morning teaching session. All the residents and attendings are there for critical appraisal and discussion. She was up late the previous night, finalizing the presentation assigned to her just the day before. Despite her best efforts, she misses some critical points in her work and gets thoroughly grilled for that. She is not discouraged. It's 9am; when most of the civilized people are just beginning to reach their offices, Amna quickly grabs a cup of coffee and a sandwich from the hospital cafeteria and runs towards the clinic to see patients. Time flies, and suddenly it is 2pm. The morning clinic has ended early that day, but Amna is not lucky enough to get some downtime. The emergency case her attending has to operate on is waiting in the pre-operative area. She quickly runs to the Operating Room (OR) and changes into scrubs. While the patient is being anesthetized, she plans the surgery and has a quick cup of tea. The surgery ends at 7pm. After updating her attending about her patient's uneventful recovery, Amna heads back to the ward to check on the admitted patients' morning round orders. By the time the hand-over to the on-call team is complete, it is 9 pm. Tired but determined, Amna strolls towards the car park, drives back home, and has a quick dinner. It is her OR day tomorrow, and she must read about the procedures. It is already 1 am when she dozes off to sleep. This is a typical day in the life of a surgical trainee.

Residency is hard. And arguably, surgery training is one of the most challenging jobs in the world. It physically drains even the strongest athletes, emotionally depletes the strongest of hearts, and mentally exhausts even the most composed and organized personalities. It is their passion and goal of becoming a surgeon that drives them to strive hard and overcome all the difficulties. There are specific attributes pivotal to survive and excel during a surgery residency – those residents who have it make a great resident and make the best of their residency training.

What follows is a discussion on those attributes. The narrative below is based on the senior author's (Syed Ather Enam) association with surgical training spanning three decades, and his lectures and motivational talks that he gives to residents.

## Prioritize, prioritize, prioritize - get the critical things done first!

Henry David Thoreau, a 19th-century American philosopher, once said, *"It is not enough to be busy. So are the ants. The question is: What are we busy about?"*

A resident is on-call when suddenly multiple tasks appear that demand her attention: two new consultation requests have been forwarded from the emergency room; a patient's son who has just arrived from abroad wants to meet to get an update on his father's condition; the intern calls he is having difficulty drawing a blood sample of a neonate, and there is a rush-call for a very sick patient having difficulty breathing on the floor. With all these issues landing one after another within 5 minutes, and the pager continuously going off, there is only one thing that will make that resident a winner in the end: prioritization.

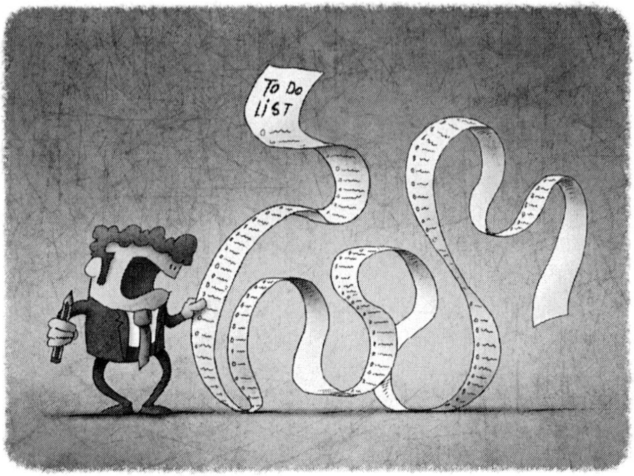


Fig. 27-1: Checklist (Casas 2021). *See centrefold for this image in colour.*

You may be on call with a long to-do list handed down to you during the sign-off in the evening. You have to chase the labs, check the computerized tomography (CT) scan report, change a dressing, see a post-op patient with shortness of breath, check up on all the post-op patients, and talk to the cardiologist about an unfinished consult, and so on. Taking care of all the tasks handed down to you simultaneously is impossible. A junior resident's usual mistake is to start from the top of the list, hoping to finish them all overnight. This strategy often leads to delays in paying attention to urgent issues.

Learn to prioritize.

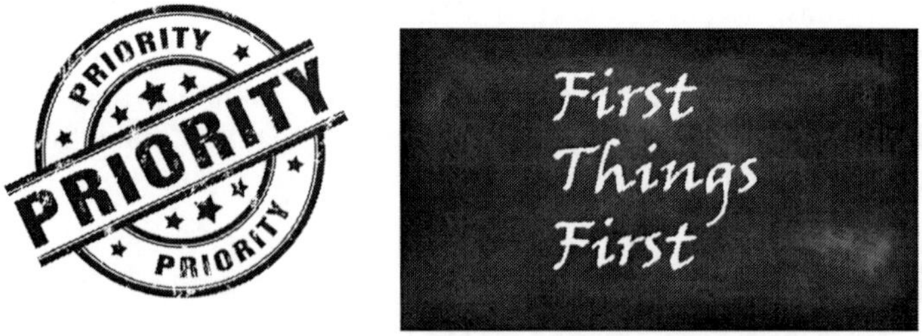


Fig. 27-2: Prioritize (Mstan 2021). *See centrefold for this image in colour.*

You will be pulled into serious matters anyway; the issues that are not serious but have the potential to get worse if delayed, are going to bite you in the end. Make a habit of paying attention to those issues; prioritize these issues after pure emergencies. This comes with practice. You must master this strategy until it becomes second nature. And it's not just patient care. Academic assignments, personal reading, and many other essential things in life all get scrambled together. On such occasions, prioritizing work will undoubtedly help manage all of it within the stipulated time and will let you avoid missing crucial responsibilities. Thoughtful prioritization allows effective time management and accomplishing a lot in a short amount of time.

A famous American executive, designer, and technology geek, John Maeda, once said, *"People who can focus, get things done. People, who can prioritize, get the right things done."*

## Manage your time - get rid of your time vampires!

Personal and professional time management is a continuous challenge for surgeons. Anxious patients with numerous questions related to their disease; concerned parents of sick children; disturbed children of elderly parents admitted with serious illnesses; unforeseen complications that prolong surgical procedures; all add a significant amount of unpredictability. Without a thoughtful time management strategy, this strain can have a substantial toll on the surgeon's physical and emotional well-being and on the trainee.

One cannot manage time if one does not know what is important and what is not necessary. Anything which takes one closer to one's vision is important; everything which does otherwise is unimportant. It must be correct and independent of time. Surgery residencies are quite overwhelming, and it is quite easy for trainees to lose focus and indulge in activities that eat up their time. Formulating clear visions at the start of a residency will make one stay focused on the essential tasks. As the old saying goes, "plan your work, and then work your plan."

The Eisenhower Matrix shown below simplifies tasks into four different categories.

| | URGENT | NOT URGENT |
|---|---|---|
| IMPORTANT | 1<br>**Urgent and important DO** | 2<br>**Not urgent but important PLAN** |
| NOT IMPORTANT | 3<br>**Urgent but not important DELEGATE** | 4<br>**Not urgent and not important ELIMINATE** |

Fig. 27-3: The Eisenhower Matrix

In the first quadrant – urgent and essential will get done – a patient with a gunshot wound to the chest lands in the ER. You will take care of the situation and learn to take care of it more efficiently over time. The second quadrant – urgent but not important - should be delegated. For example, follow-up of labs of all post-op patients can be delegated to an intern, but you must make sure you have taught the intern to do it right and the intern is dependable. The fourth quadrant - not urgent, not important - needs to be eliminated as much as possible. You don't need to spend hours in a chat group to get your points across about a political party you favour. You can do it when you have finished your residency. The third quadrant is not urgent, but important, and is the most important quadrant for your career. This typically gets pushed back because quadrant 2 and quadrant 4 were not managed appropriately. You have been thinking about writing a paper for which data has been collected, or about initiating a research project in your senior years but have been putting it off regularly. Those who pay attention to this quadrant and are disciplined about it are the ones with a better chance of a brighter career and excelling. Don't mistake putting your limited but essential recreation in quadrant 4; it also goes into the third quadrant.

It is often seen that improper prioritization and lack of time management put trainees under undue stress, which leads to burnout. The absence of this crucial aspect of training in the undergraduate and postgraduate curricula results in many residents missing important personal and professional obligations during the highly stressful years of training. Multi-tasking is a skill that not every resident is aware of before starting their residency. Therefore, dedicated education on time management for surgical trainees will undoubtedly increase productivity and motivation and lessen errors. Multi-tasking is good but try to avoid it when you can. Multi-tasking decreases efficiency. If you have four 15-minute tasks, do them sequentially, don't start all of them together; you will perform better if you do them successively. However, there are times when multi-tasking is indispensable. Practise multi-tasking whenever possible.

Try to perform necessary tasks when they are not yet urgent, when one can schedule work and achieve the maximum output with optimum effort. A punctual person who fulfils his/her commitments timely is considered dependable, trustworthy, responsible, and organized. The first step is to estimate time correctly, then avoid taking on more work than you can fulfil, and finally always keep a buffer. Unlike in non-medical professions, doctors carry an additional burden of temporarily dropping what is important for them to interact compassionately with patients to ease their fears and make them feel better. This cannot be put off and requires a buffer period when you plan the day.

Lord Chesterfield, a 17th-century British statesman, very rightly said, *"I recommend you to take care of the minutes, for the hours will take care of themselves."*

## Resourcefulness: the art of knowing who's who, what's where, and who can do what!

According to Napoleon Hill, *"A resourceful person will always make an opportunity fit his or her needs."*

An urgent magnetic resonance imaging (MRI) scan on a patient, a stat blood test, a quick medicine consult, and an early clinic appointment can be managed promptly by a resourceful resident. This is only possible if one knows instinctively who does what and maintains a cordial relationship with everyone who can be a potential messiah someday.

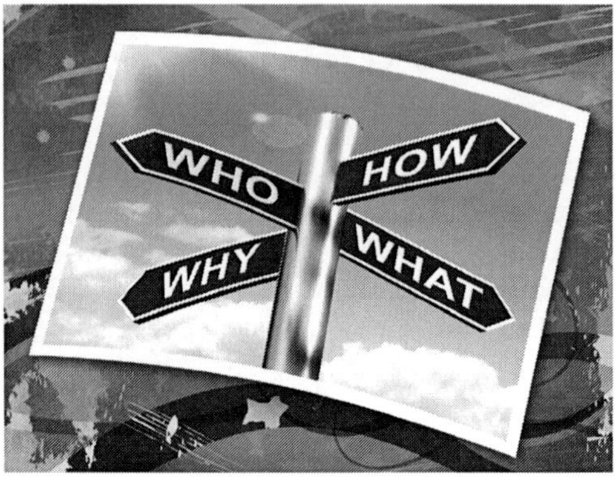


Fig. 27-4: Get to know (Miles 2021). *See centrefold for this image in colour.*

A resident should not hesitate to ask for help. Your ability to ask for help reflects your resourcefulness. If one knows what number to call, which person can do what, who can help you schedule cases in the OR correctly, and who to call if you need an MRI right away, you will find your life much easier. Systems are there to get everything done but knowing the right person and the proper method helps you get the job done efficiently and leaves you time to breathe and focus on other things. On the other extreme, I have encountered individuals abusing this capacity. They end up being loathed and despised. That is why this aptitude should be considered an art - use it, but don't overdo it.

## Call your senior - it is not a sign of weakness

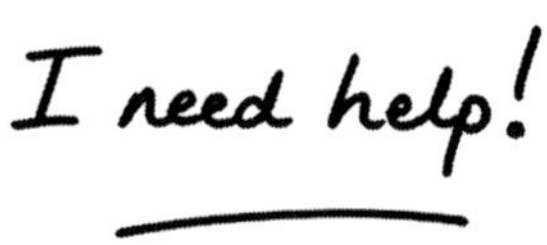


Fig. 27-5: Ask for help (Dorney 2021)

Expectations from a surgical trainee are extraordinarily high, and sometimes these expectations can make one reluctant to ask for help when it is genuinely needed. A surgical trainee should not forget that he is in a training programme and should learn; he should be eager to learn and ask for help whenever it is required. Err towards calling a pass on the buck.

When in doubt, call. I learned it the hard way as a resident. When I came across situations where I was not sure what to do, I would rather be called weak and face annoyance from my senior resident or faculty for waking them up in the middle of the night, than let a potential disaster become real. The other reason a resident may not ask for help from a senior is over-confidence or arrogance. Don't be a cowboy out of a movie. Conceit in a trainee may halt their progress. One might find themselves in a predicament when help is needed in something quite simple and basic tasks. A trainee should never hesitate to accept his limitations and seek support.

Benjamin Hendricks, an American neurosurgery resident, mentioned in one of his articles, *"Residents earn the trust of the attending surgeon only if they are aware of their own limitations and consistently know when to call for help."*

## Independent learning, self-discipline, humbleness and eagerness – learn to learn

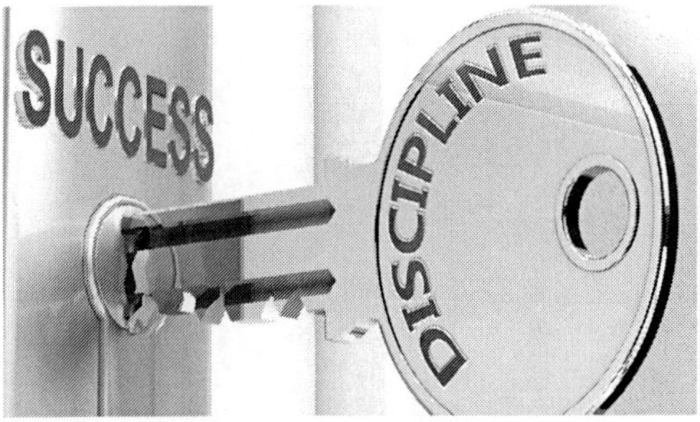


Fig. 27 6: Discipline leads to success (Suszycki 2021). *See centrefold for this image in colour.*

Exhibiting self-motivation and proactiveness in reading and learning is an attribute of a great resident, requiring discipline. Discipline is vital to achieving any goal in life. It also means staying emotionally intelligent and confident. Every resident faces a difficult time during their residency. So, learn to show restraint and develop perseverance and resilience. A disciplined resident translates into a better surgeon. Independent learners are aware of their limitations and do not wait for anyone to make them overcome gaps in their knowledge and skills. Set aside time to read every day and every weekend. Everyone will find their own best time to do so. Find the schedule that suits you the best, and discipline yourself to stick to that schedule. Slow and steady wins the race—over time, you will find that you have done a lot of reading.

Albert Einstein, arguably one of the greatest physicists of all time, once said, *"I never teach my pupils, I only provide the conditions in which they can learn."*

The widespread online availability of educational resources has made the path to learning quite feasible and more accessible and has created favourable conditions for everyone. There is an increasing trend of webinars and virtual conferences. The resident, who does not depend on motivation from peers or faculty to learn, excels much earlier in surgical training and career than those who lack the drive and impetus for acquiring experience and knowledge.

Punctuality is discipline and professionalism; it leaves a good impression on people around you and earns you respect. It also enhances your learning experience and helps you learn more.

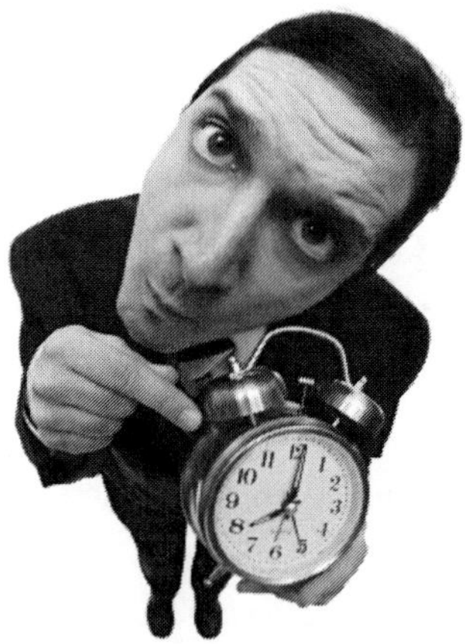

Fig. 27-7: Strategic time management is crucial for success (Image from website, "Everyone a Leader" 2013). *See centrefold for this image in colour.*

Another attribute that is central during the learning years is a humble attitude. My first rotation in my preliminary surgery residency training was in an ICU in Erie County Medical Centre in Buffalo. I had not done any house job or internship before that, and I had not learned much during clinical rotations during my medical school years. I had taken time off for a Ph.D. right after medical school which worsened things. On my first day on call, I was as clueless as one could be. A senior, frail nurse named Sue watched me and realized how inept I was. She took pity on me and taught me all the basics about taking care of ICU patients. I realized that I needed to learn from all the possible sources, and I needed to learn fast. This attitude also helped me when I started my neurosurgery training. Hermann was the name of the gentleman who taught me how to position the patient during surgery, how to balance the microscope, and many other things.

Arrogance is detrimental to learning. Develop genuine humbleness and eagerness to learn. A surgical trainee needs to have a humble attitude to learning. He must learn from everyone, including faculty, fellow residents, nursing staff, technical staff, administrative staff, or anyone in the work environment. This positive attitude will take him a long way in his career.

## See one, do one, teach one - repeat until you master it

Practice makes perfect. A common discontent for surgery residents is that they do not get enough hands-on training. They grumble and complain about not having enough practical experience. Little do they realize that the surgery residency is much more than a hands-on experience. Holding the knife, dissecting the tissue, manipulating the pathology, and closing the wound represent only a small component of training. This is a complaint I hear frequently. But I also hear frequently from residents who have been in practice for a few years after graduation that how well they were trained. It was not because they got to do the surgeries independently, but because they were prepared to carry out the surgery with the proper thought process. There may be much more hands-on experience in some institutions, but without much supervision. This is worse than a no hands-on experience. Anybody can cut. One of my mentors in neurosurgery used to repeat the euphemism, "you can teach a monkey to operate," and then he would add, "we teach you judgment and decision-making." It is easy to learn how to operate, it takes several years of training to know when to operate, and it takes a significant period of your career to gain the wisdom of when not to operate.

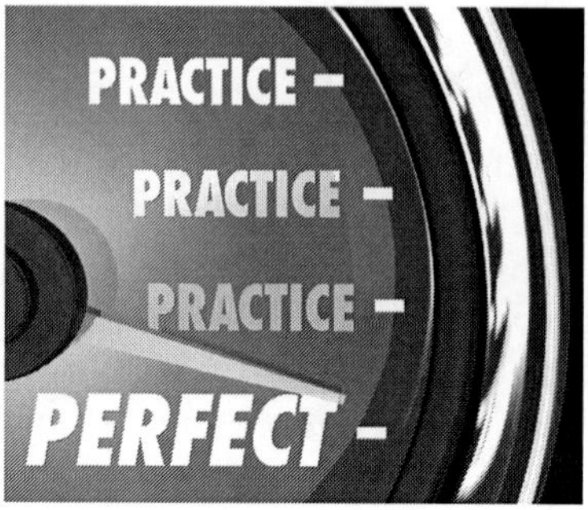


Fig. 27-8: Practice makes one perfect (Iqoncept 2021). *See centrefold for this image in colour.*

Try to perform every operation thrice on the same patient. First, imagine all the steps when planning the surgical approach in your mind. Next, do the actual surgery on the patient (it's OK if you assist or only observe), and then find a few minutes of solitude to go over it again in your mind after the surgery is done.

Some trainees come with superior hand-eye coordination and surgical skills, whereas some have to struggle in the beginning to develop psychomotor skills. It is not uncommon to see someone struggle through their early residency years to develop surgical skills, only to blossom suddenly in the last year and develop an excellent surgical hand. It is not a linear graph; it is a curve; everyone's curve is as unique as the individual. The good thing is, with sincere efforts, that almost all the curves end up excellent.

## God is in the details

Atul Gawande, a US-based general surgeon, wrote in his book, *The Checklist Manifesto*, *"...under conditions of complexity, not only are checklists a help, they are required for success."*

If a resident does not pay attention to details, round orders are missed, wrong blood tests and radiological exams are performed, and even wrong side surgeries are carried out. Missing even the tiniest details can have serious consequences for a patient. Most residents understand this concept, but often do not realize it until they fail to be attentive and make a blunder. It can shatter a resident's confidence and an attending's trust.

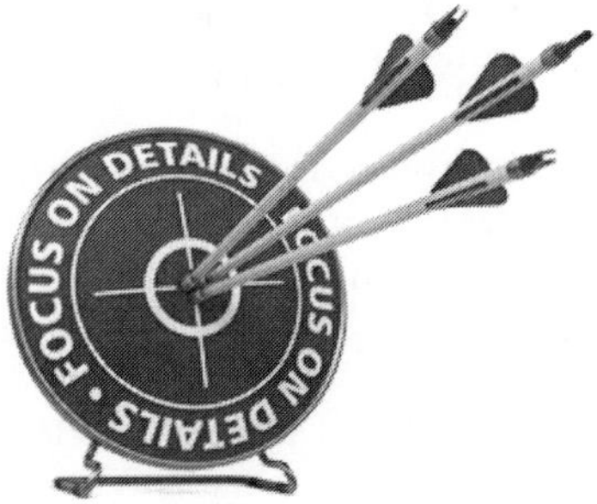


Fig. 27-9: Attention to details (Tushatuvango 2021). *See centrefold for this image in colour.*

Attention to detail is essential in any profession but is particularly crucial in surgery. The outcome of a surgery depends on how you position a patient, where you make an incision, how deep you go with your first cut, how you identify different tissues as you go deeper, how you study the details of the pathology when you reach it, and what manoeuvres you use to tackle the pathology. Attention to detail starts to play its role long before the surgery. Pay attention to the patient's history, the expression on the patient's face, subtle signs during the examination, and observations in the imaging studies. These all culminate in a better decision. Paying attention to detail guarantees your success.

"The difference between mediocrity and excellence is attention to details."

*- S A Enam*

A checklist is part of attention to detail. The human brain can make an error. You may think you have followed all the details, but you might have missed one; everyone is prone to making errors. Memory can also be faulty. Comprehension can be limited. A checklist will always rescue you and save the day. Make it a habit to use the checklist, whether preparing a patient for surgery or writing admission orders. Did you write all the medications the patient was taking at home? Did you stop anti-platelets five days before surgery? Did you write a blood draw for electrolytes in the morning? Did you register for DVT prophylaxis? There are so many "did you" questions that you are bound to miss one now and then, and then one of those misses will end up in a disaster.

## Professionalism – dress for success, write perfect, speak confidently

Dr James Ausman (former Chair of Neurosurgery, Henry Ford Hospital) always insisted the resident present a professional appearance. Chronic fatigue, especially after an on-call night, makes you look shabby. You do not exude confidence when your semblance is unkempt. Dressing professionally (meaning decent, clean, and appropriate attire) displays poise; it also indicates you respect the patient. Try to speak confidently, logically, and to the point; practice doing it. When you write, your writing should also reflect that you are an educated person. Not paying attention to grammar, syntax, and punctuation can be a big turn-off, even in an informal email. If you want your colleagues and mentors to take you seriously, learn to speak confidently and write well.

Professionalism goes beyond dressing, speaking, and writing. Epstein and Hundert comprehensively defined professionalism in a paper published in JAMA in 2002: "*Professional competence is the habitual and judicious use of communication, knowledge, technical skills, clinical reasoning, emotions, values, and reflection in daily practice for the benefit of the individual and community being served.*"

It means maintaining the highest ethical standards and moral values, managing conflicts of interest, keeping patient information confidential, disclosing errors and morbidities, and always putting patients' interests first. Responsibility, maturity, communication skills, and respect can all be grouped under professionalism. Professionalism is a lifelong quest, it's an attitude, and the attitude starts with your dressing, speech, and writing.

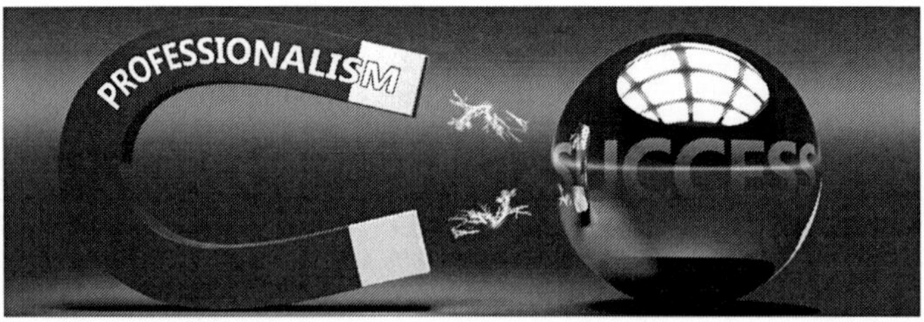


Fig. 27-10: Professionalism attracts success (Suszycki 2021). *See centrefold for this image in colour.*

## Communicate efficiently - prevent a disaster

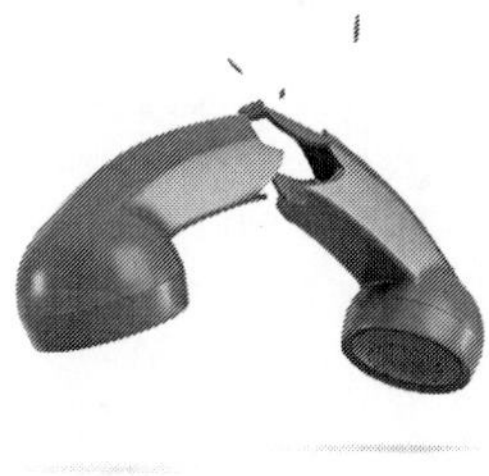

Fig. 27-11: Ineffective communication is a recipe for disaster (Gearstd 2021)

As the old saying goes, "good communication is the bridge between confusion and clarity." Communication is not only getting the message across. Listening is equally important. No one can remember all that is being said, so jot down whatever important things are being communicated. In the earlier days, keeping a pocket diary was recommended; now, most residents have smartphones to maintain a checklist of all the tasks.

Of all the mishaps in a hospital, lack of good communication is a leading cause.

Communication is a skill that you develop over time. This skill needs practice too. Practise good communication during your residency years. Learn to communicate well with your colleagues, subordinates, seniors, patients, and their families. Chapter 7, "The Ethnic Theory of Plane Crashes," in the book *Outliers* by Malcolm Gladwell, is worth reading in this context. If you communicate well, you have practically averted many disasters.

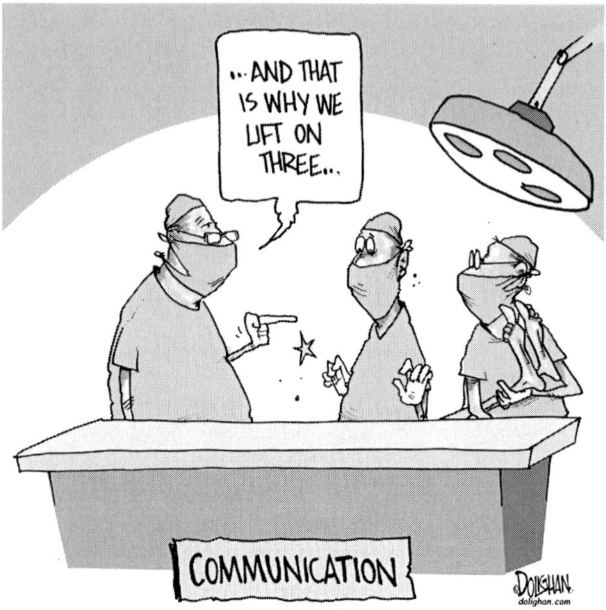
...AND THAT IS WHY WE LIFT ON THREE...
COMMUNICATION
DOLIGHAN
dolighan.com

Fig. 27-12: Communication (The Reel Newsletter 2010). *See centrefold for this image in colour.*

## Give respect to gain respect

Residency is also learning how to build new relationships, win over friends, influence people, and most important of all, work as a team. But love and respect must be earned by giving them to others. Respect everyone, including fellow residents, interns, nursing staff, housekeeping staff, faculty, admin staff, patients, and their families. Doing this earns you respect for yourself and helps you maintain good links with the staff. Showing regard and maintaining a cordial work environment is vital to the efficiency of your team. On a hectic night call, when a resident doesn't get a minute to rest, the one who always greeted everyone with a smile and esteem will have everyone on the floor ready to help.

Anger is a common phenomenon among surgery residents. Surgery residents are the hardest working lot, and with the most stressful job in the hospital, and a more than 12-hour rigorous work shift can intensify negative feelings. A minor spat with the nurse or a short row with a fellow resident from another specialty heightens the tension, aggravates the atmosphere, and becomes an energy vampire. If you forgive and forget, you will be cherished by the team, you will enjoy your work, and you will be more productive.

Residencies are filled with difficult days when nothing falls into place. The patients aren't well, the attendants are not satisfied, the professor isn't happy, the case presentation doesn't go well, and it gets late at the hospital. And then someone comes along and rubs you the wrong way. Repeatedly giving in to anger, showing spite, or making snide comments will eventually wear you down. Being friendly to everyone and keeping a few very close friends is always a good strategy. Discussing all the frustration with a good friend at work can be very therapeutic.

Dr. Mark Rosenblum (former Chair of Neurosurgery at Henry Ford Hospital) taught me that the key to a successful career in neurosurgery is to master the three A's: Ability, Availability, and Affability.

## Trustworthiness and integrity are achieved when you know and admit your limitations

Honesty and truthfulness are fundamental to any job. When patients seek treatment, they place their lives in the hands of their doctors. And when the attendings let the residents manage their patients in wards, clinics, and operating rooms, and transfer their knowledge to them, they are bestowing their trust onto them. One incident is enough to shatter years of trust.

Integrity is everything in residency training. When a patient, an attending, a resident, or a nurse asks a question or seeks information, and the resident is not aware of the answer, the resident should be ready to say, I don't know. Not knowing something which is important shows carelessness. But there is one thing worse than a careless resident, and that is a dishonest resident.

A famous Russian playwright, Anton Pavlovich Chekhov, once said, *"Medical profession is a feat, it requires self-sacrifice, purity of soul and purity of thoughts."* I learnt this from my mentor in neurosurgery, Dr. Ghaus Malik

## Work-life balance - you will have enough time to balance it out eventually

Until recently, the lives of most surgeons, let alone surgical residents, had been devoid of work-life balance, resulting in frequent examples of burnout. The term refers to the proportional time spent at work and in one's private life, to the equilibrium sought when dividing one's time among the two. This can be subjective, depending on the person's priorities and abilities. In real life, a work-life balance is not an absolute static thing. It is a dynamic practice, changing its proportion from time to time during a surgeon's career.

This means that a surgical resident's work-life balance will tilt heavily towards work because of the limited time one has for training. When preparing for an exam the next day, you do not seek a work-life balance that day. When the exam is done, you take a break. The idea is that it balances over time. As one completes training and starts their practice, the balance slowly begins to shift. While one nears retirement, leisure time and personal time become a more prominent component.

Many studies on work-life balance for surgery residents have mentioned physician burnout, mental stress, lack of motivation, and low productivity. These studies have been used to advocate a reduction in the working hours of trainees. However, very few have considered that trainees spend only 4 to 5 years in residency training, shaping their lifelong surgical practice. Training is bound to be brutal and hectic. This does not mean residents should just have a robotic life. As the old saying goes, “All work and no play, makes Jack a dull boy.” The surgical training prepares a trainee to cope with many challenges. Learning how to maintain a well-organized, professional life while experiencing an enjoyable personal life is essential. One should not plan all the fun for the future, but one should not compromise the training years with an unrealistic and short-sighted work-life balance; it is vital to keep an eye on the destination but enjoy the process and journey.

“Life is what happens to you while you're busy making other plans.” That line is from John Lennon's song “Beautiful Boy” on his last album “Double Fantasy”, with Yoko Ono (1980, Geffen Records). It is not uncommon for us to believe that we will settle down and start our life once we are done with our training. By the time you are done with all the training, including residency and fellowships, you might already be in your mid - or late thirties, or even early forties, in some cases. Keeping in mind the skewed work-life balance during residency years, one must remember to enjoy the years as one plans for the future. My wife instilled this sense in me. We went through our residency training during the same period and managed our lives with two children. The concept of quality versus quantity comes into play strongly here.

The tricky topic of getting married and pregnancy (for female residents) during residency must be thought out in this context. Unfortunately, the culture in many surgical residency programmes has still not matured enough to help those who want to get married or have a child. The decision to get married or have a child should be thought out well, because stress from work may strain relationships. It does not mean that one should put off these important life matters. This is a personal decision, and everyone will have unique circumstances. A good understanding with my better half, solid teamwork in the residency programme, prioritizing what was essential, and avoiding low-quality time-consuming activities helped me manage those tough years.

Work-life balance for surgery residents effectively means maintaining healthy activities alongside work that refreshes the mind now and then. This can be a regular schedule of physical activity in the gym or early morning or late-night walk, hanging out with friends and family over the free weekends, going on a short annual vacation, or indulging in extra-curricular activities and hobbies, such as writing blogs, reading fiction, painting - whatever soothes your mind and soul.

## Don't make one person your role-model - it takes a village to raise a child

Nobody is perfect. You will come across many individuals whose footsteps you would like to follow, but look closely; none of them are perfect. This is important for an apprentice. Residency years are formative years. Your fundamental nature develops in your pre-teen years, but the habits and style you carry in your practice as a surgeon form during these years of training. Avoid the mistake of making one person your exclusive role model. No matter how good a mentor is, he or she has flaws.

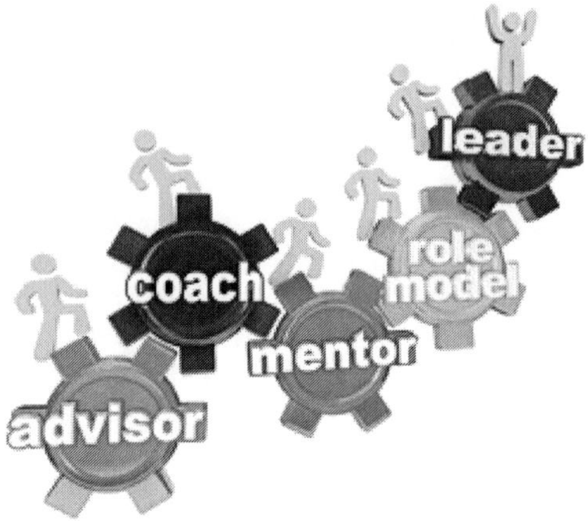


Fig. 27-13: Mentors (Iqoncept 2021). *See centrefold for this image in colour.*

One may be compassionate but disorganized; another may be disciplined and stoic but lacks interpersonal skills; yet another may be good clinically but does not have a solid academic base. Try to figure out the habits and traits you like about that senior, that faculty member, or that mentor, and try to emulate those characteristics. Try to pick up only those attributes that you admire; don't try to become that person.

Look around, and you will find everyone with a certain quality, a particular distinction. Observe, absorb, and build your own collection of good habits. Just like it takes a village to raise a child (an African proverb), it takes a group of mentors to create an excellent surgeon.

## Build up research during residency years - the key to excel

Lack of sleep and tiredness when you get home will ensure that research and academic activities are the last things on your mind. Research is in the not urgent, but essential category in the Eisenhower matrix. You must remind yourself daily of this non-urgent but essential activity, because it is very easy to be pushed onto the back burner. Paying attention to this and managing it in a disciplined manner will make you excel during your residency. For those residents who have not had any research experience before starting their residency, it is best to keep things simple and start with case reports. A case report can be written and submitted quickly. Finishing a case report can give a lot of confidence to someone who has never published a scientific paper. From there, start to pick more complex projects. Look for opportunities to sharpen your statistics and writing skills. Don't spread yourself out too much. Pick two to three solid projects, collaborate with your colleagues, and focus on these. As one project ends, pick up another one. There will be some who will be outliers and successfully juggling multiple tasks. For most of us close to the median, it is best to stay realistic and focus on a few; complete, write, and submit them, and then take more. From case reports, move on to case series and other experimental studies. It will be challenging to conceptualize a randomized controlled trial and conclude it during your residency. Review papers and systemic analysis papers are also good options.

## Show empathy - put yourself in their shoes

Empathy is to understand, feel and share the feelings of others. Treating patients with similar diseases can frequently decrease empathy among residents, which they may not regain once training is completed. It takes a conscious effort to keep compassion alive. Remind yourself at every encounter with a patient. Make a habit of trying to feel how that person is feeling. For you, it may be the hundredth brain tumour case, but for that patient and that family, it is news that has devastated them.

Try to see the patient beyond the surgical problem the patient sees you for: the socioeconomic difficulties, the social structure, the co-morbidities, the psychological pressures - all these things need to be factored in when you devise a plan for the patient. Whether it is haemorrhoids in a patient with chronic constipation or glioblastoma in an octogenarian being taken care of by a son with a large family and limited resources, don't treat the images and numbers; treat the patient.

Empathy adds humanity to surgical practice. It elevates the efforts towards patient care from being just an act to a noble virtue. It results in higher patient satisfaction and better outcomes; prevents the physician from malpractice; protects a surgeon from a lawsuit; and fosters a sense of satisfaction in the healthcare provider. The famous writer and speaker Stephen Covey sums it up well: *"When you show deep empathy toward others, their defensive energy goes down, and positive energy replaces it. That's when you can get more creative in solving problems."*

## Have a tender heart but a thick skin

Working in a hospital as a trainee, you will find yourself in situations where stakes are high, everybody is stressed, and the environment is emotionally charged. This may happen routinely, and you will come across all kinds of people. You will come across bullies, across egocentric, narcissistic, and mean individuals. You will have to deal with demands, rebukes, criticism, admonishes and beratement. There will be times when you will feel small, neglected, dejected, crestfallen. Someday you will make a mistake for which you will be chided, berated, admonished. You will feel worthless. But pick yourself up; remember, one day you will become a surgeon, you will attain your dream: do not let somebody's inability to act maturely hurt you deeply.

You also need to be aware that in most institutions across the world, harassment is no more tolerated. If someone repeatedly harasses you, don't be afraid to report it to the proper authorities. Don't be intimidated by the position or stature of the person harassing you. Don't let your wrong decision make you think too low of yourself.

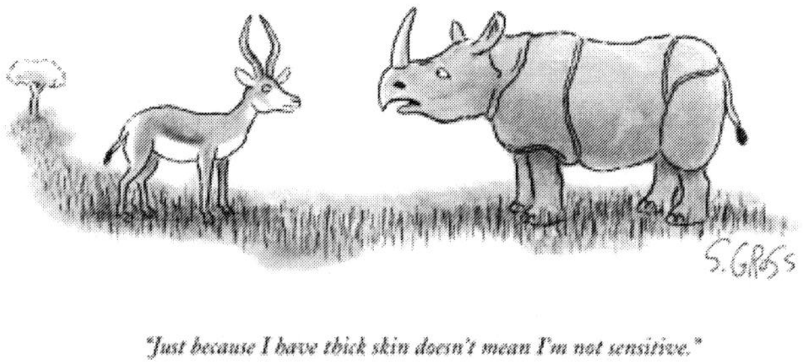
S.GROSS
"Just because I have thick skin doesn't mean I'm not sensitive."

Fig. 27-14: Have a tender heart but a thick skin (Gross 2014)

Learn from your mistake, make sure you don't do it again; learn the habit of healthy introspection, but avoid negative self-criticism. Move on if somebody yells at you, criticizes you, or shames you. In other words, have thick skin. Don't take it personally when someone vents their emotional distress on you. Stay focused; your goal is to get through residency. Lace yourself with armour-plates, but don't lose your compassion for the patients and those around you. This is hard to do when you are feeling down in the dumps. Remind yourself how to detach yourself from somebody's negative behaviour and connect to those who need you.

## The U-curve - keep your head above the water

Whenever you start on an endeavour, the chances are you will go through a U-curve. Surgical residencies are typically like that. When you begin an arduous journey, you start with certain expectations. You start with hankering, aspirations, and ambition, mixed with some apprehension, but hope overshadows the concerns. You are looking forward to a great experience. You have worked hard to get onto that programme and are psyched up. These positive feelings carry you along for a while, but then the reality starts to set in. No matter how realistic you were, you did not expect these problems and issues you face every day on the ward, in the OR, or on rounds. They start to bear down on you, wear you out. The excitement begins to fade away, and the daily chores become intolerable. Long tiring hours begin to seem longer. You notice that you are not performing well. You are facing too much criticism. The training programme is much more gruelling than you expected, and you find yourself failing at many points. You start to think maybe you were not cut out for this. You will not finish it after all. Angst replaces anxiety. Thoughts of giving it up start looming in your mind; everything looks gloomy. When all these negative thoughts crowd in your brain, you are hitting the bottom of the U-curve.

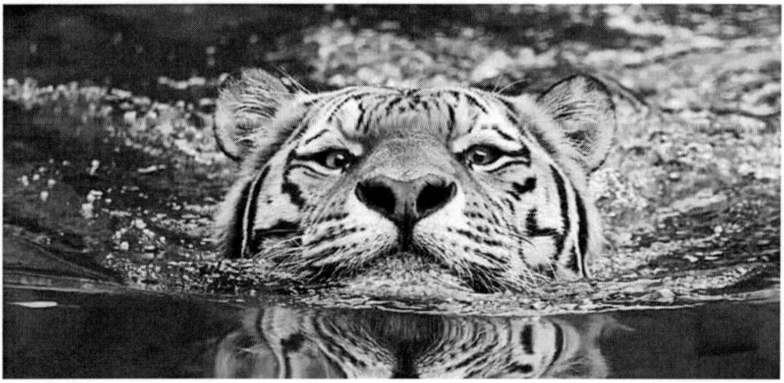

Fig. 27-15: Keep your head above the water (Blah 2020). *See centrefold for this image in colour.*

The only strategy is to focus on one thing: keep your head above the water; don't drown. During these moments, you don't have to excel; you just have to survive. All you have to do is cross the river—no matter what. And then, things start to look positive. Your outlook slowly starts to become sanguineous. You have crossed the lowest of the lows, and now you see the light at the end of the tunnel. Hope and a feeling of accomplishment start to displace the desperation and gloom. Your pride and confidence begin to grow taller. And before you know it, you have done it. You have graduated from a surgical residency programme. That was the other limb of the U-curve.

My father told me about the U-curve when I went to a boarding high school. He quoted it from a lecture at Cornell for his graduate studies, undertaken before I was even born. But my awareness of this phenomenon helped me through my residency in neurosurgery. Throughout my career of mentoring residents, I find this happening to almost everyone. For some, the U-curve is narrow; for some, the U-curve is shallow. Their ties with the surgical career snapped for a very small number, because I failed to pull them up from the bottom of the U- curve. I have found that focusing on keeping your head above the water when everything looks dark and depressing helps the residents cross the abyss.

## Surgery is not just cutting and suturing - think beyond that!

Surgical skills can be acquired by anyone who wants them and can be polished with practice. But an outstanding surgery resident thinks beyond all this. An outstanding surgery resident is also a creative individual, a thoughtful person, a sincere mentor, and a diligent researcher.

"A good surgeon must have an eagle's eye, a lion's heart, a lady's hand." Thus runs the old English proverb (The Journal of the American Medical Association 1924). But an exceptional surgeon also has a passion for teaching and training, and an enthusiasm for academia. This trajectory develops during one's residency years. During training, a surgery resident should train himself to become a competent surgeon, a critical thinker, an innovator, and a true leader. It is not easy to achieve all these qualities and skills if we do not pay attention and make sincere efforts persistently.

As residents progress and become senior, they are also required to learn and carry out administrative responsibilities. They learn how to manage people, resolve conflicts, build a team, mentor the juniors, work in an organization, lead a group. Look at your mentors and see how they do it.

To sum it all up, a great surgery resident is dedicated and committed. and strives to attain the best possible level of professionalism, honesty, academic excellence, and empathy. Residency training equips the residents with all the attributes necessary for embarking on their careers. The traits and features mentioned above will not just let the residents survive their residency training. Instead, it would surely help them excel and do wonders.

Enrich your mind by reading on all topics. The five books recommended below are pertinent to the experience that starts during the surgical residency years. Try to read them in the first year of your residency:

- Atul Gawande, *Complications: A Surgeon's Notes on an Imperfect Science* (London: Profile Books, 2002)
- Atul Gawande, *The Checklist Manifesto: How to Get Things Right* (London: Profile Books, 2010)
- Malcolm Gladwell, *Outliers: The Story of Success* (London: Penguin, 2013)
- Henry Marsh, *Do No Harm: Stories of Life, Death and Brain Surgery* (London: Orion, 2014)
- Haider Warraich, *Modern Death: How Medicine Changed the End of Life* (New York: St Martin's Press, 2017)

## Bibliography

Blah, Capitao. "Uploaded by Capitao Blah". *Pinterest.* Accessed 2nd August 2021 URL: https://www.pinterest.com/pin/509258670360744169/.

© Can Stock Photo / Lyolya1, "Silhouettes of Business People". CanStockPhoto. Accessed 2nd August 2021. URL: https://www.canstockphoto.com/silhouettes-of-business-people-6565797.html.

Casas, Jr. "Businessman holds a long list of scroll or tasks". Dreamstime. Accessed 2nd August 2021. URL: https://www.dreamstime.com/businessman-hold-long-list-scroll-tasks-man-suit-manager-image101696777.

Dorney, Chris. “I need help! Handwritten on a white background.” Dreamstime. Accessed 2nd August 2021. URL: https://www.dreamstime.com/i-need-help-handwritten-white-background-image215882965
ID 181848135

Gearstd. “3D rendering of a red retro phone receiver broken in half on a white background.” Dreamstime. Accessed 2nd August 2021. URL: https://www.dreamstime.com/d-rendering-red-retro-phone-receiver-broken-half-white-background-important-call-stop-communication-line-image127367947.

Gross, Sam. "Just because I have thick skin doesn't mean I'm not sensitive." *New Yorker.* 12 May 2014. URL: https://www.newyorker.com/cartoons/random/share/1559471

Iqoncept. “Practice word repeated on a speedometer or gauge and needle hitting word Perfect to illustrate improving your performance with constant practicing.” Dreamstime. Accessed 2nd August 2021. URL: https://www.dreamstime.com/stock-illustration-practice-makes-perfect-speedometer-gauge-measure-performance-per-word-repeated-needle-hitting-word-to-illustrate-image49155055.

Iqoncept. “Coach Advisor Mentor Leading You To Achieve Goals”. CanStockPhoto. Accessed 2nd August 2021. URL: https://www.canstockphoto.com/coach-advisor-mentor-leading-you-to-13471338.html.

Miles, Stuart. “Who How Why What Questions Sign Meaning Researching And Investigating”. Dreamstime. Accessed 2nd August 2021. URL: https://www.dreamstime.com/stock-illustration-who-how-why-what-questions-sign-mean-researching-investigati-meaning-investigating-image41432523.

Mstan. “Priority rubber stamp illustration isolated on white background.” Dreamstime. Accessed 2nd August 2021. URL: https://www.dreamstime.com/stock-illustration-priority-rubber-stamp-illustration-isolated-white-background-image78071748.

NG, TITUS. “Leadership and Punctuality: Must Leaders Always Be Late?” Everyone a Leader (February 2013). URL: https://titusng.com/2013/02/18/leadership-and-punctuality-must-leaders-always-be-late/.

Suszycki, Michal. “Discipline and success - pictured as word Discipline on a key, to symbolize that Discipline helps achieving success and prosperity in life and business, 3d illustration.” Dreamstime. Accessed 2nd August 2021. URL:

https://www.dreamstime.com/discipline-success-pictured-as-word-key-to-symbolize-helps-achieving-prosperity-life-business-d-illustration-image181848135.

Suszycki, Michal. "Professionalism leads to success, attracts achievements and progress - this abstract idea and relation pictured as two objects, magnet attracting a ball, labelled with English words, 3D illustration." Dreamstime. Accessed 2nd August 2021. URL: https://www.dreamstime.com/professionalism-leads-to-success-attracts-achievements-progress-abstract-idea-relation-pictured-as-two-objects-magnet-image164603639.

The Journal of the American Medical Association." The Surgery of the Heart". JAMA 83, no. 20 (November 1924): 1590-1591. doi:10.1001/jama.1924.02660200042014

The Reel Newsletter. "Communication/Persuasion". 9 February 2010. URL: https://thereelteamnewsletter.wordpress.com/2010/02/09/communicationpersuasion/.

Tushatuvango. "Focus on details concept. three arrows hit in blue target." CanStockPhoto. Accessed 2nd August 2021. URL: https://www.canstockphoto.com/focus-on-details-concept-hit-target-19427057.html.

# CHAPTER 28

# FOSTERING GENDER DIVERSITY IN SURGICAL TRAINING

MAHIM MALIK AND JENNIFER LAWTON

"We cannot succeed when half of us are held back."
—Malala Yousafzai

## Introduction

Gender inequality remains a pervasive problem in Pakistan's workforce, where women account for only 24% of the country's labour force, receiving a mere 18% of the country's labour income. These disparities increase along the ladder to leadership, with only 5% of senior leadership positions being held by women.

Over the last two decades, the number of women in medical schools has reached parity globally, and in the case of Pakistan, has become a significant majority (Lautenberger, Dandar and Raezer 2014; Zakaria 2013). Data published by the Pakistan Medical Council (formerly known as Pakistan Medical and Dental Council) in 2017 shows that despite a large majority of female medical students (over 70%), only 48% of the registered physicians are women, with a staggeringly lower number (30%) registered as specialists (Pakistan Council for Science & Technology 2017). In the field of surgery and its surgical sub-specialties, female representation remains subpar. The College of Physicians and Surgeons of Pakistan (CPSP) lists 327 women out of 2,319 (14%) fellows who have completed surgical and surgical subspecialty training in Pakistan since 1967 (Malik et al. 2020). While these numbers have improved in Pakistan and globally, much work needs to be done until gender equity is reached. This undoubtedly benefits society as a whole, and has been identified as one of the United Nation's Sustainable Developmental Goals. Evidence from other sectors has shown that gender diversity in organizations results in better decision-making and in achieving better outcomes (Badal and Harter 2014; Nishii 2013). In the particular context of medicine, gender disparity has been shown to be negatively associated with patient outcomes (Greenwood, Carnahan and Huang 2018; Tsugawa 2017).

A number of areas require urgent attention. While holding a majority in medical schools, the number of women in surgical training programmes continues to lag behind. The absence of women in senior academic positions is striking, and even more impactful since academic leaders play an instrumental role in shaping the futures of aspiring surgeons. Research has shown that working conditions need to be improved to cater for gender-specific needs for women, such as pregnancy and lactation. Changing paradigms have brought increasing focus on parenthood and attaining a work-life balance in surgeons' lives, and this needs to be incorporated in surgical training programmes.

To strive towards gender parity, we must develop a better understanding of gender-specific barriers. In this chapter, we will examine and study these barriers in surgical training while discussing possible strategies to overcome these challenges, in the specific context of lower-middle-income countries (LMICs).

## Start early: medical students entering surgery

### Are we reaping what we sow?

A considerable demographic shift in the field of medicine has occurred and continues to manifest, as more women enter medical schools. In fact, in Pakistani medical schools, women have been in the majority since the last decade. However, the corresponding increase in the field of surgery, and surgical subspecialties in particular, is still sluggish. According to publically available data, women form only 4.5% of professors in the field of surgery (Figure 28-1).

According to the data available from CPSP, only 30% of currently enrolled surgical trainees are women. Western literature has shown similar results, with women accounting for 10-39% of the trainee population (Borman 2007; McAleese 2013; Shemin and Ikonomidis 2012). Also interesting to note is that while the women in general surgery training are increasing, in surgical subspecialties, particularly orthopaedic surgery, cardiothoracic surgery, and neurosurgery, they continue to lag behind significantly (Myers et al. 2018; O'Connor 2016; Renfrow et al. 2018;

Shemin and Ikonomidis 2012). Additionally, there has been a recent global trend of fewer medical students wishing to pursue a surgical career (Al-Heeti et al. 2012; Are et al. 2017). This growing lack of interest in surgery, compounded with the gender gap, will have profound consequences, particularly in LMICs that already face a significant shortage in terms of the available surgical workforce (Dall et al. 2015; Siddiqi et al. 2020). These statistics cannot be explained by preference of specialty alone, but rather a host of multiple social and systemic factors that have been shown to deter women from pursuing surgical careers (Inam et al. 2020; Larsen 2019).

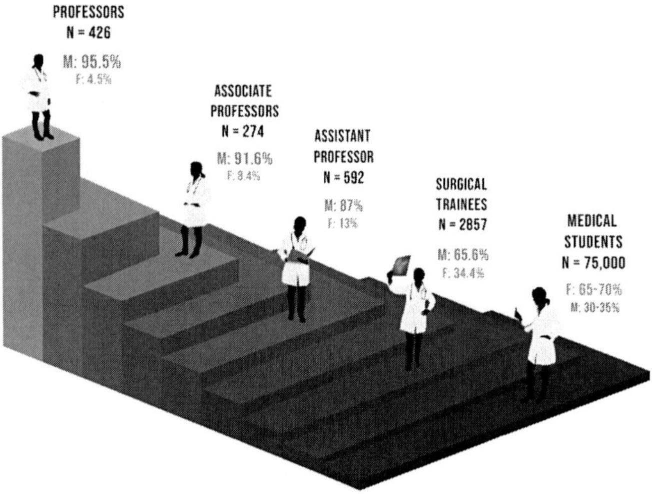


Figure 28-1: Female representation in surgery in Pakistan (data collected from PMC and CPSP website and direct communication with universities). *See centrefold for this image in colour.*

Medical school education is a critical period and experiences during that time have been shown to impact multiple facets in young physicians' lives. During this time, medical students interact with current practitioners, get involved in clinical activities, and understand the lifestyle implications of various subspecialties. Extra-curricular activities, finding mentors, and witnessing or being involved in negative experiences, have all been shown to have a critical impact on choosing a career (Cronin et al. 2019; Stratton 2005). Thereof, it is of critical importance that interest in these fields needs to be nurtured at an early stage, forming the premise of devising interventions that help to sustain this interest and encourage women to pursue their goals.

## Mentorship and role models

Effective mentoring is a key contributor to academic and career success, and results in increased overall productivity. Mentoring relationships have been shown to help in recruiting and retaining students from groups in under-represented STEM (science, technology, engineering and math) fields (Brown II, Davis and McClendon 1999; Eby 2008; Hund et al. 2018), and reduce stress, anxiety and depression amongst students (Levecque et al. 2017; Panger and Janell 2014). A study by Cochran and colleagues (2005) showed that identification of a surgical mentor correlated significantly with medical students' choice to pursue a career in surgery (Cochran, Melby and Neumayer 2005). Conversely, studies have shown that women are more likely to perceive lack of mentors as a barrier to career success (Sanfey, Hollands and Gantt 2013; Zhuge et al. 2013). Similarly, a recent qualitative study aimed to understand the roles of gender and mentoring in choosing and continuing a surgical education (Bettis et al. 2019). This study demonstrated that while it was not important to receive mentoring *by* a woman to have a successful surgical career, it was important to *see* a female surgeon role model (Bettis et al. 2019). This belies the importance and the influence of recent social media movements such as #ilooklikeasurgeon and #youcantbewhatyoucantsee. Additionally, this study also highlighted that women were more comfortable with discussing lifestyle, personal and child-related issues with other women (Bettis et al. 2019). Another important factor is the mentorship provided by surgical trainees, who have more interaction with students and are directly able to influence medical students' perceptions of surgical training. Based on these studies and the large corpus of literature we make the following recommendations:

1. Medical schools should maintain and circulate names and panels of surgeons, with women surgeons in particular, who are willing to address medical students to provide career advice. Formal visiting lectures should be arranged to provide information and opportunities to discuss gender-specific subjects.
2. Formal information sessions should be established for medical students interested in surgical training with both male and female trainees to discuss lifestyle, work hours, and other issues.
3. Develop surgical interest groups and surgical clubs that encourage first and second year medical students to become members.

### Exposure to surgical subspecialties

As mentioned earlier, the proportion of women in surgical subspecialties remains critically low, particularly in the fields of orthopaedic surgery, cardiothoracic surgery and neurosurgery. As students decide on these careers early in medical school or even before, it is of critical importance that interest in these fields needs to be fostered early. Studies in these male-dominated fields have shown that there is limited exposure in the preclinical years, and early exposure may increase interest (Baldwin et al. 2011; Foote et al. 2017), provided through literature, lectures and shadowing. Interventional outreach programmes in these fields, such as summer research or internship programmes may also increase interest and the likelihood of applying for a residency. We therefore make the following recommendations:

1. Increase promotion of postgraduate programmes to medical students, highlighting training and career progression opportunities.
2. Develop and offer nationwide outreach programs for students to gain exposure in these fields across institutions, such as summer research programmes and elective rotations.
3. Create surgery clubs or interest groups for first and second year medical students.

### Clinical rotations experience

The importance of clinical clerkships in students' intentions to pursue surgical careers has been well studied and established (Cochran, Paukert and Neumayer 2003; Hagopian et al. 2015; Schmidt, Cooper and Guo 2016). Students who have had early and positive exposures during medical school are more likely to pursue surgical careers, while negative experiences serve as deterrents. Additionally, more practical exposure to the realities of a surgical career, including integration with the clinical team through electives, student-selected modules and apprenticeships should be developed. Surgical clerkships must be designed to foster these interests and not primarily to serve as presenting only the difficult aspects of a surgical career.

### Deciding on a career in surgery

Choosing a specialty is a complex process that may be influenced by multiple factors. Studies in other countries have shown considerable variations, identifying gender, prestige and income as influencing factors

(Deutsch et al. 2013; Enoch et al. 2013; Puertas, Arosquipa and Gutierrez 2013). Undoubtedly, perceived gender discrimination plays a major role in shaping these decisions. Although the experience of gender discrimination is not unique to surgical specialties (Ku et al. 2011), several surveys have shown that the perception of gender bias is frequently reported during surgical experiences and has been shown to decrease interest in the pursuit of further surgical training (Gargiulo, Hyman and Hebert 2006; Sanfey et al. 2006). Therefore, it is important to target gender discrimination not only to protect trainees but also to ensure the future of surgical training.

An important factor that has been shown to influence career choice is verbal discouragement experienced by medical students. Significantly more women report being discouraged by peers than males and appear to be more susceptible to this discouragement. Larsen and colleagues (2019), like others, reported that the majority of the discouragement was based on family aspirations. While achievement of work-life balance and lifestyle choices is now equally important to both genders, women students have shown a higher level of concern regarding ability of find time to have children, spend time with family and take maternal leave (Inam et al. 2020; Janjua et al. 2020; Larsen et al. 2019; Sanfey et al. 2006). To counteract these issues, we suggest the following:

1. Additional and explicit support must be offered to medical students and trainees regarding parental leave and family life so as to mitigate these fears.
2. Clear institutional policies regarding parental leave and options for child support must be developed and shared with medical students early on during clerkships.
3. Herein, the role of mentors and role models again becomes extremely important to demonstrate and help with balancing work and family life.
4. Support nationwide surgical career information sessions with medical students interested in a career in surgery so they have an opportunity to meet male and female trainees at various stages of their careers.

**Table 28-1: Summary of recommendations. Adapted from the Royal College of Surgeons of Ireland Working group guidelines.**

| **Area of focus** | **Recommendations** | **What does success look like?** |
|---|---|---|
| Undergraduate interest in surgical and surgical subspecialties<br><br>Role modelling and mentorship<br><br>Clinical clerkship experience<br><br>Early exposure to surgery during medical school<br><br>Intent to apply for residency in surgical specialties | 1.1.1 Medical schools should maintain and circulate names and panel of surgeons willing to provide mentorship<br><br>1.1.2 Invite both male and female surgeons to provide information and opportunities to discuss gender specific subjects<br><br>1.2.1 Arrange Information sessions with surgical trainees to discuss lifestyle, working hours, and other issues<br><br>1.2.2 Provide explicit and additional support to medical students regarding parental leave and family related issues<br><br>1.2.3 Clear institutional policies regarding parental leave and options for child support must be developed and shared with medical students early on during clerkships.<br><br>1.3 Encourage early exposure by developing surgical interest groups and clubs and open membership to 1st and 2nd year medical students | An increase in the overall numbers and gender parity of direct and graduate entry medical students applying for surgical training.<br>Reduction in perceived barriers for female medical students considering a career in surgery. |

## The next step: where are the women in surgical training?

In Pakistan, despite being the majority in medical schools, women comprise only 34% of trainees in general surgery and are significantly underrepresented in surgical subspecialties. Multiple factors can be attributed to these numbers, but the issues seem to be at both ends of the pipeline: fewer women are attracted to surgical careers and a higher percentage of women leave surgical training prior to completion (Forel et al. 2018; Walsh and Meyer 2011). Quantitative studies attempting to elucidate the contributing factors have identified a number of possibilities: insufficient female role models, lack of institutional support, gender discrimination and harassment (Khoushhal et al. 2017), pregnancy and child-bearing (Cochran et al. 2013), and child-rearing duties (Dyrbye et al. 2011). Several studies from the West have suggested a higher dropout of women from surgical training programmes (27% versus 17%) (Bergen, Turnage and Carrico 1998; Yeo et al. 2010), which is mirrored in developing countries (Nadeem, Effendi and Ather 2014). Herein, we will examine factors behind attrition of women trainees in surgical programmes and strategies to increase retention.

### The counter-culture: building a culture that supports female trainees

While it is important to encourage more women to enter surgical training, we should also be asking ourselves what needs to be done to make the workplace a more equitable, hospitable place where women would *want* to work. Encouraging women to enter surgery is not enough if the workplace actively excludes or discriminates against them.

The surgical workplace has long been identified as a "boys' club" in spite of the recent "feminization of medicine." Qualitative studies exploring why women leave surgical training have identified misogynistic attitudes and sexism as a major contributing factor (Liang, Dornan and Nestel 2019). While overt gender discrimination has become uncommon and unacceptable, women continue to face implicit or unconscious bias, impacting career satisfaction, selection of specialty and leading, attrition and burnout (Janjua et al. 2020; Park et al. 2005). Such behaviour and so-called "micro aggressions," start early on from medical school and are pervasive throughout surgical training (Barnes et al. 2019). During training, women are often faced with inappropriate comments and behaviours. The perpetrators range from peers, to mentors, to patients. Comments about their appearances, mannerisms and conduct are frequent and make women uncomfortable and feel inadequate. However, any objections are brushed off as women being too "touchy," or patients' comments being innocent or harmless. Frequently, women physicians are mistaken for nurses and not given the kind of respect that their position demands. Prior research has indicated that gender stereotypes depress the professional performance of women (Schmader, Johns and Forbes 2008). A recently published study by Myers and colleagues (2020) demonstrated this via a well-designed randomized control trial, eloquently concluding that

> "[N]egative stereotypes about women and pro-male gender bias affect career engagement and technical performance among individuals pursuing careers in academic surgery."

Based on the vast body of literature and experiences of women surgical trainees, we recommend the following steps to promote a culture of change:

1. Hospitals need to take a tougher stance on misogynistic attitudes and behaviours. Zero-tolerance policies need to be developed and any observed or reported behaviour should not be ignored. As suggested by Mello and Jagsi (2020), sexual discrimination should be recognized as an ethical issue that doctors should have an obligation to object. This should also include patients, who if observed making such comments, should be called out for it.
2. In situations of sexual harassment, the perpetrator should be held criminally responsible, as if they had harassed someone outside the hospital.
3. Like in the corporate world, hospitals and organizations need to take active steps to improve awareness of sexist language and behaviour. What is deemed acceptable and what is not should be clearly defined and reporting of harassment should be actively encouraged. Training can occur through guest lectures by experts in grand rounds, focus groups, and interactive lectures.
4. Active engagement programmes by organizations (as in the United Kingdom and the United States of America [Michigan Medicine, University of Michigan 2021; Royal College of Surgeons of England 2021]) to counter misconceptions about women surgeons, should be set up. A recently established organization in Pakistan, Association of Women Surgeons of Pakistan (Figure 28-2), aims to set up such programmes in institutions to educate and improve awareness.

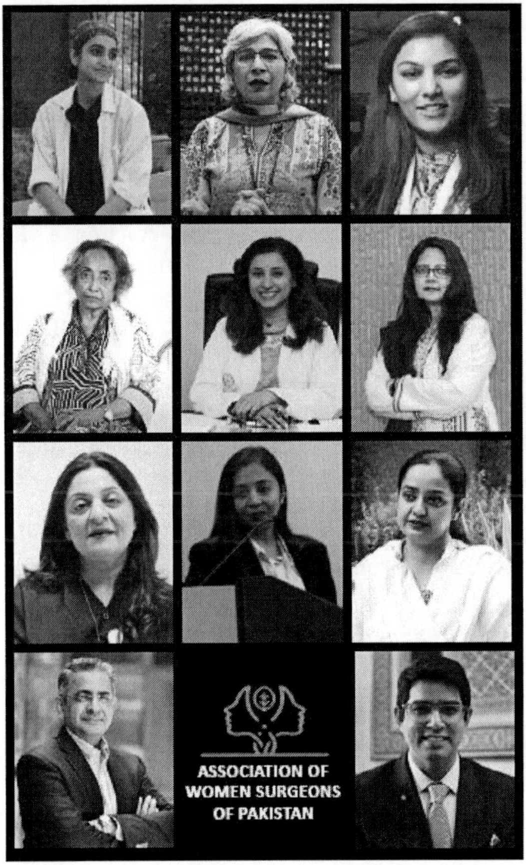


Figure 28-2: Members of the Association of Women Surgeons of Pakistan (established in 2019). *See centrefold for this image in colour.*

Top row (left to right): Dr Hina Inam (Treasurer), Dr Sadaf Khan (President), Dr Mahim A. Malik (General Secretary); second row from top (left to right): Dr Shaista Khan, Dr Aneela Darbar, Dr Nuzhat Faruqui (Founding Members); third row from top (left to right): Dr Sharmeen Akram, Dr Sajida Qureshi, Dr Abida Sattar (Founding Members); and bottom row (left to right): Dr Ather Enam, Chair Department of Surgery AKUH, Pakistan (Patron), and Dr Adil H. Haider, Dean, Medical College, AKU, Pakistan (Patron).

## Impact of the surgical lifestyle: family life, pregnancy and child rearing during training

Surgeons of both genders are growing to expect a balance between their personal and professional lives, with increasing importance placed upon lifestyle and family life. Additionally, women are attaching more importance to lifestyle considerations including prolonged working hours, work-life balance, and quality of patient interactions. Multiple studies have shown that lifestyle factors play a significant role in choosing to embark upon or quit a career, and surgical careers are not always considered compatible with a healthy work-life balance (Grigg, Arora and Diwan 2014; Park et al. 2005). In the past women were more likely to delay having children until after their residency (Troppmann et al. 2009), but more are choosing to have children earlier (Turner et al. 2012). Studies of residents in general surgery and other surgical specialties have shown that women faced bias from their surgical programmes regarding having children during training (Todd, Cawthorn and Temple-Oberle 2020). An alarmingly high number of residents continued with unmodified schedules until birth, despite the concerns for their own and foetal well-being (Mulcahey et al. 2019; Rangel et al. 2018). These fears are not unfounded, since studies suggest that complications of pregnancy occur with higher frequencies in surgical residents (Todd, Cawthorn and Temple-Oberle 2020). Additionally, a survey of general surgery programme directors in the USA found that more than 60% believed that motherhood adversely affects a trainee's work (Sandler et al. 2016). Moreover, difficulties faced by pregnant residents place them at high risk for attrition, and also jeopardize their role as positive role models for younger residents and students.

Persistent gender stereotypes and gender schema place women with the primary responsibility for child-rearing and family care. Despite being in dual-professional relationships, studies have shown that household responsibilities fall primarily on women (Baptiste 2017; Dyrbye et al. 2011). Particularly in patriarchal social settings more common in the developing world, these stereotypes become more pronounced, placing additional pressure on women trainees (Inam et al. 2020; Malik et al. 2020).

An interesting analogue to the problem of women leaving surgical careers proposed by Liang and colleagues (2019) is a tower of blocks (Figure 28-3), where each block represents a factor contributing to the decision to leave, and the toppling of the tower represents the decision to leave (Liang, Dornan and Nestel 2019).

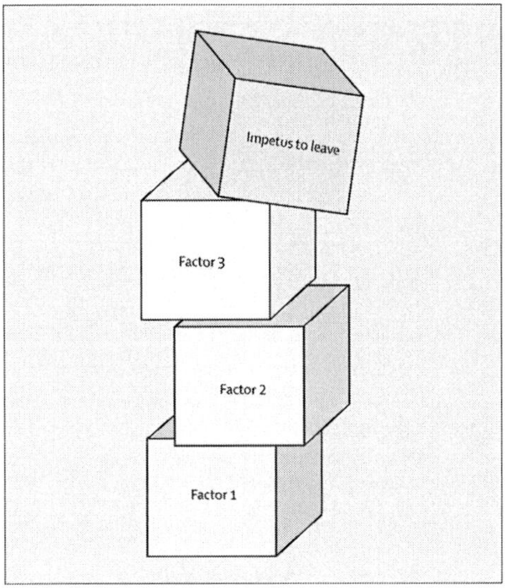


Figure 28-3: Lancet tower of blocks.

This emphasizes the need to move beyond single factor interventions and work in a more complex, multi-dimensional and contextual manner to improve retention of women in the academic surgical profession. While the contributing factors might differ according to context and need local research for better elucidation, the approach of single factor intervention is going to be partially effective at best. Evidence suggests that women might be better served by interventions that do not focus solely on so-called "*female factors*" and gender. In fact, amplification of gender differences may inhibit male mentorship and socialization, perpetuating the exclusion of women from the traditional structures of surgery.

In conclusion, women leave surgery for reasons that are complex, intersectional and contextual. Interventions need to be designed keeping social contexts in mind and should address multiple factors. Institutions need to be alert to the possibility of unplanned negative effects, and not focus unduly on gender. When discussing support of women trainees, attention needs to not only be focused on provision of childcare, but also take a more feminist view, where women are not just trying to fit into an institution created by men, but one that has embedded gender-congruent roles.

**Table 28-2.1: Recommendations adapted from a Royal College of Surgeons of Ireland (RCSI) gender equality report and RCSI working group guidelines.**

| **Area of focus** | **Recommendations** | **What does success look like?** |
|---|---|---|
| Build a culture that supports female surgical trainees. | 2.1 Institutions should ensure gender neutrality in their training processes and standard operating procedures<br><br>2.2 A governing body should ensure trained mentors are available for all trainees, including both male & female surgeons, and encourage trainees to avail of a network of mentors<br><br>2.3 The governing body should report annually on the rate of progression of training programme alumni to surgical training fellowships and to consultant posts by gender and practice settings<br><br>2.4 The governing body should work with stakeholders, including PGME for each institution, to improve surgical training fellowship options for female surgeons<br><br>2.5 Work with residency programmes to develop part time training options, while mapping out clearly the effect of these options on training duration<br><br>2.6 Active engagement with organizations such as AWSP, WINS and AWS to counter misconceptions about women surgeons | • Trainees receive the information and support they need to have a good training experience<br>• Male and female trainees have equal opportunities to do high quality surgical training fellowships<br>• Male and female alumni are equally likely to be appointed consultants<br>• Decrease in overall attrition of residents<br>• Increase in female trainees in surgical subspecialties |

**Table 28-2.2: Recommendations, continued: adapted from an RCSI gender equality report and RCSI working group guidelines.**

| Area of focus | Recommendations | What does success look like? |
|---|---|---|
| Combat and prevent gender discrimination and bias | 2.6 Institutions should develop clear zero tolerance policies towards gender discrimination and bias and ensure their implementation<br><br>2.7 Develop and maintain a system that supports safe disclosure by trainees without fear of repercussion<br><br>2.8 Hospitals and organizations will institute mandatory training to promote awareness about sexist behaviour and implicit gender bias<br><br>2.9 A national training body should track whether training programmes on gender appropriate behaviour are conducted at institutions | • Female trainees feel safe and protected in the environment<br>• Formal feedback from graduating trainees regarding their experience with gender related issues during training<br>• Institutions and hospitals develop systems that follow up and track outcomes of complaints of inappropriate behaviour |

| | | |
|---|---|---|
| Consider the needs of trainees who are parents | • Protected time for research and study: ensure all trainees receive information required to protect pregnant trainees, especially as it relates to exposure to radiation and other potential hazards including on-call duties, shift length and working conditions (e.g., prolonged standing)<br>• Develop recommendations and SOPs regarding training contacts during and after pregnancy and will standardize back-to-work reintegration for trainees returning from a period of leave through development of SOPs applying to all specialties | • Pregnant trainees will receive information, support and advice in a consistent way<br>• Policies in relation to periods of leave for surgical trainees will be consistent and will support trainees in returning to work after such periods<br>• Adequate notice of future post allocations to enable trainees to combine their career with their personal and family responsibilities<br>• Trainees have the information they require to have a healthy pregnancy and experience<br>• Trainees on career leave are treated consistently and receive the support they require to recommence their career upon completion of their leave |

## Setting an example: fix the broken pipeline

Though the number of women in surgical training continues to increase, their rise through institutional hierarchy remains a daunting process. By recent estimates of publicly available data, less than 5% of professors of surgery in Pakistan are women. The number of women in academic leadership in the West is not much different, with a study by the Association of Women Surgeons predicting that not until 2136, will half of all professors of surgery be women. Although many early career surgeons desire a career in academia, the rate of attrition remains high. In fact, it was estimated in 2000 that women at the assistant professor level were almost six times more likely than their male colleagues to intend to leave academia within two years (Colletti, Mulholland and Sonnad 2000). A wait of 115 years to reach gender parity in leadership is indeed too long a time, underscoring the importance of addressing the issue now.

Perceived barriers to career advancement can lead to dissatisfaction and burnout, impeding career development. Several studies have examined these perceived barriers, which differ between various stages of a woman surgeons' career as it progresses from medical school to residency to early faculty positions. It remains of utmost importance to recognize that there are contextual risks at each stage that need to be understood and managed intersectionally. This is particularly important since these women at every stage are role models to aspiring surgeons and may play a significant role in shaping the emerging surgical workforce.

**Role models and mentoring**

As mentioned in earlier sections, appropriate role models and mentors continue to play a significant role in the early career years of young surgeons. A lack of role models affects both genders at this stage, although for men it appears to be due to a generational divide, whereas for women it is likely due to a paucity of female role models in leadership roles (Bickel and Brown 2005; Cochran et al. 2013). A study by Schroen and colleagues (2004) showed that women tend to believe that inadequate mentoring was an impetus for attrition and led to feelings of isolation (Schroen, Brownstein and Sheldon 2004). Central to the concept of mentoring is "the ability to network," which is an important component of the retention and promotion of junior faculty. While residents in many programmes may have formally assigned mentors or seek out mentors in their field of interest, academic programmes rarely have structured programmes for junior faculty. Additionally, the nature of certain practice models may not be conducive to accessing senior faculty members who may serve as effective role models.

**Gender discrimination**

Previous research has shown that there is an increase in perception of gender discrimination among female faculty when compared to residents (Bruce et al. 2015; Cochran et al. 2013). A study by Janjua and colleagues (2020) reported similar rates of gender discrimination in Pakistan, ranging from 16.1% in medical school to almost 43% during practice (Janjua et al. 2020). One possible cause for this may be the perpetuation of implicit bias and unspoken gender norms within academia, which goes unrecognized during training years. Or perhaps, on a more optimistic note, this may represent an actual improvement in culture that has lessened these experiences for residents. Even so, these experiences have been shown to have an impact on job satisfaction and negatively impact patient care (Malik et al. 2020). This may also make women faculty less likely to encourage aspiring surgeons to pursue careers in academic surgery.

**The gender salary gap**

Women have a long-standing history of receiving unequal pay for equal work, which has been slow to reverse inspite of labour protection laws being passed. Women surgeons, on average, make 8% less than their male counterparts when adjusted for age, rank, specialty, and other metrics for clinical and academic productivity (Ash et al. 2004; Jena, Olenski and Blumenthal 2016). Evidence shows that this disparity begins on entry into the workforce and widens over time, with women making about 82% of what their males colleagues make after the age of 35 (Sanfey et al. 2017). Several theories have been proposed to explain this pay gap. Men may be more proactive than women in seeking offers and counter offers, thereby driving up their salaries at the onset. Employers may leverage the fact that women are less likely to negotiate as an excuse to offer lesser salaries. Additionally, cultural stereotypes continue to characterize women as deficient in "agentic" traits, which in turn promotes the assumption that women are less competent and less likely to succeed in leadership roles. This becomes a self-fulfilling prophecy where women feel that they constantly have to do more to prove themselves and get rated consistently lower by evaluators (Engineering, Committee on Maximizing the Potential of Women in Academic Science 2007; Hamel et al. 2006).

Based on the above and further evidence, the Association of Women Surgeons developed a set of recommendations, which have been modified to our context below:

- Identify the policies, procedures, leadership, and culture that promote equity in some specialties in order to determine best practices and remedy the disparity that exists in surgery.
- Encourage department and institutional policies that promote transparency in defining the criteria for initial and subsequent physician salaries.
- Establish programmes to empower women to understand their worth and negotiate appropriately. These should be extended to

residents and medical students so that essential negotiation skills are fostered early in training.
- Provide implicit bias training for all department chairs, deans, search committees, and private practice employers. This would increase awareness of how subtle differences exist in the evaluation of male and female candidates.
- Increase efforts to promote women into senior leadership positions.
- Evaluate the organizational culture to promote equal access to opportunities and resources, value work-life balance for both men and women, and create a supportive environment.

## Conclusion

While women have reached parity in medical schools and more women are entering the field of surgery, there still remains a significant gender gap, especially in surgical subspecialties. Women trainees represent an at-risk population for attrition from residencies, and need a multifactorial approach to encourage retention. Women remain underrepresented in academia and are slow to progress through the academic ranks. They remain vulnerable to both explicit and implicit bias, which has far-reaching implications. Organizational culture needs to be examined in terms of how men and women are treated differently. A multifactorial approach needs to be developed and implemented at every level so as to counteract these effects and provide an environment that is equitable to both men and women.

## Bibliography

Al-Heeti, Khalaf N. M., Aussama K. Nassar, Kara DeCorby, Joanne Winch, and Susan Reid. "The Effect of General Surgery Clerkship Rotation on the Attitude of Medical Students towards General Surgery as a Future Career." *Journal of surgical education* 69, no. 4 (July-August 2012): 544-49. DOI: 10.1016/j.jsurg.2012.04.005.

Are, Chandrakanth, Hugh Stoddard, Lauren A. Carpenter, Brigid O'Holleran, and Jon S. Thompson. "Trends in the Match Rate and Composition of Candidates Matching into Categorical General Surgery Residency Positions in the United States." *The American Journal of Surgery* 213, no. 1 (January 2017): 187-94. DOI: 10.1016/j.amjsurg.2016.03.015.

Ash, Arlene S., Phyllis L. Carr, Richard Goldstein, and Robert H. Friedman. "Compensation and Advancement of Women in Academic

Medicine: Is There Equity?" *Annals of internal medicine* 141, no. 3 (August 2004): 205-12. DOI: 10.7326/0003-4819-141-3-200408030-00009.

Badal, Sangeeta, and James K. Harter. "Gender Diversity, Business-Unit Engagement, and Performance." *Journal of Leadership & Organizational Studies* 21, no. 4 (September 2014): 354-65. DOI: https://doi.org/10.1177/1548051813504460.

Baldwin, Keith, Surena Namdari, Andrea Bowers, Mary Ann Keenan, L. Scott Levin, and Jaimo Ahn. "Factors Affecting Interest in Orthopedics among Female Medical Students: A Prospective Analysis." *Orthopedics* 34, no. 12 (December 2011): e919-e32. DOI: 10.3928/01477447-20111021-17.

Baptiste, Dadrie, Alison M. Fecher, Scott C. Dolejs, Joseph Yoder, C. Maximillian Schmidt, Marion E. Couch, and DuyKhanh P. Ceppa. "Gender Differences in Academic Surgery, Work-Life Balance, and Satisfaction." *Journal of Surgical Research* 218 (October 2017): 99-107. DOI: 10.1016/j.jss.2017.05.075.

Barnes, K. Lauren, Lauren McGuire, Gena Dunivan, Andrew L. Sussman, and Rohini McKee. "Gender Bias Experiences of Female Surgical Trainees." *Journal of Surgical Education* 76, no. 6 (November-December 2019): e1-e14. DOI: 10.1016/j.jsurg.2019.07.024.

Bergen, Patricia C., Richard H. Turnage, and C. James Carrico. "Gender-Related Attrition in a General Surgery Training Program." *Journal of Surgical Research* 77, no. 1 (June 1998): 59-62. DOI: 10.1006/jsre.1998.5335.

Bettis, Jessica, Carol R. Thrush, Rachel L. Slotcavage, Krista Stephenson, Erika Petersen, and Mary Katherine Kimbrough. "What Makes Them Different? An Exploration of Mentoring for Female Faculty, Residents, and Medical Students Pursuing a Career in Surgery." *The American Journal of Surgery* 218, no. 4 (October 2019): 767-71. DOI: 10.1016/j.amjsurg.2019.07.029.

Bickel, Janet, and Ann J. Brown. "Generation X: Implications for Faculty Recruitment and Development in Academic Health Centers." *Academic Medicine* 80, no. 3 (March 2005): 205-10. DOI: 10.1097/00001888-200503000-00003.

Borman, Karen R. "Gender Issues in Surgical Training: From Minority to Mainstream." *The American Surgeon* 73, no. 2 (February 2007): 161. DOI: https://doi.org/10.1177/000313480707300215.

Brown II, M. Christopher, Guy L. Davis, and Shederick A. McClendon. "Mentoring Graduate Students of Color: Myths, Models, and Modes." *Peabody Journal of Education* 74, no. 2 (July 1999): 105-18. DOI:

https://doi.org/10.1207/s15327930pje7402_9.
Bruce, Adrienne N., Alexis Battista, Michael W. Plankey, Lynt B. Johnson, and M. Blair Marshall. "Perceptions of Gender-Based Discrimination during Surgical Training and Practice." *Medical education online* 20, no. 1 (February 2015): 25923. DOI: 10.3402/meo.v20.25923.
Cochran, Amalia, Spencer Melby, and Leigh A. Neumayer. "An Internet-Based Survey of Factors Influencing Medical Student Selection of a General Surgery Career." *The American journal of surgery* 189, no. 6 (June 2005): 742-46. DOI: 10.1016/j.amjsurg.2005.03.019.
Cochran, Amalia, Judy L. Paukert, and Leigh A. Neumayer. "Does a General Surgery Clerkship Influence Student Perceptions of Surgeons and Surgical Careers?" *Surgery* 134, no. 2 (August 2003): 153-57. DOI: 10.1067/msy.2003.216.
Cochran, Amalia, Tricia Hauschild, William B. Elder, Leigh A. Neumayer, Karen J. Brasel, and Marie L. Crandall. "Perceived Gender-Based Barriers to Careers in Academic Surgery." *The American Journal of Surgery* 206, no. 2 (August 2013): 263-68. DOI: 10.1016/j.amjsurg.2012.07.044.
Cochran, Amalia, William B. Elder, Marie Crandall, Karen Brasel, Tricia Hauschild, and Leigh Neumayer. "Barriers to Advancement in Academic Surgery: Views of Senior Residents and Early Career Faculty." *The American Journal of Surgery* 206, no. 5 (November 2013): 661-66. DOI: 10.1016/j.amjsurg.2013.07.003.
Colletti, Lisa M., Michael W. Mulholland, and Seema S. Sonnad. "Perceived Obstacles to Career Success for Women in Academic Surgery." *Archives of surgery* 135, no. 8 (August 2000): 972-77. DOI: 10.1001/archsurg.135.8.972.
Cronin, Ciara, Mairi Lucas, Andrea McCarthy, Fiona Boland, Raghu Varadarajan, N. Premnath, and Peter Gillen. "Are We Reaping What We Sow? Gender Diversity in Surgery: A Survey of Medical Students." *Postgraduate medical journal* 95, no. 1121 (April 2019): 119-24. DOI: http://dx.doi.org/10.1136/postgradmedj-2018-136136.
Dall, Tim, Terry West, Ritashree Chakrabarti, William Iacobucci, and Peter Brunec. *The Complexities of Physician Supply and Demand: Projections from 2013 to 2025.* Washington DC: Association of American Medical Colleges, 2015.
DOI: 10.13140/RG.2.2.13111.57764.
Deutsch, Tobias, Petra Hönigschmid, Thomas Frese, and Hagen Sandholzer. "Early Community-Based Family Practice Elective Positively Influences Medical Students' Career Considerations–a Pre-Post-Comparison."

*BMC family practice* 14, no. 1 (February 2013): 24. DOI: 10.1186/1471-2296-14-24.

Dyrbye, Liselotte N., Tait D. Shanafelt, Charles M. Balch, Daniel Satele, Jeff Sloan, and Julie Freischlag. "Relationship between Work-Home Conflicts and Burnout among American Surgeons: A Comparison by Sex." *Archives of surgery* 146, no. 2 (February 2011): 211-17. DOI: https://doi.org/10.1001/archsurg.2010.310.

Eby, Lillian T., Tammy D. Allen, Sarah C. Evans, Thomas Ng, and David L. DuBois. "Does Mentoring Matter? A Multidisciplinary Meta-Analysis Comparing Mentored and Non-Mentored Individuals." *Journal of vocational behaviour* 72, no. 2 (April 2008): 254-67. DOI: 10.1016/j.jvb.2007.04.005.

Engineering, Committee on Maximizing the Potential of Women in Academic Science. *Beyond Bias and Barriers: Fulfilling the Potential of Women in Academic Science and Engineering.* Washington, DC: National Academies Press, 2007.

Enoch, Lindsey, John T. Chibnall, Debra L. Schindler, and Stuart J. Slavin. "Association of Medical Student Burnout with Residency Specialty Choice." *Medical education* 47, no. 2 (February 2013): 173-81. DOI: 10.1111/medu.12083.

Foote, Darci C., James M. Meza, Vikram Sood, and Rishindra M. Reddy. "Assessment of Female Medical Students' Interest in Careers in Cardiothoracic Surgery." *Journal of surgical education* 74, no. 5 (September-October 2017): 811-19. DOI: 10.1016/j.jsurg.2017.02.013.

Forel, Deanne, Meegan Vandepeer, Joanna Duncan, David R Tivey, and Stephen A. Tobin. "Leaving Surgical Training: Some of the Reasons Are in Surgery." *ANZ journal of surgery* 88, no. 5 (May 2018): 402-07. DOI: 10.1111/ans.14393.

Gargiulo, Debra A., Neil H. Hyman, and James C. Hebert. "Women in Surgery: Do We Really Understand the Deterrents?" *Archives of Surgery* 141, no. 4 (April 2006): 405-08. DOI: 10.1001/archsurg.141.4.405.

Greenwood, Brad N., Seth Carnahan, and Laura Huang. "Patient–Physician Gender Concordance and Increased Mortality among Female Heart Attack Patients." *Proceedings of the National Academy of Sciences* 115, no. 34 (August 2018): 8569-74. DOI: doi.org/10.1073/pnas.1800097115.

Grigg, Megan, Manit Arora, and Ashish D. Diwan. "Australian Medical Students and Their Choice of Surgery as a Career: A Review." *ANZ journal of surgery* 84, no. 9 (September 2014): 653-55. DOI: 10.1111/ans.12389.

Hagopian, Thomas M., Gerardo A. Vitiello, Alexandra M. Hart, Sebastian D. Perez, John F. Sweeney, and Barbara J. Pettitt. "Does the Amount of Time Medical Students Spend in the Operating Room During the General Surgery Core Clerkship Affect Their Career Decision?" *The American Journal of Surgery* 210, no. 1 (July 2015): 167-72. DOI: 10.1016/j.amjsurg.2014.10.031.

Hamel, Mary Beth, Julie R. Ingelfinger, Elizabeth Phimister, and Caren G. Solomon. "Women in Academic Medicine—Progress and Challenges." *N. Engl. J. Med.* 355, no. 3 (July 2006): 310-312. DOI: 10.1056/NEJMe068143.

Hund, Amanda K., Amber C. Churchill, Akasha M. Faist, Caroline A. Havrilla, Sierra M. Love Stowell, Helen F. McCreery, Julienne Ng, Cheryl A. Pinzone, and Elizabeth S. C. Scordato. "Transforming Mentorship in Stem by Training Scientists to Be Better Leaders." *Ecology and evolution* 8, no. 20 (October 2018): 9962-74. DOI: doi.org/10.1002/ece3.4527.

Inam, H., M. Janjua, R. S. Martins, N. Zahid, S. Khan, A. K. Sattar, A. Darbar, et al. "Cultural Barriers for Women in Surgery: How Thick Is the Glass Ceiling? An Analysis from a Low Middle-Income Country." [In eng]. *World J. Surg.* 44, no. 9 (September 2020): 2870-78. DOI: https://doi.org/10.1007/s00268-020-05544-9

Janjua, Mahin B., Hina Inam, Russell S. Martins, Nida Zahid, Abida K. Sattar, Shaista M. Khan, Sadaf Khan, et al. "Gender Discrimination against Female Surgeons: A Cross-Sectional Study in a Lower-Middle-Income Country." *Annals of Medicine and Surgery* 57 (September 2020): 157-62. DOI: https://doi.org/10.1016/j.amsu.2020.07.033.

Jena, Anupam B., Andrew R. Olenski, and Daniel M. Blumenthal. "Sex Differences in Physician Salary in Us Public Medical Schools." *JAMA internal medicine* 176, no. 9 (September 2016): 1294-304. DOI: 10.1001/jamainternmed.2016.3284.

Khoushhal, Zeyad, Mohamad A. Hussain, Elisa Greco, Muhammad Mamdani, Subodh Verma, Ori Rotstein, Andrea C. Tricco, and Mohammed Al-Omran. "Prevalence and Causes of Attrition among Surgical Residents: A Systematic Review and Meta-Analysis." *JAMA surgery* 152, no. 3 (March 2017): 265-72. DOI: 10.1001/jamasurg.2016.4086.

Ku, Manwai C., Yan E. Li, Charles Prober, Hannah Valantine, and Sabine C. Girod. "Decisions, Decisions: How Program Diversity Influences Residency Program Choice." *Journal of the American College of Surgeons* 213, no. 2 (August 2011): 294-305. DOI: 10.1016/j.jamcollsurg.2011.04.026.

Larsen, A. M. Giantini, Susan Pories, Sareh Parangi, and Faith C. Robertson. "Barriers to Pursuing a Career in Surgery: An Institutional Survey of Harvard Medical School Students." *Annals of Surgery* 9 (October 2019). DOI: 10.1097/SLA.0000000000003618.

Lautenberger, Diana M., Valerie M. Dandar, and Claudia L. Raezer. "The State of Women in Academic Medicine: The Pipeline and Pathways to Leadership," 2013-2014. Data and Reports: Association of American Medical Colleges, 2014.

Levecque, Katia, Frederik Anseel, Alain De Beuckelaer, Johan Van der Heyden, and Lydia Gisle. "Work Organization and Mental Health Problems in PhD Students." *Research Policy* 46, no. 4 (May 2017): 868-79. DOI: doi.org/10.1016/j.respol.2017.02.008.

Liang, Rhea, Tim Dornan, and Debra Nestel. "Why Do Women Leave Surgical Training? A Qualitative and Feminist Study." *The Lancet* 393, no. 10171 (February 2019): 541-49. DOI: doi.org/10.1016/S0140-6736(18)32612-6.

Malik, Mahim, Hina Inam, Mahin B. N. Janjua, Russell S. Martins, Nida Zahid, Sadaf Khan, Abida K Sattar, Adil H. Haider, and Syed Ather Enam. "Factors Affecting Women Surgeons' Careers in Low–Middle-Income Countries: An International Survey." *World Journal of Surgery* 45 (October 2020): 1-7. DOI: https://doi.org/10.1007/s00268-020-05811-9.

McAleese, Sara. "'The Humanisation' of Medicine? The Feminisation of Medicine: A Qualitative Study of the Career Experiences of Female Doctors and Implications for Human Resources Management in Ireland." Repository: Royal College of Surgeons in Ireland, 2013.

Mello, Michelle M., and Reshma Jagsi. "Standing up against Gender Bias and Harassment-a Matter of Professional Ethics." *The New England journal of medicine* 382, no. 15 (April 2020): 1385. DOI: 10.1056/NEJMp1915351.

Michigan Medicine, University of Michigan. "Michigan Women's Surgical Collaborative." Accessed January 14, 2021. URL: https://mwsc.med.umich.edu/.

Mulcahey, Mary K., Chelsea Nemeth, Jeffrey D. Trojan, and Mary I. O'Connor. "The Perception of Pregnancy and Parenthood among Female Orthopaedic Surgery Residents." *JAAOS-Journal of the American Academy of Orthopaedic Surgeons* 27, no. 14 (July 2019): 527-32. DOI: 10.5435/JAAOS-D-18-00216.

Myers, Sara P., Mohini Dasari, Joshua B. Brown, Stephanie T. Lumpkin, Matthew D. Neal, Kaleab Z. Abebe, Nicole Chaumont, et al. "Effects of Gender Bias and Stereotypes in Surgical Training: A Randomized Clinical Trial." *JAMA Surgery* 155, no. 7 (Jul 2020). 10.1001/jamasurg.2020.1127.

Myers, Sara P., Katherine A. Hill, Kristina J. Nicholson, Matthew D. Neal, Megan E. Hamm, Galen E. Switzer, Leslie R. M. Hausmann, et al. "A Qualitative Study of Gender Differences in the Experiences of General Surgery Trainees." *Journal of Surgical Research* 228 (August 2018): 127-34. DOI: 10.1016/j.jss.2018.02.043.

Nadeem, Mehwash, M. Shahrukh Effendi, and M. Hammad Ather. "Attrition in Surgical Residency Programmes: Causes and Effects." *Arab journal of urology* 12, no. 1 (March 2014): 25-29. DOI: 10.1016/j.aju.2013.07.002.

Nishii, Lisa H. "The Benefits of Climate for Inclusion for Gender-Diverse Groups." *Academy of Management Journal* 56, no. 6 (October 2013): 1754-74. DOI: doi.org/10.5465/amj.2009.0823.

O'Connor, Mary I. "Medical School Experiences Shape Women Students' Interest in Orthopaedic Surgery." *Clinical Orthopaedics and Related Research®* 474, no. 9 (September 2016): 1967-72. DOI: 10.1007/s11999-016-4830-3.

Pakistan Council for Science & Technology. "Women in Health." December 31, 2017. Accessed February 10, 2021. URL: http://pcst.org.pk/wst/wst_whea.php.

Park, Jason, Sam Minor, Rebecca Anne Taylor, Elena Vikis, and Dan Poenaru. "Why Are Women Deterred from General Surgery Training?" *The American Journal of Surgery* 190, no. 1 (July 2005): 141-46. DOI: 10.1016/j.amjsurg.2005.04.008.

Panger, Galen, and T. Janell. *Graduate Student Happiness & Well-Being Report*. Berkeley, CA: Graduate Assembly, University of California Berkeley, 2014. Accessed February 10, 2021. URL: ga.berkeley.edu/wellbeingreport.

Puertas, E. Benjamín, Carlos Arósquipa, and Daniela Gutiérrez. "Factors That Influence a Career Choice in Primary Care among Medical Students from High-, Middle-, and Low-Income Countries: A Systematic Review." *Revista Panamericana de Salud Pública* 34, no. 5 (November 2013): 351-58. URL: https://scielosp.org/pdf/rpsp/v34n5/a08v34n5.pdf.

Rangel, Erika L., Douglas S. Smink, Manuel Castillo-Angeles, Gifty Kwakye, Marguerite Changala, Adil H. Haider, and Gerard M. Doherty. "Pregnancy and Motherhood during Surgical Training." *JAMA surgery* 153, no. 7 (July 2018): 644-52. DOI: 10.1001/jamasurg.2018.0153.

Renfrow, Jaclyn J., Analiz Rodriguez, Taylor A. Wilson, Isabelle M. Germano, Aviva Abosch, and Stacey Quintero Wolfe. "Tracking Career Paths of Women in Neurosurgery." *Neurosurgery* 82, no. 4 (April 2018): 576-82. DOI: 10.1093/neuros/nyx251.

Royal College of Surgeons of England. "Women in Surgery (Wins)." Accessed January 14, 2021. URL: https://www.rcseng.ac.uk/careers-in-surgery/trainees/foundation-and-core-trainees/women-in-surgery/.

Sandler, Britt J., John J. Tackett, Walter E. Longo, and Peter S. Yoo. "Pregnancy and Parenthood among Surgery Residents: Results of the First Nationwide Survey of General Surgery Residency Program Directors." *Journal of the American College of Surgeons* 222, no. 6 (June 2016): 1090-96. DOI: 10.1016/j.jamcollsurg.2015.12.004.

Sanfey, Hilary, Celeste Hollands, and Nancy L. Gantt. "Strategies for Building an Effective Mentoring Relationship." *The American Journal of Surgery* 206, no. 5 (November 2013): 714-18. DOI: 10.1016/j.amjsurg.2013.08.001.

Sanfey, Hilary A., Alison R. Saalwachter-Schulman, Joyce M. Nyhof-Young, Ben Eidelson, and Barry D. Mann. "Influences on Medical Student Career Choice: Gender or Generation?" *Archives of surgery* 141, no. 11 (Nov 2006): 1086-94. 10.1001/archsurg.141.11.1086.

Sanfey, Hilary, Marie Crandall, Elizabeth Shaughnessy, Sharon L. Stein, Amalia Cochran, Sareh Parangi, and Christine Laronga. "Strategies for Identifying and Closing the Gender Salary Gap in Surgery." *Journal of the American College of Surgeons* 225, no. 2 (August 2017): 333-38. DOI: https://doi.org/10.1016/j.jamcollsurg.2017.03.018.

Schmader, Toni, Michael Johns, and Chad Forbes. "An Integrated Process Model of Stereotype Threat Effects on Performance." *Psychological review* 115, no. 2 (April 2008): 336. DOI: 10.1037/0033-295X.115.2.336.

Schmidt, Lauren E., Clairice A. Cooper, and Weidun Alan Guo. "Factors Influencing US Medical Students' Decision to Pursue Surgery." *Journal of Surgical Research* 203, no. 1 (June 2016): 64-74. DOI: doi.org/10.1016/j.jss.2016.03.054.

Schroen, Anneke T., Michelle R. Brownstein, and George F. Sheldon. "Women in Academic General Surgery." *Academic Medicine* 79, no. 4 (April 2004): 310-18. DOI: 10.1097/00001888-200404000-00006.

Shemin, Richard J., and John S. Ikonomidis. "Thoracic Surgery Workforce: Report of Sts/Aats Thoracic Surgery Practice and Access Task Force—Snapshot 2010." *The Journal of Thoracic and Cardiovascular Surgery* 143, no. 1 (January 2012): 39-46. e6. DOI: 10.1016/j.athoracsur.2011.10.036.

Siddiqi, S., M. S. Khan, N. Rizvi, I. Naeem, S. Rozi, A. Enam, and S. Khan. "Are Rural Hospitals in Pakistan Responding to the Global Surgery Movement? An Analysis of the Gaps, Challenges and Opportunities." [In eng]. *World J. Surg.* 44, no. 4 (April 2020): 1045-52. DOI: https://doi.org/10.1007/s00268-019-05327-x.

Stratton, Terry D., Margaret A. McLaughlin, Florence M. Witte, Sue E. Fosson, and Lois Margaret Nora. "Does Students' Exposure to Gender Discrimination and Sexual Harassment in Medical School Affect Specialty Choice and Residency Program Selection?" *Academic Medicine* 80, no. 4 (April 2005): 400-08. DOI: 10.1097/00001888-200504000-00020.

Todd, A. R., T. R. Cawthorn and Claire Temple-Oberle. "Pregnancy and Parenthood Remain Challenging During Surgical Residency: A Systematic Review." *Acad. Med.* 95, no. 10 (October 2020): 1607-1615. DOI: 10.1097/ACM.0000000000003351.

Troppmann, Kathrin M., Bryan E. Palis, James E. Goodnight, Hung S. Ho, and Christoph Troppmann. "Women Surgeons in the New Millennium." *Archives of Surgery* 144, no. 7 (July 2009): 635-42. DOI: 10.1001/archsurg.2009.120.

Tsugawa, Yusuke, Anupam B. Jena, Jose F. Figueroa, E. John Orav, Daniel M. Blumenthal, and Ashish K. Jha. "Comparison of Hospital Mortality and Readmission Rates for Medicare Patients Treated by Male Vs Female Physicians." *JAMA internal medicine* 177, no. 2 (February 2017): 206-13. DOI: 10.1001/jamainternmed.2016.7875.

Turner, Patricia L., Kimberly Lumpkins, Joel Gabre, Maggie J. Lin, Xinggang Liu, and Michael Terrin. "Pregnancy among Women Surgeons: Trends over Time." *Archives of surgery* 147, no. 5 (May 2012): 474-79. DOI: 10.1001/archsurg.2011.1693.

Walsh, U., and F. J. Meyer. "Awareness and Impact of Wins on Female Surgical Trainees." *The Bulletin of the Royal College of Surgeons of England* 93, no. 3 (March 2011): 1-5. DOI: https://doi.org/10.1308/147363511X558155.

Yeo, Heather, Emily Bucholz, Julie Ann Sosa, Leslie Curry, Frank R. Lewis Jr, Andrew T. Jones, Kate Viola, Zhenqui Lin, and Richard H. Bell Jr. "A National Study of Attrition in General Surgery Training: Which Residents Leave and Where Do They Go?" *Annals of Surgery* 252, no. 3 (September 2010): 529-36. DOI: 10.1097/SLA.0b013e3181f2789c.

Zakaria, Rafia. "The Doctor Brides." *Dawn*, 2013. Accessed February 10, 2021. URL: https://www.dawn.com/news/1032070.

Zhuge, Ying, Joyce Kaufman, Diane M. Simeone, Herbert Chen, and Omaida C. Velazquez. "Is There Still a Glass Ceiling for Women in Academic Surgery?" *Annals of Surgery* 253, no. 4 (April 2011): 637-43. DOI: 10.1097/SLA.0b013e3182111120.

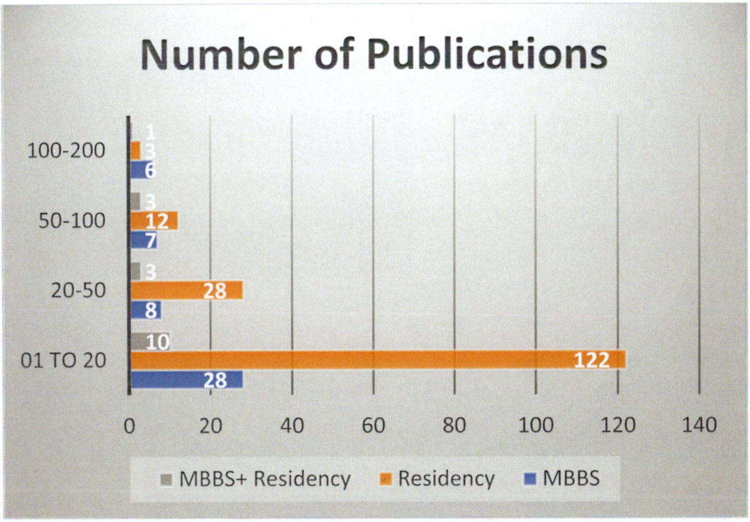


Figure 26.1: Number of publications in research and medical sciences by AKU alumni.

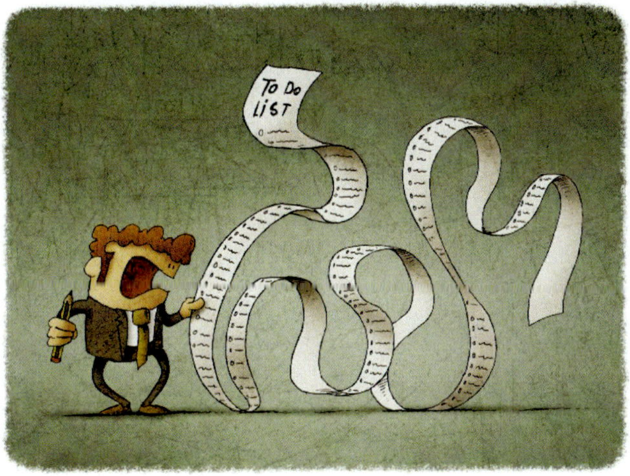


Fig. 27-1: Checklist (Casas 2021).

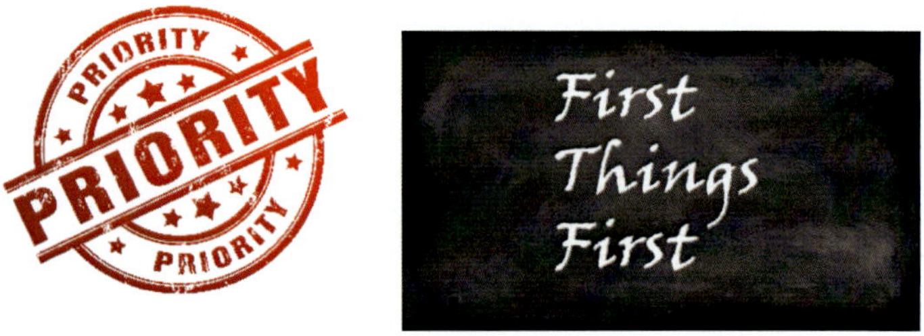


Fig. 27-2: Prioritize (Mstan 2021).

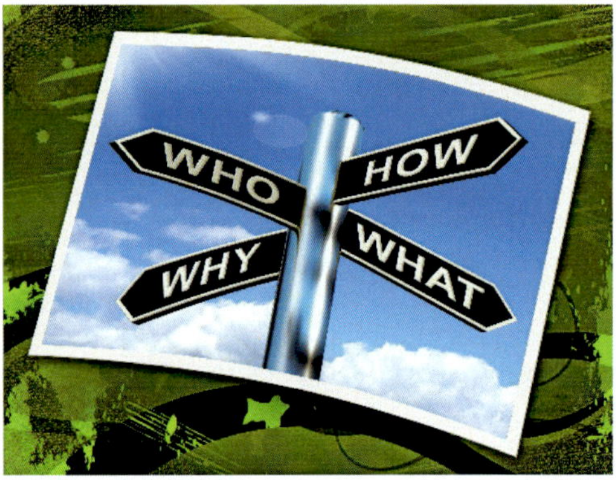


Fig. 27-4: Get to know (Miles 2021).

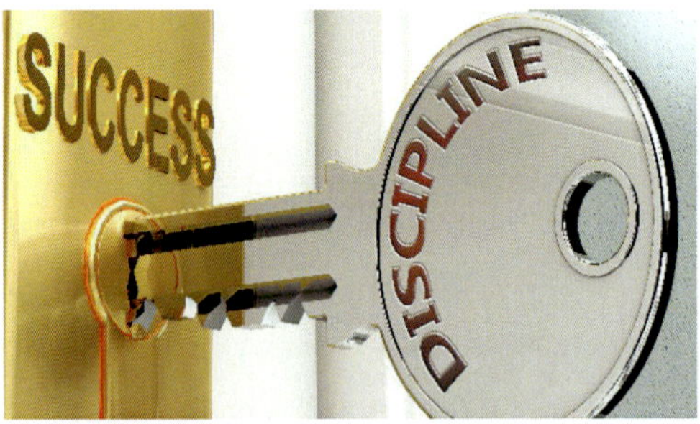


Fig. 27-6: Discipline leads to success (Suszycki 2021).

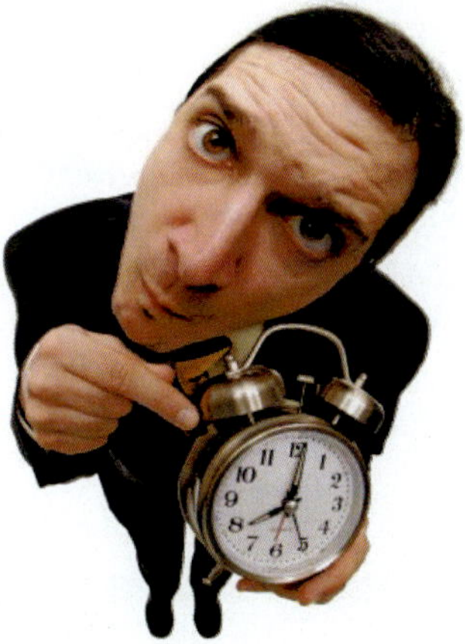

Fig. 27-7: Strategic time management is crucial for success (Image from website, "Everyone a Leader" 2013).

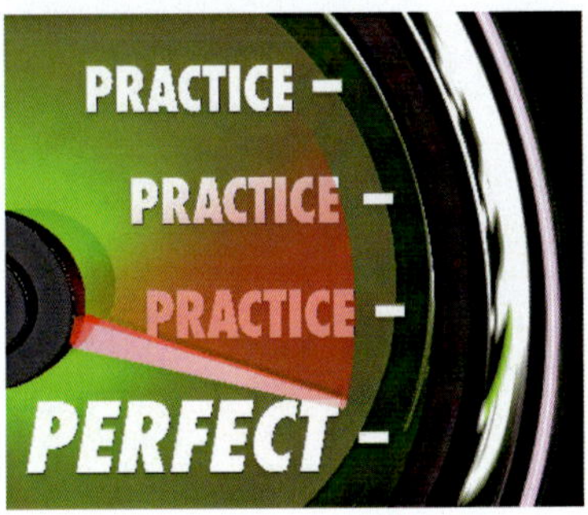


Fig. 27-8: Practice makes one perfect (Iqoncept 2021).

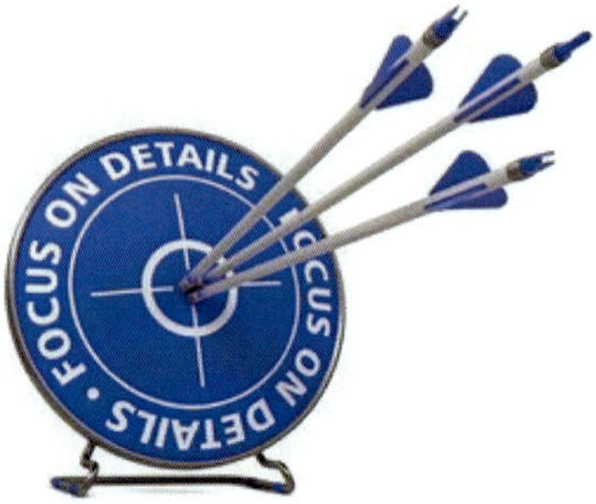


Fig. 27-9: Attention to details (Tushatuvango 2021).

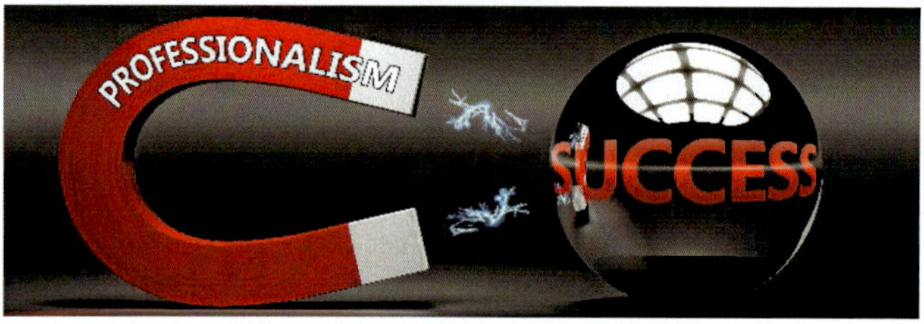


Fig. 27-10: Professionalism attracts success (Suszycki 2021).

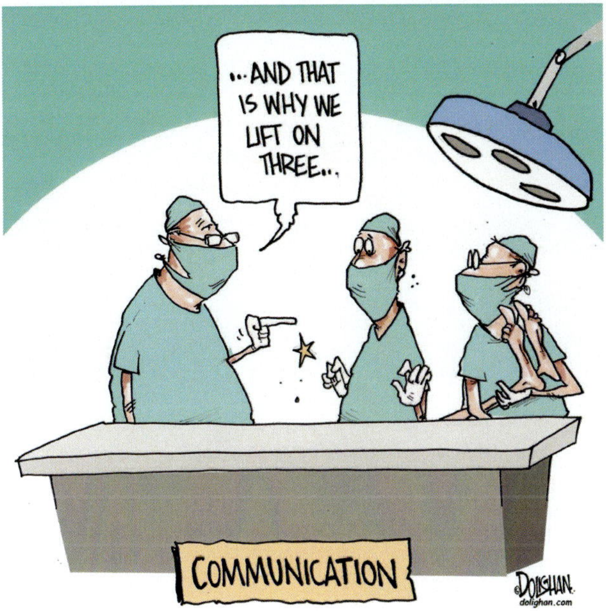


Fig. 27-12: Communication (The Reel Newsletter 2010).

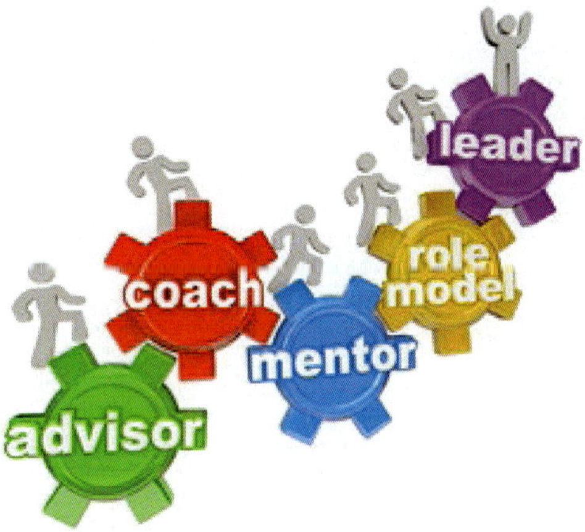


Fig. 27-13: Mentors (Iqoncept 2021).

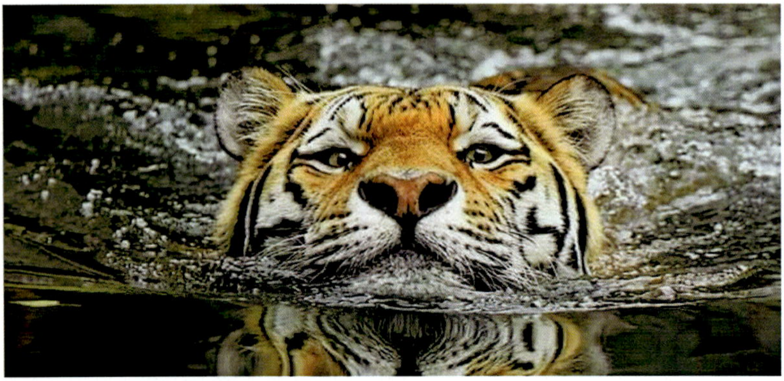

Fig. 27-15: Keep your head above the water (Blah 2020). *See centrefold for this image in colour.*

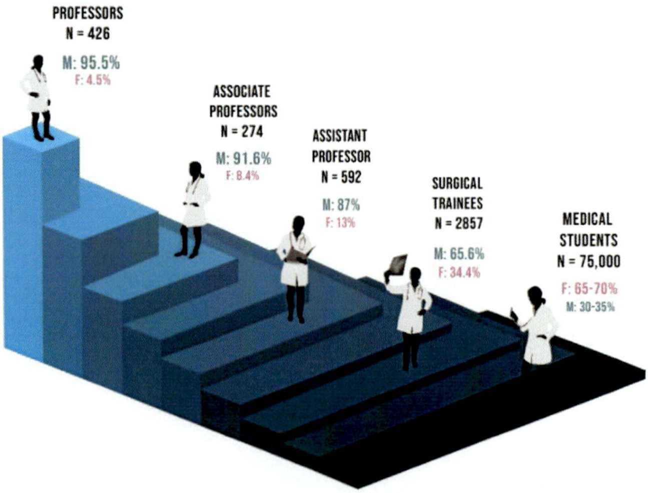


Figure 28-1: Female representation in surgery in Pakistan (data collected from PMC and CPSP website and direct communication with universities).

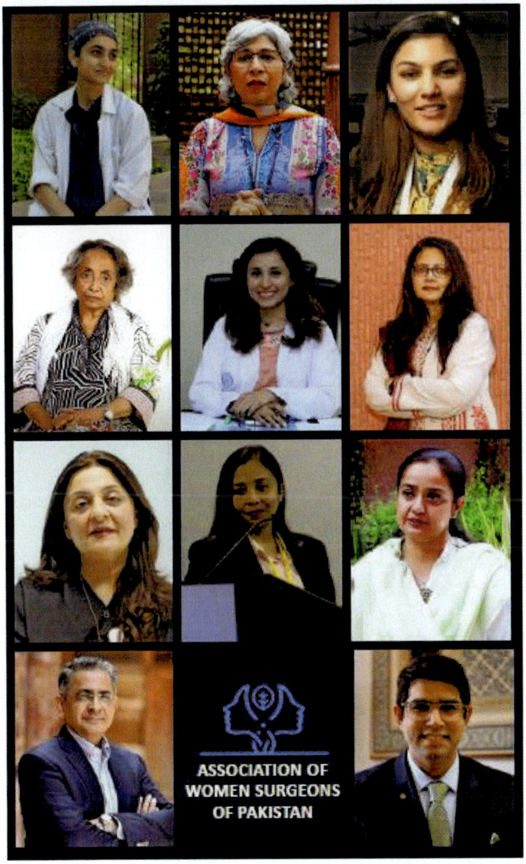


Figure 28-2: Members of the Association of Women Surgeons of Pakistan (established in 2019).

# CHAPTER 29

# THE NEW NORMAL

MUNAWAR SHAH, NIKHIL A KHADABADI,
DANIAL SHAH AND KISHEN PAREKH

We live in an age where modern phones are easily accessible to all. Many students are now using social media platforms which are slowly gaining recognition in medical learning. A large number of medical students are now labelled as the Net Generation (Kennedy, Gray and Tse 2008). They may not be experts, but are exposed to it and apply it in various walks of life. The modern student has an earlier and more vigorous exposure to the digital world and leans to use them increasingly. This is the same all over, irrespective whether one lives in an urban and well developed environment or in remote and less developed parts of the world.

Education is becoming cheaper and more accessible by e-learning. Today's students are very different than from the past when the net was not easily accessible in education in general and medical education in particular. E-learning platforms are now freely put to great use by schools and universities around the world. It encompasses video tutorials, audio-visual learning and virtual modules. The new use of media possesses superiority over long established gold standard education norms. It provides live update in real time. This method has been shown to be as successful as traditional methods, and is a great instrument in promoting self-learning. It stimulates students to control their learning by allowing flexibility. Teachers can assess projects and provide personalized feedback online.

In a survey long before COVID times, 234 students filled in an anonymous questionnaire. 80% were utilising the internet to complete projects and educate themselves in medical sciences, 60% of students were using social media platforms more than once during a single day (Dar et al. 2017). E-learning would have evolved eventually as time progressed and would have had a major influence in education. The COVID times have exaggerated this role and it has, as a result, evolved exponentially. 1992 was the landmark year where web based education took shape (Chumley-Jones, Dobbie and Alford 2002). This first appeared as computer-assisted instructions. The experts proposed computer-assisted instruction was better than text books, lecture and traditional methods as there was customised control by the recipient over when and where to access learning along with some form of control in self-learning (Chumley-Jones, Dobbie and Alford 2002).

I have personal experience of dissemination of education through media based tools since 2015. I have used Whatsapp application to successfully train and teach students of the Fellow of the College of Physicians & Surgeons (FCPS) exam in Pakistan. I have also introduced Zoom based webinars since 2017 in Pakistan, on education in sports injuries with a group of trainers who are UK based. I have also used Zoom to do live video teaching for exams and various current topics including a surgeon's response to the COVID Pandemic. This was a combination of my wanting to teach and give back to my country, combined with the fact that I was located in a different location; so electronic media based education was a happy middle. With the on-going COVID Pandemic, term "The New Normal" has come to be recognised. It cannot be more applicable to deliver medical education, in a more acceptable way. (The New Normal)

There is opportunity in adversity, as quoted by Benjamin Franklin. The new normal is an amazing chain of events and circumstances for the development of surgical sciences. As COVID-19 creates havoc, education has evolved, and compelled us into thinking out of the box and adapting teaching techniques to further surgical education and training. Surgical placements play vital in transferring skills to student's perusing a surgical career. This has been largely affected, as medical schools have stopped their students from all clinical placements, as part of social distancing to stop viral transmission. This situation has further compounded already diminished time devoted to surgical training within the medical syllabus and thus has hindered surgical education.

In the environment of decreased volume trying to limit COVID-19 infection there has been an unprecedented reorganising of surgical teaching over the past year. Social distancing measures have disrupted traditional ways of teaching which earlier mandated congregation of trainees. A recent study carried out in the UK, using an electronic survey to assess the effect of COVID-19 on cardiothoracic surgical training, noted that 78% of trainees noticed decreased exposure in the surgical theatre, with 88% showing concerns about the detrimental effect on their training and 71% felt that they may need special measures such as more time in training (Caruana et al. 2020).

There is now the opportunity to think out of the box and look into overhauling methods of providing surgical education. There has been an explosion in the amount of didactic content available for training. Virtual platforms have been implemented widely which has helped create new frontiers not considered possible before the COVID-19 Pandemic (Villamizar and Nguyen 2020). Use of telemedicine and virtual reality software provides a trainee real time experience, which can augment surgical training. In the current environment it may be a way out but as the COVID-19 Pandemic restrictions ease, this can be used to provide additional mode of training and surgical experience. It is a well-known fact surgical acumen can only be consolidated in the surgical theatre (Greenfield et al. 2018).

In spite of efforts made to streamline training in difficult times, there has been increasing concern about decreased hands on training among program directors and trainees. Shafi and colleagues (2020) in their study noted that not only the volume of surgical procedures during the Pandemic was low; the trainee being first surgeon was also drastically reduced (Shafi et al. 2020). To address these detrimental effects due to paucity of procedures, clinical encounter needs to be utilised to its fullest, and robust assessment tools made available to highlight where change is needed.

It may take a while before case volumes increase to the levels that preceded the COVID times. Till it happens, a robust plan must be in place to maximize the training experience of the trainees to make available the right environment to feel comfortable about their skills, to start independent work at the completion of their residency, as well as provide them with the desired knowledge at their stage of career.

## Electronic media in teaching

Computer- and phone-based technologies have facilitated teaching via electronic media providing availability to case based video data, virtual reality surgical room simulations, and other interactive surgical programmes. These platforms are freely on hand and have the resources to fulfill the training requirement of surgical trainees as set out in their curriculum. A variety of virtual reality video based interaction programmes and apps have been used. Those which have a wide variety inclusive are Zoom, Whatsapp, Microsoft Skype, Microsoft Teams, and Cisco based web application. Virtual education via electronic media has shown to be more than viable alternatives and has evolved, augmented, adapted and adopted by almost all organisations for virtual education.

## Social media

Social media by definition is a highly interactive digital platform that allows users to produce and share a wide range of content via virtual communities and networks.

It is a very powerful tool in this modern day and age for providing various aspects of robust surgical learning due to its fluidity, ease of use universal availability, affordability, immense popularity and worldwide audience, and feeling of being involved. These provide platform for trainees for discussion of topics of interest, enable sharing of knowledge and allow them to collaborate on research projects. It enables sharing of educational video banks, articles and books making them easily accessible and engaging. Use of social media as a teaching and training platform has its own limitations which include dissemination of non- peer reviewed materials, interaction with non-negotiable pre-set knowledge within a closed environment, selective display of information due to applied filters on devices and difficulty in differentiating valid information due to questionable source (Johannsson and Selak 2020; Pariser 2012). They also lack the credibility and structure to robustly organise a structured educational programme. Numerous measures have been advocated to address these limitations, including use of established professional forums, clear identification of information source and declaration of conflicts of interest (Chan et al. 2020). One must not forget that the impact medical students and trainees can have on the public at large via the social media and they should use this medium to not only influence the behaviour of the public in a positive way but at the same time educate them.

**Table 29-1: Social media groups and examples in surgery**

| Group | Definition | Examples |
|---|---|---|
| Blogs and microblogs | Informational website where the author shares his or her opinion and experiences with possibility to share images, videos and polls | RCS England JCST |
| Social networking site | Online platform which people use to build social networks or social relationships with other people who share similar personal or career interests, activities, backgrounds or connections | Facebook Twitter Whatsapp Telegram |
| Employment based social networking site | An online platform that focuses on building employment based networks or relations. | LinkedIn |
| Smartphone/tablet apps | Computer program designed specifically for handheld hardware, using features such as Navigation, touchscreen and Magnetometer | Touch Surgery BMJ app NEJM image app |
| Podcast and video cast | Digitally recorded material that can be downloaded or streamed by users in the form audio and video files | BOA Podcasts Websurg AIS Channel |

## Virtual learning

Before the COVID-19 Pandemic virtual learning was gradually creeping into educational methods, creating blended learning (traditional and e-learning combined), as trainees are becoming more in control of their learning. Lindeman and Colleagues (2015) in their study comparing blended online curriculum and traditional curriculum observed significantly improved student satisfaction and non-inferior academic outcomes with blended online curriculum (Hew and Lo 2018). Due to the Pandemic, the integration of e-learning in surgical training has exploded in a good way, thus diminishing the impact of COVID-19 on knowledge deficit (Lindeman et al. 2015). Surgical field is inundated with web based information that is always produced for the requirement of students and trainees. Virtual learning platforms are increasingly being used to maximize virtual learning. These platforms not only impart clinical skills but also help in developing making decisions and help students prepare for their clerkships to further enhance their surgical experience.

There are, at the present time, more than 20 virtual platforms, for over nine surgical specialties resources online and can be accessed from home. Example of one such interactive platform is Aquifer-Wise MD, which provides walkthroughs in surgical procedures, surgical anatomy reviews, mock assessment quizzes and case based assessment and discussions (Ehrlich, McKenney and Elkbuli 2020). Hangout, provided by American College of Surgeons, is another virtual learning platform which provides virtual lectures, study modules, and educational virtual data for trainees to follow along each week (American College of Surgeons 2021). Vargo and colleagues have used virtual learning effectively to create a structured framework with the use of online platforms to provide educational activity for each day of the week, which included discussing updates in urology, virtual journal clubs, virtual guest lectures, cases discussions and review of textbooks (Vargo et al. 2020).

Though virtual learning helps in familiarizing residents in the surgical procedures, it cannot help in fulfilling the surgical quotas, nor does it help a trainee completely immerse in the surgical specialty. In current times, virtual learning continues to provide nonstop ever accessible interactive medium for online materials to augment surgical learning. Also, virtual education provides means to improve surgical education by making resources easily accessible and is not a substitute of gold standard teaching. Taking the roll out of COVID-19 vaccine as an example, enough financing was redirected to provide the finished article in record times. I feel education progress will be no different and all teachers will combine to embrace and develop out of the box methods for learning and teaching. The virtual education and training has improved exponentially and made easily accessible, hence should be endorsed, embraced and made part of training and try to keep pace with the ever changing and improving methodology and resources.

## Virtual exam preparations

We are experiencing new and somewhat unusual methods, which are progressive and adaptive in education and knowledge transfer in the COVID-19 Pandemic, which were certainly not seen before in the recent past. There has been profound disruption of in-person educational activities with a massive switch to virtual platforms. There have been cancelling and rescheduling of in-person didactics and examination. Preparation for exams is now commonly done online in small groups who convene in virtual team settings. Mock in-person oral examinations have been used traditionally to prepare medical students and surgical trainees.

Teaching activities such as lectures and grand rounds have made smooth transition on to the virtual platform. Shebrain and colleagues (2020) have demonstrated virtual mock oral examinations as viable and a more than acceptable substitute for face to face mock viva examination for American Board of Surgery certifying exam (Shebrain et al. 2020). In reality virtual assessments have shown benefits in transfer to home and familiar environment. Some can argue that it results in prolonged isolation, over use of social media, and sometimes it is difficult to define boundaries, thus affecting students in particular and supporting staff and educators in general (Rose 2020).

## Virtual assessments

The Pandemic has created many new challenges for assessment of surgical education and training. Assessment of projects, learning and understanding of course work are at the forefront and a conundrum. They have been swiftly adapted to be accessed online. There are many positives of online teaching over gold standard forms of assessment, where in it enables the provision of continuous and real-time feedback, and it can be presented at the convenience of the teacher and student and at a place of choosing (Cantillon, Irish and Sales 2004). A second, and no less vital feature, that is evolving is that e-assessment will start to avail maximum benefit and even outgrow what current technology offers. For example, it will enable learners to listen to heart murmurs, look at clinical investigations or access a clinical scenario online and then use the multimedia resources to answer questions (Dennick, Wilkinson and Purcell 2009; Walsh, Rafiq and Hall 2007).

Many surgical training programs are now adopting virtual assessments with virtual interviews, including the Royal College of Surgeons England. The traditional in-person interviews are put on hold for the current unprecedented COVID times.

Virtual e-assessment is now developed and streamlined to conduct oral table assessment and virtual clinical examinations with the examiner assessing and scoring from the comfort of his home or office. In traditional exams, there is an overhead for designated assessment halls; printed paper, accommodation and travel which are surplus for this setup (Lewiss et al. 2014). In the recent past e-assessment used to take place in separate learning rooms with computer aids. However, the Pandemic has forced the assessment to be conducted within the confines of one's personal space with strict regulations. This has helped with significant savings as a result (Walsh 2015).

Evidence to compare cost effectiveness in virtual training and gold standard face to face teaching is sparse. In summary it can be said that, like online learning, online assessment will help reduce overhead cost in printing. However, for it to work secure and reliable software needs to be utilised and that will have its own overhead cost (Fawcett and Oldfield 2016). The very real shortcomings of virtual assessment would be assessing technical and surgical operative skills. A major drawback for such an undertaking would be the major initial setup cost and dependency on technology. In times of Pandemic, virtual assessments supplement all other forms of assessment. However, the reality is, very little evidence is available to support validity of self-assessment and their limitations are for all to see (Walsh ed. 2010). Virtual assessment is still in its infancy as time moves on this ultimately will be the mainstay of assessments. Currently, virtual assessment is mainly utilised to assess applied knowledge; however, the days to incorporate simulated clinical skills virtually are not far.

## Webinars

The norm of the time is to organise or attend webinars and make it easily accessible. They are one such example which is well suited to impart knowledge to a widely distributed and international cohort of students. There are many applications available which are available to all with new platforms being developed and promoted effortlessly. Zoom (San Jose, California) already present has evolved leap and bounds and is way ahead of its contemporary software in these difficult times.

Microsoft Teams, the flag bearer of Microsoft, is now one of the main medium used in the National Health Service (NHS) and many other allied national institutions. They usually work in the following way in which after registration, students are sent a link via e mail and access can be gained via clicking the link. This allows the tutor to see which participants have signed in. A key advantage of webinar is that it lends itself to interaction and dialogue by exchange of messages which have known to make these more interactive and enjoyable (Walsh et al. 2010). Messages can be exchanged allowing one to ask questions on these forums, concurrently listening to the tutors. These also allow the syllabus to be saved and shared. The content is then available online for all so it can be used regularly and repeatedly. This further allows students and trainees to use the information to revise, save for future use and to go into virtual breakout rooms to discuss and develop further. This also helps to enhance ones presenting skills by sharing with peers and non-peers.

These sessions are of tremendous benefits to international students, whose first language is not the same as the presenting language, by allowing them to listen repeatedly to recorded videos which are made available after the completion of live webinars. Besides being accessible to wide cohort of students, these allow large number of participants to partake in these meetings (Fonseka et al. 2020; Jeong et al. 2020). The real benefit of this system of education is it is easily and freely available and can be stored and used repeatedly and is accessible from the comfort of one's personal environment and at their convenience and time of choosing.

## Virtual specialty meetings

With the pandemic taking a turn for the worse, social distancing was recommended and many conferences were called off. Many considerations were made to postponing numerous conferences to next year. As fear dawned into reality, many organisations realised that next year might be no different. With many applications and software available like Zoom, Teams and many more in the pipeline being made available to us in the future, the meetings were converted to virtual conferences. This was the light bulb moment in education and distance learning, with education becoming more easily accessible between the first world and third world, and there was no limitation to where we could take it. The organisers made available openly accessible educational platforms for all (Ma and Vervoort 2020; Vervoort et al. 2020).

The norm has been to plan meetings in advance, organise finances and try to fit it into study leave and work commitment, then to make arrangements to travel and find a suitable accommodation especially into high profile speciality meetings. It was even more cumbersome for trainees who were keen to attend but due to the meetings being held in different parts of the world, and also with them being in different stages of their career, it was difficult for one to attend. Virtual meetings have totally changed the dynamics of these meetings, with now anyone having access to such privileged meetings at short notice with very little rejigging of life and work commitments. It has also made it possible for the previously under represented group to be now present, network and speak up.

The scaling of virtual conferences will support more efficient training of surgeons in third world underprivileged countries where there is hard work and talent in abundance, but limitation of training and resources and access to new evidence. This amazing change will set a new precedence and will be healthy for making education easily and freely at nominal cost available to all. Many annual surgical meetings have taken place virtually during the Pandemic including British Elbow and Shoulder Society and annual British Orthopaedic Association conference. Some of the important lessons learned from these conferences are summarised in the table below (Table 29-2).

**Table 29-2: Lessons learned from virtual conferences in the COVID-19 Pandemic**

| | |
|---|---|
| Whole Audience Participation | Online chat boxes enable increased interaction compared to reduced participation due to absence of limiting factors such as constrained time limits and social stigmas |
| Scaling of Medical Education | Wider access of content to participants all across the world by using platforms with high volume access |
| Research Presentations | Provide opportunity for research work to be presented both in the form Papers and e posters with wider dissemination of information |
| Streamline Networking | Individual profiles can be created allowing information to be readily available about oneself on discussion forums |
| Innovation and Industry Immersion | Easy navigation among stalls in possible virtually |
| Social Media and Data Analytics | Evolving role of social media in discussions and connectivity complementing conferences is noted Also data collection about participation, demographics and engagement is easier. |

Virtual meetings are fraught with numerous limitations with foremost concern being that they are impersonal with mere text based interaction. Issues due to connectivity and technological shortcomings have forced many such meetings to adapt a recorded route. Interaction with presenters is via merely through the chat boxes and feels quite remote and distant compared to live in-person discussions. These platforms also lack a common networking area, such as a lobby, which is one of the major incentives in attending a conference for many for career progression, job opportunities and to broaden knowledge. The ultimate answer would be a fusion of both virtual and live conferences thus complementing shortcomings of one another.

## What the future holds?

The pandemic has resulted in a fundamental change in approach or underlying assumptions in the methodology of training. The tried and tested ''see one, do one, teach one'' is for ever changing and adapting to the present needs (Gillinov et al. 2016). We have learnt and evolved very quickly to utilise what is available and overcome obstacles from this crisis. Training has evolved and changed into a more efficient, adaptable method and process for training tomorrow's surgeon.

Virtual modalities for training and education will not substitute the conventional ways completely but ways to incorporate them into the gold standard methods need to be devised in order to promote a hybrid approach. It is absolutely vital that the educators adapt from this experience and implement an educated, open minded approach and think outside the box. We would like to conclude by stating that the environment and available resources has forced the current training program to evolve in a short space of time offering robust, scalable, authentic, and auditable solutions to the decision makers and institutions. Necessary steps need to be taken to incorporate evolving advancements to usher in a new era of virtual digital education.

## Bibliography

American College of Surgeons. "RAS-ACS Hangouts". Accessed January 17, 2021. URL: www.facs.org/memberservices/ras/hangout#covid.

Cantillon, P, B Irish and D Sales. "Using computers for assessment in medicine". *BMJ* 329, no. 7466 (September 2004): 606-9. DOI: 10.1136/bmj.329.7466.606.

Caruana E J, A Patel, S Kendall and S Rathinam. "Impact of coronavirus 2019 (COVID-19) on training and well-being in subspecialty surgery: a national survey of cardiothoracic trainees in the United Kingdom". *J Thorac Cardiovasc Surg*. 160, no. 4 (October 2020): 980-987. DOI: https:// doi.org/10.1016/j.jtcvs.2020.05.052.

Chan, A K M, C P Nickson, J W Rudolph, A Lee and G M Joynt. "Social media for rapid knowledge dissemination: early experience from the COVID-19 pandemic". *Anaesthesia* 75, no. 12 (December 2020): 1579-1582. DOI: 10.1111/anae.15057.

Chumley-Jones, Heidi S, Alison Dobbie and Cynthia L Alford. "Web-based learning: sound educational method or hype? A review of the evaluation literature'. *Academic Medicine* 77, Suppl 10 (October 2002): S86-S93. DOI: 10.1097/00001888-200210001-00028

Dar, Q A, F Ahmad, M Ramzan, S H Khan, K Ramzan, W Ahmed and Z Kamal. "Use of Social Media Tool "Whatsapp" in Medical Education". *Annals of King Edward Medical University* 23, no. 1 (January-March 2017): 2541-2547. DOI: https://doi.org/10.21649/akemu.v23i1.1497.

Dennick, R, S Wilkinson and N Purcell. "Online eAssessment: AMEE guide no. 39". *Med Teacher* 31, no. 3 (March 2009): 192–206. DOI: 10.1080/01421590902792406

Ehrlich, H, M McKenney and A Elkbuli. "We Asked the Experts: Virtual Learning in Surgical Education During the COVID-19 Pandemic—Shaping the Future of Surgical Education and Training". *World Journal of Surgery* 44, no. 7 (July 2020): 2053-2055. DOI:10.1007/s00268-020-05574-3.

Fawcett, Hannah, and Jeremy Oldfield. "Investigating expectations and experiences of audio and written assignment feedback in first-year undergraduate students". *Teaching in Higher Education* 21, no. 1 (January 2016): 79-93. DOI: 10.1080/13562517.2015.1115969

Fonseka, T, R Ellis, H Salem, P Brennan and T Terry. "The effects of COVID-19 on training within urology: Lessons learned in virtual learning, human factors, non-technical skills and reflective practice". *Journal of Clinical Urology* 14, no. 1 (August 2020): 29-35. DOI: 10.1177/2051415820950109.

Gillinov, M, S Mick, T Mihaljevic and R M Suri. "Watch one, do one, teach one". *J Thorac Cardiovasc Surg*. 151, no.6 (June 2016): 1506-7. DOI: 10.1016/j.jtcvs.2016.02.033.

Greenfield, M J, J Luck, M L Billingsley, R Heyes, O J Smith, A Mosahebi, A Khoussa, G Abu-Sittah and N Hachach-Haram. "Demonstration of the Effectiveness of Augmented Reality Telesurgery in Complex Hand Reconstruction in Gaza". *Plast Reconstr Surg Glob Open* 6, no. 3 (March 2018): e1708. DOI: 10.1097/GOX.0000000000001708.

Hew, K F, and C K Lo. “Flipped classroom improves student learning in health professions education: a meta-analysis”. *BMC Med Educ* 18, no.1 (March 2018): Article no. 38. DOI: https://doi.org/10.1186/s12909-018-1144-z.

Jeong, L, Z Smith, A Longino, S E Merel and K McDonough. “Virtual Peer Teaching During the COVID-19 Pandemic”. *Med.Sci.Educ.* 30 (September 2020): 1361–1362. DOI: https://doi.org/10.1007/s40670-020-01065-1.

Johannsson, H, and T Selak. “Dissemination of medical publications on social media - is it the new standard?” *Anaesthesia* 75, no. 2 (February 2020): 155–7. DOI: 10.1111/anae.14780

Kennedy G, Kathleen Gray and Justin Tse. “'Net Generation' medical students: technological experiences of pre-clinical and clinical students”. *Med Teach* 30, no. 1 (February 2008):10-6. DOI: 10.1080/01421590701798737.

Lewiss, R E, B Hoffmann, Y Beaulieu and M B Phelan. “Point-of-care ultrasound education: the increasing role of simulation and multimedia resources”. *J Ultrasound Med.* 33, no. 1 (January 2014): 27–32. DOI: 10.7863/ultra.33.1.27

Lindeman, B M, J K Law, P A Lipsett, T Arbella, M Stem and A O Lidor. “A blended online curriculum in the basic surgery clerkship: a pilot study”. *Am J Surg*. 209, no. 1 (January 2015): 145-51. DOI: 10.1016/j.amjsurg.2014.10.003.

Ma, X, and D Vervoort. “Leveraging e-learning for medical education in low- and middle-income countries”. *Cardiol Young* 30, no. 6 (June 2020): 903–904. DOI: 10.1017/S1047951120001109

Pariser, E. *The Filter Bubble: How The New Personalized Web Is Changing What We Read And How We Think*. New York: Penguin Books, 2012.

Rose, S, “Medical Student Education in the Time of COVID-19”. *JAMA.* 323, no. 21 (June 2020): 2131–2132. DOI: 10.1001/jama.2020.5227.

Sandars, J. “Cost-effective e-learning in medical education”. In *Cost effectiveness in medical education* edited by K Walsh, 40-47. Abingdon: Radcliffe Publishing, 2010.

Shafi, A M A, A E Atieh, A Harky, A M Sheikh and W I Awad. “Impact of COVID 19 on cardiac surgical training: our experience in the United Kingdom”. *J Card Surg.* 35, no. 8 (August 2020): 1954-1957. DOI: https://doi.org/10.1111/jocs.14693

Shebrain, S, K Nava, G Munene, C Shattuck, J Collins and R Sawyer. “Virtual Surgery Oral Board Examinations in the Era of COVID-19

Pandemic. How I Do It!" Journal of Surgical Education. Accessed January 21, 2021. DOI: 10.1016/j.jsurg.2020.09.012.
Vargo, Ethan, Marwan Ali, Fabrice Henry, Daniel Kmetz, David Drevna, Jayram Krishnan and Raymond Bologna. "Cleveland Clinic Akron general urology residency program's COVID-19 experience". *Urology* 140 (June 2020): 1-3. DOI: 10.1016/j.urology.2020.04.001
Vervoort, D, B Meuris, B Meyns and P Verbrugghe. "Global cardiac surgery: access to cardiac surgical care around the world". *J Thorac Cardiovasc Surg*. 159, no. 3 (March 2020): 987–996. DOI: 10.1016/j.jtcvs.2019.04.039.
Villamizar, N, and D M Nguyen. "Enhancement in virtual learning cannot substitute for hands-on training in cardiothoracic surgery". *Journal of Cardiac Surgery* 35, no. 12 (December 2020): 3449-3450. DOI: 10.1111/jocs.14956
Walsh, K. "Online assessment in medical education-current trends and future directions". *Malawi Med J.* 27, no. 2 (June 2015): 71-2. DOI: 10.4314/mmjv27i2.8.
Walsh, K, I Rafiq and R Hall. "Online educational tools developed by Heart improve the knowledge and skills of hospital doctors in cardiology". *Postgraduate medical journal* 83 no. 981 (August 2007): 502–503. DOI: 10.1136/pgmj.2007.059501
Walsh, K, A Rutherford, J Richardson and P Moore. "NICE medical education modules: an analysis of cost-effectiveness". *Educ Prim Care.* 21, no. 6 (November 2010): 396-8. DOI: 10.13140/RG.2.2.28104.62724

# CHAPTER 30

# TRAINING OF COMMUNITY SURGEONS

MAHNOOR NAWAB, HIRA KHALID ZUBERI, IRUM FATIMA, MOHAMMAD SALMAN KHALIL, SADAF KHAN, ASAD LATIF AND LUBNA SAMAD

## I. Introduction

Global surgery was linked to health equity and social justice for the first time in 1980 by Dr Halfdan Mahler, the Director General of the World Health Organization (WHO) at the time. He brought to light the fact that the vast majority of the world's population has little or no access to skilled surgical care. Almost three decades later, Paul Farmer and Jim Kim described global surgery as the "neglected stepchild" of global health (Farmer and Kim 2008). Despite being an integral component of any robust and comprehensive healthcare delivery system, the discussion around development and advancement in surgical care had largely been absent from mainstream global health discourse. Slowly but surely, this has started to change.

The year 2015 was a landmark year in the history of global surgery. The World Bank published the 3rd edition of Disease Control Priorities (DCP3) (Jamison et al. [eds] 2017). The first volume focuses on *Essential Surgery,* defining 44 surgical procedures as "*essential on the basis that they address substantial needs, are cost-effective, and can feasibly be implemented.*" Later the same year, the report of The Lancet Commission on Global Surgery (LCoGS) was published (Meara et al. 2015). It emphasized the need to focus on developing surgical systems and stated that *"Surgery is an integral, indivisible component of a properly functioning health system, and all people should have access to safe, high-quality surgical and anaesthesia care with financial protection when needed.*" This momentum reached a pinnacle in May 2015 when the World Health Assembly (WHA) passed Resolution 68.15 ('Strengthening emergency and essential surgical care and anaesthesia as a component of universal health coverage') and urged member states to improve surgical systems, integrate surgical care and include surgical indicators in their health plans to ensure universal health coverage (Price, Makasa and Hollands 2015).

## A. Global burden of surgery

The LCoGS estimated that *five billion people worldwide are without access to safe, affordable, and timely surgical care*, of which two-thirds reside in low- and middle-income countries (LMICs) (Meara et al. 2015). It further stated that of the estimated 313 million surgical procedures taking place worldwide each year, only 6% are performed in LMICs. An additional 143 million procedures are needed in LMICs each year to bridge this gap. In 2010, it was estimated that 16.9 million people died from conditions requiring surgical interventions, which is far more than deaths due to HIV/AIDS, TB, and malaria combined. Between 28-32% of the global disease burden is estimated to be due to surgically treatable conditions (Shrime et al. 2015).

Cost is a significant barrier for populations that need to pay out of pocket for surgical care. Catastrophic health expenditures due to medical and non-medical costs of accessing surgical care are faced by 81 million individuals annually. Therefore, investing in surgical services in LMICs is "*affordable, saves lives, and promotes economic growth*" (Shrime et al. 2015).

In Pakistan, almost a quarter of the disease burden is attributable to surgical causes. This translates into a deficit of 17 million surgical procedures annually and results in 187 deaths per 100,000 of the population due to acute surgical illnesses, compared to 164 per 100,000 for all infectious diseases combined (Zafar and McQueen 2011). This deficit mainly affects the nearly 63% of the community that resides in rural areas, and are unable to access surgical services. This rural community also faces an acute shortage of surgical services as a result of the biased allocation of healthcare resources. Last but not the least, more than 90% of the population living below the poverty line also resides in these rural areas (World Bank 2018).

### B. Essential surgical care in Pakistan

The LCoGS defined essential surgical care as

> any and all procedures, contextually and culturally dependent, that are deemed by that region, society, or culture to promote individual and public health, wellbeing, and economic prosperity. The Bellwether Procedures—caesarean delivery, laparotomy and open fracture treatment—serve as a proxy for surgical systems that have the ability to provide a broad range of procedures.

Timely access to safe affordable surgical care is still a distant ideal for the majority of Pakistanis. Healthcare delivery in Pakistan is offered by two parallel systems: the public sector that mostly offers free-of-cost services, and the unregulated private sector, where the patient has to bear out-of-pocket (OOP) expenses to receive healthcare services. Charitable organizations provide healthcare services in many parts of the country, but other than a few notable exceptions, they do not address surgical care, usually due to the high infrastructure costs and required expertise. Public sector secondary facilities (DHQ and THQ) are meant to provide essential surgical care in smaller towns and rural areas, but due to inadequate infrastructure and staffing, they are unable to provide care to those in need. Therefore, tertiary care hospitals in metropolitan cities are left to provide the bulk of surgical care in the country. Not surprisingly, the public sector hospitals in large cities are invariably overburdened and urban private sector hospitals step in to fill the gap. The private sector is the first point of contact for around 70% of the population to receive healthcare (Shaikh 2015), and therefore must be involved if any strategy for surgical care is to prove successful.

In addition to the inadequate surgical care delivery platforms, a key challenge is the lack of trained surgical workforce. The LCoGS recommends a minimum of 20 surgeons, anaesthesiologists, and obstetricians (SAO) per 100,000 of the population; in Pakistan there are only an estimated six per 100,000 (Meara et al. 2015).

## II. Need for surgical care as a part of National Health Plans and Universal Health Coverage (UHC)

### A. National Health Vision (2016-2025)

Pakistan's Ministry of National Health Services, Regulation and Coordination (MoNHSRC) published an overarching policy document to provide a common direction to achieve desired health outcomes across the country. This policy commits

> to improve the health of all Pakistanis, particularly women and children, through universal access to affordable quality essential health services, and delivered through resilient and responsive health system, ready to attain Sustainable Development Goals and fulfil its other global health responsibilities.

Surgical care is not explicitly stated as a priority area in this document, even though Pakistan became a signatory to the World Health Assembly Resolution 68.15 in May 2015, through which it committed to acknowledge and resolve the global health challenge of inequitable access to surgical care.

An initiative was taken at the national level by the MoNHSRC in collaboration with the Indus Hospital and Health Network to address this priority area. In November 2018, a wide range of national and international stakeholders were brought together at a conference where the importance of providing safe and timely surgical care was recognized and the gaps and challenges in current surgical care in Pakistan were acknowledged. A National Vision for Surgical Care (NVSC) 2020-2025 was proposed to provide a strategic approach for improved surgical care delivery within the country. The NVSC provides a framework covering different domains like workforce issues, infrastructure, service delivery, information management and finance in addition to the provincial perspectives, specialty focus, a monitoring framework, and a governance framework to streamline surgical care delivery across the country; this policy document also recognizes that surgery is an integral component of UHC.

**B. UHC in Pakistan**

MoNHSRC introduced the "Essential Package of Health Services" (EPHS) in October 2020 to be implemented across all five service delivery platforms: community, primary, secondary, tertiary and population levels. EPHS follows the UHC approach and addresses causes of disease, mortality, and morbidity through the provision of preventive, promotive, curative and rehabilitative services. Surgical interventions have been prioritized, budgeted and mapped for delivery, developing a comprehensive and integrated surgical system across all healthcare levels.

In this context, emergency and essential surgical services need to be made available as close to the community as possible in order to be utilized optimally. The dearth of a trained surgical workforce, which includes anaesthetists, obstetricians, nursing staff and technicians, is a key challenge especially at primary (Rural Health Centre—RHC) and secondary (Tehsil/Taluka Headquarter (THQ) Hospital) levels (Abdullah et al. 2014). The inability to provide essential surgical care at these levels has led to increased patient flow at tertiary care facilities, with patients traveling to cities for even minor surgical problems. Recruitment of SAOs is required at the primary and secondary levels of care. With the implementation of EPHS, surgical care can be brought closer to the communities and a key component of UHC may be provided.

## III. Pakistan's Healthcare system

The provision of healthcare is ultimately the responsibility of the government, particularly in countries with poorer populations. This is especially relevant to rural areas since the private sector tends to focus on urban centres where financial returns are higher and staffing is easier. Pakistan's public sector healthcare delivery system was designed to provide healthcare services close to the community through a three-tiered system featuring primary, secondary and tertiary care levels (Kumar and Bano 2017).

**A.** The primary healthcare level delivers the services through a network of Basic Health Units (BHUs) and Rural Health Centres (RHCs) covering a population of up to 25,000 and 100,000 respectively. The primary healthcare level covers two different healthcare structures:

1. The BHUs provide preventive and out-patient services. By design, no surgical services are provided at this level of care.

2. The RHCs provide promotive, preventive, curative, diagnostic, and referral services along with in-patient services. It is supposed to provide medico-legal, "basic surgical and dental," and ambulance services.

**B.** The secondary healthcare level includes the Tehsil/Taluka Headquarter (THQ) hospitals, and District Headquarter (DHQ) hospitals, covering a population of up to one million and three million respectively (Abdullah et al. 2014).

1. THQ hospitals provide promotive, preventive, curative, diagnostic, and specialist care, as well as in-patient and referral services. THQ hospitals are supposed to provide basic and comprehensive Emergency Obstetric and New-born Care (EmONC). Each THQ has positions for nine standard specialists including a surgeon, anaesthetist, physician, obstetrician and gynaecologist, paediatrician, eye specialist, orthopaedic surgeon, pathologist and radiologist, and thus are designed to provide essential surgical services.

2. The DHQ hospitals provide promotive, preventive, curative, advanced diagnostic, and advanced specialist care, as well as in-patient and referral services, including basic and comprehensive EmONC. They also act as a recipient of referrals from the BHUs, RHCs and THQs along with Lady Health Workers (LHWs) and other primary care facilities. In addition to the specialists at THQ hospitals, positions include specialists in urology, physiotherapy, cardiology, neurosurgery, psychiatry, chest diseases, dermatology, and paediatric surgery. In addition to essential surgical procedures, they are meant to provide a broader spectrum of specialized surgeries (Punjab Healthcare Commission 2021).

**C.** Tertiary healthcare services are primarily provided by teaching hospitals located in large cities and are meant to provide all basic as well as advanced surgical services, including cardiac surgery, orthopaedic surgery, cancer surgery and organ transplantation.

In theory, the three-tiered health system of Pakistan has been well designed to provide appropriate levels of care as close to the population as possible. However, the implementation of this model has faced significant challenges. In the past few decades, the burgeoning population of the country has added additional strain to the system. There is an acute shortage in the workforce in Pakistan with a physician density of 0.473 per 1,000 of the population against the standard of two. The nurse, midwife, and LHW density is 0.25 per 1,000 people (Abdullah et al. 2014). The existing infrastructure is sub-standard, with most secondary care facilities lacking the minimum infrastructure needed for comprehensive EmONC services, general surgical care, and trauma care (Brückmann et al. 2019).

Although more than a third of the country's population is under-15 years of age (UNSD Statistics Division 2021), specialist paediatric surgical services are not available in most rural areas. The inadequate quality of services results in the suboptimal utilization of these services. A large percentage of the population is left with no option but to seek private sector services, even though the out-of-pocket expenditure invariably leads to financial impoverishment or catastrophe.

A comprehensive and integrated approach is required to address these fundamental deficiencies and ensure improvement in surgical services across Pakistan. Specialists and paramedical staff have gravitated to urban centres over the past few decades, leaving most secondary level facilities deficient both in terms of the number and quality of surgical care providers. A key pillar of this strategy is a well-trained surgical workforce that can meet the specific needs of our population, especially at the RHC, THQ and DHQ hospital levels. The minimum service delivery standards set forth by the provincial governments provide explicit requirements in terms of surgical infrastructure, SAO workforce requirements and surgical service delivery. These standards can be used as a framework to achieve our goal (Kumar and Bano 2017).

## IV. Training surgeons and serving the community

In order to address this gap in Pakistan's surgical system, interventions are needed at both the policy and service delivery levels. Surgeons, obstetricians and anaesthetists across the country must be sensitized to think "beyond the OR" and start exploring and documenting access and service delivery challenges across the country. This input will inform the development of locally relevant solutions. It is not a surprise that since the leaders of the medical (and specifically, surgical) community are based at urban centres, they are often unable to understand the countless barriers to accessing surgical care that are faced by the rural population. Training programmes must be adapted to be able to address the surgical needs of our marginalized populations, thinking beyond tertiary hospitals in cities.

At present, no defined training tracks exist in Pakistan to bridge these gaps. We present some existing strategies that have successfully been adopted in different parts of the world, and have the potential to be adapted for our national needs as well as some innovative strategies to bridge this gap. Before going into the details of these strategies it is important to define them and lay out a clear and precise understanding of the different approaches. We propose the following definitions for the surgeon workforce:

*The **global surgeon** is a trained surgeon (general or sub-specialist) with an additional academic qualification in global/public health with practical experience of the challenges in the delivery of surgical services in resource constrained settings.*

*The **rural surgeon** is a trained surgeon and physician looking after the promotive, preventive and curative healthcare needs of the target community and is able to perform a selected range of surgical procedures in a resource constrained setting.*

*The **community surgeon** is a surgeon trained with a broader horizontal knowledge base, is able to perform procedures relevant to the country's needs for the surgical component of universal health coverage, and is able to provide these surgical services to the target community in a resource constrained setting.*

### A. *I want to be a global surgeon*

Perhaps one of the biggest achievements over the past five years has been the increasing awareness among SOAs that they must play a critical role in the global health arena if surgical services are to improve. Similar to the way paediatricians have led the vaccination and childhood nutrition initiatives worldwide, SOAs must push for meaningful improvement in surgical care delivery at all levels of the service spectrum. In order to equip SOAs to affect this change, a strong understanding of both policy and implementation sciences is required.

In addition to a sound training in the surgical specialty of choice, a global surgeon should have the skills to initiate and develop new surgical programmes, conduct research and advocate for evidence-based improvements in surgical care.

In the past decade, multiple "global surgery" programmes have been established. In general, these programmes are directed towards postgraduate doctors, and their goal is to provide them with the opportunities to acquire the skills necessary for informed policy development and effective implementation of these policies. The focus of these programmes ranges from research fellowships to the development and formulation of global health structures. Most programmes are housed in universities and span two years. Prospective students include surgeons-in-training or students enrolled in health-related degrees. Most programmes focus on research, innovation, and advocacy.

### i. Master's in Public Health

This degree programme is offered by numerous internationally accredited universities in many countries, including several institutions in Pakistan. It is an interdisciplinary degree aimed at developing the capacity to build healthy and resilient communities. The course of study covers a wide range of subjects, including epidemiology, health education, environmental health, population science, biostatistics, research, and health services administration. Enrolment in the degree programme can be during or after medical degree studies or postgraduate training. For a surgeon, these programmes allow a comprehensive understanding of public health principles and facilitate the acquisition of the skillsets required to be effective public health managers, in addition to being a surgeon.

### ii. Master's in Science in Global Surgery

This postgraduate degree is offered by many universities across the globe. It is a two-year specialized programme designed to prepare surgical care providers to bridge gaps, address challenges, and contribute to finding solutions to providing surgical care in low resource settings globally. These programmes are designed for graduate medical students, postgraduate trainees, surgical faculty, or surgery-related allied healthcare workers across the globe.

The programmes seek to train surgeons within the field as experts on the subject of global surgery. This allows them to become leaders and innovators in the field by providing several research opportunities in LMICs to better understand the challenges faced by these populations. This approach aims to inculcate a sense of larger responsibility within practitioners and trains them as academics even as they continue with their clinical practice.

### iii. Programme in Global Surgery and Social Change (PGSSC 2021)

This Harvard University programme focuses on a two-year research fellowship that seeks to train the individual to educate, advocate and develop policies for global surgery in resource-poor countries, along with a one-year research assistant option for anyone pursuing a health-related degree.

### iv. Other global surgery programmes offered by universities

Many universities offer the chance to work closer to the affected community by providing options for educational or research rotations in collaboration with agencies such as the WHO. For instance, the programme in the Department of Surgery at the Washington University School of Medicine offers a multitude of options, ranging from 2, 3, or 5 year rotations that one can pursue in accordance with their interest (Washington University School of Medicine 2021). All these rotations include field projects, coursework, certifications, and—most importantly—obtaining a master's degree in public health during those rotations is a requirement. This allows for candidates to harmonize the education they garner as part of the programme with developing implementable models. These courses are designed to manifest the results of research and seek to inculcate the various elements that comprise global surgery.

## B. Rural surgery: a well-established track

Rural surgery is an increasingly popular approach for addressing the surgical component of universal health coverage. Rural surgeons not only perform various surgical procedures across multiple surgical disciplines, but they are also general practitioners who promote preventive medicine including maternal and child health. Thus, although they are trained as surgeons, they follow a holistic approach to healthcare according to the needs of the community. This model of healthcare delivery is common in some parts of Africa, India and even the US. While the average general surgeon performs 23 different operations, the spectrum is wider for surgeons who practise in rural environments. It requires expertise in surgical areas essential to small community practice, including endoscopies/colonoscopies, ENT, orthopaedics, urology and gynaecology. It also provides a significant focus on trauma and emergency general surgery.

### Global experiences in rural surgery

i. Africa: In Africa, the Pan-African Academy of Christian Surgeons (PAACS) is the only international, rural-based, surgical training programme. It started an initiative in 1997 to provide surgical training to African surgeons in rural centres across various African countries (Essen et al. 2019). It consists of a rigorous five-year curriculum, designed on an American, competency-based training model. A study of the basic sciences is integrated into the expected reading, rounds, patient care, and operating room teaching and is reinforced by weekly didactic conferences and required reports, presentations, and formal papers. After graduation from the training programme, residents are bonded for one year of service for each year of training and are placed in carefully selected rural hospitals (Pollock et al. 2011). 100% of practising PAACS surgeons stay in Africa and 79% remain in their home country. PAACS bases training mostly in underserved, rural areas, using curricula specifically matched to meet the diverse rural and underserved healthcare needs, a method which has also been emphasized by other training programmes in LMICs. PAACS has shown that a multifaceted approach, which recruits motivated trainees, uses a rural education model, incorporates financial incentives, and supports on-going professional development can improve the short- and long-term retention of surgeons working in rural African settings (Essen et al. 2019).

ii. India: In 1992 the Association of Rural Surgeons of India (ARSI) was formed, which focused on providing and expanding surgical resources in Rural Indian communities (Association of Rural Surgeons of India 2021). The group devised a multidisciplinary course in rural surgery for practising community surgeons and medical graduates in association with the Indira Gandhi National Open University, New Delhi. In 2007, the National Board of Examination started three-year training courses in rural surgery in association with the Ministry of Health. The course includes rotations in general surgery, orthopaedics, obstetrics and gynaecology, ENT and ophthalmology. The curriculum was designed to train doctors with the necessary surgical skills in these specialties and develop administrative skills to set up and run surgical centres in rural parts of the country and meet most of the surgical needs of the community. Based on the LCoGS report, "Global Surgery 2030," the ARSI provided recommendations that now comprise the Karad Consensus Statement (KCS) which details short and medium-term solutions to surgical access for India's poor, from the perspective of the clinicians serving them (The Association of Rural Surgeons of India: Lancet Commission on Global Surgery Consensus Committee 2019).

iii. United States: In the United States, special training programmes are provided to residents interested in rural surgery, focusing on building a broad-based surgical capacity in residents, enabling them to perform various resource appropriate surgical tasks not limited to general surgery. Exposure to rural training experiences during medical school and residency seems to be associated with an increased likelihood of

> pursuing a rural practice, either by facilitating training in these practice areas or by building a clinical or personal interest (Deveney et al. 2013). Several centres have established rural surgery training tracks for general surgeons to meet rural communities' current and future workforce needs (Mercier et al. 2019).

Many countries are now trying to implement strategies to create rural surgery residency tracks. These include rural rotations for medical students and residents. However, rural surgery as a separate entity still remains to be explored in Pakistan. Aggressive measures need to be taken to create a training curriculum for surgeons, allocate resources, and develop a functional referral system for patients who urgently require higher-level care.

### C. Proposing a community surgery track for Pakistan

According to World Bank data, Pakistan's surgical workforce capacity is much higher than most low- and middle-income countries including many African countries such as Sudan, Kenya and Rwanda. The College of Physicians and Surgeons Pakistan is the main regulatory body responsible for the training and certification of surgical specialists across the country. While the increasing number of specialty and subspecialty training tracks have led to a greater number of surgeons graduating each year, this has not necessarily translated into an increase in the surgical workforce's capacity at the secondary hospital level. The minimum service delivery standards in the public sector recommend hiring multiple specialists at the secondary level in order to function, which is a challenge in itself as these surgeons do not have the resources to perform advanced surgical procedures in their own field (Punjab Healthcare Commission 2021). This inevitably leads to surgeons opting to relocate to large, mostly urban, tertiary care centres which are better equipped and allow more opportunities for the surgeons to advance in their respective fields.

We propose a "*community surgeon*" with a broader horizontal knowledge base, who can safely and competently perform surgical procedures along with their team (which includes anaesthetists, OT assistants, nurses and other support staff). DCP3 has recommended the implementation of *44 essential surgical procedures* across primary, secondary and tertiary healthcare levels to be a part of the WHO's universal health coverage agenda. In Pakistan, through a consultative provincial and national process, this list of essential procedures has been adapted for local needs, and 19 addenda specific to children's requirements have been included.

To train these community surgeons there is an urgent need to establish a well-rounded surgical curriculum that will enable surgeons to perform a broader spectrum of procedures in rural and resource-constrained settings.

**i. Training of community surgeons**

These community surgeons should be equipped with the skills of a good manager as well as a professional surgeon. The focus should be directed towards providing relevant surgical and procedural skills to competent trainees to allow them to deal with a wide variety of surgical procedures across multiple specialties as well as the most commonly faced obstetric, orthopaedic, trauma, and abdominal emergencies at the THQ and DHQ hospital levels. This is the concept of "essential surgical care" that is now gaining traction; it can also be adapted locally to overcome the gap in our surgical service delivery (Taylor and Hollaar 2005).

An additional training programme needs to be considered by the CPSP for "surgeons in general," providing comprehensive and well-structured training for surgcons committed to working in communities. The community surgeon should additionally have intersectional skills in the basics of anaesthesia, infection control, nursing, storage and administration of medicines etc., to develop a better understanding and capacity for integrated practice.

**ii. Recruitment and retention**

Most practitioners opt for large urban hospitals for better career prospects, higher-level training opportunities, and a better family and social life. This increases the health equity gap between urban and rural communities even further. According to WHO recommendations, measures should be taken to increase the retention of doctors in these areas by compulsory service requirements in rural and remote areas accompanied with appropriate support and financial incentives (World Health Organization 2021). Professional isolation and lack of access to continuing medical education/continuing professional development (CME/CPD) have been identified as another key deterrent to rural practice (Curran, Rourke and Snow 2010). Distance learning programmes can be initiated to help overcome this issue. These programmes can enable community surgeons to remain connected with their peers, learn new skills and keep themselves updated with the advances in surgical techniques.

### iii. Career development and credentialing as a community surgeon

There should be a clear career development programme to provide health workers with opportunities to move up the career path based on professional experience, education and training (WHO 2021). Better living conditions for health workers and their families and investment in infrastructure and services are also essential to improve outcomes (Buykx et al. 2010).

### iv. Supervision and monitoring

In order to ensure effective supervision, oversight, and in-service training for community surgeons, a mentoring and monitoring system can be devised where surgical specialists can be made available to provide training and direct supervision to community surgeons. Simultaneously, web-based learning can also be incorporated to teach surgical procedures through off-site observation (Boghdady, Ewalds-Kvist and Afshin Alijani 2019).

Pakistan is in dire need of a well-coordinated strategy where a combination of the above training tracks can improve surgical care for the end user. NVSC2025 provides a strong platform for all stakeholders to actively engage and develop a strategy for surgical training that is relevant to the needs of the Pakistani population, particularly the rural majority. A generation of "Pakistani global surgeons" attuned to the surgical needs of the population can make much-needed changes at the level of policy—from strategies developed at federal and provincial health ministries and departments on the one hand, to the accreditation of surgeons and the adaptation of the curricula for residents and medical students to meet the needs of the growing population on the other. Ensuring that infrastructure and incentives are provided is an essential part of the strategy. The next steps of the implementation of this surgical strategy will require trained community and/or rural surgeons to provide surgical care in remote areas under a strong monitoring and evaluation umbrella, ensuring that easier access goes hand in hand with safe and high-quality care.

## Bibliography

Abdullah, Muhammad Ahmed, Fatima Mukhtar, Salim Wazir, Irum Gilani, Zulfikar Gorar and Babar Tasneem Shaikh. "The Health Workforce Crisis in Pakistan: A Critical Review and the Way Forward." *World Health & Population* 15, no. 3 (June 2014): 4-12. DOI: doi:10.12927/whp.2015.24031.

Association of Rural Surgeons of India. "Rural Surgery". Accessed March 26, 2021. URL: https://www.arsi-india.org/rural_surgery.htm.

Boghdady, Michael El, Béatrice Marianne Ewalds-Kvist and Afshin Alijani. "A Review of Online Platforms in Training and Surgical Education". *European Surgery* 51, no. 2 (April 2019): 41–48. DOI: https://doi.org/10.1007/s10353-019-0569-x.

Brückmann, Peter, Ashfa Hashmi, Marina Kuch, Jana Kuhnt and Ida Monfared. "Public Provision of Emergency Obstetric Care: A Case Study in Two Districts of Pakistan." *BMJ Open* 9, no. 5 (May 2019): e027187. DOI: https://doi.org/10.1136/bmjopen-2018-027187.

Buykx, Penny, John Humphreys, John Wakerman and Dennis Pashen. "Systematic Review of Effective Retention Incentives for Health Workers in Rural and Remote Areas: Towards Evidence-Based Policy." *Australian Journal of Rural Health* 18, no. 3 (June 2010): 102–9. DOI: https://doi.org/10.1111/j.1440-1584.2010.01139.x.

Curran, Vernon, Leslie Rourke and Pamela Snow. "A Framework for Enhancing Continuing Medical Education for Rural Physicians: A Summary of the Literature." *Medical Teacher* 32, no. 11 (November 2010): e501-508. DOI: https://doi.org/10.3109/0142159X.2010.519065.

Deveney, Karen, Mark Deatherage, David Oehling and John Hunter. "Association between Dedicated Rural Training Year and the Likelihood of Becoming a General Surgeon in a Small Town." *JAMA Surgery* 148, no. 9 (September 2013): 817–21. DOI: https://doi.org/10.1001/jamasurg.2013.2681.

Essen, Caleb Van, Bruce C Steffes, Keir Thelander, Beryl Akinyi, Hsin-Fang Li and Margaret J Tarpley. "Increasing and Retaining African Surgeons Working in Rural Hospitals: An Analysis of PAACS Surgeons with Twenty-Year Program Follow-Up." *World Journal of Surgery* 43, no. 1 (January 2019): 75–86. DOI: https://doi.org/10.1007/s00268-018-4781-9.

Farmer, Paul E., and Jim Y. Kim. "Surgery and Global Health: A View from Beyond the OR." *World Journal of Surgery* 32, no. 4 (April 2008): 533–36. DOI: https://doi.org/10.1007/s00268-008-9525-9.

Jamison, Dean T., Hellen Gelband, Susan Horton, Prabhat Jha, Ramanan Laxminarayan, Charles N. Mock, and Rachel Nugent (eds). *Disease Control Priorities: Improving Health and Reducing Poverty*, 3rd edn. Washington (DC): The International Bank for Reconstruction and Development / The World Bank, 2017.

Kumar, Santosh, and Suria Bano, "Comparison and Analysis of Health Care Delivery Systems: Pakistan versus Bangladesh." *Journal of Hospital & Medical Management* 3, no. 1 (January 2017). DOI: https://doi.org/10.4172/2471-9781.100020.

Meara, John G., Andrew J. M. Leather, Lars Hagander, Blake C. Alkire, Prof Nivaldo Alonso, Prof Emmanuel A. Ameh, Prof Stephen W. Bickler, et al. "Global Surgery 2030: Evidence and Solutions for Achieving Health, Welfare, and Economic Development - The Lancet." *The Lancet Commissions* 386, no. 9993 (August 2015): 569-624. DOI: https://doi.org/10.1016/S0140-6736(15)60160-X.

Mercier, Phillip J., Steven JSkube, Samantha L. Leonard, Ashley N. McElroy, Tyler G. Goettl, Melissa M. Najarian, Paula M. Termuhlen and Jeffrey G. Chipman. "Creating a Rural Surgery Track and a Review of Rural Surgery Training Programs." *Journal of Surgical Education* 76, no. 2 (March 2019): 459–68. DOI: https://doi.org/10.1016/j.jsurg.2018.09.004.

null On Behalf of The Association of Rural Surgeons of India-Lancet Commission on Global Surgery Consensus Committee. "The Lancet Commission on Global Surgery - Association of Rural Surgeons of India Karad Consensus Statement on Surgical System Strengthening in Rural India." *Healthcare (Amsterdam, Netherlands)* 7, no. 2 (June 2019): 7–9. DOI: https://doi.org/10.1016/j.hjdsi.2018.10.003.

PGSCC. "Program in Global Surgery and Social Change | Harvard Medical School." Accessed March 26, 2021. URL: https://www.pgssc.org.

Pollock, Jonathan D., Timothy P. Love, Bruce C. Steffes, David C. Thompson, John Mellinger and Carl Haisch. "Is It Possible to Train Surgeons for Rural Africa? A Report of a Successful International Program." *World Journal of Surgery* 35, no. 3 (March 2011): 493–99. DOI: https://doi.org/10.1007/s00268-010-0936-z.

Price, Raymond, Emmanuel Makasa and Michael Hollands, "World Health Assembly Resolution WHA68.15: 'Strengthening Emergency and Essential Surgical Care and Anesthesia as a Component of Universal Health Coverage'–Addressing the Public Health Gaps Arising from Lack of Safe, Affordable and Accessible Surgical and Anesthetic Services." *World Journal of Surgery* 39, no. 9 (August 2015): 2115-2125. DOI: https://doi.org/10.1007/s00268-015-3153-y.

Punjab Healthcare Commission. "WELCOME TO : Punjab Healthcare Commission". Accessed March 26, 2021. URL: https://phc.org.pk/catI_HCE.aspx.

Shaikh, Babar. "PRIVATE SECTOR IN HEALTH CARE DELIVERY: A REALITY AND A CHALLENGE IN PAKISTAN," *Journal of Ayub Medical College, Abbottabad: JAMC* 27, no. 2 (July 2015): 496–98. URL: https://pubmed.ncbi.nlm.nih.gov/26411151/.

Shrime, Mark G., Anna J. Dare, Blake C. Alkire, Kathleen O' Neill and John G. Meara. "Catastrophic Expenditure to Pay for Surgery: A Global Estimate." *The Lancet. Global Health* 3, no. 2 (April 2015): S38–44, DOI: https://doi.org/10.1016/S2214-109X(15)70085-9.

Shrime, Mark G., Stephen W. Bickler, Blake C. Alkire and Charlie Mock. "Global burden of surgical disease: an estimation from the provider perspective." The Lancet Global Health 3, Special Issue (April 2015): S8-S9. DOI: https://doi.org/10.1016/S2214-109X(14)70384-5.

Taylor, Robert H., and Gwen Hollaar, "Review of a Canadian Forum on International Surgery: The Bethune Round Table." *Canadian Journal of Surgery. Journal Canadien De Chirurgie* 48, no. 6 (December 2005): 479–84. URL:

UNSD Statistics Division. "UNSD — Demographic and Social Statistics." Accessed March 26, 2021. URL: https://unstats.un.org/unsd/demographic-social/products/dyb/dyb_2019/.

Washington University School of Medicine in St Louis. "International Surgery. General Surgery Residency." Accessed March 26, 2021 URL: https://gsres.wustl.edu/clinical-education/international-surgery/.

World Bank. "When Water Becomes a Hazard | Other Poverty Study". Accessed February 23, 2021. URL: https://elibrary.worldbank.org/doi/abs/10.1596/30799.

World Health Organization. "WHO | Increasing Access to Health Workers in Remote and Rural Areas through Improved Retention." Accessed March 26, 2021. URL: https://www.who.int/hrh/retention/guidelines/en/.

Zafar, Syed Nabeel, and K A Kelly McQueen. "Surgery, Public Health, and Pakistan." *World Journal of Surgery* 35, no. 12 (December 2011): 2625–34. DOI: https://doi.org/10.1007/s00268-011-1304-3.

# CHAPTER 31

# 21ST CENTURY LEADERS IN SURGERY

HASAN BADRE ALAM
AND UMAR FAROOQ BHATTI

*"If your actions inspire others to dream more, learn more, do more, and become more, you are a leader."*
John Quincy Adams (1767–1848)

## Surgical leadership and the changing landscape

Leadership is not about titles, seniority, or one's position in the hierarchy of an organization. In reality, it is a process of social influence, which maximizes the efforts of others, towards the achievement of a goal (Kruse 2013). Successful leaders are good at predicting future needs, and in successfully aligning the efforts of others towards the achievement of meaningful goals. The delivery of healthcare is a complex process where leaders have to deal with numerous competing priorities. Not only are the needs of the aging patient population becoming more challenging, but treatment options are also multiplying at a dizzying pace. This is further complicated by the rapidly evolving financial and regulatory landscape and the changing needs of the healthcare workforce. To address these transformations, the surgical leaders of the 21st century will need to acquire a skillset that has not been part of their traditional training. Historically, leaders in surgery needed to display excellence in three areas: patient care, education, and research, along with some basic administrative skills. However, as a result of the spectacular advancements in science and technology in the latter half of the 20th century, many things that were once considered pure fantasy are now taken for granted—cross-sectional imaging, organ transplantation, endovascular stents/grafts/valves, extracorporeal circulation, robotic surgery, telemedicine, to name just a few. These spectacular advancements in knowledge and rapid innovations in technology have created a need for multi-disciplinary collaboration, changes in the working roles of surgeons and other team members, financial challenges for surgeons and institutions, and changes in training requirements. In many ways, the ecosystem has also become more complex, interdependent, costly, and fragile. To cope with this new reality, surgical leaders of the future will have to master skillsets that were not that critical for their predecessors to possess (Souba 2003).

Their key responsibilities still include setting a compelling and appealing direction for the team (*vision*), selecting the right people (*talent*), and creating and embracing the right set of guiding core values (*culture*), but now they also need to focus on a much longer list of characteristics (Patel et al. 2010):

1. Professionalism
2. Technical competence
3. Motivation
4. Innovation
5. Teamwork
6. Communication skills
7. Decision-making
8. Business acumen
9. Emotional competence
10. Resilience
11. Effective teaching

## Various styles and evolving needs

Not surprisingly, leadership and its various conceptual models are among the most studied sociological concepts. Leadership, at its core, is the accomplishment of goals through the coordinated efforts of the team members. The person who successfully marshals their collaborators to achieve particular ends is a leader; and a great leader is one who can do so day after day, and year after year, in a wide variety of circumstances (Prentice 2004). While some theorists have argued that great leaders are born with innate natural leadership skills, most contemporary experts agree that leadership consists of a series of well-defined skills and behaviours, that can be learned, taught, and refined through practice, experience, feedback, and coaching. In other words, most of us who want to become better leaders can do so with the help of appropriate training, expert coaching, effective mentoring, and ongoing learning/feedback. Good leaders develop through a continuous process of self-improvement and they refine their skills and styles through training and practical experience. It is also important to better understand the relationship of leaders to their followers (Table 31.1), and how this has evolved. Historically, surgical leaders were chosen based upon quantitative measures of their achievements, but nowadays skills related to team building and how to best develop others are much more critical (Figure 31.1). To be successful in the 21st century, the level of emotional intelligence (Figure 31.2) that a surgical leader brings to the table is (and will continue to be) more relevant than their academic accomplishments.

**Table 31.1: Comparison of transactional and transformational leadership (Gopee and Galloway 2009)**

| Transactional leadership | Transformational leadership |
|---|---|
| • Aims to maintain balance and current situation<br>• Task-centred and organized<br>• Compassionate and focuses on present issues<br>• Performs tasks meticulously and does not deviate from policies and guidelines<br>• Teaches and promotes sheltered learning<br>• Rewards extrinsically<br>• Egotistical<br>• Views home and work as distinct entities | • Motivates followers and organizations to focus on common goals<br>• Arouses emotions in followers so that they believe they have the ability to do exceptional things<br>• Creates learning opportunities to stimulate growth and development<br>• Challenges followers<br>• Rewards intrinsically<br>• Possesses good insight, communication and management skills to develop strong emotional bonds with followers<br>• Views home and work on a continuum |

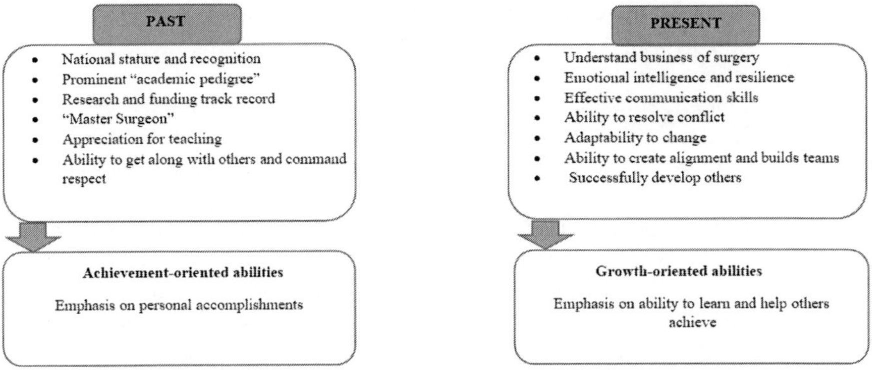


Figure 31.1: Traditional and contemporary leadership styles in surgery

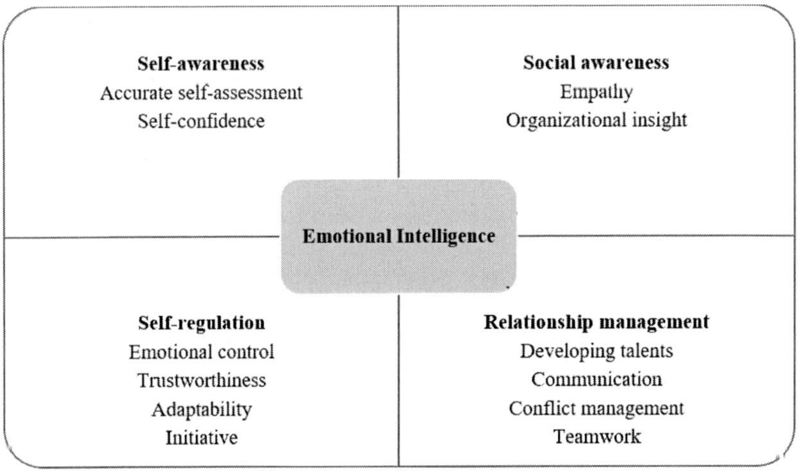


Figure 31.2: Emotional intelligence (Gewertz 2006)

The US Institute of Medicine, in their landmark report "Crossing the Quality Chasm: A New Health System for the 21st Century," outlined six areas where the leaders in the healthcare system should be held accountable (Wolfe 2001). These six domains can act as a guide for aspiring leaders if they hope to improve the quality of patient care through effective leadership. The recommendations suggest being:

1. Effective: avoiding overuse, underuse, and wrong services
2. Safe: avoiding injuries to patients
3. Patient-centred: respects the need of the individual
4. Timely: reducing harmful waits and delays
5. Efficient: avoiding waste
6. Equitable: gender, ethnicity, geographic, and socioeconomic status

Many of these domains were not high priority areas for the surgical leaders of the past. However, to succeed in the 21st century, and to remain relevant in the new and interconnected healthcare system, the next generation of surgical leaders have to acquire skills that would allow them to understand and be effective in these new areas. As opposed to the "command and control" style of the traditional department of surgery chair, the next generation of leaders may or may not be chair, and their approach is likely to be more about "adding value" to the institutional mission, rather than focusing on what they can control. As surgical leaders develop their teams to remain effective in the 21st century, they are also likely to face many new challenges. Here we would like to highlight just a few.

***Generational and gender issues***

Today, generations X and Y compose most of the surgical workforce, with millennials soon to follow. In contrast, most of the leadership positions are still held by the baby boom generation. Although generalizations are imperfect, much has been written about how these generations differ in their value systems and priorities, which can create misalignments and worsen job satisfaction. Physicians between the ages of 40 and 54 seem to be more vulnerable than younger or older physicians. Nearly half of generation X physicians reported feeling burned out, compared to 38% amongst millennials (ages 25 to 39) and 39% of baby boomers (55 to 73 years), with roughly half of those surveyed willing to take a substantial pay cut to achieve a better work-life balance (The Wall Street Journal 2020).

Nevertheless, there is a desire on the part of the newer generations (Millennials and Gen Z) to have a better work-life balance, and what the surgeons expect from their work-life in the future is likely to be quite different from the expectations of past generations. At the same time, more than half of medical graduates are women, and an increasing number of them are going into surgical specialties. Despite the increasing number of women in the surgical workforce, they face disparities and biases in compensation, mentorship, and advancement in leadership positions (Morris et al. 2018; Singletary 2005; Sorouri et al. 2021; Thompson-Burdine et al. 2019). This is a multi-faceted and complex problem that requires a comprehensive and thoughtful approach. Nevertheless, as the global agenda towards equality progresses, this pressing issue must be addressed head-on by the surgical leaders of the 21st century (Lim et al. 2021).

### *Burnout*

*"Aus der Kriegsschule des Lebens. — Was mich nicht umbringt, macht mich stärker."*
*("Out of life's school of war — What doesn't kill me, makes me stronger.")*
Friedrich Nietzsche (1844–1900)

This aphorism from the "Maxims and Arrows" section of the German philosopher Friedrich Nietzsche's *Twilight of the Idols* may just as well be describing the traditional surgical training mantra. In our minds, and the imagination of the public, surgeons are brilliant, highly skilled, and iron-willed individuals who calmly make life and death decisions. They are mentally and physically tough, emotionally inexhaustible, highly dexterous, and their superhuman personalities have been forged in the fires of the surgical residency, where only the fittest can survive.

The reality is a lot more nuanced. While most surgeons are indeed highly skilled individuals with "take-charge" personalities, and are driven, task-oriented, motivated, passionate, and competitive, these same traits can create blind spots and unique susceptibilities. For example, high achievers often disregard opposing viewpoints, and they tend to delegate poorly. Competitive and passionate individuals are prone to evolve into micromanagers and perfectionists. A laser-like focus on excellent patient care can easily coexist with a lack of focus on self-care and family life, and an attempt to excel at everything can instead lead to failure at things that truly matter. Nowhere else is this tension more obvious than the recent data about surgeon burnout. Physicians in general, and surgeons in particular (including trainees), seem to be suffering from burnout at truly alarming rates. Here we highlight the potential reasons behind this pressing issue and summarize the findings from some of the key studies.

#### Definitions

American physiologist Herbert Freudenberger was the first to coin the term "burnout" in 1974 to describe the "consequences of severe or prolonged stress and anxiety experienced by people working in healing professions" (Freudenberger 1974). Maslach and Jackson subsequently refined the definition as being "a syndrome of emotional exhaustion and cynicism" (1981). The Maslach Burnout Inventory (MBI) is considered the current gold standard tool for burnout assessment. It consists of 22 items (score range 0–54) that measure (based upon self-reported frequency) three domains: *emotional exhaustion*, *depersonalization*, and *sense of reduced personal accomplishment*. Although emotional exhaustion has been considered to be the dominant domain of burnout, depersonalization may align better with the negative consequences of this syndrome (Maslach and Leiter 2008; West, Dyrbye and Shanafelt 2018). Burnout is often complicated by disruptive behaviours, depression, substance abuse, interpersonal conflicts, and even suicidal ideations. For example, in a survey of more than 7,000 members of the American College of Surgeons (ACS), alcohol abuse/dependence was reported by 15.4% (males 13.9%; females 25.6%), and the odds ratios were significantly higher in surgeons that were either burned out (OR 1.25; $p=0.01$) or depressed (OR 1.48; $p<0.01$) (Oreskovich et al. 2012). A striking 6.3% of the surgeons reported suicidal ideations (SI), but only a quarter of them sought psychiatric care (Shanafelt et al. 2011). Importantly, recent surgical internships have had a large, statistically significant adverse relationship with all the 3 domains of burnout, and symptoms of depression. It is important to point out that burnout is distinct from other similar constructs such as job dissatisfaction, fatigue, job stress, and depression. Although there is a correlation, burnout may be present in their absence or absent in their presence.

## Scope of the problem

Burnout appears to be very common among surgeons, and it may be the single greatest predictor of surgeons' satisfaction with career and specialty choice. Members of the ACS were sent an anonymous, cross-sectional survey in June 2008. The survey evaluated demographic variables, practice characteristics, career satisfaction, burnout, and quality of life (QOL) (Shanafelt et al. 2009). Out of the 7,905 surgeons who returned the survey, 40% were burned out, 30% screened positive for symptoms of depression, and 28% had a mental QOL score >1/2 standard deviation below the population norm. Factors independently associated with burnout included younger age, having children, area of specialization (trauma surgeons were more commonly affected), number of nights on call per week, hours worked per week and having compensation determined entirely based on billing. On a positive note, despite the high burnout rates, surgeons continue to find their work personally meaningful and rewarding, as 75% would become a surgeon again if given a choice.

**Reasons for the increasing burnout**

The problem is multifactorial, and potential reasons include high workload, financial strains, administrative hassles, job inexperience, the conflict between work and family obligations, fear of litigation, certain surgical practices, new technologies/expanding information, decreasing academic resources/funding, increasing patient expectations, decreasing surgeon autonomy, and cumbersome electronic medical records (Dimou, Eckelbarger and Riall 2016; Money 2017; Patti, Schlottmann and Sarr 2018; Shanafelt et al. 2016). Issues related to the work environment are equally important, and these seem to affect more junior individuals and women disproportionately. For example, in a recent study of 7,409 surgical residents from 262 surgical residency programmes, 16.6% reported racial discrimination, 30.3% reported verbal or physical abuse (or both), and 10.3% reported sexual harassment (Hu et al. 2019). Rates of all the mistreatment measures were higher among women: 65.1% of the women surveyed reported gender discrimination and 19.9% reported sexual harassment. Weekly burnout symptoms were reported by 38.5% of the residents and 4.5% reported having had suicidal thoughts during the past year. This is unacceptable, and much-needed cultural changes are already underway at many institutions (The Michigan Daily 2019).

**Consequences**

Physician burnout can harm multiple fronts, including patient care, physician wellbeing, and healthcare system viability. For example, we know that each one-point increase in depersonalization score (scale range, 0–33) is associated with an 11% increase in the likelihood of reporting an error, while each one-point increase in emotional exhaustion (scale range, 0–54) is associated with a 5% increase (Shanafelt 2010). Shanafelt's study also showed that burnout and depression remained independent predictors of reporting a recent major medical error by using a multivariate analysis that controlled for other personal and professional factors. In contrast, the frequency of overnight calls, practice setting, method of compensation, and the number of hours worked were not associated with errors on the multivariate analysis. Critical ingredients to making progress include prioritization by leadership, physician involvement, organizational science/learning, metrics, structured interventions, open communication, and promoting cultural change at the work unit, leader, and organizational level.

**Potential solutions/strategies**

The fact that half of our surgical trainees and practising surgeons are reporting burnout represents a public health crisis, with negative impacts on individual physicians, patients, and healthcare organizations and systems. Drivers of this epidemic are largely rooted within the healthcare systems and include excessive workloads, inefficient work processes, clerical burdens, work-home conflicts, lack of input or control for physicians for issues affecting their work lives, organizational support structures, and leadership culture. Individual physician-level factors also play a role, with higher rates of burnout commonly reported in female and younger/mid-career physicians. Effective solutions should align with these drivers. For example, organizational efforts such as locally developed practice modifications and increased support for clinical work have demonstrated benefits in reducing burnout. Individually focused solutions such as mindfulness-based stress reduction and small-group activities to promote community, connectedness, and meaning have also been shown to be effective. Cognitive, behavioural, and mindfulness-based approaches are effective in reducing stress and may also contribute to lower levels of burnout (Regehr et al. 2014). Regardless of the specific approach taken, the problem of physician burnout is best addressed when viewed as a shared responsibility of both healthcare systems and individual physicians (Panagioti et al. 2017; Ruotsalainen et al. 2014). It is gratifying to note that many professional organizations are now addressing this issue head-on. For example, the ACS is not only acknowledging the magnitude of the problem but has made surgeon well-being a high-priority area (American College of Surgeons 2021). The ACS is not only providing surgeons the tools for measuring burnout and tracking wellness, but also promoting free access to national and local resources that span multiple categories and topics. The good news is that the increased focus on physician burnout may finally be having the desired effect. Burnout and satisfaction with work-life integration among US physicians have shown some improvement between 2014 and 2017, with burnout dropping down to the 2011 levels (Shanafelt et al. 2019).

## Time management

To be an effective leader while balancing a clinical practice or an academic interest is tough, especially when you also throw in work-life balance, personal fulfilment, and competing family priorities. Countless books have been written about time management, and about ways to enhance your effectiveness. Some of these are very good (Covey 2004; Mackenzie and Nickerson 2009). However, there is no replacement for learning directly from the individuals who do it well; from those that have figured out how to achieve the perfect balance, setting up the correct priorities, maintaining a healthy (not all-consuming) clinical practice, finding time to teach, being effective leaders, and somehow still finding time for important family events. This is never easy, and there is no magic formula, but here are some simple suggestions based on my own experience. You must make sure not only that there is no time wastage, but that your time is allocated appropriately to high-priority areas. Defining what is "high priority" is uniquely personal, and often evolves as one goes through different life and career phases. However, this is an area that needs your utmost attention. Do not leave it to others to decide where your time should be spent. On a personal front, optimal time utilization has been an ongoing quest. I am ferociously protective of my time as this is the only resource in my life that I just can't generate. Simply stated, you can always make more money but wasted time is gone forever. One must know exactly where their time goes.

There are 168 hours in each week—you should be able to account for all of it and be in control of its allocation. It is often tough for a junior person to set their priorities appropriately. A significant portion of discretionary time must be dedicated to acquiring leadership skills, through formal courses/mentorship programmes or self-education. This is one area where advice from a seasoned mentor is invaluable. Set clear priorities, delegate what you can, learn to say no and revisit your priorities frequently. During these deliberations, set aside time for issues that are important for your happiness, health, family, and personal growth. Remember that you will be in this field for 30 years, and nobody can be successful over such a long time with self-deprivation as their main strategy. As mentioned above, mid-career burnout is a real problem for surgeons (Spickard Jr, Gabbe and Christensen 2002). Make time for hobbies, family, exercise, travel, vacations, and other things that make life worth living. Your goal is not to achieve academic success at any cost, but to do so while leading a meaningful, productive, and fulfilling life.

## Some lessons to go by

At an individual level, we must remind ourselves to focus on the positive aspects of our careers and to fully appreciate the rewarding things in our lives. It should be emphasized that despite recent economic stresses, physicians and especially surgeons remain extremely well compensated. Their salaries place them in the top few percentiles of the US socioeconomic strata. They also have the unique privilege of positively impacting the lives of their patients consistently through their daily work, which few other professions can claim. Another possible approach has been very well described by Stephen Covey in his highly influential book, *7 Habits of Highly Effective People* (1998). Covey introduces the concept of a paradigm shift and helps the reader understand that different perspectives exist, i.e., that two people can see the same thing and yet react very differently. The first habit that he recommends is to "be proactive," which emphasizes taking responsibility for your life, "Instead of reacting to or worrying about conditions over which they have little or no control, proactive people focus their time and energy on things they can control" (Covey 2004). The problems, challenges, and opportunities we face fall into two areas: the circle of concern and circle of influence. Proactive people focus their efforts on their circle of influence. They work on the things they can do something about (circle of influence): adopting a healthy lifestyle, better time management, setting the right priorities, family, children, optimal patient care/professional excellence. In contrast, reactive people focus their efforts on things over which they have little or no control (circle of concern): the national debt, tort reform, terrorism, violent crimes, national health care policies, etc. Gaining an awareness of the areas in which we choose to expend our energies is a major step in becoming proactive. How we respond to any stimulus is our greatest strength, and also our biggest vulnerability, or as Covey described it, "I am not a product of my circumstances. I am a product of my decisions."

It is also important to understand what motivates us. Daniel Pink in his book *Drive: The Surprising Truth About What Motivates Us*, and in a TED talk that has been watched more than 25 million times, argues that human motivation is largely intrinsic and that the aspects of this motivation can be divided into *autonomy*, *mastery*, and *purpose* (TEDGlobal 2009). Once again, surgeons are in an enviable position of being the practitioners of a highly sophisticated healing art that builds upon all of these key drivers of motivation. Interestingly, what makes us happy in the short term often has no bearing on long-term happiness and satisfaction. In many articles and a hugely popular TED talk, Daniel Gilbert describes how people who win a lottery are no happier 1 year later compared to people who became paraplegic (TED 2004). Both of these groups essentially reverted to their baseline levels of happiness following the acute "life-changing" episode.

There will always be things that disturb our equilibrium. However, the key is to keep the focus on things that give meaning to our lives: find mentors, build relationships, and be there for your patients, but also connect deeper with your family, develop your teams and watch your mentee thrive, hug your kids, go for a run, pick up a new hobby, enjoy good food, give to your favourite charity, or do a difficult operation that tests your surgical skills. None of these will fix the problems of the world, but all of them are highly likely to make you happier, feel more fulfilled, and possibly less stressed.

## Conclusions

The surgical world is rapidly changing and becoming more complex, and to be successful the surgical leaders of the 21st century must evolve. Our training programmes have to adapt to this new reality by training surgeons who can be effective leaders in this new environment. Traditional surgical leadership skills will remain essential, but these alone will not be enough to succeed. The leaders of tomorrow will need to have additional capabilities such as better business acumen, emotional competence and resiliency; better team building, mentorship, conflict resolution, communication and listing skills; and an ability to focus on others rather than the self. While some of the traits may be innate, there is good evidence that most of these can be learned (and improved) through education, practice, and feedback. Also, while building the workforce of tomorrow, we have to pay special attention to eliminate biases (gender, race, socio-economic status, etc.) to ensure that the leadership ranks are open to all the deserving candidates, and to implement strategies to protect against burnout. The last century is widely regarded as the "golden era" for surgery. However, we firmly believe that this century is likely to be even better, though it will clearly require a different skillset to succeed.

## Bibliography

American College of Surgeons. "Surgeon Well Being". Accessed Feb 10, 2021. URL: https://www.facs.org/member-services/surgeon-wellbeing.

Covey, Stephen R. *The 7 habits of highly effective people: Powerful lessons in personal change.* United States of America: Simon and Schuster, 2004.

Dimou, Francesca M., David Eckelbarger, and Taylor S. Riall. "Surgeon burnout: a systematic review." *Journal of the American College of Surgeons* 222, no. 6 (Mar 2016) DOI: 1230. 10.1016/j.jamcollsurg.2016.03.022.

Freudenberger, Herbert J. "Staff burn-out." *Journal of social issues* 30, no. 1 (1974): 159-165. DOI: 10.1111/j.1540-4560.1974.tb00706.x.

Gewertz, Bruce L. "Emotional intelligence: impact on leadership capabilities." *Archives of Surgery* 141, no. 8 (Aug 2006): 812-814. DOI: 10.1001/archsurg.141.8.812.

Gopee, Neil, and Jo Galloway. *Leadership and Management in Healthcare*. London: Sage, 2009.

Hu, Yue-Yung, Ryan J Ellis, D. Brock Hewitt, Anthony D. Yang, Elaine Ooi Cheung, Judith T. Moskowitz, John R. Potts III et al. "Discrimination, abuse, harassment, and burnout in surgical residency training." *New England Journal of Medicine* 381, no. 18 (Oct 2019): 1741-1752. DOI: 10.1056/NEJMsa1903759.

Kruse, Kevin. "What is leadership?" *Forbes*. Accessed Apr 9, 2013 URL: https://www.forbes.com/sites/kevinkruse/2013/04/09/what-is-leadership/?sh=1d1c4c115b90.

Lim, Wen Hui, Chloe Wong, Sneha Rajiv Jain, Cheng Han Ng, Chia Hui Tai, M. Kamala Devi, Dujeepa D. Samarasekera, Shridhar Ganpathi Iyer, and Choon Seng Chong. "The unspoken reality of gender bias in surgery: A qualitative systematic review." *Plos one* 16, no. 2 (Feb 2, 2021): e0246420. DOI: 10.1371/journal.pone.0246420. E-Collection 2021.

Mackenzie, Alec, and Pat Nickerson. *The time trap: The classic book on time management*. California, USA. Amacom, 2009.

Maslach, Christina, and Michael P Leiter. "Early predictors of job burnout and engagement." *Journal of applied psychology* 93, no. 3 (Nov 2008): 498. DOI: 10.1037/0021-9010.93.3.498.

Maslach, Christina, and Susan E. Jackson. "The measurement of experienced burnout." *Journal of organizational behaviour* 2, no. 2 (Apr 1981): 99-113. DOI: 10.1002/job.4030020205.

Money, Samuel R. "Surgical personalities, surgical burnout, and surgical happiness." *Journal of vascular surgery* 66, no. 3 (Sep 2017): 683-686. DOI: 10.1016/j.jvs.2017.04.034.

Morris, Melanie, Herb Chen, Martin J. Heslin, and Helen Krontiras. "A structured compensation plan improves but does not erase the sex pay gap in surgery." *Annals of surgery* 268, no. 3 (Sep 2018): 442-448. DOI: 10.1097/SLA.0000000000002928.

Oreskovich, Michael R., Krista L. Kaups, Charles M. Balch, John B. Hanks, Daniel Satele, Jeff Sloan, Charles Meredith, Amanda Buhl, Lotte N. Dyrbye, and Tait D. Shanafelt. "Prevalence of alcohol use disorders among American surgeons." *Archives of surgery* 147, no. 2 (Feb 2012): 168-174. DOI: 10.1001/archsurg.2011.1481.

Panagioti, Maria, Efharis Panagopoulou, Peter Bower, George Lewith, Evangelos Kontopantelis, Carolyn Chew-Graham, Shoba Dawson, Harm Van Marwijk, Keith Geraghty, and Aneez Esmail. "Controlled interventions to reduce burnout in physicians: a systematic review and meta-analysis." *JAMA internal medicine* 177, no. (2 Feb 2017): 195-205. DOI: 10.1001/jamainternmed.2016.7674.

Patel, Vanash M., Oliver Warren, Penny Humphris, Kamran Ahmed, Hutan Ashrafian, Christopher Rao, Thanos Athanasiou, and Ara Darzi. "What does leadership in surgery entail?" *ANZ journal of surgery* 80, no. 12 (Dec 2010): 876-883. DOI: 10.1111/j.1445-2197.2010.05530.x.

Patti, Marco G., Francisco Schlottmann, and Michael G. Sarr. "The problem of burnout among surgeons." *JAMA surgery* 153, no. 5 (May 2018): 403-40. DOI: 10.1001/jamasurg.2018.0047.

Prentice, W. C. H. "Understanding Leadership. 1961." *Harvard Business Review* 82, no. 1 (Jan 2004): 102-109. URL: https://hbr.org/2004/01/understanding-leadership#:~:text=Prentice%20defined%20leadership%20as%20%E2%80%9Cthe,interests%20to%20the%20group's%20purpose.

Regehr, Cheryl, Dylan Glancy, Annabel Pitts, and Vicki R. LeBlanc. "Interventions to reduce the consequences of stress in physicians: a review and meta-analysis." *The Journal of nervous and mental disease* 202, no. 5 (May 2014): 353-359. DOI: 10.1097/NMD.0000000000000130.

Ruotsalainen, Jani H., Jos H. Verbeek, Albert Mariné, and Consol Serra. "Preventing occupational stress in healthcare workers." *Cochrane Database of Systematic Reviews* 11, no. 13 (Nov2014). DOI: 10.1002/14651858.CD002892.pub3.

Shanafelt, Tait D., Charles M. Balch, Gerald J. Bechamps, Thomas Russell, Lotte Dyrbye, Daniel Satele, Paul Collicott, Paul J. Novotny,

Jeff Sloan, and Julie A. Freischlag. "Burnout and career satisfaction among American surgeons." *Annals of surgery* 250, no. 3 (2009): 463-47. DOI: 10.1097/SLA.0b013e3181ac4dfd.

Shanafelt, Tait D., Charles M. Balch, Gerald Bechamps, Tom Russell, Lotte Dyrbye, Daniel Satele, Paul Collicott, Paul J. Novotny, Jeff Sloan, and Julie Freischlag. "Burnout and medical errors among American surgeons." *Annals of surgery* 251, no. 6 (Jun 2010): 995-1000. DOI: 10.1097/SLA.0b013e3181bfdab3.

Shanafelt, Tait D., Charles M. Balch, Lotte Dyrbye, Gerald Bechamps, Tom Russell, Daniel Satele, Teresa Rummans et al. "Special report: suicidal ideation among American surgeons." *Archives of surgery* 146, no. 1 (Jan 2011): 54-62. DOI: 10.1001/archsurg.2010.292.

Shanafelt, Tait D., Lotte N. Dyrbye, Christine Sinsky, Omar Hasan, Daniel Satele, Jeff Sloan, and Colin P. West. "Relationship between clerical burden and characteristics of the electronic environment with physician burnout and professional satisfaction." *Mayo Clinic Proceedings* 91, no. 7 (Jul 2016): 836-848. DOI: 10.1016/j.mayocp.2016.05.007.

Shanafelt, Tait D., Colin P. West, Christine Sinsky, Mickey Trockel, Michael Tutty, Daniel V. Satele, Lindsey E. Carlasare, and Lotte N. Dyrbye. "Changes in burnout and satisfaction with work-life integration in physicians and the general US working population between 2011 and 2017." *Mayo Clinic Proceedings* 94, no. 9 (Sep 2019): 1681-1694. DOI: 10.1016/j.mayocp.2018.10.023.

Singletary, S. Eva. "Mentoring surgeons for the 21st century." *Annals of Surgical Oncology* 12, no. 11 (Nov 2005): 848-860. DOI: 10.1245/ASO.2005.04.035.

Sorouri, Kimia, Shawn Khan, Sylvie Bowden, Stephanie Searle, Lauren Carr, and Jory S. Simpson. "The Glaring Gender Bias in the Operating Room: A Qualitative Study of Factors Influencing Career Selection for First-Year Medical Students." *Journal of Surgical Education* S1931-7204(21)00014-3 (Feb 2021). DOI: 10.1016/j.jsurg.2021.01.014.

Souba, Wiley W. "The new leader: new demands in a changing, turbulent environment." *Journal of the American College of Surgeons* 197, no. 1 (Jul 2003): 79-87. DOI: 10.1016/S1072-7515(03)00335-1.

Spickard Jr, Anderson, Steven G. Gabbe, and John F. Christensen. "Mid-career burnout in generalist and specialist physicians." *Jama* 288, no. 12 (Sep 2002): 1447-1450. DOI: 10.1001/jama.288.12.1447.

TED 2004. "Dan Gilbert: the surprising science of happiness." Apr 26, 2012. Video, 02:54 URL: http://www.ted.com/talks/dan_gilbert_asks_why_are_we_happy.

TEDGlobal 2009. “Dan Pink: The puzzle of motivation.” Aug 23, 2009. Video, 04:00 URL: https://www.ted.com/talks/dan_pink_the_puzzle_of_motivation/transcript?language=en.

The Michigan Daily. “Michigan Medicine joins the #MeToo conversation with new study, #MedToo.” Accessed Feb 12, 2021. URL: https://www.michigandaily.com/section/research/michigan-medicine-joins-metoo-conversation-new-study-medtoo.

The Wall Street Journal. “Physician burnout widespread, especially among midcareer.” Accessed Feb 14, 2021. URL: https://www.wsj.com/articles/physician-burnout-widespread-especially-among-those-midcareer-report-says-11579086008.

Thompson-Burdine, Julie A., Dana A. Telem, Jennifer F. Waljee, Erika A. Newman, Dawn M. Coleman, Hadley I. Stoll, and Gurjit Sandhu. "Defining barriers and facilitators to advancement for women in academic surgery." *JAMA network open* 2, no. 8 (Aug 2019): e1910228-e1910228. DOI: 10.1001/jamanetworkopen.2019.10228.

West, Colin P., Liselotte N. Dyrbye, and Tait D. Shanafelt. "Physician burnout: contributors, consequences and solutions." *Journal of internal medicine* 283, no. 6 (Mar 2018): 516-529. DOI: 10.1111/joim.12752.

Wolfe, A. “Institute of Medicine Report: crossing the quality chasm: a new healthcare system for the 21st century.” *Policy, Politics, & Nursing Practice* 2, no. 3 (Jan 2001): 233-235. DOI: 10.17226/10027.

# CHAPTER 32

# REFLECTIONS OF SURGEON LEADERS (MONOLOGUES)

## THE FIRST CARDIAC SURGEON OF THE GOVERNMENT OF SINDH

ABDUL BARI KHAN

I am a cardiac surgeon. However, my career path took a slightly altered yet, relevant path and I ended up becoming the founder of Pakistan's first and the largest free-of-cost hospital and healthcare network.

I chose healthcare as it is aligned with my inner calling and resonated with my sense of purpose.

I graduated from Dow Medical College (DMC), Karachi, in 1986. In 1995, I did a Fellow of College of Physicians and Surgeons Pakistan (FCPS) diploma in Cardiac Surgery from College of Physicians and Surgeons, Pakistan. After completing it, I was commissioned as Assistant Professor in Cardiac Surgery in 1999. Later, I became the Professor and Head of the Cardiac Surgery Department at the Civil Hospital, Karachi.

When I started my career, the National Institute of Cardiovascular Diseases (NICVD) was the only public sector Cardiac Surgery Centre in Sindh. There was no place for the poor cardiac patients to go for treatment. During my residency, the surgeon Mohammad Rehman was heading NICVD. He was a source of inspiration for me. That year, eight residents joined NICVD for training but there were only two operating theatres and a 10-bed ICU. It was not enough to train eight residents; as a result there was a years-long waiting list of patients. I knew that most of them would not survive to see their turns. Therefore, while training, I facilitated the expansion of the operating facilities and ICU.

I had a background of social work. While working for the Faculty of Science at Adamjee Science College I was awarded "Best Social Worker Gold Medal," while as a medical student in Dow Medical College I was associated with the Patient Welfare Association (PWA) and a project in-charge of the Blood Bank and Blood Fractionation Unit. The dire situation at NICVD compelled me to take action and I started fundraising to add two more theatres and 10 more beds to the existing ICU. The expansion resulted in better training facilities for us and the future residents, and a shorter waiting list.

After completing the fellowship, I joined Civil Hospital, Karachi, as a Cardiac Surgeon. Unfortunately, there was no Cardiac Surgery Department at that time. I again, had to use my fundraising skills. I formed a group, "Friends of Cardiac Surgery," and in a span of merely two years, we were able to raise 30.5 million rupees. We established the Department of Cardiac Surgery in 1998. The unit served as the model Cardiac Surgery Centre for the country, providing "free-of-cost cardiac surgery" to those in need.

I was the first Cardiac Surgeon of the Government of Sindh, which was the first Department of Cardiac Surgery of the province, *and* it was established without the government's support.

We started performing surgeries in 2000. It was a life-changing period where we not only treated patients but worked as administrators, teachers, workers, et cetera. During the day we used to do surgeries and after that we used to teach and train nurses and other staff. These were trying times. The workload was excessive and stressful, leaving too little time for family responsibilities and recreation. However, the passion to help people kept me moving. In 2005, we started the Cardiac Surgery residency programme at the Civil Hospital.

As a cardiac surgeon I often saw immediate and life-changing results which provided me with a source of satisfaction and joy. Cardiac diseases are a major cause of mortality throughout the world, so when you restore a patient's life you feel happy.

The specialty has seemingly limitless challenges and opportunities. Extraordinary progress and remarkable achievements have occurred in every aspect of the specialty over the past decades. Technological advancement can be assimilated into practice. Learning to apply new discoveries and technological advancements are crucial in order to succeed in cardiac surgery.

I find the future of the treatment of cardiac diseases bright, as surgeons are evolving and learning new skills to complement conventional surgical skills. However, I think that the cost of such procedures will increase and become a challenge for the already poverty-stricken Pakistani population. I therefore, as usual, advocate the idea of free healthcare for all.

My innate desire to create a health sector where patients are not treated like customers had not yet been satiated. I was simultaneously working to make this dream come true. So in 2007, I and some of my friends were able to lay the foundations of a hospital which later on became Pakistan's first absolutely free hospital in the private sector.

Although I'm now focusing more on the management of the Indus Hospital and Health Network, cardiac surgery is still my passion, and I am part of many professional forums including the Pakistan Society of Surgeons and the Pakistan Society of Cardiovascular and Thoracic Surgeons. I am on the Board of Governors at Peshawar Institute of Cardiology and an Examiner for FCPS II Cardiac Surgery for the College of Physicians and Surgeons Pakistan. I also hold the position of Honorary General Secretary, Friends of Cardiac Surgery.

# MY JOURNEY: ORTHOPAEDIC TEACHING AND TRAINING PROGRAMME

MOHAMMAD UMAR

Getting accepted into Government College, Lahore was a matter of great celebration for me. The college, with its impressive and historic building and incomparable "Oval," has the reputation of a premier institution for learning, with a dignified and very capable teaching faculty. The student body had an aura of freedom and strength as shown by fearless debates and activities, along with the student union. However, life as part of the pre-medical group was very demanding, and there was no such thing as enjoyment. The two years from 1961 to 1963 were the most difficult years of my student life. There was always the fear of the unknown, of not making it to medical college.

Despite the uncertainties, I got admission into King Edward Medical College; at a mere walking distance from Government College, Lahore. In the days of "One Unit" (1963), to be admitted to King Edward Medical College was a dream come true: the grand and majestic Patiala Block and iconic historical Mayo Hospital has no equal; the medical faculty consisted of senior, mostly British trained Professors with decades of experience, which was overwhelming as well as inspiring; and the knowledge on display so relevant that you could touch and feel it.

Medical education and training meant a new and unique experience. It required hard work and dedication, but it seemed like a very fulfilling endeavour, and the final destination was assured. The days in medical college were my happiest, turning a teenager into an adult with a limitless desire for learning. I was blessed with sincere friends and travelled extensively during summer vacations to every nook and corner of this beautiful country for five years. I graduated from medical college (in 1968) and passed my ECFMG exam, starting surgical house job which I would not finish.

President Kennedy's Commission on "Health and Human Services" reported that the USA needed 30% more medical professionals to provide adequate care to the American public. This opened the flood gates of the USA for easy travel and training opportunities in numerous specialties with adequate scholarships. There was even an incentive to work in the USA as a specialist and eventually get immigration and citizenship.

I was fortunate to start training in a tertiary care hospital in New York City. I had the opportunity to rotate through several surgical specialities. I was most impressed by orthopaedic rotation, which had a high level of orthopaedic trauma, managed by surgical intervention which resulted in quick recovery and early mobilization of the patients. I was sold on orthopaedics, and at the same time I came to know that the orthopaedic residency was one of the hardest to get onto for training.

I applied to nearly all of the university orthopaedic training programmes in the country, one and a half years ahead of time. The *Journal of Surgery* and *Journal of Bone & Joint Surgery* were a must read for me every month.

I was fortunate to get a general surgery residency at Downstate Medical Centre (Downstate University of New York). Most of my time was spent in the trauma unit, which consisted of thoracic, abdominal and musculoskeletal trauma). Professor Gerry Shafton was chair of trauma service, which consisted of two units. Professor Shafton was outstanding in these multiple fields including clinical research and publications.

He was the most pivotal person in guiding me about true learning and the principles of training. It was his strong support and guidance which made it possible for me to be admitted onto an outstanding orthopaedic training programme at Albert Einstein College of Medicine, New York. This four year training programme was very organized with perfect ascending education and training, and a balanced coverage of all disciplines of orthopaedics. In the end, it became very challenging to choose a field for fellowship training. It was a matter of great pride and delight to be admitted to the Adult Reconstructive Surgery Fellowship at the Hospital for Special Surgery (University of Cornell) under Professor John Insall (1974–1975).

He was recognized as a world authority in this field, who ultimately with his team designed the first successful total knee implant (total condylar knee) which came into clinical use in early 1974. All other subsequent designs were modifications of this main design.

He was a scientist par excellence and a strict disciplinarian. His fellowship programme was one of the most sought after. He influenced me greatly as a mentor. It was easy to talk to him and he inspired fellows to achieve bigger and better things through hard work, dedication, passion and compassion. His teachings and dealings with patients were worthy of emulating in medical ethics, patient advocacy and excellence of medical care. As a young consultant at the University of Rochester (1975), I was very active in teaching and training assignments of orthopaedic residents and an active member of the team which reviewed and updated the orthopaedic curriculum.

Here, Professor Mac Everts, the chairman of the orthopaedic department, was the guiding light and under his leadership I learned how to be independent, self-critical and self-confident, and became dedicated to patient care. After several years at the University of Rochester, I was an integral part of the teaching programme and considered as a mature, safe surgeon capable of excelling in managing complex reconstructive procedures.

Right at this time (1989) a modest desire changed into an intense determination to return to Pakistan, to an environment where I could participate in the teaching and training of orthopaedic residents, in addition to specialized orthopaedic practice. But there was no clear pathway. However, I trusted that one of the options would work. Maneeza, my wife, was equally enthusiastic about returning to Pakistan. Here, responsibilities as a homemaker and a mother of two young children were very challenging. She, however, persevered and did a great job single-handedly in keeping things together.

I desired part time association in orthopaedic service at The Aga Khan University Hospital (AKUH). However, it ended up being a full time job. Orthopaedic service was a new-born and stepping towards infancy. Dr Phillip D'Souza was my senior and we dreamed of developing a modern orthopaedic service and training programme. We worked very diligently to prepare an orthopaedic training curriculum of a four-year duration, and got it approved from the College of Physicians and Surgeons Pakistan (CPSP) in a short duration of time. AKU's orthopaedic curriculum followed the guidelines of the American Academy of Orthopaedic Surgeons, and two universities where I trained and worked, along with additions considered suitable for Pakistani graduates. The residents were required to have two years of general surgery training prior to joining the orthopaedic training programme.

**Training programme**

I truly believe in the following sayings attributed to great men of philosophy and science. I benefitted enormously from these principals during various stages of my own training and forty odd years as a trainer:

> *"You cannot teach a man anything, you can only help him find it within himself." (Galileo Galilei)*

> *"I never teach my pupils, I only attempt to provide the conditions in which they can learn." (Albert Einstein)*

> *"Excellence is never an accident, it is always the result of high intention, sincere effort, and intelligent execution, it represents the wise choice of many alternatives – choices, not chance determines your destiny." (Aristotle)*

Our immediate challenge was to recruit two first year residents in orthopaedics. As luck would have it, I knew two fully trained general surgery residents (Dr Riaz Hussain and Dr Masood ur Rehman) who were preparing for a general surgery exam. They frequented the AKU library and were often available to assist me in orthopaedic procedures. I requested they look for residents interested in orthopaedic training. I was shocked to learn that both of them had decided to join orthopaedic training. I tried to convince them that they were already trained surgeons and starting all over again at first year level would not be fair. But they were sold on training in orthopaedics. Orthopaedic service was very fortunate to have such a fantastic start.

Orthopaedic training became well reorganized at AKU, and the orthopaedic rotation of medical students created a very positive energy. We inducted several orthopaedic residents with good potential from all over the country over a few years, in addition to AKU graduates.

First year training consisted of a working knowledge of musculoskeletal system anatomy and physiology, classification of fractures, manipulative reduction and immobilization in plaster casts; learning about dislocation of extremity joints and their closed reduction; the evaluation of open fractures and their severity; and learning the principles of debridement. Hands on training of first year residents is always under the supervision of senior residents and consultants. Junior residents assist seniors in carrying out open reductions and internal fixations, percutaneous internal fixations, and open reductions of old and complex dislocations. All senior residents are involved in learning orthopaedic history and physical exams of all joints, including neurovascular status, especially the effect of cervical nerves on upper limbs and lumber nerves on the lower limbs.

During the second year, routine open reductions and internal fixations are to be done under the supervision of senior residents and an assigned consultant. Examination of the spine and a paediatric orthopaedic examination are stressed. Junior residents are asked to act as 1st assistant and 2nd assistant in complex cases and carry out closures after major procedures. First and second year residents must be part of the morning rounds and, when possible, the evening rounds, to monitor the progress of in-care patients and the detection of any complications at the earliest stage possible.

A resident at third year level is expected to make correct diagnoses after workups and exams in most cases and carry out surgical procedures under supervision. Teaching and supervising junior residents are their important undertakings. Standard primary total knee and hip replacement under consultant supervision is the hallmark of their training. They also treat acute hand injuries with flexor tendon laceration and nerve injuries, as well as performing muscle flap and myocutanous flap reconstruction for soft tissue defects.

The fourth year resident, the chief resident, should be on the hunt for all challenging cases. This may mean an infected non-union with soft tissue and bone loss, complex primary joint replacement, revision total joint shoulder and elbow arthroplasty; tendon transfer for failed treatment of nerve injuries or corrective osteotomies for deformities; deformity correction and limb lengthening using the Ilizarov method, participation in wide margin excision of soft tissue, bone sarcomas and reconstruction with special implants; and surgical treatment of neglected DDH.

It is very important for senior residents (third and fourth years) to learn administrative skills, learn how to organize group activities, such as academic meetings of the department, and learn how to resolve problems of their fellow residents. Our residents have participated with distinction in national orthopaedic meetings.

The cardinal principle of training is that it must be supervised. Increasing their level of responsibility is passed on to residents as their knowledge and skills permit. At no time are training activities allowed to compromise the quality of care. In the present day and age, there is no place for ghost surgery (surgery without the presence of a consultant). The critical part(s) of surgery must be done by the consultant, as determined by him.

**Clinical meetings**

The weekly meetings are a critical part of teaching and training, organized by residents under the leadership of the chief resident and supervised by consultants.

**1. Weekly Indication Conference**

All-important elective cases are discussed including rationales and justifications of choices of procedure. Residents learn how to apply theoretical knowledge in decision-making resulting in successful treatment. This may make some chief residents and consultants uncomfortable.

**2. Weekly Review Conference**

It is mandatory for all residents and consultants. All major procedures, emergency and elective, are presented along with x-rays with special attention paid to any difficulty and complications encountered. Residents present cases of their services. Residents learn how to avoid complications and medical action to correct the problems.

**3. Orthopaedic Oncology Conference**

A multi-disciplinary conference consisting of orthopaedics, radiology, histopathology, medical oncology and radiotherapy. A monthly meeting, discussing cases of last month and cases under work-up being processed for treatment.

**4. Morbidity and Mortality Conference**

A monthly meeting, as a combined conference, of the Department of Surgery.

**5. Annual Musculo-Skeletal Applied Anatomy Course**

A systematic review of anatomy is presented and demonstrated on cadavers. Surgical approaches to important procedures are demonstrated on cadavers. This is the most important course for first and second year residents. One cannot be a good surgeon without mastery of applied anatomy. It is a one week course; mostly weekend time is utilized.

**6. Fellowship Training Academic Pathway**

Most promising residents are retained as senior instructors after their training. We have been able to arrange fellowship training at the centre of excellence in all subspecialties of orthopaedics including spine surgery, hand surgery and micro surgery, orthopaedic oncology and Illizarov fellowships. Such surgeons were inducted in our faculty and at other academic institutions. Dr Masood Umar and Dr Haroon have made excellent contributions to teaching Ilizarov techniques and its various applications through workshops all over the country.

**7.** The orthopaedic department that I wanted to develop always had a desire to excel in basic and clinical research. We were able to send Dr Tashfeen to Karloinska Institute to do a PhD in research after 2 years of orthopaedic training. He successfully completed his PhD and returned to complete orthopaedic training and start research work in addition to clinical practicc but most of lab research work was stopped after a very promising beginning. Possibly it was not the right time for basic and applied research. This can be considered a work in progress.

Reflecting on my own training, the advice and input of my mentors was most critical. I was encouraged to set higher goals and remained determined to overcome all hurdles to achieve those goals. As the saying goes, “great minds have purpose, others have wishes.”

As a mentor, I have endeavoured to stress medical ethics, patient advocacy and excellence of care, and the continuing advancement of professional competence. When hard work and dedication are combined with passion, it is like a ladder with a limitless loft and one’s aspirations become loftier. As I have benefitted tremendously from my mentors, I have tried to give back to my residents and young colleagues wholeheartedly. I believe our people have great potential to perform beyond expectations. Our great philosopher and poet Allama Iqbal had high hopes for the Muslim “Ummah” to rise and take its rightful place in world leadership.

ذرا نم ہو تو, یہ مٹی بہت زرخیز ہے ساقی

# My Journey

## Mohammed Saeed Quraishy

My journey started at Dow Medical College in January 1983, on achieving the coveted MBBS degree. I then completed my internship at the Civil Hospital, Karachi, unaware that this would be where I would spend most of my professional life.

I flew to the UK in mid-1984, and enrolled on Professor Slome's primary course. The next three months were mostly spent studying and enjoying central London. My accommodation was centrally placed in Nuffield College, Lincoln's Inn Fields. Here I developed an appetite for West End shows and British medical history. This was a fortunate time for me as I was successful not only in the Primary FRCS but I passed the PLAB exam as well!

Initially I wanted to train in Orthopaedics and secured a position at the Royal Edinburgh Infirmary, but my career-defining move was to Cardiff. Here I was appointed as SHO to Mr Gordon Heard, an extraordinary, exemplar surgeon of my times. He dissuaded me from pursuing orthopaedics. I then moved on to the Professorial Unit to work with Professor Hughes and Mr Mansell. It was indeed the most memorable and golden period in my academic surgical training career. I recognised this and took full advantage of this opportunity.

Thereafter, Mr Heard organised a job for me in South London with Mr John Dormandy to learn about peripheral vascular disease, where I simultaneously became exposed to the intricacies of research and publishing.

The next stop for me was Guildford. Here with the assistance of the entire surgical team, I was transformed into a conventional general surgeon and subsequently into a laparoscopic surgeon.

My knowledge of the art and science of surgery was further refined by Paddy Boulter (President of the Edinburgh College), Tony Giddings, Chris Marks and Mike Bailey. I returned to Pakistan briefly but my desire to complete my research was overwhelming. So I returned to the UK for a further two years. In England, I worked as a Research Fellow looking at electron microscopic changes and absorption in the gut in patients with obstructive jaundice. Yet again, serendipity prevailed and in tandem I was able to learn laparoscopic surgery from none other than Mr Mike Bailey. For me, he remains one of the best teachers of keyhole surgery. Visits during my later career were paid to Dundee, Liege and Strasbourg to refine my knowledge of laparoscopic surgery.

I returned to Karachi and progressed through a surgical career at Dow Medical College. Here I put knowledge into practice in my unit, and in addition to laparoscopic surgery I developed a sub speciality interest in oesophago-gastric surgery and widened the sphere to pancreatico-biliary surgery. However the real impact in patient surgical outcomes was attained once I was promoted to Professor, first at Lyari, and thereafter at Civil Hospital, Karachi. I needed this autonomy to implement my training from the UK. Both Lyari and Civil Hospital benefitted from the development of endoscopy services in particular. I am proud to admit that my unit at Civil Hospital remains probably the most versatile endoscopy service in Pakistan. All its trainees and postgraduate students have been trained to the required safe and competent standards, which I set to international levels. The reputation of the unit is such that it has consistently attracted the best residents and graduates. My services to training and medical education have been recognised and I was promoted to Meritorious Professor. Meanwhile, I was also elected President of the Pakistan Gastroenterology and GI Endoscopy Society, and the Pakistan Chapter of IHPBA. I was also nominated to the Boards of Primary Healthcare Initiative and the Sindh Health Care Commission.

I have been the longest serving Medical Superintendent of Civil Hospital. This gave me the much awaited golden opportunity to create improvements across the hospital. The hospital was radically modernised and services were improved and expanded in every department. Specific to surgery, the theatres were brought up to date (including the addition of a da Vinci Robot). Perhaps the most significant contribution is the Trauma Centre, a 500-bed facility.

I am contributing this piece as the incumbent Vice Chancellor of Dow University. Last year, I was nominated for the Tamgha-e-Imtiaz for services rendered to health sciences and medical education. My legacy shall be education, training and recognition for Dow as an institution of international repute.

# It Cuts Both Ways: Caring and Craft in Surgery

## Mumtaz Maher

In 1972, I had just started my house job in medicine at Liaquat Medical College, Jamshoro, when I received a letter that would fundamentally affect the course of my career. Like many doctors my age, I had been conscripted into the army. I would serve for 3 years, and in 1975 I was posted to Guddu. It was an incident here that led to my decision to take up surgery.

One day, an old man came into the emergency room with a broken forearm, and cuts and bruises, after his turban got caught in a conveyor belt. I plastered his arm and stitched his lacerations. At every point, the old man uttered *duas* (prayers) for me. It gave me a feeling of gratification. I had never realized surgery had this aspect to it, that it could bring instant results and relief in that way. That was the day I decided to become a surgeon.

After I left the army, I decided that studying anatomy would give me a good start to a life in surgery. From 1975 to 1976, I taught anatomy at Sindh Medical College, Karachi, Pakistan. I then travelled to England for my FRCS.

I didn't give in to the temptation, as many around me did, to do the PLAB to get the work permit and start earning. Instead, I finished the Part I and then did the PLAB.

I was lucky enough to get into a 3 year registrar rotation at the prestigious Royal Victoria Hospital, Belfast. These were turbulent times in Ireland's history, and that exposed me to a lot of trauma and vascular surgery. One surgeon who left a lasting impression on me, a great teacher and human being, was Aires Barros D'Sa. It was here at the Royal Victoria Hospital in 1979, that I cleared my FRCS Part II. During these years, my seniors came to like me as they saw me as a hard worker. But I worked hard because I never wanted them to find fault in my work or me lacking in my duties.

I learned a saying that would come to be a guiding principle: *"Speed in surgery is not rushing; it is economy of movement."*

I observed that Dr Barros D'Sa would operate on a leaking abdominal aortic aneurysm in half the time that other surgeons would take. I wanted to be as good, if not better, than surgeons like him.

By 1979, I came back to Pakistan and realised there was a great deal more to learn. I returned to the UK and, for the next 5 years, I focused on thyroid, breast and plastic surgery. Working at the Derriford General Hospital, Plymouth, a regional centre for head and neck surgery and burns, I developed a respect for tissue and the art of the perfect stitch. For instance, when I closed a wound with stitches, a consultant would point out the ones that did not look right—the skin had blanched, he showed me. My advice to young surgeons, even now, would be to hone their craft through vascular and plastic surgery: both will give your work finesse.

In 1984, I had returned to Pakistan and joined Dow Medical College, Karachi, as Assistant Professor of Surgery. In 1987, I joined Jinnah Postgraduate Medical Centre (JPMC) as Assistant Professor of Surgery. My pursuit of liver and biliary surgery led me to a month-long attachment at the Vienna General Hospital with Professor Josef Funovics. This enabled me to perform complex biliary procedures, which were uncommon in Pakistan at the time. In 1989, I went to Houston for a month-long attachment with Dr Frank Moody. He generously gave me access to his library of videos of his surgeries, and I spent hours poring over each detail, rewinding or pausing to commit his technique to memory.

By 1991 I had been introduced to laparoscopic surgery at the National University Hospital in Singapore. That year, I performed the first laparoscopic cholecystectomy in Karachi, Pakistan.

One lifetime is not enough to learn everything you need to about surgery. In the 15 years from the start of my career, I worked with almost 50 surgeons around the world to hone my craft. My advice to surgeons: make the time and effort to learn from the best in the field. In Pakistan, we need general surgeons, but moreover, we need specialists and specialised equipped units. Right now, we lag behind when compared with the rest of the world. In 2002, as unit in-charge and professor of surgery at JPMC, I established the divisions of colorectal, thyroid, breast and laparoscopic surgery with separate out-patients and theatres. Since then, every year, we have invited leaders in colorectal surgery to Karachi at the JPMC. Surgeons from all over Pakistan are given the chance to watch these masters operate and teach for one week. Within Pakistan's health system, a government-employed doctor is treated no different than a bureaucrat, promoted or transferred once they have served a number of years rather than on the basis of their specialisation. There is little incentive to invest time and expertise in one place.

Above all, we must remember that as doctors, we are given the privilege of restoring that which only Allah can grant us: health and well-being. The blessings of that old man in Guddu gave me a sense of purpose and gave meaning to my work. You may be a highly skilled doctor, but remember that a kind word, a gentle touch, and a reassuring bedside manner, are hallmarks of a humane caregiver.

# My Career in the Department of Surgery, The Aga Khan University (AKU), Karachi from 1985 to 2020

Murad Ali Bana

It gives me immense pleasure to write of the past, moving towards the developments that have taken place in this span of time. It seems like a miracle to see how the Surgery Department has evolved over the years.

I started as a volunteer typist in Employee Relations & Public Administration (ER/PA), Human Resources (HR), in December 1985. This was a temporary/volunteer job, with a pay of Rs 1000, and no benefits. All the work was done manually, on paper. One manual typewriter was a shared resource across the HR staff in the department. This was my first office job, and I had been working with honesty in the attempts to secure a full time permanent job. However, I was not given an opportunity in HR.

As The Aga Khan University Hospital (AKUH) was fully functional in November 1985, I kept searching for more opportunities across the institution, and was selected as a Filing Clerk/Typist in May 1986, in the Department of Surgery (DoS). Besides me, there were 2 secretaries, one for the Chairman and another for the faculty (DoS).

There was only one IBM typewriter shared between 2 secretaries. After days passing by, a Canon typewriter was provided. There were no computers in the early days. Later, individual computers (type DX 1) were introduced in 1990.

We routinely used dictation machines, transcribing patient referral letters, memos, letters for referees, M&Ms, on-call rotas and all office correspondence first in draft format, and then finalizing the documents—some by retyping, and some using Blanco (a correction fluid).

Presentations were made and enlarged on photocopy machines, and displayed on overhead projectors. Later, I was responsible for making

PowerPoint presentation slides for lectures on a desktop computer, along with sizing the fonts and requesting the Information System Department (Mr Zulfiqar Meghani) for a laser print out. These were then handed over to the Audio-Visual Department (Late Mr Amir Tariq) to develop slides for presentation. There was only one laser printer available at AKU. Slides were developed through a studio and were on x-ray films.

From the beginning, I was actively involved in the undergraduate, postgraduate and academic activities of the DoS, which included scheduling examinations; short and long cases; organizing internal and external examiners; and typing question papers for MBBS examinations on a typewriter, with full proof security.

From Day 1, I have been actively involved in the on-call rota, academic activities and tumour board. I am honoured to have typed approximately more than 70 dissertations (for FCPS II) of all specialties of surgery including anaesthesia and obstetrics & gynaecology.

I worked as an Administrative Officer and Secretary for surgery specialties, along with being an organizer/coordinator for conferences and workshops.

In 1994, we were able to obtain email access. This connection was only available for 30 minutes every day. We had only one designated desktop computer for this purpose. We were taught by Dr Talati about its usage, and learned how to get connected with the rest of the world. All correspondence was done manually and filed.

There was complete dedication towards undergraduate and postgraduate education right from the beginning. I routinely conducted and organized examination and skills workshops. Patients with basic diagnoses were brought from Civil and Jinnah Hospital for examination by Aziz Hayder.

From my experience and knowledge, from colleagues, faculty and residents, I have learnt many good things in my life. I feel proud and honoured to see our alumni revisit AKU and meet me wholeheartedly.

I am thankful to my mentors Dr Jamsheer Talati, Dr Farhat Moazam, Dr Sohaila Mohsin Ali, Dr Mushtaq Ahmed, Dr Shaista Khan, Dr Rizwan Azami, Dr Shahid Sami and Dr Asad Jamil Raja.

Something about myself: I have spent days and nights working to the best of my abilities to run the activities of the Surgery Department. My reporting relationship is with all full time and part time faculty, residents and medical officers, management and staff. There is no limit to my job responsibilities. Many managers have been recruited, but my workload never seems to be ending.

In the end, I should mention the names of some of the staff members who worked for the DoS and are well remembered by faculty and alumni: Aziza Lalani, Martha Travas, Greta Sequeria, Daphne D'souza, Amyn Laasi, Syed Hameeduddin, Aneeta Anwarali and Riaz Contractor.

With the blessings of Allah, my parents, family members and all my colleagues, I have completed 35 years of service in the Department of Surgery, The Aga Khan University.

Murad Ali Bana
Associate
Department of Surgery
December 2020

# My Journey

Nasir Ahmad

## Part 1

When asked why they want to become a doctor, most students will blurt out the clichéd phrase, "to serve humanity." My reason was simple: an "order" from my father.

"Your brother has gone for engineering, so you have to become a doctor."

I was very good at maths and physics, and wanted to pursue a career in these fields. But, no; it simply had to be medicine.

I was born and grew up in Malaysia. As a newly independent country (the British left in 1957), there was only one medical school and most of my classmates were headed to Australia or the UK. Pakistan in those days, under the government of Ayub Khan, was the model of a very progressive and fast developing country. It was offering scholarships in various fields of higher education to less developed (so called "third world") countries like Jordan, Nepal, East Africa, Malaysia and Singapore. Because of geographical proximity, most students from the Far East were placed in East Pakistan.

I landed there and found the curriculum extremely challenging. There was an outstanding Professor of Anatomy, Dr SIMG Mannan, who had a PhD from Oxford University. The clinical years were exhilarating and our teachers were simply brilliant. One Professor of Internal Medicine, S. M. Rab, was a genius. Years later, when I was in the US and saw and met brilliant physicians, I thought Dr Rab was head and shoulders above them. He was the personification of bedside teaching, and in the mould of Sir William Osler, one of the founders of clinical medicine at Johns Hopkins School of Medicine in Baltimore, over a century ago.

Another was the Professor of Surgery, Dr K. S. Alam, who although he had trained in the UK, was like another famous Hopkins surgeon, Dr William Halstead (it was at Hopkins that the concept of a structured "residency" training programme was started). Even for American surgeons today, their surgical training is called "Halstead training."

With such a solid background, many of us were able to sit for, and pass the ECFMG (Educational Council for Foreign Medical Graduates) exam (today known as the USMLE).

The US was in the throes of a brutal war in Vietnam, and there was a compulsory military draft. There was an extreme shortage of American physicians and thus, the doors were opened to foreign doctors.

Because a friend was already there, I landed in Baltimore to begin my internship and residency. Those days were brutal: on-call every other day, and weekend call meant being in the hospital from Saturday, 8AM, till Monday, 5PM (a whopping 60 hour stretch).

After the internship and a year of surgical residency, it was time to either stay in general surgery or choose a speciality. My Chief called one morning to ask what I really wanted to do.

"My classmate is Dr Denton Cooley in Houston, and just a phone call can get you in!"

Wow! To train under one of the world's renowned cardiac surgeons. But the more I thought about it, the more I realised this speciality was non-existent in countries like Malaysia and Pakistan. So I thanked him and decided to opt for ENT.

I did this at McGill University in Montreal, and then a friend suggested going into private practice in Flint, Michigan.

**Part 2**

Flint, Michigan, was the headquarters of the Buick division of General Motors and was a very prosperous city in the '70s when I moved there. General Motors (it was then the world's largest auto maker) and its workers were highly paid and medical insurance reimbursement was phenomenal.

Private practice had its own charm; we were fortunate to have medical students from Michigan State University rotate with us, and this carried some academic load.

I got a call one freezing winter day from someone in Boston telling me if I had heard of a new medical school in Karachi, Pakistan, called the Aga Khan University (AKU). Frankly, I had never ever lived in West Pakistan, but my wife was from Karachi, so I knew something about the city.

“But why are you calling me, a Malaysian born US citizen to discuss an academic appointment?”

Dr David Ulmer, the then Dean was straightforward, in that this new medical college was to be based on a curriculum inspired by medical schools based in the US, and he was trying to recruit US physicians. The offer of an expatriate pay was on the table and my wife and I decided to give it a try.

I joined AKU as the Head of the ENT/Head & Neck Division, under the then Chair of Surgery, Dr Farhat Moazzam, a paediatric surgeon with impeccable academic credentials. Although we were all (the subspecialties) under the umbrella of the Department of Surgery, the Chair gave us full responsibilities for our sections.

I was fortunate enough to recruit two very dedicated, smart, intelligent and superb residents to help out. One was Dr Najeeb Shirwany, who today is living in California with his AKU graduate wife Dr Mobina. The other was Dr Ausaf Khan, who today is the Professor and Head of ENT/Head & Neck Surgery, at Hamdard University. He is a dedicated professional and academician and it makes me profoundly happy that I trained him.

One thing about AKU is that it has the very best and brightest medical students, all admitted on merit. At the first convocation the chief guest was the President of Pakistan, Ghulam Ishaq Khan. I remember him saying that even his own “*sifarish*” (referral) wouldn’t be able to help any student get admission at AKU!

The sad part is that almost *all* our graduates who land up in the US, Canada or the UK, never return; and this massive brain drain is simply shameful. The aim of the AKU, then and today, is to produce doctors who can serve this country. When asked why the vast majority do not return, the answer is that they are all so highly trained and well paid abroad that coming back is dreadful; there are no institutions except The Aga Khan University Hospital, where they can utilize their talents.

The Aga Khan University Hospital was to be *the* centre of medical excellence for the people of Pakistan. Today it is considered to be the most expensive health care facility in the country. A small number of poor patients are accommodated under a welfare scheme but the overwhelming numbers are the rich and the uber rich.

The key to the greatness of any institution is the faculty. Not only their recruitment of brilliant staff members, but their retention of them too.

In the six years I spent at AKU we set up a unique curriculum for undergraduate students and at the hospital I was appointed the first director of the residency programme (with guidelines for all specialities from the American Boards). We were able to do an amazing amount of clinical work, especially Head and Neck cancer surgeries, and I was able to recruit a second full time faculty member, Dr Jamil Hyder who is now in Oman.

I returned to the US in 1993 because my children were going to the US for a college education, and it was becoming impossible to finance them on an academic salary. Those who followed me also left for very similar reasons and unless this inability to retain faculty is not resolved, I fear the good name and reputation of this unique institution will be sullied.

A final note: medicine today is *big* business. We don't treat patients; they are simply “clients”. The overriding aim is profitability, sometimes at the expense of outcome, care and compassion. But we as physicians must always remember we took an oath to serve our fellow humans who bare their soul and body to us.

# MY JOURNEY

RIZWAN AZAMI

The beginnings of my journey and some of the milestones along the way have been lost in the haze of time. Some mundane milestones are presented for the record.

There is not much of my admission to Dow Medical College in 1967 that I remember, other than two incidents. One in which senior students attempting to indulge in ragging promptly abandoned me as a victim when they learnt that I was born in Bannu, and the other when I was thrown out of the first anatomy class (of women, really no fault of mine) because of a typographical mistake. The admissions office changed my gender by adding the "A" in my surname, to the end of my first name; thus placing me in the female group.

My failure in several first year subjects was as a consequence of many factors; essentially disillusionment and anxiety at the way the cadavers were treated, and the uninspiring attitude of some teachers amongst other things.

I was to return to anatomy twice after graduation, to reassure myself that it was not the subject that I disliked.

In my tenure as a surgical trainee I was to experience the frightening bravado and bluster of young consultants and learnt to ask questions of myself. A great deal of reflection resulted (regarding when and why not to do surgery) while managing morbidities and mortalities, thanks to these consultants.

After nine years in the service of the Sindh Government, a resignation became essential in 1983. I passed the FCPS and joined the Anatomy Department of the Aga Khan University (AKU), then located on the third and fourth floors of the College of Physicians and Surgeons, in Karachi, Pakistan. Among the many things that one is responsible for when setting up a new facility, the one thing that comes to mind is the change in name of a department. A presentation was made by the AKU Public Relations

Department and I couldn't help laughing by the time the third slide was projected. The effort to control myself was so prodigious that I became tearful and the speaker noticed this. At the end of the presentation he asked me if everything was alright and I said, "NO! The department name and the abbreviation, so liberally used in the presentation and accompanying talk, were liable to be misinterpreted."

He could not understand why. So it was explained what the abbreviation "PR" stood for in medical parlance. The presentation faded from memory, but a few days later the department came to be known as the Public Affairs Department.

When the Surgery Department began to take shape in early 1985, I moved to it and enjoyed setting up (with the help of others) the operating room systems, the packs, the Central Sterilization and Supply Department, finally developing the Emergency Room (ER) in the Community Health Centre (CHC), and then in the actual location. As no specialties existed, the ER handled everything (ENT, medicine, neurosurgery, obstetrics & gynaecology, orthopaedics, paediatrics, surgery and trauma). This can only be described as an amazing clinical and administrative experience.

No matter how well thought out a design, there is always opportunity for improvement. When the ER shifted from the CHC to its location in the main building, the ambulance trolley could not be rolled directly into the ER. The trolley had to be lifted off the road, placed on the pavement and then rolled in. The numerous ramps that today permit the rolling of wheelchairs and trolleys did not yet exist; kerb stones existed everywhere and the architect would not allow their removal and a change in design. Maintenance (with whom I had a special bond) was convinced to create overnight a prototype ramp at the entrance of the maintenance workshop. This was begrudgingly accepted by the architect and that is how all the ramps in the institution came into being.

In 1987, Surgical Team Two came into existence and that is where I stayed till 2014. After twelve years as Assistant Professor, I was promoted to Associate Professor. Meanwhile numerous residents' dissertations were completed and submitted, instead of papers.

In 2007, when I happened to be elected to the Council of the College of Physicians and Surgeons of Pakistan, the rule of the dissertation being the property of the College was abolished (as were a host of other strictures) and supervisors and trainees were allowed to publish their dissertation work as papers.

It is to the credit of the residents and other consultants of Surgical Team Two, that they were from the very beginning of the team's existence able to create a volume of surgical work that can best be described as awesome. It was responsible for honing the surgical and clinical skills of every level of resident that came to the team.

The consultants of the team believed that without surgical work, the training of residents was not possible and the residents in turn ensured that care was optimal and morbidity and mortality were kept to a minimum. The blistering pace of surgical work was maintained, despite the occasional jeering and perhaps the envy of other consultants over a period of two and a half decades.

In 2015 winds of administrative change began to blow and I left the Aga Khan University Hospital (AKUH) and joined the Memon Medical Institute Hospital, which was wishing to start postgraduate training. The programmes were created and the supervisors recruited. I held various positions starting with the Chair of Surgery, Medical Director, and Chief Executive Officer (all synchronously) till December 2018, when I unceremoniously left the place.

In January 2019, the Liaquat College of Medicine and Dentistry, and Darul Sehat Hospital appointed me as Consultant Surgeon and Director of Medical Services.

This account has been limited to a specific word count and it is not possible to expound on the reasons and rationale for various moves in the allotted quota of words. The reader may be left hungering for the why and how about various decisions that were taken at different times, which I have no hesitation or shame in sharing; for what good is an experience and a story with perhaps a lesson in it if it cannot be shared?

# SIUT:
# A JOURNEY OF HOPE AND COMMITMENT

S. ADIBUL HASAN RIZVI
AND S. A. ANWAR NAQVI

In the early 1960s when Dr Rizvi was in training at the Civil Hospital, the plight of patients could be seen among the outpatients where prescriptions were not honoured at the hospital. The situation was not too dissimilar for admitted patients. Investigation and medicines had become the responsibility of patients. When he returned from the UK in 1970, after an 8 year exposure to the National Health Service, the situation had not changed and was not likely to. He found it unacceptable and rose to the challenge of altering the status quo so that the poor did not have to look to their pockets for treatment.

**The Beginning**

Sindh Institute of Urology and Transplantation (SIUT) started as an 8-bed department of urology in the Civil Hospital, the largest in the province. Stone disease was the most common clinical ailment. Urethral stricture, mostly following trauma, became the first specialized clinic. A small departmental laboratory was also a first.

The great floods in the summer of 1973 inundated vast areas of lower Sindh. A relief team of the Pakistan Medical Association (PMA) headed by Dr Rizvi was sent to Chuhar Jamali about 100 miles south east of Karachi. I joined Dr Rizvi, a house surgeon, at the camp which was literally under a huge bunyan tree. Dr Zafar Hussain, Dr Altaf Hashmi and Dr Manzoor Hussain joined the team a few years later. This exposure of rural poverty and almost non-existent medical facilities were so profound that SIUT's mission of providing free medical care with dignity and compassion, irrespective of ethnicity and religious belief, became the clarion call for the future.

## Growing influx of the underprivileged

Free treatment increased the number of patients coming from the interior of Sindh, the majority harbouring stones. To cater to these patients a lithotripter was purchased through donations, the first in a public sector hospital, which successfully treated stones as a day care procedure. Initially peritoneal dialysis was started in response to patients with renal failure and later haemodialysis machines were added. In November 1985, the first living donor kidney transplantation was performed. The lifetime care of the recipients and of their donors has since become SIUT's long term commitment.

## Autonomy and independence

The exponentially growing volume of patients prompted the Government of Sindh to give SIUT autonomy in financial and operational matters as an independent entity. A board of governors headed by the Minister of Health and several members from the civil society was set up and the Government of Sindh started an annual grant. A trust was set up to formalize the donation and zakat collections.

## Continuing expansion of the services

Presently SIUT treats over 3 million patients yearly. SIUT is now more than a 1000-bed facility in Karachi and Sukkur, providing a variety of health services in the fields of urology, nephrology, transplantation, paediatrics and gastroenterology.

A dedicated oncology unit with 100 beds equipped with radiotherapy, chemotherapy and brachytherapy started its services in 2006. A paediatric urology department was set up with the support of Prof Philip Ransley and Dr Jeeta Dhillon, and the unit was named after Philip Ransley in recognition of his enormous contributions.

The nephrology department has grown into the largest dialysis and transplant centre of the region. SIUT has performed around 6,300 transplants and now regularly performs over 350 a year, adding laparoscopic removal of the kidney to its procedures—a first in the country. Paediatric nephrology was added in 2004 with a separate paediatric dialysis and transplant units (again the only centre in the country where this is present).

The hepatogastroenterology department evolved with a focus on transplantation. A living donor programme was embarked upon with initial help from Dr Nigel Heaton and Dr Mohamed Rela from Kings College Hospital London, and later by the team from Shiraz led by Prof Malek Hosseini and Dr Saman Nikeghbalian, who trained two of our surgeons. Thus far 40 live related donor liver transplants have been done.

**Dialysis at the door step**

Since transportation became increasingly difficult, dialysis centres were required at many places. SIUT considered these, "dialysis at the doorstep." SIUT responded by increasing the number of dialysis beds at Shah Faisal Colony, 12 miles from SIUT. More satellite centres were opened at Bara Maidan Nazimabad and Garden East with the help of the community.

**SIUT Chablani and Mehrunnisa Hospitals**

SIUT's model of success motivated the government to support establishing another centre 300 miles away in Sukkur, which is manned and run by indigenously trained staff at SIUT. By the 1990s almost 60% of patients came from the rural areas of Sindh, Baluchistan and lower Punjab. The hospital was named after a gynaecologist, Dr Chablani, who had started it selflessly for the poor.

A businessman, Mr Haroon, donated a 200-bed hospital on 10 acres in Korangi. It was named after his wife Ms Mehrunnisa. It started with a dialysis unit and has now expanded to surgery and PET CT facilities.

**Rising to the challenges of organ sales**

By 2000, the country was hit by steeply rising unethical transplants in the form of sale of kidneys. At the height of commercial transplant activity, there were an estimated 1,500 transplants for foreigners coming from richer countries. These individuals received transplants where kidneys were vended by the poorest donors from Punjab. SIUT spearheaded the campaign for legislation which was successfully promulgated into law in 2010.

**Footprints of deceased donation**

In 1994 the first deceased donor transplant in the country was performed at SIUT. Naveed, a university student, met with a road traffic accident and became brain dead and the family agreed to donate his organs. Two kidneys and two corneas were given to deserving patients. Up till now, eight deceased donors have donated their organs including kidneys, liver and corneas.

**SIMS and degree awarding status**

In the eighties, SIUT initiated Master of Surgery (MS) and Doctor of Medicine (MD) research degrees, with the collaboration of Karachi University, and a PhD in Biomedical Sciences. The number of programmes and the growing student community necessitated a formal degree awarding status which was given to SIUT by the Higher Education Commission in the form of Sindh Institute of Medical Sciences (SIMS).

A four year Bachelor of Science (BS) programme in intensive care, dialysis, laboratory sciences, radiology, nuclear medicine and operative surgery started in 2005. After their internship, the students become physician assistants, a cadre unique to this country. SIUT established the School of Nursing in 2006 which runs a 3-year general nursing diploma.

**Strengthening ethical frontiers**

The Centre of Biomedical Ethics and Culture (CBEC) came into being as a first in the country. Teaching ethics to healthcare providers, CBEC became the first centre as part of SIUT's initiative. A mid-level 1-year postgraduate diploma programme began in 2005, with candidates from all over the country. Its success led to development of a Master's programme attracting students from across the country and also from South Asia and Africa. In 2018 CBEC became a WHO collaborating centre.

**Opening SIUT to school children**

The student volunteer programme at SIUT began in the year 2005, to help students in their finishing years become exposed to the plight of poor patients. They interacted with patients, especially children, reading to them and teaching them how to draw and paint. A red-crescent basic course was arranged and a certificate was awarded after completing 30 hours spread over 5 days. More than 6,500 student volunteers have graduated up to now.

**Research**

Research has been an integral part of education and training since the inception of SIUT. The first research paper on the study of 400 cases of stone disease was published in the *Journal of Pakistan Medical Association* (JPMA), as early as 1975. Since then, over 1,400 articles conducted by faculty, graduate and postgraduate students in clinical and basic laboratory sciences, as well as biomedical ethics, have been published in national and international indexed journals.

**Responding to natural calamities**

The great floods of 1973 were an example of how timely the beginning of SIUT was. Years later, after the great earthquake of 2005 in Northern Pakistan, the first team deployed from SIUT included 20 members, who went to Abbottabad. The Abbas Institute of Medical Sciences became a hub of patient surgery and dialysis support for crush victims. Moreover, SIUT donated a centre for dialysis on a permanent basis.

**Epilogue**

In the nearly 50 years of its journey, SIUT has touched the lives of over tens of millions of patients and treated them free with dignity and compassion, irrespective of any differentiation of caste, religious belief or class divide. Today, SIUT—with 73 departments and over 3,000 employees—provides quality tertiary care to the poorest of the poor. It performs 33% of the dialyses and 80% of the ethical transplants in the country. Robotic surgery is also offered to the most underprivileged, again a first in the country. This model has now been replicated in hospitals across the country. In nearly 50 years, SIUT has solidified a new paradigm of community-government partnership in tertiary healthcare and SIUT's forte will be remembered for posterity.

# Development of a Profession: Dentistry with emphasis on Oral and Maxillofacial Surgery

Syed Mahmood Haider

Historically speaking, the de'Montmorency College of Dentistry, Lahore, is the second oldest dental college in Pakistan, having been founded in 1934. It was preceded by Calcutta Dental College, which opened its doors in 1920. The de'Montmorency College is named after the then Governor of Punjab, Sir Geoffrey Fitzhervey de'Montmorency. The first Principal of this newly founded college was Dr Peter Gillies, and a two years dentistry course was offered to medical graduates through Punjab University. In 1949, on the recommendation of Prof Bradlaw (later Lord Bradlaw), who inspected the institution on behalf of the Dental Council of Great Britain, de'Montmorency College and Dental Hospital was recognized. Dr Muhammad Abdul Haq, a first batch graduate of 1936 was elected as a Fellow of the newly created Dental Faculty of the Royal College of Surgeons of England. He later rose to the rank of the Principal in 1953 (Obituary 1986).

Thereafter, when the government was prompted to further develop the dental profession, dental colleges were established in existing medical colleges in Hyderabad (1951), Peshawar (1964), Quetta (1971) and Multan (1974) through the untiring efforts of a few individuals. The first dental college in the private sector was established at Baqai Medical University in 1991; thereafter there was a stream of successive colleges being established in the public and private sector, with the numbers presently standing at 46 nationwide with a capacity nearly for 2,496 graduates annually (Pakistan Medical Commission 2021).

Specialty education and training was grossly neglected until 1994, when the College of Physicians & Surgeons of Pakistan (CPSP) initiated a 3-year FCPS (Fellowship of College of Physicians and Surgeons, Pakistan) diploma in some of the important dental disciplines. The delay was partly due to the incapacity of the existing dental educationists to lead the development of structured formal specialty training programmes at the university level. The actual inception of the FCPS programmes in dental specialties by the CPSP was prompted by the Royal College of Surgeons of England holding the first Primary FDSRCS exams in Karachi in 1994. The Oral & Maxillofacial Surgery unit at the Abbasi Shaheed Hospital, Karachi, was the first beneficiary of this new found status and the department was recognized for FCPS training following its inspection and approval for training by the Royal College of Surgeons of England in 1994. Earlier, the CPSP had been delving into postgraduate dental education since 1981. It initiated the minor diploma of the MGDS, then the MFD, moved on to the MCPS, and finally established the major qualification of the FCPS in four major clinical dental disciplines. These were orthodontics, prosthodontics, operative dentistry and oral & maxillofacial surgery. Much later the fifth discipline of periodontology was added.

Within dentistry, oral & maxillofacial surgery (OMFS) has seen a manifold increase in trained manpower, following the adoption of the fellowship programme by the CPSP in 1994. Prior to that, there was the Master's in Dentistry qualification offered by the University of Punjab. The establishment of the FCPS diploma by the CPSP provided the much-needed impetus that was missing to let the specialty flourish. Today, the CPSP has produced over 300 indigenously trained and qualified fellows in OMFS; all because of the untiring efforts of the founders, and almost twice that number are currently undergoing training throughout various institutions in the country.

OMFS stands out as a unique blend of dentistry, medicine, orthopaedics and trauma surgery, general surgery, plastic surgery, neuro surgery and ENT surgery, all into one part of human anatomy. An OMF surgeon is called upon to provide their expertise which ranges from bone mending, gland removal, and scar revision to tumor excision, tooth removal and repairing frontal sinus fractures, to name just a few. So, our next generation OMF surgeons have to be well armed by all accounts (Haider and Latif 2018).

Like all surgical specialties, OMFS demands great expertise. Hence, its specialty training programmes are focused on the careful selection of candidates who can undergo the vigour of years of training to develop into good clinicians. But unlike other surgical specialties, which are clearly medically based, OMFS is unique in the sense that it tends to fashion a surgeon from a dentist, and that predominantly remains the case in

Pakistan. However, there is a strong medical and surgical component to the training.

There have been changes made to the OMFS training over the years: the length of the residency programme was extended to 4 years, an e-log was established and an intermediate module examination was introduced amongst other changes. There are other university-based Master's degree programmes also offered, but generally it is the FCPS that is more in demand. There is now a need to focus on the enhanced residency programme with a strong medical component in line with the international guidelines.

The difference in training standards in specialties of medicine and dentistry among various education systems throughout the world is a well-known problem. What works well in the United States of America or Europe may not be applicable to Pakistan's healthcare system or for that matter to any other developing country. An interesting assessment of the integration of the medical degree in OMFS was done by Herford, Pulsipher and Sinn in the USA in 2001. They concluded that there had been a trend towards a broader spectrum of surgical privileges over the 10 years prior to the study for both single and dual-degree OMFS. The results emphasized a need to continually assess the influence the medical degree has on the OMFS specialty (Herford, Pulsipher and Sinn 2001).

As a rapidly evolving specialty, OMFS in Pakistan should inculcate formal medical training as part of the specialty training curriculum and this should be facilitated on an urgent basis. This should not take a great deal of time to complete. Mouth diseases, and more importantly oral cancer, will continue to stress the already stretched resources in Pakistan and we need to train surgeons quickly as a matter of priority for the emerging threat.

## Bibliography

Haider, S. M. and W. Latif. "Oral & Maxillofacial Surgery; A historical review of the development of the surgical discipline." *Int. J. Surg.* 55 (July 2018): 224-6. DOI: 10.1016/j.ijsu.2018.02.051.

Herford, A. S., D. A. Pulsipher and D. P. Sinn. "Integration of the medical degree in oral and maxillofacial surgery: A 10-year follow-up." *J. Oral Maxillofac. Surg.* 59, no. 12 (December 2001): 1471-6; discussion 1477-8. DOI: 10.1053/joms.2001.28285.

"Obituary: Dr. Mohammad Abdul Haq [(MBBS, BDS (Pb.), LDSRCS (Ed.), FDSRCS (Eng.), FICD)]". *J. Pak. Med. Assoc.* 36, no. 4 (April 1986): 95-9. URL: https://jpma.org.pk/PdfDownload/6041.

Pakistan Medical Commission. "Recognized colleges and qualifications." Accessed: 14th Feb 2021. URL: https://www.pmc.gov.pk/Colleges.